THE CIBA COLLECTION OF MEDICAL ILLUSTRATIONS

VOLUME 3

A Compilation of Paintings on the
Normal and Pathologic Anatomy of the

DIGESTIVE SYSTEM

PART II

LOWER DIGESTIVE TRACT

Prepared by

FRANK H. NETTER, M.D.

Edited by

ERNST OPPENHEIMER, M.D.

Commissioned and published by

C I B A

OTHER PUBLISHED VOLUMES OF
THE CIBA COLLECTION OF MEDICAL ILLUSTRATIONS

By
FRANK H. NETTER, M.D.

NERVOUS SYSTEM

REPRODUCTIVE SYSTEM

UPPER DIGESTIVE TRACT

LIVER, BILIARY TRACT AND PANCREAS

ENDOCRINE SYSTEM AND
SELECTED METABOLIC DISEASES

HEART

KIDNEYS, URETERS, AND
URINARY BLADDER

RESPIRATORY SYSTEM

(See page 244 for additional information)

First Printing, 1962
Second Printing, 1969
Third Printing, 1973
Fourth Printing, 1975
Fifth Printing, 1979

ISBN 0-914168-04-5
Library of Congress Catalog No.: 53-2151

Printed in U.S.A.

Original Printing by Colorpress, New York, N.Y.
Color Engravings by Embassy Photo Engraving Co., Inc., New York, N.Y.
Offset Conversion by R. R. Donnelley & Sons Company
Fifth Printing by R. R. Donnelley & Sons Company

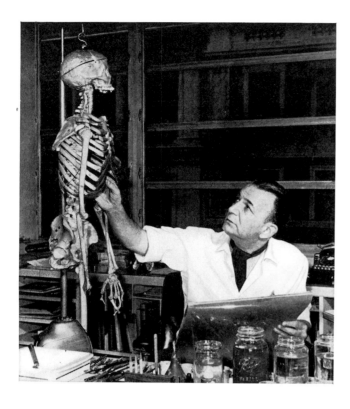

THE ARTIST

Many readers of the CIBA COLLECTION have expressed a desire to know more about Dr. Netter. In response to these requests this summary of Dr. Netter's career has been prepared.

Frank Henry Netter, born in 1906 in Brooklyn, New York, received his M.D. degree from New York University in 1931. To help pay his way through medical school and internship at Bellevue, he worked as a commercial artist and as an illustrator of medical books and articles for his professors and other physicians, perfecting his natural talent by studying at the National Academy of Design and attending courses at the Art Students' League.

In 1933 Dr. Netter entered the private practice of surgery in New York City. But it was the depth of the depression, and the recently married physician continued to accept art assignments to supplement his income. Soon he was spending more and more time at the drawing board and finally, realizing that his career lay in medical illustration, he decided to give up practicing and become a full-time artist.

Soon, Dr. Netter was receiving requests to develop many unusual projects. One of the most arduous of these was building the "transparent woman" for the San Francisco Golden Gate Exposition. This 7-foot-high transparent figure depicted the menstrual process, the development and birth of a baby, and the physical and sexual development of a woman, while a synchronized voice told the story of the female endocrine

system. Dr. Netter labored on this project night and day for 7 months. Another interesting assignment involved a series of paintings of incidents in the life of a physician. Among others, the pictures showed a medical student sitting up the night before the osteology examination, studying away to the point of exhaustion; an emergency ward; an ambulance call; a class reunion; and a night call made by a country doctor.

During World War II, Dr. Netter was an officer in the Army, stationed first at the Army Institute of Pathology, later at the Surgeon General's Office, in charge of graphic training aids for the Medical Department. Numerous manuals were produced under his direction, among them first aid for combat troops, roentgenology for technicians, sanitation in the field, and survival in the tropics.

After the war, Dr. Netter began work on several major projects for CIBA Pharmaceutical Company, culminating in THE CIBA COLLECTION OF MEDICAL ILLUSTRATIONS. To date, five volumes have been published and work is in progress on the sixth, dealing with the urinary tract.

Dr. Netter goes about planning and executing his illustrations in a very exacting way. First comes the study, unquestionably the most important and most difficult part of the entire undertaking. No drawing is ever started until Dr. Netter has acquired a complete understanding of the subject matter, either through reading or by consultation with leading authorities in the field. Often he visits hospitals to observe clinical cases, pathologic or surgical specimens, or operative procedures. Sometimes an original dissection is necessary.

When all his questions have been answered and the problem is thoroughly understood, Dr. Netter makes a pencil sketch on a tissue or tracing pad. Always, the subject must be visualized from the standpoint of the physician; is it to be viewed from above or below, from the side, the rear, or the front? What area is to be covered, the entire body or just certain segments? What plane provides the clearest understanding? In some pictures two, three, or four planes of dissection may be necessary.

When the sketch is at last satisfactory, Dr. Netter transfers it to a piece of illustration board for the finished drawing. This is done by blocking the back of the picture with a soft pencil, taping the tissue down on the board with Scotch tape, then going over the lines with a hard pencil. Over the years, our physician-artist has used many media to finish his illustrations, but now he works almost exclusively in transparent water colors mixed with white paint.

In spite of the tremendously productive life Dr. Netter has led, he has been able to enjoy his family, first in a handsome country home in East Norwich, Long Island, and, after the five children had grown up, in a penthouse overlooking the East River in Manhattan.

ALFRED W. CUSTER

CONTRIBUTORS AND CONSULTANTS

The artist, editor and publishers express their appreciation
to the following authorities for their generous collaboration:

WILLIAM H. BACHRACH, M.D., Ph.D.

Associate Clinical Professor of Medicine, University of Southern California School of
Medicine; Associate Chief, Gastroenterology Section, Wadsworth General Medical and
Surgical Hospital, Veterans Administration Center, Los Angeles; Chief, Gastroenter-
ology Service A, Mount Sinai Hospital, Los Angeles, Cal.

E. S. CRELIN, Ph.D.

Associate Professor of Anatomy, Yale University School of Medicine, New Haven,
Conn.

MICHAEL E. DE BAKEY, M.D.

Professor and Chairman, Cora and Webb Mading Department of Surgery, Baylor
University College of Medicine, Houston, Tex.

R. V. GORSCH, M.D., F.I.C.S., F.A.P.S., D.A.P.B.

Director of Proctology, Midtown Hospital, New York; Consultant Proctologist, New
York Polyclinic Hospital and Medical School, New York; Consultant Proctologist,
Monmouth Memorial Hospital, Long Branch, N. J.

JOHN FRANKLIN HUBER, M.D., Ph.D.

Professor and Chairman of the Department of Anatomy, Temple University School of
Medicine, Philadelphia, Pa.

ALFRED H. IASON, M.D.

AND BEN PANSKY, Ph.D.

New York Medical College, New York, N. Y.

SAMUEL H. KLEIN, M.D.

Attending Surgeon, The Mount Sinai Hospital, New York, N. Y.

AND ARTHUR H. AUFSES, JR., M.D.

Assistant Attending Surgeon, The Mount Sinai Hospital; Adjunct Attending
Surgeon, Montefiore Hospital, New York, N. Y.

C. EVERETT KOOP, M.D., Sc.D. (Med.)

Professor of Pediatric Surgery, School of Medicine and Graduate School of Medicine,
University of Pennsylvania; Surgeon-in-Chief, The Children's Hospital of Philadelphia, Pa.

H. E. LOCKHART-MUMMERY, M.D., M.Chir., F.R.C.S.

Surgeon, St. Thomas' Hospital, London, and St. Mark's Hospital, London, England.

NICHOLAS A. MICHELS, M.A., D.Sc.

Professor of Anatomy, Daniel Baugh Institute of Anatomy, Jefferson Medical College, Philadelphia, Pa.

G. A. G. MITCHELL, O.B.E., T.D., M.B., Ch.M., D.Sc.

Professor of Anatomy and Director of the Anatomical Laboratories, University of Manchester, England.

SÃO PAULO UNIVERSITY GROUP:

JOSÉ FERNANDES PONTES, M.D.

Head of Department of Gastroenterology, Hospital das Clínicas, Faculty of Medicine, University of São Paulo; Director of the Instituto de Gastroenterologia de São Paulo, Brazil.

VIRGILIO CARVALHO PINTO, M.D., F.A.C.S.

Professor of Pediatric Surgery, Catholic University of São Paulo; Head of Section of Pediatric Surgery, Hospital das Clínicas, Faculty of Medicine, University of São Paulo, Brazil.

DAHER E. CUTAIT, M.D., F.A.C.S.

Head of Section of Proctology, Third Surgical Clinic of the Hospital das Clínicas, Faculty of Medicine, University of São Paulo, Brazil.

MITJA POLAK, M.D.

Department of Gastroenterology, Hospital das Clínicas, Faculty of Medicine, University of São Paulo, Brazil.

JOSÉ THIAGO PONTES, M.D.

Department of Gastroenterology, Hospital das Clínicas, Faculty of Medicine, University of São Paulo, Brazil.

SHEPPARD SIEGAL, M.D.

Associate Attending Physician (Allergy), The Mount Sinai Hospital, New York, N. Y.

GERHARD WOLF-HEIDEGGER, M.D., Ph.D.

Professor and Director of the Anatomical Institute, Faculty of Medicine, University of Basle, Switzerland.

INTRODUCTION

The general outline for THE CIBA COLLECTION OF MEDICAL ILLUSTRATIONS calls for eight to ten volumes, each of which is designed to cover the anatomy, pathology and essential physiologic aspects of one of the various systems of the human organism. When planning the volume on the digestive system, it was decided that, because of its scope, the volume should be divided into three separate parts. Part I was to deal with the upper alimentary tract from the mouth through the duodenum; Part II, with the lower alimentary tract from the jejunum through the anal canal, the abdominal cavity and the fetal development of the gastro-intestinal pathway; Part III, with the liver, biliary tract and pancreas. For various reasons I did not undertake these sequentially but first prepared Part III and then Part I. When these two books were completed, I thought that the most difficult problems were behind me. Consequently, as I began this second part of Volume 3, I felt the relief of a long-distance swimmer who, having battled perseveringly against a strong current, senses the tide turning in his favor and believes that, despite his fatigue, the remainder of the course will be relatively easy. Imagine my chagrin to find, as I "paddled" furiously among the conflicting eddies of knowledge dealing with the lower digestive tract, that the "swimming" here was even more difficult than it had been in the upper alimentary canal.

Fortunately, however, in this portion of the course I had the support of a valiant "team", who had struggled with me through Part I of this volume. In the Introduction to that part, I wrote about the personal pleasure and scientific help received from my contacts with Professor G. A. G. Mitchell of Manchester, England; Dr. John Franklin Huber of Temple University, Philadelphia; Dr. Nicholas A. Michels of Jefferson Medical College, Philadelphia; Professor Gerhard Wolf-Heidegger of the University of Basle, Switzerland; and Dr. William H. Bachrach of the Veterans Administration Center, Los Angeles. In working on this book, my appreciation of these men and of the tremendous help they have given has been multiplied many times.

In addition, I have had the good fortune to make new associations which have proved equally enjoyable and advantageous. Notable in this respect was my collaboration with the São Paulo (Brazil) University Group — Dr. José Fernandes Pontes, his brother Dr. José Thiago Pontes, Dr. Mitja Polak, Dr. Daher E. Cutait and Dr. Virgilio Carvalho Pinto.

To Dr. Polak, in particular, I must express my sincerest appreciation, not only for his work in connection with those plates for which he was specifically the consultant, but also for his coordinating activities on behalf of the entire group. The spirit of cooperation among this group was exemplified by the way other members of the Faculty of Medicine of the University of São Paulo generously contributed of their time and knowledge. Specifically, I must mention Dr. Mario R. Montenegro of the Department of Pathology, Dr. Luis Rey of the Department of Parasitology, Dr. Fernando Teixeira Mendes of the Section of Hematology and Cytology, and Dr. Godofredo Elejalde, Bacteriologist.

From the Brazilian group I learned much about the diseases of the gastro-intestinal tract. I learned also to admire their knowledge and their sound and progressive medical thinking. In particular, I was gratified by their devotion to the project we had in hand and by the assiduity with which they pursued it.

Finally, I am grateful to Dr. Pontes and his associates for their efforts to acquaint me with the many wonderful cultural and social features of Brazil. In particular, its architecture and its music will remain among my most treasured memories.

In preparing those plates concerned with congenital anomalies and those demonstrating the anatomic complexity of the peritoneum, it became strikingly evident that, for a better understanding of these topics, a short review of the essential steps and phases in development would be indispensable. The next problem, naturally, was centered around the question as to how deeply we would have to go into detail to present a coherent narrative of the normal developmental processes and to clarify the deviations which lead to the most frequent congenital anomalies. Dr. E. S. Crelin, thanks to his many years of teaching experience and his acquaintance with the mentality of student and physician alike, knew exactly what and how much embryology we would need in order to provide the basic background for all the topics touching upon intestinal development and its anomalies. It was a rare pleasure to have Dr. Crelin as consultant, not only because of his interest in the task before us and the stimulation he conveys, but also because his critical attitude did not permit the omission of any important detail, in spite of the inevitable condensation.

As the specialty of proctology developed during the past few decades, it became important to obtain a more exact knowledge of the anatomy of the anorectal region. The older anatomic concepts did not suffice either for an understanding of the pathology of the region or for the development of improved operative techniques based on physiologic principles. This led to new investigations of the subject, undertaken by a number of men, largely spearheaded by the group at St. Mark's Hospital in London. In this country, Dr. Rudolph V. Gorsch of New York City was one of the pioneers in this work and is one of the leading students of the subject. His painstaking and meticulous studies were always carried out with an eye to practical application of the knowledge gained. It was through perusal of his publications, particularly of his classic book, *Proctologic Anatomy,* that I came to the conclusion that he was the man who could best help with this subject. This decision proved to be correct, and I enjoyed unraveling with him the most modern concepts of the anorectal regions, the perineopelvic spaces, the sphincters and the various related structures.

In the section dealing with the diseases of the small and large intestine, I encountered topics which, because of their almost totally surgical character, required special handling. For certain of these — volvulus, intussusception and the surgical aspects of ulcerative colitis — Dr. Cuthbert E. Dukes, the distinguished pathologist at St. Mark's Hospital in London, recommended to us the brilliant young surgeon, Dr. H. E. Lockhart-Mummery. His knowledge of the conditions on which we worked is all-encompassing, and his ability to restrict the discussion to its essentials was illuminating.

The enormous progress made in the handling of infants with serious congenital anomalies of the digestive tract similarly required the cooperation of a surgical expert. Dr. C. Everett Koop of The Children's Hospital in Philadelphia has made emergency surgery of the newborn his special field of endeavor. The benefit derived from discussing with him, and preparing under his guidance, the plates which appear at the beginning of Section XII was indeed remarkable, and I can only hope that his clarity in describing the pathophysiologic situations and the essential points of the surgical procedures is adequately reflected in the paintings.

When we came to "hernia", though it is, strictly speaking, a disease of the abdominal wall, the editor and I decided to devote a special section to it, because it is so important and so much of an entity. The consultant for this topic was Dr. Alfred H. Iason, a man who has studied the subject in all its phases, who has written voluminously concerning it, and who has had vast operative experience in the field. His monumental volume, *Hernia,* is widely known.

Intestinal obstruction and the "acute abdomen" proved to

be unique subjects because of the vastness of the fields they encompass. These two topics touch on almost every condition covered in this book, but what was needed was a cross-sectional view, a reclassification of the material in such a manner as to be helpful to the student and practitioner. For aid in these problems I called on a close friend, Dr. Samuel H. Klein of New York City. Because of his vast surgical experience and knowledge, his keen analytical mind and his understanding of the teaching approach, he was ideally suited for the task at hand. In order to get another point of view for the task of abridgment, Dr. Klein called in an associate, Dr. Arthur H. Aufses, Jr. Together, we worked out the plates which appear on pages 188 to 192.

Paroxysmal peritonitis is an entity of relatively recent recognition, and for the plate on this subject I fortunately was able to obtain the collaboration of Dr. Sheppard Siegal of New York City, who had much to do with the identification of this condition.

Gastro-intestinal physiologists and clinicians have for some time suspected that the ileocecal junction acts not purely as a flap valve but as a physiologic sphincter or pylorus. It remained for Dr. Liberato J. A. Di Dio of the University of Minas Gerais, Belo Horizonte, Brazil, to demonstrate a more appropriate concept of the structure of this valve and its function. Dr. Di Dio, who was in New York at the time I was working on this subject with Professor Wolf-Heidegger, most graciously explained to us his findings and showed us drawings and photographs of his dissections and also his remarkable motion picture of the function of the valve in vivo. The illustrations on page 52 are based on his material.

Our concept of the structure of the epithelial cells of the intestine has been greatly modified in recent years, and the help of an expert in this field was needed when it came to the making of the illustration on page 50. This subject is most important today because of the interest in absorption and malabsorption. I am therefore most grateful to Dr. S. L. Palay of the Laboratory of Neuro-anatomical Sciences, National Institutes of Health, Bethesda, Maryland, who has personally made most extensive electron microscopic studies of these cells and who graciously gave me of his time and his knowledge.

A number of illustrations in this volume were originally made in consultation with Dr. Jacob Buckstein of New York. They were first issued in individual brochures and later in THE CIBA COLLECTION OF MEDICAL ILLUSTRATIONS, published in 1948. These plates appear in Section X, Plates 1, 2, 3, 6, 7, 8, 25, 28 and 29; in Section XII, Plates 16, 18, 23, 30, 34, 44, 45, 46 and 49; in Section XIII, Plate 4; and in Section XIV, Plate 11. Some of them are reproduced here in their original form; others with modifications. I wish to thank Dr. Buckstein for his help with these plates.

Also from an older series of pictures stem Plates 9 to 14 in Section XIII, dealing with abdominal injuries. I am most grateful to Dr. Michael E. De Bakey, under whose guidance these pictures were developed in 1945, for his kindness in checking the correctness of both pictures and texts.

I should also like to express appreciation for the generous aid and advice given me by the following: Dr. Robert A. Nordyke, now of the Straub Clinic, Honolulu, Hawaii, for his aid in planning the illustration of the use of radio-isotopes in tests of absorption (Plate 22, Section XI); Dr. Robert J. Matthews of Van Nuys, California, for demonstrating to me the test for occult blood in the stool (Plate 24, Section XI); and Dr. Paul K. McKissock of Veterans Administration Center, Los Angeles, California, for his advice in connection with the sketch of reversal of an intestinal loop (Plates 1 and 2, Section XI).

For the Plates in Sections IX and X, dealing with the blood vessels of the abdominal wall and of the intestine, Dr. Michels and I were helped a great deal by Paul Kornblith, a medical student at Jefferson Medical College, and by Dr. Padmanabhan Siddharth of Madras Medical College, India, presently a teaching fellow at the Daniel Baugh Institute of Anatomy.

Throughout this project there has been to me one source of encouragement and stimulation, one fountainhead of counsel and advice, my very dear friend, the editor of these volumes, Dr. Ernst Oppenheimer, to whom I shall be forever grateful. I cannot here recount the multitudinous ways in which he has helped. Suffice it to say that his devotion to the work, his confidence in me and his tireless attention to organization and detail have been an inspiration.

FRANK H. NETTER, M.D.

*   *   *   *   *

The editor wishes to express his special gratitude to the consultants for their fine cooperation and for their meticulous care in writing the texts. The renewal of the pleasant relationships with those consultants who contributed also to Part I of this volume has been most enjoyable, and the ready understanding shown by those who encountered, for the first time, the various difficulties we face in producing these books has been deeply appreciated.

I wish to add my own expression of thanks to Dr. Mitja Polak for his successful efforts to make my task much easier by assuming the rôle of coordinator for the five São Paulo University contributors who, as a group, were responsible for the greatest number of plates.

We are deeply indebted to my good friend, Dr. Samuel R. M. Reynolds, Professor and Head of the Department of Anatomy of the University of Illinois School of Medicine, for supplying the very rare slides of the intestinal plexuses of the human being, which appear in the plate on page 78. To Dr. Jack Crane, formerly of the University of California Medical School, now Professor and Head of the Department of Pathology of the University of Oregon Medical School, we extend our thanks for making the three photomicrographs from the slides supplied by Dr. Reynolds. Our thanks go also to Dr. Leo Kaplan, Director of the Clinical and Anatomic Laboratories of Mount Sinai Hospital in Los Angeles, for the very difficult-to-obtain photomicrographs of human stools (page 108). Dr. Kaplan also kindly supplied us with the photomicrograph, on page 55, depicting the longitudinal section through the colon wall. The photomicrograph of the argentaffine cells (on the same page), as well as information regarding the function of these cells, we owe to Dr. Bernard J. Haverback, Chairman of Gastroenterology Service, University of Southern California School of Medicine.

Many other persons contributed generously of their time and energy to make this volume possible. In particular, I would like to mention Mrs. L. A. Oppenheim and her associates on the CIBA staff in Summit, N. J., and our literary consultants, Wallace and Anne Clark of Buttzville, N. J. Many thanks go also to Harold B. Davison of Embassy Photo Engraving Co., Inc., and to the staff of Colorpress for their devotion and effective support of our desire to improve, with each new book, the high standard we set for ourselves when we embarked on this project.

Finally, to Dr. Hans H. Zinsser, Assistant Clinical Professor of Surgery at the College of Physicians and Surgeons, Columbia University, I would like to express my appreciation and thanks for his cooperation and help in his capacity of associate editor.

E. OPPENHEIMER, M.D.
(DECEASED 1962)

CONTENTS OF COMPLETE VOLUME 3
DIGESTIVE SYSTEM

CONTENTS

Section VIII

DEVELOPMENT OF THE DIGESTIVE TRACT

by

FRANK H. NETTER, M.D.

in collaboration with

E. S. CRELIN, Ph.D.

Development of Gastro-intestinal Tract

The flat entodermal roof of the yolk sac underlying the embryonic disk [1, 2]* becomes incorporated within the human embryo in the form of a tube, the primitive gut, as the embryonic disk folds into a cylindrical embryonic body. The cranial end of the yolk sac roof invaginates into the developing embryonic *head fold* to become the *foregut* [3]. Then the caudal end of the yolk sac roof invaginates into the developing *tail fold* to become the *hindgut*. Another tubular diverticulum of the caudal end of the yolk sac roof, the *allantois,* originally invaginates into the *body stalk* before the hindgut develops [1]. It is drawn into the tail fold along with the hindgut to become a hindgut diverticulum [3, 5]. Within the body of the embryo, the roof of the yolk sac intervening between the fore- and hindguts, the *midgut,* originally has a wide communication with the extra-embryonic portion of the yolk sac [3, 4]. Along the periphery of this midgut and yolk sac communication, the body of the embryo becomes bounded by definite folds, which increase in depth and undercut the embryo, gradually to decrease the size of the midgut and yolk sac communication [6, 7]. Before the communication is ultimately lost, it is reduced to a long, slender tube, the *yolk stalk* [8], passing from the tubular midgut into the umbilical cord [11-13]. The approximation of the body folds forms the ventral body wall and is associated with the formation of the umbilical cord [8, 11, 12].

The blind cranial end of the foregut forms the inner entodermal layer of the *buccopharyngeal membrane,* the outer layer of which is the ectodermal floor of a surface depression in the oral region, the *stomodeum* [5]. Disintegration of this membrane establishes the cranial gut opening [8]. The blind caudal end of the hindgut forms the inner entodermal layer of the cloacal membrane, the outer layer of which is the ectodermal floor of a surface depression in the anal region, the *proctodeum* [5, 8, 11]. Disintegration of the cloacal membrane establishes the caudal gut opening [13].

The gut entoderm gives rise to the mucosal lining (and the secretory cells of the glands derived from it) of various structures: *foregut* — pharynx, respiratory tract, esophagus, stomach, first part and upper half of the second part of the duodenum; *midgut* — lower half of the second part and the third and fourth parts of the duodenum, jejunum, ileum,

*Numbers in brackets refer to the individual pictures in the six following plates.

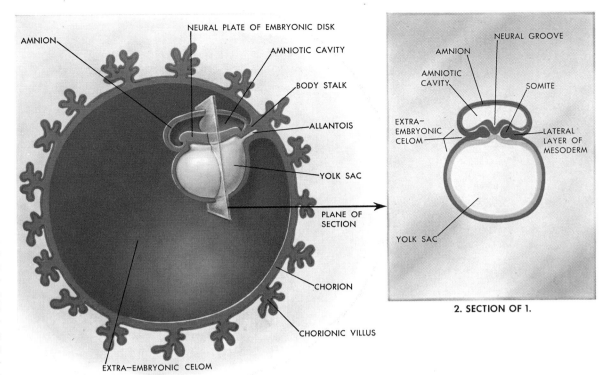

1. FOURTEEN DAYS

2. SECTION OF 1.

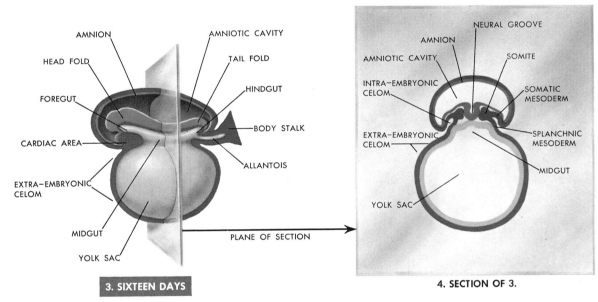

3. SIXTEEN DAYS

KEY

ENTODERM
MESODERM
ECTODERM

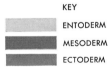

4. SECTION OF 3.

cecum, appendix, ascending colon, right and middle thirds of the transverse colon; *hindgut* — left third of the transverse colon, descending and sigmoid colon, rectum, upper part of the anal canal and a greater part of the urogenital system from its allantoic diverticulum.

Before the primitive gut develops into a tube, a flat layer of mesoderm, continuous with the somites located on each side of the midsagittal plane of the embryonic disk, intervenes between the disk ectoderm and the entodermal yolk sac roof [2]. A split occurs in each of these lateral mesodermal layers throughout their length within the boundaries of the embryonic disk to produce a slitlike cavity, the *intra-embryonic celom* [4]. It communicates with the relatively large chorionic cavity, the *extra-embryonic celom,* beyond the boundaries of the embryonic disk [1, 2, 4]. The intra-embryonic celom becomes the

pericardial, pleural and peritoneal cavities. The dorsal sheets of intra-embryonic mesoderm, the somatic (parietal) mesoderm, resulting from the split in the lateral mesodermal layers to form the intra-embryonic celom, become closely associated with the disk ectoderm and ultimately give rise to the parietal peritoneum of the abdominal cavity [4, 6, 7, 9, 10]. The ventral sheets of the intra-embryonic mesoderm, the splanchnic mesoderm, resulting from the split in the lateral mesodermal layers, become closely associated with the primitive gut. They give rise to the musculature of the gut, its serosal covering (visceral peritoneum) and its primary ventral and dorsal mesenteries.

When the body folds at the periphery of the midgut and yolk sac communication completely undercut the embryo and form the ventral abdominal wall and umbilical ring, the communication between the intra-

(Continued on page 3)

2

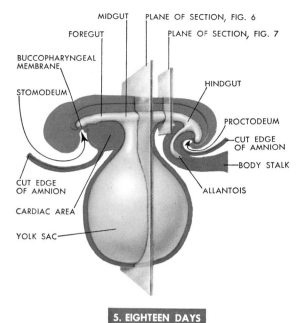

MIDGUT
FOREGUT
BUCCOPHARYNGEAL MEMBRANE
STOMODEUM
CUT EDGE OF AMNION
CARDIAC AREA
YOLK SAC
PLANE OF SECTION, FIG. 6
PLANE OF SECTION, FIG. 7
HINDGUT
PROCTODEUM
CUT EDGE OF AMNION
BODY STALK
ALLANTOIS

5. EIGHTEEN DAYS

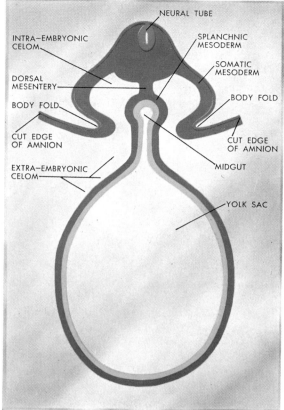

NEURAL TUBE
INTRA-EMBRYONIC CELOM
SPLANCHNIC MESODERM
SOMATIC MESODERM
DORSAL MESENTERY
BODY FOLD
BODY FOLD
CUT EDGE OF AMNION
CUT EDGE OF AMNION
EXTRA-EMBRYONIC CELOM
MIDGUT
YOLK SAC

6. SECTION OF 5.

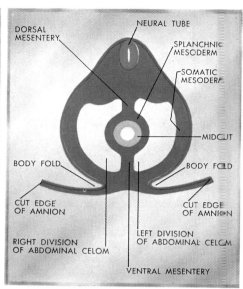

DORSAL MESENTERY
NEURAL TUBE
SPLANCHNIC MESODERM
SOMATIC MESODERM
MIDGUT
BODY FOLD
BODY FOLD
CUT EDGE OF AMNION
CUT EDGE OF AMNION
RIGHT DIVISION OF ABDOMINAL CELOM
LEFT DIVISION OF ABDOMINAL CELOM
VENTRAL MESENTERY

7. SECTION OF 5.

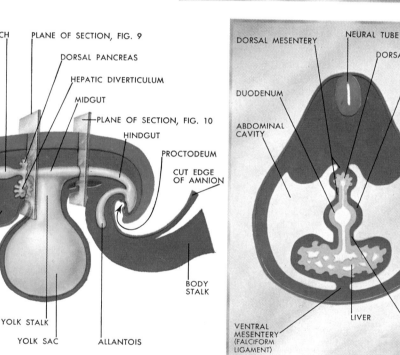

STOMACH
ESOPHAGUS
LUNG BUD
THYROID GLAND
PHARYNX
STOMODEUM
CARDIAC AREA
CUT EDGE OF AMNION
PLANE OF SECTION, FIG. 9
DORSAL PANCREAS
HEPATIC DIVERTICULUM
MIDGUT
PLANE OF SECTION, FIG. 10
HINDGUT
PROCTODEUM
CUT EDGE OF AMNION
BODY STALK
YOLK STALK
YOLK SAC
ALLANTOIS

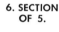

8. ONE MONTH

NEURAL TUBE
DORSAL MESENTERY
DORSAL PANCREAS
VISCERAL PERITONEUM
PARIETAL PERITONEUM
DUODENUM
ABDOMINAL CAVITY
VENTRAL MESENTERY (FALCIFORM LIGAMENT)
LIVER
VENTRAL MESENTERY (LESSER OMENTUM)

9. SECTION OF 8. (ANTERIOR)

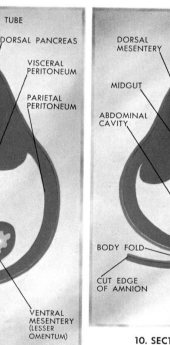

NEURAL TUBE
DORSAL MESENTERY
VISCERAL PERITONEUM
PARIETAL PERITONEUM
MIDGUT
ABDOMINAL CAVITY
BODY FOLD
BODY FOLD
CUT EDGE OF AMNION
CUT EDGE OF AMNION
PERSISTING EDGES OF VENTRAL MESENTERY

10. SECTION OF 8. (POSTERIOR)

SECTION VIII—PLATE 2

DEVELOPMENT OF GASTRO-INTESTINAL TRACT

(*Continued from page 2*)

and extra-embryonic celoms is greatly reduced in size as the extra-embryonic celom becomes a tubular cavity within the umbilical cord [12]. Faulty closure of the body folds to form the umbilical ring can result in most of the abdominal viscera developing outside of the body cavity in a transparent sac of amnion. The sac is directly attached to the placenta, with only a portion or no true ventral abdominal wall present. This is one type of omphalocele (see page 125),

also known as eventration of the abdominal viscera or abdominal hernia. During the closure of the body folds, the two layers of splanchnic mesoderm approach each other and come into direct contact at the midline of the embryonic body. In so doing, they enclose the now tubular gut and form the dorsal and ventral divisions of the primary mesentery, which suspends the gut from the dorsal and ventral body walls [4, 6, 7, 9, 10]. This mesentery completely separates the celomic cavity into right and left divisions in the abdominal area. However, each of the two abdominal divisions of the cavity at this developmental stage extends as a pleural canal, one on each side of the esophagus dorsal to the transverse septum, to become continuous with the single pericardial celom surrounding the developing heart [11]. The pericardial celom is later subdivided into

the pleural and pericardial cavities as the lungs develop.

The *transverse septum* is a shelf of somatic mesoderm extending from the ventral body wall, which partitions off the pericardial region from the abdominal region [11]. It becomes the *ventral part of the diaphragm* [16]. The pleural canals become closed by folds of somatic mesoderm, the pleuroperitoneal membranes, arising from the posterolateral body wall on each side. They extend toward the midline of the body, being continuous during this process with the dorsal border of the transverse septum, to meet and *fuse with the midline visceral mesoderm* in which the *esophagus* is *embedded* to complete the formation of the diaphragm [12, 13, 16]. Later, the musculature of the diaphragm deve-

(Continued on page 4)

3

DEVELOPMENT OF GASTRO-INTESTINAL TRACT

(Continued from page 5)

drawn last into the abdominal cavity its *cecal end continues its rotation in a counterclockwise direction* toward the right side of the abdominal cavity and then downward to the lower right quadrant of the abdomen [15]. This establishes the transverse colon in a position above the jejunum and ileum and the ascending colon close against the right side of the dorsal body wall. As the ascending colon approximates the dorsal body wall, the *original left side* of its *mesocolon fuses with the parietal peritoneum dorsal to it in a triangular fashion.* The base of this fusion triangle is the ascending colon from the ileocecal junction to the right colic flexure. The apex of the triangle is at the duodenojejunal flexure. The upper border of the triangle runs from the right colic flexure to its apex to form the *right half of the attachment of the transverse mesocolon* to the dorsal body wall. The lower border of the triangle passes from its apex to the ileocecal junction to form the attachment *(root) of the mesentery* of the small intestine to the dorsal body wall. In the adult the attachment or root of the mesentery of the small intestine, which is 6 or 7 in. long, runs on an angle from the level of the left side of the second lumbar vertebra to the right iliac fossa anterior to the right sacroiliac joint.

When the original left side of the serous lining of the ascending mesocolon met with the parietal peritoneum, both fused over a *triangular space,* leaving a fusion fascia, which is a double connective tissue plane remaining after the loss of the serous cells. Likewise, a layer of fusion fascia came into being between the surface of the ascending colon, which fused with the body-wall peritoneum, to constitute the bare area of the ascending colon. Since the vessels and nerves supplying the ascending colon were originally within its mesocolon, they pass to its left surface, following fusion of its mesocolon to the body wall, parallel with the plane of fusion fascia. Therefore, the ascending colon in the adult can be freed from its attachment to the body wall by first incising its visceral peritoneum as it is reflected off its lateral surface to become the parietal peritoneum all along its right border. Following the incision, blunt dissection along the plane of fusion fascia toward the midline of the body allows extensive elevation of the ascending colon, and its nerve and blood supply, away from the dorsal body wall.

When the descending colon closely approximated the dorsal body wall on the left side, as the intestine returned to

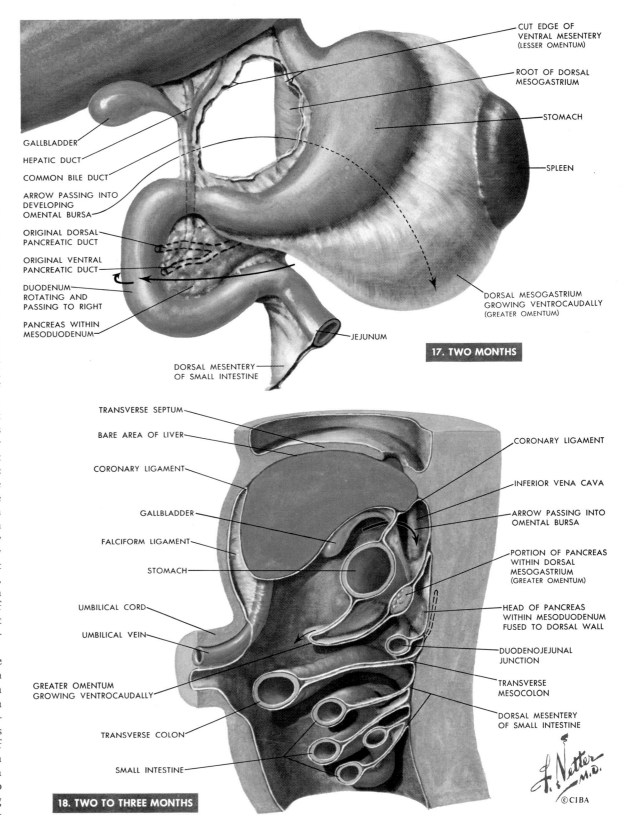

CUT EDGE OF VENTRAL MESENTERY (LESSER OMENTUM)

ROOT OF DORSAL MESOGASTRIUM

STOMACH

SPLEEN

GALLBLADDER

HEPATIC DUCT

COMMON BILE DUCT

ARROW PASSING INTO DEVELOPING OMENTAL BURSA

ORIGINAL DORSAL PANCREATIC DUCT

ORIGINAL VENTRAL PANCREATIC DUCT

DUODENUM ROTATING AND PASSING TO RIGHT

PANCREAS WITHIN MESODUODENUM

DORSAL MESOGASTRIUM GROWING VENTROCAUDALLY (GREATER OMENTUM)

JEJUNUM

DORSAL MESENTERY OF SMALL INTESTINE

17. TWO MONTHS

TRANSVERSE SEPTUM

BARE AREA OF LIVER

CORONARY LIGAMENT

CORONARY LIGAMENT

INFERIOR VENA CAVA

ARROW PASSING INTO OMENTAL BURSA

GALLBLADDER

FALCIFORM LIGAMENT

STOMACH

PORTION OF PANCREAS WITHIN DORSAL MESOGASTRIUM (GREATER OMENTUM)

HEAD OF PANCREAS WITHIN MESODUODENUM FUSED TO DORSAL WALL

UMBILICAL CORD

UMBILICAL VEIN

DUODENOJEJUNAL JUNCTION

TRANSVERSE MESOCOLON

GREATER OMENTUM GROWING VENTROCAUDALLY

DORSAL MESENTERY OF SMALL INTESTINE

TRANSVERSE COLON

SMALL INTESTINE

18. TWO TO THREE MONTHS

the abdominal cavity from the umbilical cord, the *original left side of its mesocolon fused with the parietal peritoneum of the dorsal body wall in a quadrangular fashion* [15]. The right border of this fusion quadrangle is the original attachment of the descending mesocolon along the midsagittal plane of the dorsal body wall from the level of the duodenojejunal flexure down to the rectum. The upper border of the quadrangle passes from the *duodenojejunal flexure to the left colic flexure,* to form the attachment of the left half of the transverse mesocolon to the dorsal body wall. The left border of the quadrangle is the descending colon from its left colic flexure down to its junction with the sigmoid colon. The *lower border* of the quadrangle passes from the junction of the descending and sigmoid colon to the rectum, to form the *attachment of the sigmoid mesocolon* to the dorsal body wall.

This *quadrangular fusion* of the original left side of the descending mesocolon to the dorsal wall parietal peritoneum resulted in the formation of a fusion fascia, in the same manner described for the ascending mesocolon on the right side of the abdominal cavity. A layer of fusion fascia also developed between the surface of the descending colon and the body-wall peritoneum, constituting the bare area of the descending colon. Since the vessels and nerves supplying the descending colon were originally within its mesocolon, they pass to its right surface, following fusion of its mesocolon to the body wall, parallel with the plane of fusion fascia. Therefore, the descending colon can be freed from its attachment to the body wall by first incising its visceral peritoneum as it is reflected off its lateral surface to become the parietal peritoneum all along its left border. Following the

(Continued on page 7)

DEVELOPMENT OF GASTRO-INTESTINAL TRACT

(*Continued from page 6*)

incision, blunt dissection along the plane of fusion fascia toward the midplane of the body allows extensive elevation of the descending colon, and its nerve and blood supply, away from the dorsal body wall.

Concomitant with the formation of the triangular and quadrangular fusion fasciae certain constant, and a number of inconstant, folds of peritoneum develop. Some of the folds conduct blood vessels, whereas others do not. Since a cul-de-sac type of fossa occurs under each fold, it is possible for a loop of intestine to burrow into and enlarge a fossa to form an intraperitoneal hernia. Such fossae occur chiefly at the duodenojejunal flexure (superior, inferior, retro- and paraduodenal), ileocecal junction (superior and inferior ileocecal), dorsal to the cecum (retrocecal) and between the dorsal surface of the sigmoid mesocolon and the body-wall peritoneum (intersigmoid).

The portions of the gut which protrude into the umbilical cord during development may not return to the abdominal cavity, as they normally do. This results in a type of umbilical hernia (omphalocele, see page 125) in which the proximal portion of the umbilical cord at birth is actually a sac of amnion containing nearly all or part of the small intestine and the proximal portions of the large intestine. A similar type of umbilical hernia can be the result of having the intestine return normally to the abdominal cavity only to herniate secondarily, either pre- or postnatally, through an inadequately closed umbilical ring.

The rotation of the intestine and its final positioning after it returns to the abdominal cavity from the umbilical cord may cease at any stage. If the intestine returns to the abdomen as a single mass, no rotation occurs, and the jejunum and ileum lie on the right side of the peritoneal cavity, with the large intestine on the left. More commonly, partial rotation, so-called malrotation (see page 113), occurs. If so, the loops of the small intestine occupy the right side of the abdominal cavity and the large intestine the left side, with the cecum lying high in the abdomen near the midline. In this instance the large intestine retains an extensive mesentery and is freely movable. Actually, the cecum may be located in any position between the middle portion of the upper part of the abdomen and the lower right quadrant, depending on the degree of nonrotation.

A complication of malrotation of the gut, known as volvulus (see page 113), is the result of having the cecal dilatation pass in a clockwise instead of a counter-

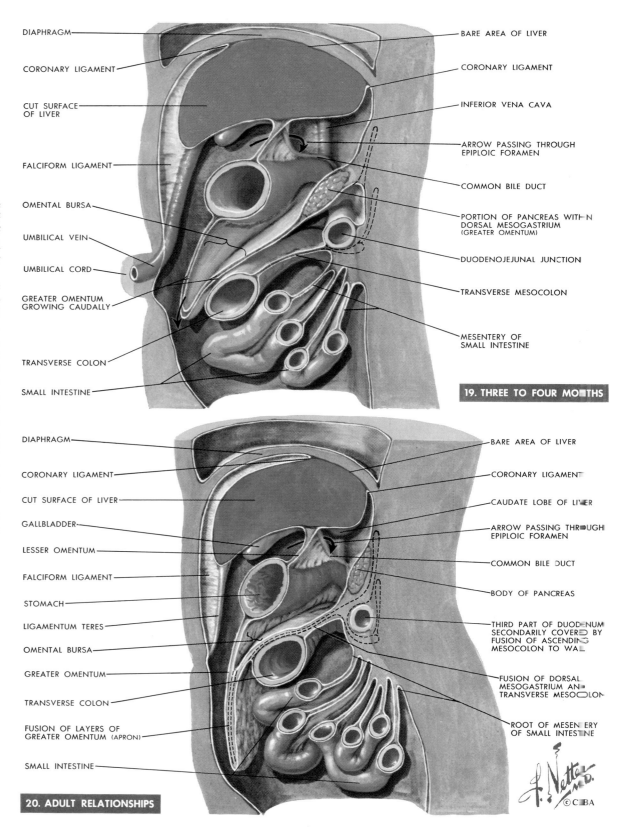

DIAPHRAGM
CORONARY LIGAMENT
CUT SURFACE OF LIVER
FALCIFORM LIGAMENT
OMENTAL BURSA
UMBILICAL VEIN
UMBILICAL CORD
GREATER OMENTUM GROWING CAUDALLY
TRANSVERSE COLON
SMALL INTESTINE

BARE AREA OF LIVER
CORONARY LIGAMENT
INFERIOR VENA CAVA
ARROW PASSING THROUGH EPIPLOIC FORAMEN
COMMON BILE DUCT
PORTION OF PANCREAS WITHIN DORSAL MESOGASTRIUM (GREATER OMENTUM)
DUODENOJEJUNAL JUNCTION
TRANSVERSE MESOCOLON
MESENTERY OF SMALL INTESTINE

19. THREE TO FOUR MONTHS

DIAPHRAGM
CORONARY LIGAMENT
CUT SURFACE OF LIVER
GALLBLADDER
LESSER OMENTUM
FALCIFORM LIGAMENT
STOMACH
LIGAMENTUM TERES
OMENTAL BURSA
GREATER OMENTUM
TRANSVERSE COLON
FUSION OF LAYERS OF GREATER OMENTUM (APRON)
SMALL INTESTINE

BARE AREA OF LIVER
CORONARY LIGAMENT
CAUDATE LOBE OF LIVER
ARROW PASSING THROUGH EPIPLOIC FORAMEN
COMMON BILE DUCT
BODY OF PANCREAS
THIRD PART OF DUODENUM SECONDARILY COVERED BY FUSION OF ASCENDING MESOCOLON TO WALL
FUSION OF DORSAL MESOGASTRIUM AND TRANSVERSE MESOCOLON
ROOT OF MESENTERY OF SMALL INTESTINE

20. ADULT RELATIONSHIPS

clockwise direction and, in so doing, loop one or more times around the superior mesenteric artery. In this type of volvulus, the ascending colon is not fused to the body wall, and the transverse colon passes dorsal to the superior mesenteric artery as it wraps around it, to cause both intestinal obstruction and occlusion of the superior mesenteric artery.

One of the commonest anomalies of the intestine, known as Meckel's diverticulum (see pages 127 and 128), is the partial persistence of the yolk stalk. It is a sacculation of the ileum, occurring about 2 to 3 ft. from the ileocecal junction in the adult. It may be a blind pouch or may extend to the umbilicus, with or without a patent lumen.

While the intestine caudal to the duodenum was undergoing changes in shape and position, the stomach and duodenum were simultaneously undergoing changes. The dorsal border of the gut dilatation,

which becomes the stomach, grows faster than its ventral border. This produces the convex greater curvature of the dorsal aspect of the stomach, in contrast to the slower-growing lesser curvature of the ventral aspect. The stomach fundus arises as a local bulge near its craniodorsal end [12]. Once the greater and lesser curvatures become established, the *stomach* undergoes a 90-degree rotation about its longitudinal axis, which results in its lesser curvature facing to the right and its greater curvature to the left [13]. The stomach rotation causes the lower end of the esophagus also to rotate. This shifts its closely associated right and left vagus nerves to dorsal and ventral positions as they pass toward the stomach. Assisting the stomach rotation is the rapid growth of the *dorsal mesogastrium*, attaching the greater curvature to the dorsal body wall, and the relatively slower growth of

(*Continued on page 8*)

the *ventral mesentery* (*lesser omentum*), attaching the lesser curvature to the liver [12, 13]. At the time of stomach rotation, the enlarging liver displaces the freely movable cranial end of the stomach to the left, whereas the caudal end is relatively anchored by the short ventral mesentery. As a result, the whole stomach extends obliquely across the abdomen from left to right [17]. While the stomach is assuming this position, the dorsal mesogastrium continues to expand to become the *greater omentum* by forming a large sac protruding to the left. The cavity developing within this increasingly voluminous greater omentum is the *omental bursa*. When the stomach has acquired its oblique position, the bursa continues to grow, but now in a caudal direction. In so doing, it encounters the transverse mesocolon, which deflects it ventrally, so that it hangs over the transverse colon and covers the underlying coils of small intestine like an apron [18-20]. While it is forming this apron, the original left side of the serous layer of the omentum dorsal to the stomach begins to fuse with the parietal peritoneum of the dorsal body wall. Also, once the apron is formed, the serous layer of the *original left side of the omentum*, which comes to lie *against the transverse colon and its mesocolon, fuses* with them. The two layers of the omentum, beyond the transverse colon forming the *apron*, then fuse with each other to obliterate the distal part of the bursal lumen. Later, when fat begins to be laid down in the body, this omental apron becomes one of the important sites of fat storage and also provides an insulating layer protecting the abdominal viscera.

During the early stages of formation of the duodenum, the *pancreas* develops from two separate primordia, which arise from the duodenal entoderm (see also CIBA COLLECTION, Vol. 3/III, page 25). The first primordium, the dorsal pancreas, appears on the dorsal duodenal wall opposite, but slightly cranial to, the hepatic diverticulum [8, 9]. The other primordium, the ventral pancreas, arises immediately caudal to the hepatic diverticulum [11]. Its cavity may communicate with that of the hepatic diverticulum, or it may open separately into the duodenum. With the growth and elongation of the common bile duct, the ventral pancreas migrates around the right side of the duodenum by passing beneath its serosal covering to extend into the mesoduodenum [12]. Simultaneously, the duodenum rotates about 90 degrees, so that its original ventral surface is then directed to the right. These growth changes bring the ventral pancreas into contact with the dorsal pancreas within the mesoduodenum, and the two merge [13, 17].

The dorsal pancreas gives rise to all of the adult gland except the caudal portion of the head and the uncinate process, which are derived from the ventral pancreas. In the coalescence of the primordial glandular tissue from the two independent sources, their duct systems fuse. The ventral duct, now communicating with the left side of the duodenum by way of the common bile duct, or in close relationship to it, persists, whereas the proximal portion of the dorsal duct usually atrophies. The distal part of the dorsal duct persists and drains the neck, body and tail of the pancreas by way of its anastomosis with the ventral duct [17]. Occasionally, the proximal portion of the dorsal duct persists as an accessory duct, opening separately into the duodenum cranial to the opening of the common bile duct (see CIBA COLLECTION, Vol. 3/III, page 27).

As the pancreas grows within the mesoduodenum at the duodenal level, it extends cranially into the dorsal mesogastrium (greater omentum), which is continuous with the mesoduodenum, toward the spleen [18]. The original left side of the part of the dorsal mesogastrium (greater omentum), now containing the neck, body and tail of the pancreas, and the original right side of the mesoduodenum, containing the head of the pancreas, fuse with the parietal peritoneum of the dorsal body wall [18-20]. Thus, part of the head, neck, body and tail of the pancreas come to lie dorsal to the stomach beneath the serosal lining of the dorsal wall of the omental bursa.

While the stomach was in its early stages of rotation, the *spleen* began to form *within* the cranial part of the *dorsal mesogastrium* (greater omentum) [11]. It grows rapidly and bulges out the left surface of the mesogastrium, forming the left lateral wall of the omental bursa [12, 13, 17]. The portion of the dorsal mesogastrium extending from the greater curvature of the stomach to the spleen becomes the gastrolienal ligament. The short portion of the dorsal mesogastrium, extending from the spleen to its point of fusion to the dorsal wall parietal peritoneum, becomes the lienophrenic ligament, where the point of fusion overlies the left dorsal aspect of the diaphragm, and the lienorenal ligament, where it overlies the left kidney.

As the ascending colon approximated the dorsal abdominal wall and its mesocolon fused with the parietal peritoneum, the upper part of its mesocolon came to overlie and fuse with the second and third parts of the duodenum, which had already fused with the original body-wall peritoneum [15, 18-20]. Thus, the original peritoneal investment of the second and third parts of the duodenum is completely resorbed when it becomes covered by this secondary peritoneal covering of mesocolon. Also, the fusion of the ascending mesocolon results in having the root of the transverse mesocolon cross the head of the pancreas and the second part of the duodenum, and the root of the mesentery of the small intestine cross the third part of the duodenum [15].

It should be restated that the original left side of the primary dorsal mesentery alone effects secondary fusions with the dorsal body wall, except for its short mesoduodenal portion, which has its right side fused to the wall.

The entrance from the main peritoneal cavity into the omental bursa is at first a broad, slitlike opening in the midsagittal body plane facing to the left [12, 17, 18]. It later becomes reduced in size to become the epiploic foramen to the right of the midsagittal body plane. This occurs when the duodenum forms a U-shaped loop and swings to the right to fuse with the body wall, as the growth of the dorsal portion of the liver extends its inferior surface to a lower body level [17-20]. Thus the cranial boundary of the completed epiploic foramen is the caudate lobe of the liver. Its dorsal boundary is the dorsal body-wall peritoneum overlying the inferior vena cava. The caudal boundary is the point where the first part of the duodenum fused with the body wall, and the ventral boundary is the free edge of the lesser omentum, enclosing the common bile duct, portal vein and proper hepatic artery.

Since the fusion to the body wall of the rotated duodenum and its mesoduodenum occurs as it does, the common bile duct, pancreatic duct or ducts, and the nerve and blood supply of the second part of the duodenum all enter it on the left pancreatic surface. This allows the right side of the second part in the adult to be elevated from the dorsal body wall by blunt dissection (see CIBA COLLECTION, Vol. 3/III, page 29) and reflected toward the midline of the body to expose the dorsal surface of the lower end of the common bile duct, which would otherwise be accessible from a direct anterior approach only with great difficulty because of the overlying head of the pancreas.

The so-called hypertrophic pyloric stenosis of infancy is a hyperplasia of chiefly the circular muscle layer and is believed to occur before birth (see CIBA COLLECTION, Vol. 3/I, page 160).

The lumen of the duodenum (and also of the jejunum and ileum) becomes occluded by masses of epithelial cells early in their development; the lumen is later recanalized. Faulty recanalization of the lumen, or its complete failure, may, in all portions of the intestine, result in localized or extensive areas of atresia (see page 112).

When the midgut first began to form its primary loop and pass out into the umbilical cord, the caudal end of the hindgut began to undergo changes. The hindgut caudal to the point of origin of the allantois becomes enlarged to form the *cloaca*. An ectodermal depression, the proctodeum, extends toward the cloaca, being separated from it by the thin *cloacal membrane* [11].

A division of the cloaca into two parts is produced by the development of a crescentic fold of its entoderm, the *urorectal fold*, which cuts into the cranial part of the cloaca in the angle where the allantois and hindgut meet. It then extends caudally toward the cloacal membrane [11, 12]. As the fold cuts deeper into the cloaca, a wedge-shaped mass of mesenchyme grows into the fold to produce the *urorectal septum*. The complete formation of the septum partitions the cloaca into a separate ventral division, the urogenital sinus, and a dorsal division, the rectum and upper part of the anal canal [13]. Once the cloaca is completely divided, the cloacal membrane disintegrates to establish a separate opening into the urogenital sinus and a separate anal opening into the anorectal cloacal division. The urogenital sinus and allantois give rise to the epithelium and secretory cells of the glandular outgrowths in the greater part of the urogenital system. The portion of the proctodeal depression of ectoderm, in continuity with the anorectal division, gives rise to the lower part of the anal canal. The lumen of the rectum, during its early stages of development, is occluded by a proliferation of epithelial cells and is later recanalized. Partial or complete failure of the lumen to recanalize results in rectal stenosis or atresia. If the union fails to take place between the rectum and the proctodeal depression, an imperforate anus (see page 115) is the result. Abnormalities in the development of the urorectal septum to divide the cloaca into two parts are responsible for an anomalous communication between the rectum and the urinary bladder, the urethra or the vagina. Many varieties are possible, but those in males are most commonly a fistula between the rectum and urethra or between the rectum and the bladder, whereas those in females are almost exclusively between the rectum and the vagina.

The basic formation and positioning of the various subdivisions of the gastro-intestinal tract and their glandular derivatives are essentially completed by the end of the fifth month of intra-uterine development.

Section IX

ANATOMY OF THE ABDOMEN

by

FRANK H. NETTER, M.D.

in collaboration with

R. V. GORSCH, M.D., F.I.C.S., F.A.P.S., D.A.P.B.
Plates 21-24

JOHN FRANKLIN HUBER, M.D., Ph.D.
Plates 1-20

NICHOLAS A. MICHELS, M.A., D.Sc.
Plates 25-28

PROF. G. A. G. MITCHELL, O.B.E., T.D., M.B., Ch.M., D.Sc.
Plates 30-34

PROF. GERHARD WOLF-HEIDEGGER, M.D., Ph.D.
Plate 29

REGIONS OF THE ABDOMEN

For the sake of convenience, the abdomen is traditionally divided into areas or regions. Of the two somewhat artificial divisions, the more simple one uses two imaginary planes, one passing vertically and the other horizontally through the umbilicus. The abdomen is thus divided into *four quadrants* — a right and a left upper quadrant and a right and a left lower quadrant.

A division of the abdomen into more and, therefore, smaller areas for descriptive purposes is accomplished by the use of two vertical and two horizontal planes, which divide the abdomen into nine regions. The zone above the upper of the two horizontal planes is divided by the two vertical planes into a centrally placed *"epigastric region"* (the epigastrium), with a "hypochondriac region" on each side of it, designated as the *right* and *left hypochondriac regions*. The zone between the two horizontal planes is divided into a centrally placed *"umbilical region"*, with a *"lumbar"* or *"lateral abdominal"* region on each side specified, of course, as *right* and *left*. The zone below the lower of the two horizontal planes has a centrally placed *"hypogastric"* or *"pubic"* (suprapubic) region, with an *"inguinal"* or *"iliac"* region on each side of it, which are labeled right and left.

Although the localization possible by the use of the nine regions named above is more specific than that possible by quadrants, the localization is still somewhat general, and it is not surprising that much difference of opinion exists concerning the best position to choose for each of the four lines or planes used in this scheme. If a general localization is all that is being accomplished, the shifting of a plane a few centimeters in one direction or another is of little significance. In the following the more common ways of locating each line will be given.

The upper horizontal (superior transverse) line, or plane, may be drawn halfway between the upper border of the sternum and the upper border of the symphysis pubis. This plane has been considered as passing through the pylorus and has thus been called the *"transpyloric plane"*, which also has been described as being halfway between the xiphisternal junction and the umbilicus, and passing through the tip of the ninth costal cartilage, the fundus of the gallbladder and the lower part of the body of the first lumbar vertebra. The other common way of locating the upper horizontal plane is at the most caudal part of the costal margin (usually the most caudal part of the tenth costal cartilage). This plane is called the *"subcostal plane"*.

The lower horizontal (inferior trans-

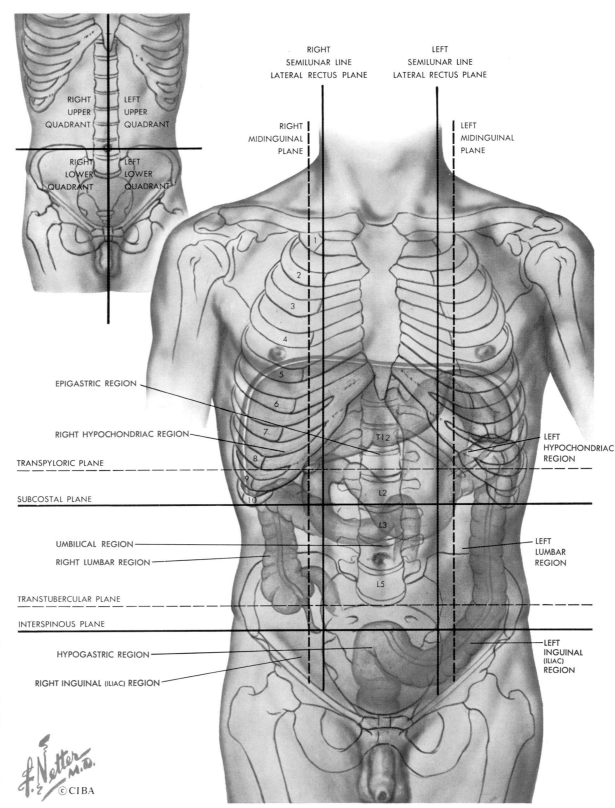

verse) line, or plane, may be assigned to the levels of the tubercles of the iliac crests and is called the *"transtubercular plane"*, which usually passes through the lower part of the fifth lumbar vertebra, or it may be located at the level of the anterior superior spine of the ilium and called the *"interspinous plane"*. It has also been located at the highest points of the iliac crests and called the "supracristal plane".

The two vertical planes, or lines, one on each side, may be located halfway between the median plane and the anterior superior spine of the ilium (or halfway between the pubic tubercle and the anterior superior spine of the ilium or the midpoint of the inguinal ligament, *right* and *left midinguinal planes*). The other common way of locating the vertical plane on each side uses the lateral border of the rectus abdominis muscle or the semilunar line,* which, if followed inferiorly and medially toward the pubic

tubercle, brings the entire inguinal canal into the inguinal region.

In attempting to use either quadrants or the smaller-sized nine regions in the localization of viscera, one finds that a goodly number of individual organs are not confined to any one region.

Attention should be called to the fact that, since the diaphragm is the upper limit of the abdomen, most of the hypochondriac (as the name indicates) regions and parts of the epigastric region are under cover of the ribs. As these three regions make up a good portion of the right and left upper quadrants, these quadrants also extend well up under the ribs.

*This imaginary line serving to divide the abdominal surface into regions is not quite identical with the anatomic "semilunar line" of Spigel, which has been described to coincide with the junction of the muscular and aponeurotic fibers of the transverse abdominal muscle (see page 14).

BONY FRAMEWORK OF ABDOMINOPELVIC CAVITY

The skeletal framework which affords attachments for the muscles that help make up the parietes of the abdominopelvic cavity consists of the lower ribs and, particularly, their costal cartilages, the five lumbar vertebrae and the bony pelvis. The costal cartilages of the 5th, 6th and 7th ribs angle obliquely upward and medially to join the sternum above and lateral to the xiphisternal junction. The terminal portion of each of the 8th, 9th and 10th costal cartilages tapers to a point and is attached to the lower border of the costal cartilage above. The 11th and 12th costal cartilages are quite short, with pointed tips, neither of which is attached to the cartilage above it. The lower border of the 10th costal cartilage is commonly the most inferior part of the caudal margin of the thoracic cage. From the beginning of the 10th costal cartilage to the junction of the 7th costal cartilage with the sternum, a cartilaginous border is formed, which is frequently referred to as the "costal arch" (costal margin), although this term is perhaps more correctly used to refer to the arch formed by the right and left cartilaginous borders as they are connected by the lower end of the sternal body. From the "infrasternal", or "subcostal", angle formed between the right and left costal margins, the quite variable *xiphoid process* of the sternum projects. The latter serves as a landmark for the level of the body of the 10th (or 11th) thoracic vertebra.

The five *lumbar vertebrae* present the parts described for a typical vertebra-body (centrum) and vertebral (neural) arch, supporting the two transverse processes, the spinous process and the superior and inferior articular processes.

The bony pelvis is made up of the two hip bones, with the sacrum and coccyx wedged between them posteriorly. For descriptive purposes the bony pelvis is divided into the major or false pelvis above the plane passing through the sacral promontory and the crest of the pubis and the minor or true pelvis below this plane. This plane lies roughly in the inlet of the true pelvis, which is bounded by the bony structures just mentioned, the anterior margin of the *ala of the sacrum,* the *arcuate line of the ilium* and the *pecten pubis,* all of which could be considered as forming the linea terminalis.

The hip bone (os coxae or innominate bone) is made up of the *ilium, pubis* and *ischium,* which are separate bones in the

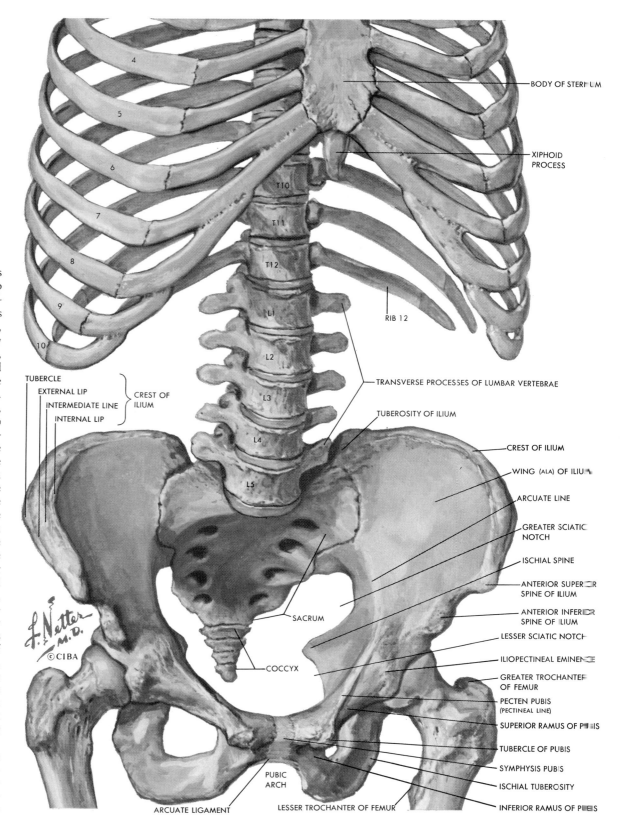

young subject but fused at the acetabulum in the adult. On the inner surface of the ilium, the arcuate line indicates the inferior border of the ala of the ilium, which ends superiorly in the usually readily palpable *crest of the ilium,* stretching from the anterior superior spine of the ilium to the posterior superior spine. The crest also presents an external (lateral) lip, an internal (medial) lip, an intermediate line or area and a thickening on its lateral aspect a short distance posterior to the *anterior superior spine,* which is called the tubercle of the crest. The body of the pubis joins, by means of a fibrocartilaginous lamina, with the one of the opposite side in the formation of the *symphysis pubis.* The upper border of the body, which is thick, roughened and turned antero-inferiorly, is called the crest, and at its lateral end is a prominence named the pubic tubercle (spine). The *superior ramus of the pubis,* coursing superiorly and

posterolaterally, enters into the formation of the acetabulum (acetabular portion, sometimes called body) and presents a prominent pecten or pectineal line which is continuous with the *arcuate line of the ilium.* The inferior ramus courses inferiorly and posterolaterally, to join the ramus of the ischium and help complete the margins of the obturator foramen. The main portion of the ischium extends inferiorly and posteriorly from the acetabulum, to expand into the *ischial tuberosity,* which presents mostly posteriorly. From the posterior border of the inner side of the lower part of the acetabular portion of the ischium, the *ischial spine* projects posteromedially between the greater and lesser sciatic notches. A ramus of the ischium courses anteriorly from the lower end of the main portion of the bone, to become continuous with the *inferior ramus of the pubis,* forming what is often referred to as the ischiopubic ramus.

ANTEROLATERAL ABDOMINAL WALL

Before describing the "abdominal parietes", or the walls (limits) of the abdomen, it is necessary to mention different ways in which the word abdomen is used. Some authors use "abdomen" as synonymous with "abdominopelvic cavity", while others use it in a more specific sense to refer to that portion of the body cavity between the diaphragm and the pelvis minor (true pelvis). "Abdomen" is also used more loosely to refer to a general region of the body.

For purposes of specific description, it seems advisable to name that portion of the body cavity below the diaphragm the "abdominopelvic cavity" and then to divide this into the abdominal cavity proper and the pelvic cavity (pelvis minor), separated from each other by the plane of the pelvic inlet (the plane passing through the sacral promontory and the pubic crests). It must be remembered, however, that certain structures which are ordinarily referred to as abdominal structures (some of the coils of small intestine, for example) usually hang into the pelvic cavity, and that the inferior and postero-inferior (dorsocaudal) support of the abdominal viscera is furnished by the parietes of the pelvic cavity and not by the theoretical plane at the pelvic inlet. It is convenient to divide the parietes of the abdominopelvic cavity into four general parts — the anterolateral abdominal wall, the posterior wall (see page 20) of the abdominal cavity, the diaphragm (see page 21) (superior wall or roof of the abdominal and the abdominopelvic cavities) and the parietes of the pelvic cavity (see page 22), which can be loosely called the floor of the abdominopelvic cavity. However, the limits of the portions of the parietes just named are not all sharp, since we are dealing with curved contours, and certain arbitrary limits need to be defined for descriptive purposes. This has been done in part above and will be completed as necessary at appropriate places in the following descriptions.

The *anterolateral abdominal wall* (called simply "abdominal wall" by some authors) fills in the gap in the bony-cartilaginous framework between the costal margin above and the hip bones below. Anterolateral, as used here, really means anterior and lateral instead of the usual meaning of the word, inasmuch as this part of the wall is anterior and lateral and, as a matter of fact, follows the curve of the wall for a distance onto the posterior aspect. (In this description the quadratus lumborum muscle and the structures medial to it are included with the posterior wall of the abdominal cavity.) Owing to its muscular components, the

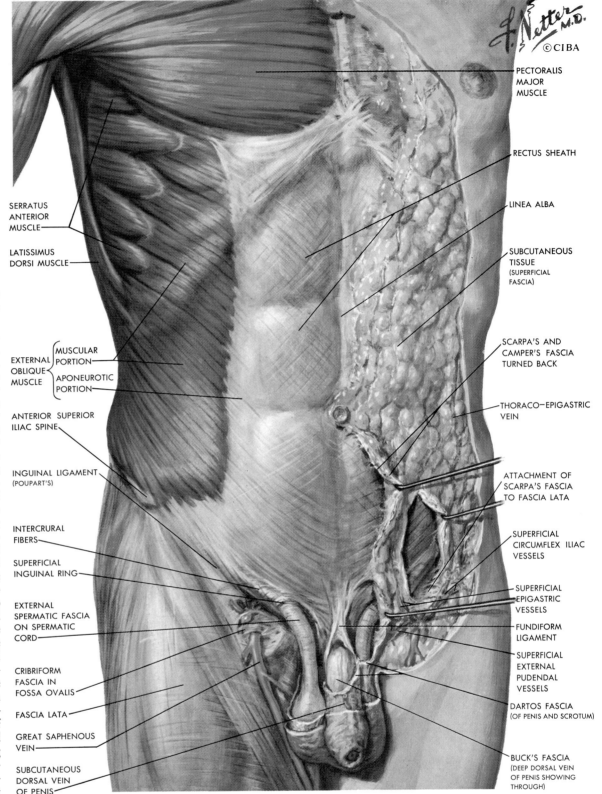

SERRATUS ANTERIOR MUSCLE

LATISSIMUS DORSI MUSCLE

EXTERNAL OBLIQUE MUSCLE — MUSCULAR PORTION / APONEUROTIC PORTION

ANTERIOR SUPERIOR ILIAC SPINE

INGUINAL LIGAMENT (POUPART'S)

INTERCRURAL FIBERS

SUPERFICIAL INGUINAL RING

EXTERNAL SPERMATIC FASCIA ON SPERMATIC CORD

CRIBRIFORM FASCIA IN FOSSA OVALIS

FASCIA LATA

GREAT SAPHENOUS VEIN

SUBCUTANEOUS DORSAL VEIN OF PENIS

PECTORALIS MAJOR MUSCLE

RECTUS SHEATH

LINEA ALBA

SUBCUTANEOUS TISSUE (SUPERFICIAL FASCIA)

SCARPA'S AND CAMPER'S FASCIA TURNED BACK

THORACO–EPIGASTRIC VEIN

ATTACHMENT OF SCARPA'S FASCIA TO FASCIA LATA

SUPERFICIAL CIRCUMFLEX ILIAC VESSELS

SUPERFICIAL EPIGASTRIC VESSELS

FUNDIFORM LIGAMENT

SUPERFICIAL EXTERNAL PUDENDAL VESSELS

DARTOS FASCIA (OF PENIS AND SCROTUM)

BUCK'S FASCIA (DEEP DORSAL VEIN OF PENIS SHOWING THROUGH)

anterolateral abdominal wall can contract and relax and, thus, help to accommodate the size of the abdominopelvic cavity to changes in volume of the contained viscera and to control the intra-abdominal pressure. Surgical approach to the abdominopelvic cavity is commonly made through this wall.

The general layers of the anterolateral abdominal wall from the outside in are skin, superficial fascia, outer investing layer of deep fascia, the muscles with their related fasciae, transversalis fascia, extraperitoneal fascia and parietal peritoneum (described on pages 23 to 25).

The skin is of average thickness (thicker dorsally than ventrally and laterally) and rather loosely attached to the underlying layers, except in the area of the umbilicus.

The *superficial fascia* (tela subcutanea) is soft and movable and contains a variable amount of fat,

depending mostly on the state of nutrition of the individual and varying to some extent in distribution. The thickness of this layer can be roughly estimated by picking up a fold, the thickness of which, minus the double thickness of the skin, would be about twice the thickness of the layer. The superficial fascia, particularly of the part of the wall inferior to the level of the umbilicus, has been classically described as having a superficial fatty layer, called *Camper's fascia,* and a deep membranous layer (to some extent discontinuous), called Scarpa's fascia. This classical description is somewhat of a simplification of the actual situation, in which the layering is not always as clear cut as indicated, but it serves as a means of description if this is kept in mind. Camper's layer is continuous with the fatty layer of surrounding areas, *e.g.,* with the fatty layer of the thigh. *Scarpa's layer fuses with*

(Continued on page 13)

ANTEROLATERAL ABDOMINAL WALL

(Continued from page 12)

the fascia lata along a line parallel to and just below the inguinal ligament. Medial to the pubic tubercle, both layers continue into the urogenital region. This is significant in relation to the path extravasated urine takes, *e.g.,* after rupture of the bladder neck. When entering the proper layer of the urogenital region, the urine may escape upward into the anterolateral abdominal wall. In the male the two layers continue into the scrotum and blend into a single smooth muscle-containing layer, the fat being rather abruptly lost as they enter into the formation of the scrotum. Just above the symphysis pubis a considerable addition of closely set strong bands to Scarpa's fascia form the *fundiform ligament of the penis,* which extends down onto the dorsum and sides of the penis.

The outer investing layer of the deep fascia (not readily distinguished from the muscular fascia on the *external surface of the external abdominal oblique muscle* and its *aponeurosis*) is easily demonstrable over the fleshy portion of the muscle but is much more difficult to separate from the aponeurotic portion of the muscle. This layer is attached to the *inguinal ligament* and blends with the fascia coming out from under this ligament to form the fascia lata. It also joins with the fascia on the inner surface of the external oblique at the *subcutaneous inguinal ring* to form the *external spermatic fascia.* External to the lower end of the *linea alba,* the outer investing layer is thickened into the *suspensory ligament of the penis,* which anchors the penis to the symphysis and arcuate ligament of the pubis. It is also continuous with the deep fascia investing the penis.

The *external abdominal oblique muscle* arises by eight fleshy digitations from the external surfaces of the lower eight ribs lateral to the costochondral junction, the middle group of digitations arising at a greater distance lateral to the junction than the ones above and below them. The digitations form an oblique line from above downward and backward. The upper five slips interdigitate with the *serratus anterior* (magnus) *muscle,* and the lower three slips interdigitate with the *latissimus dorsi muscle.* The general direction taken by the fibers of this muscle is downward and forward, and this leads the fibers from the lower two or three digitations to a fleshy insertion on the anterior half of the outer lip of the crest of the ilium, this portion of the muscle having a free posterior border which forms the anterior side of the lumbar triangle (see Plate 6). The muscular portion from the remainder of the origin becomes the strong *aponeurosis* of this muscle along a line which

courses almost vertically downward through about the tip of the ninth costal cartilage to almost the level of the anterior superior iliac spine, where it curves rather sharply laterally to course toward this spine. The aponeurosis passes in front of the rectus muscle (where it partly fuses with the aponeurosis of the internal oblique) to blend with the one of the opposite side in the midline linea alba, gaining attachment to the xiphoid process at the upper end of the linea alba and to the pubis at the lower end. The lower margin of the aponeurosis is folded backward and slightly upward upon itself between the anterior superior iliac spine and the pubic tubercle. The folded edge, together with an extremely variable number of fibrous strands running along it, is called the *inguinal ligament.* The detailed description of the pubic attachment of the external oblique aponeurosis and the split in this aponeurosis, known as the subcu-

taneous inguinal ring, is given, with the description of the inguinal canal, on pages 17 and 18.

The nerve supply of the external abdominal oblique muscle (see also page 41) is derived from the anterior primary divisions of the (fifth) sixth to twelfth thoracic spinal nerves. The (sixth) seventh to the eleventh are intercostal nerves, which continue from the intercostal spaces into the anterolateral abdominal wall to lie in the plane between the internal oblique and transversus muscles. The twelfth is the subcostal nerve and follows a course similar to the nerves above. The iliohypogastric nerve from T12 and L1 also contributes to the supply. The nerves probably have a segmental distribution corresponding to the primitive segmental condition of the muscle, with the tenth thoracic extending toward the umbilicus and the twelfth toward a point about halfway between

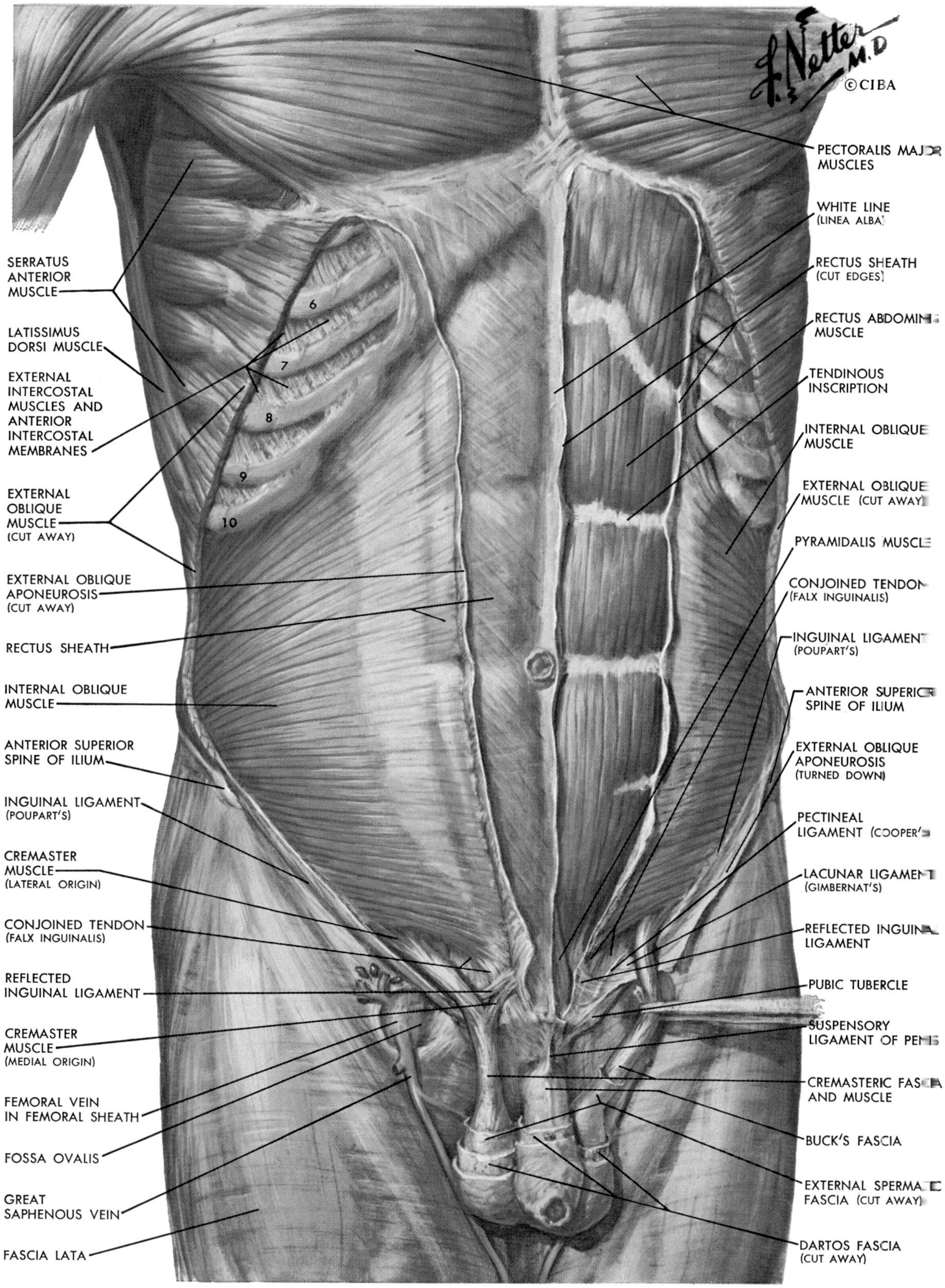

(Continued on page 14)

Figure labels (left side):
SERRATUS ANTERIOR MUSCLE
LATISSIMUS DORSI MUSCLE
EXTERNAL INTERCOSTAL MUSCLES AND ANTERIOR INTERCOSTAL MEMBRANES
EXTERNAL OBLIQUE MUSCLE (CUT AWAY)
EXTERNAL OBLIQUE APONEUROSIS (CUT AWAY)
RECTUS SHEATH
INTERNAL OBLIQUE MUSCLE
ANTERIOR SUPERIOR SPINE OF ILIUM
INGUINAL LIGAMENT (POUPART'S)
CREMASTER MUSCLE (LATERAL ORIGIN)
CONJOINED TENDON (FALX INGUINALIS)
REFLECTED INGUINAL LIGAMENT
CREMASTER MUSCLE (MEDIAL ORIGIN)
FEMORAL VEIN IN FEMORAL SHEATH
FOSSA OVALIS
GREAT SAPHENOUS VEIN
FASCIA LATA

Figure labels (right side):
PECTORALIS MAJOR MUSCLES
WHITE LINE (LINEA ALBA)
RECTUS SHEATH (CUT EDGES)
RECTUS ABDOMINIS MUSCLE
TENDINOUS INSCRIPTION
INTERNAL OBLIQUE MUSCLE
EXTERNAL OBLIQUE MUSCLE (CUT AWAY)
PYRAMIDALIS MUSCLE
CONJOINED TENDON (FALX INGUINALIS)
INGUINAL LIGAMENT (POUPART'S)
ANTERIOR SUPERIOR SPINE OF ILIUM
EXTERNAL OBLIQUE APONEUROSIS (TURNED DOWN)
PECTINEAL LIGAMENT (COOPER'S)
LACUNAR LIGAMENT (GIMBERNAT'S)
REFLECTED INGUINAL LIGAMENT
PUBIC TUBERCLE
SUSPENSORY LIGAMENT OF PENIS
CREMASTERIC FASCIA AND MUSCLE
BUCK'S FASCIA
EXTERNAL SPERMATIC FASCIA (CUT AWAY)
DARTOS FASCIA (CUT AWAY)

ANTEROLATERAL ABDOMINAL WALL

(Continued from page 13)

the umbilicus and the symphysis pubis.

The external abdominal oblique muscle has several actions in common with the other large muscles of the anterolateral abdominal wall. These are to: (1) support the abdominal viscera and, by compressing them, help to expel their contents; (2) depress the thorax in expiration; (3) flex the spinal column; (4) help in rotations of the thorax and pelvis in relation to each other. Contraction of the external oblique of one side would tend to help produce a rotation which would bring the shoulder of the same side forward if the pelvis were fixed.

The *internal abdominal oblique muscle*, smaller and thinner than the external oblique, arises from the posterior layer of the lumbodorsal (thoracolumbar) fascia, from the anterior two thirds or more of the intermediate line (lip) of the crest of the ilium and the lateral one half to two thirds of the folded-under edge of the external oblique aponeurosis, together with the immediately adjacent and closely related iliac fascia. The majority of the fibers from the lumbodorsal fascia (see Plate 6) and the iliac crest course upward and medially, which means that their direction is perpendicular to the general direction of the fibers of the external oblique. The most posterior fibers insert on the inferior borders of the lower three (or four) ribs and their costal cartilages. The rest of these fibers end in an aponeurosis along a line which extends downward and medially from the tenth costal cartilage toward the crest of the pubis. In the upper two thirds (to three fourths) of the abdomen, the aponeurosis splits at the lateral margin of the rectus into a posterior layer, which passes behind the rectus muscle, and an anterior layer passing in front of the rectus. These two layers join medial to the rectus and blend with those of the opposite side in the linea alba. In the lower one third to one fourth of the abdomen, the aponeurosis does not split but passes as a whole in front of the rectus to reach the linea alba. The fibers arising from the margin of the external oblique aponeurosis and the related iliac fascia are paler and less compact and course downward and medially, arching over the spermatic cord in the male (round ligament in the female). This portion of the internal oblique is variably closely blended with the related portion of the transversus and tends to fuse with the transversus for a common more or less aponeurotic insertion in front of the insertion of the rectus muscle on the pubic crest and for a variable distance on the pecten pubis. The name *"conjoined tendon"* can be

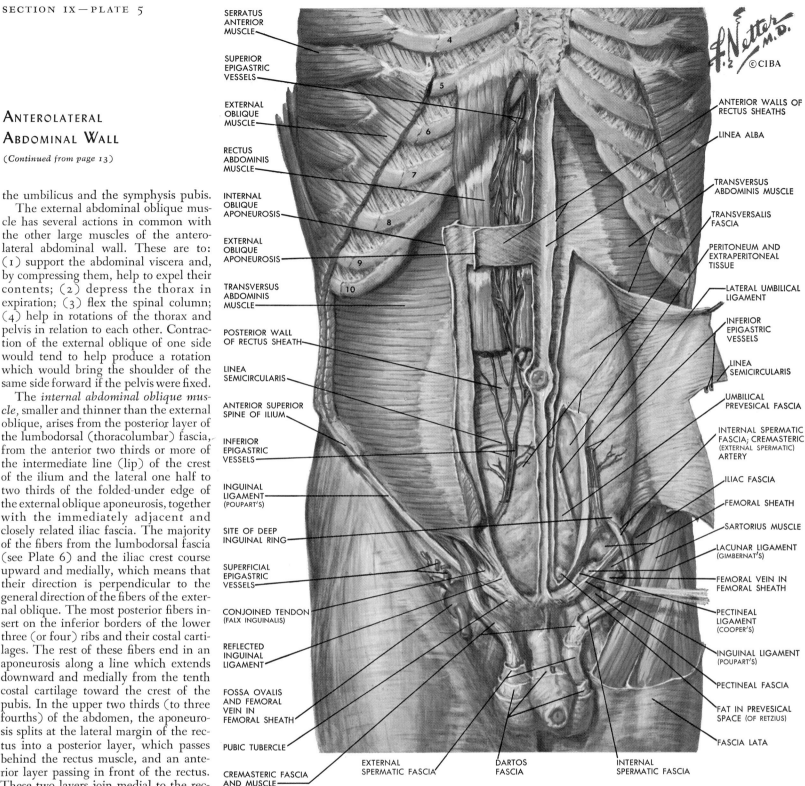

used for the medial part of the lower fibers of the internal oblique and transversus musculo-aponeurotic layers, which are fused together before their insertion. (Some authors call this same structure the inguinal falx, other authors wish to use these two terms differently, and still others decry the use of the name conjoined tendon at all.)

The nerve supply of the internal abdominal oblique is by way of the lowest two or three intercostal nerves, the subcostal nerve and the ilio-inguinal and iliohypogastric nerves (see pages 41 and 42).

The actions of the internal oblique are similar to those of the external oblique (see above), except that the muscle of one side would help to produce a rotation which would carry the shoulder of the same side posteriorly if the pelvis were fixed.

The *cremaster muscle* which is variably well developed only in the male represents an extension of the

lower border of the internal oblique (and possibly the transversus) over the testis and the spermatic cord. Laterally it is thicker and fleshier and attaches to about the middle of the turned-under edge of the external oblique aponeurosis and to the inferior edge of the internal oblique. From here the somewhat scattered fibers, with connective tissue (*cremasteric fascia*) between them, spread in loops over the spermatic cord and testis to end at the *pubic tubercle* and the anterior layer of the rectus sheath. The nerve supply of this muscle is from the genital (external spermatic) branch of the genitofemoral nerve (see pages 42 and 43) and, usually, also a branch from the ilio-inguinal nerve. The action of the cremaster muscle is to lift the testis toward the subcutaneous inguinal ring.

The *transversus abdominis* is a broad thin muscle

(Continued on page 15)

ANTEROLATERAL ABDOMINAL WALL

(Continued from page 14)

which takes nearly a horizontal course around the inner side of the antero-lateral abdominal wall. It arises from: (1) the inner surfaces of the costal cartilages of the lower six ribs by fleshy slips, which interdigitate with the slips comprising the costal origin of the diaphragm; (2) an aponeurosis formed by the union at the lateral border of the erector spinae muscle of the layer of the lumbodorsal (thoracolumbar) fascia attached to the tips of the transverse processes of the lumbar vertebrae and the layer of this fascia attached to the tips of the spinous processes of the same vertebrae (an indirect origin from the lumbar vertebrae); (3) the anterior one half to three fourths of the internal lip of the iliac crest; (4) about the lateral one third of the folded-under margin of the external oblique aponeurosis and the closely related portion of the iliac fascia. The muscular fibers terminate in a strong (for most of its extent) aponeurosis (see Plate 5) along a line that extends from well under the rectus muscle above and courses inferiorly and slightly laterally to emerge lateral to the rectus at about the level of the umbilicus and then to extend variably toward, roughly, the middle of the inguinal ligament. In the upper two thirds to three fourths of the abdomen, the aponeurosis passes posterior to the rectus muscle, fusing with the posterior layer of the aponeurosis of the internal abdominal oblique muscle, and ends by meeting the one of the opposite side in the linea alba. Insertion occurs also on the xiphoid process at the upper end of the linea alba. In the lower one fourth to one third of the abdomen, the aponeurosis passes in front of the rectus muscle to reach the linea alba. The lower fibers of the transversus have a common insertion with the lower fibers of the internal oblique, as described with the insertion of the latter muscle above (see Plate 4). The transversus is often described as having an inferior free border which arches over the spermatic cord in the male (round ligament in the female) from the origin on the external oblique aponeurosis to the pubic attachment. At the medial border of the abdominal inguinal ring, an aponeurotic band, called the interfoveolar ligament, extends between the arching lower border of the transversus muscle and the turned-under margin of the external abdominal oblique aponeurosis.

The nerve supply of the transversus muscle comes from the anterior primary divisions of the lower five or six thoracic nerves (lower intercostals and subcostal) and the iliohypogastric, ilio-inguinal and genitofemoral nerves (see page 42).

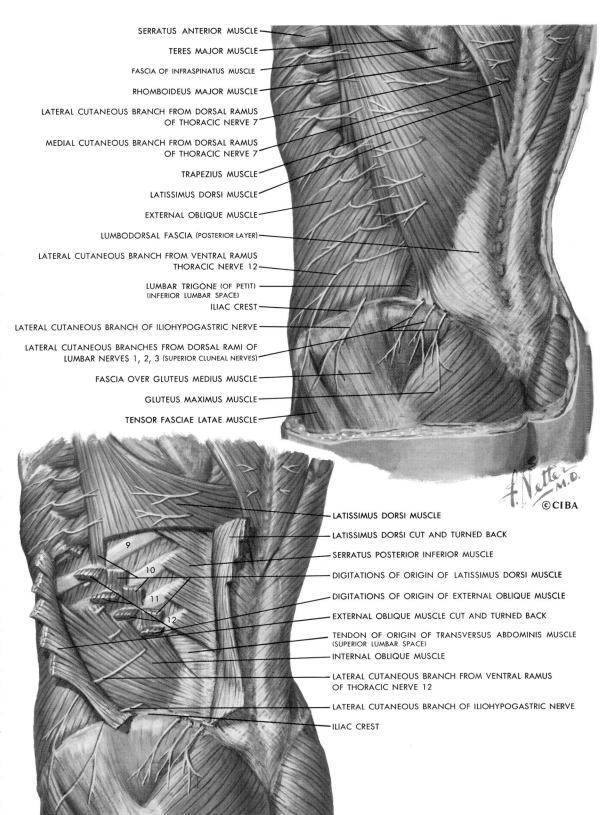

SERRATUS ANTERIOR MUSCLE
TERES MAJOR MUSCLE
FASCIA OF INFRASPINATUS MUSCLE
RHOMBOIDEUS MAJOR MUSCLE
LATERAL CUTANEOUS BRANCH FROM DORSAL RAMUS OF THORACIC NERVE 7
MEDIAL CUTANEOUS BRANCH FROM DORSAL RAMUS OF THORACIC NERVE 7
TRAPEZIUS MUSCLE
LATISSIMUS DORSI MUSCLE
EXTERNAL OBLIQUE MUSCLE
LUMBODORSAL FASCIA (POSTERIOR LAYER)
LATERAL CUTANEOUS BRANCH FROM VENTRAL RAMUS THORACIC NERVE 12
LUMBAR TRIGONE (OF PETIT) (INFERIOR LUMBAR SPACE)
ILIAC CREST
LATERAL CUTANEOUS BRANCH OF ILIOHYPOGASTRIC NERVE
LATERAL CUTANEOUS BRANCHES FROM DORSAL RAMI OF LUMBAR NERVES 1, 2, 3 (SUPERIOR CLUNEAL NERVES)
FASCIA OVER GLUTEUS MEDIUS MUSCLE
GLUTEUS MAXIMUS MUSCLE
TENSOR FASCIAE LATAE MUSCLE

LATISSIMUS DORSI MUSCLE
LATISSIMUS DORSI CUT AND TURNED BACK
SERRATUS POSTERIOR INFERIOR MUSCLE
DIGITATIONS OF ORIGIN OF LATISSIMUS DORSI MUSCLE
DIGITATIONS OF ORIGIN OF EXTERNAL OBLIQUE MUSCLE
EXTERNAL OBLIQUE MUSCLE CUT AND TURNED BACK
TENDON OF ORIGIN OF TRANSVERSUS ABDOMINIS MUSCLE (SUPERIOR LUMBAR SPACE)
INTERNAL OBLIQUE MUSCLE
LATERAL CUTANEOUS BRANCH FROM VENTRAL RAMUS OF THORACIC NERVE 12
LATERAL CUTANEOUS BRANCH OF ILIOHYPOGASTRIC NERVE
ILIAC CREST

The actions of the transversus muscle are the same as those listed as being common to the external oblique and other large muscles of the abdomen.

The *rectus abdominis* is a flat, vertically running muscle, just to the side of the anterior midline, which is wider and thinner cranially and becomes narrower and thicker caudally. It has a superior and an inferior attachment, each of which is called the origin of the muscle by some authors and the insertion by others. Several incomplete, zigzag, transversely running *tendinous bands* (inscriptions) are present in the muscle. These are better developed on the ventral surface of the muscle and are closely attached to the anterior wall of the rectus sheath. The one at the level of the umbilicus is segmentally related to the tenth rib. Two are usually present between the umbilicus and the xiphoid process, and, in about one third of the instances, one is found below the level of the umbili-

cus. The superior (cranial) attachment of the rectus muscle is to the ventral surfaces of the fifth, sixth and seventh costal cartilages, the xiphoid process and the costoxiphoid ligament. These attachments fall more or less in a horizontal line. The inferior (caudal) or pubic attachment of the rectus muscle is by a short tendon, a broader lateral portion of which ends on a roughened area on the pubic crest, extending from the pubic tubercle to the symphysis pubis. The narrower medial portion of the tendon is attached to the front of the symphysis, where it interdigitates with the one of the opposite side.

The nerve supply of the rectus abdominis muscle comes from the anterior branches of the anterior primary divisions of the lower six or seven thoracic nerves (intercostal and subcostal), which enter the deep surface of the muscle near its lateral edge

(Continued on page 6)

ANTEROLATERAL ABDOMINAL WALL

(Continued from page 15)

to send cutaneous branches obliquely through the muscle (see page 41) as muscular branches enter into the formation of an intramuscular plexus. The branch from the tenth thoracic nerve usually enters the muscle below the tendinous inscription at the level of the umbilicus.

The rectus abdominis acts, in general, in conjunction with the previously described muscles but, in particular, is involved in producing forced expiration and flexion of the vertebral column.

The *pyramidalis* is a small and apparently not very important muscle, which is quite variable and is absent in 20 to 25 per cent of the population. It arises from the crest of the pubis, just anterior to the line of attachment of the rectus muscle, and its fibers run superiorly and toward the linea alba, into which they are inserted as high as one third of the distance to the umbilicus. The pyramidalis is supplied by a branch from the subcostal nerve and, sometimes, also the iliohypogastric or ilio-inguinal nerves. No specific action is ascribed to this muscle.

The *rectus muscle* (including the pyramidalis) is wrapped in a *sheath* formed, for the most part, by the aponeuroses of the three large flat muscles of the anterolateral abdominal wall, the make-up of which differs in the lower one fourth to one third of the abdomen from the make-up for the rest of its length. In the upper two thirds to three fourths of the abdomen (see Plates 4 and 5), the aponeurosis of the external abdominal oblique muscle fuses with the anterior lamella of the aponeurosis of the internal abdominal oblique muscle to form the anterior layer of the rectus sheath, and the aponeurosis of the transversus abdominis fuses with the posterior lamella of the internal oblique aponeurosis to form the posterior layer of the rectus sheath. The anterior and posterior layers of the sheath fuse medial to the rectus muscle in the linea alba, and, at the lateral margin of the rectus muscle, the anterior and posterior layers come together at the line of the splitting of the aponeurosis of the internal oblique. The posterior layer of the sheath does not extend superior to the costal margin, so that the uppermost part of the rectus muscle lies directly on the chest wall. In the lower part of the abdomen, the aponeurosis of the internal oblique muscle does not split into two layers, and both it and the greater part of the aponeurosis of the transversus muscle pass anterior to the rectus muscle, so that the transversalis fascia (with perhaps some elements of the transversus

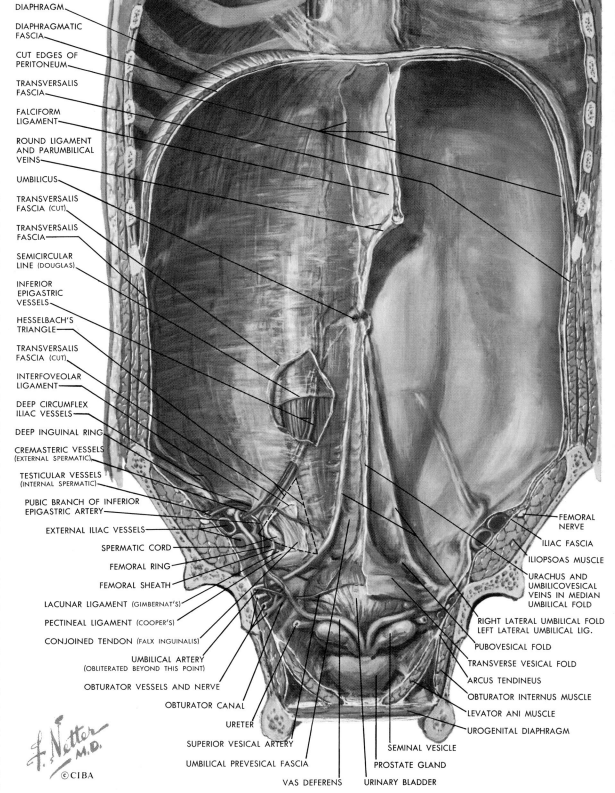

aponeurosis) forms the *posterior layer of the rectus sheath* in this area. Usually, the caudal margin of the definitely aponeurotic part of the posterior layer of the sheath is an obvious margin, called the *semicircular (arcuate) line*.

The name transversalis fascia is used by some authors specifically for the fascia on the inner surface of the transversus abdominis muscle (including its aponeurosis); others use this term to mean all of the internal investing layer of deep fascia of the abdominopelvic cavity. Whether it is all called transversalis fascia or parts of it are given names referring specifically to the muscles on whose inner surfaces it lies, an internal investing fascia does line the entire abdominopelvic cavity, and it differs greatly in different areas, being thin and adherent in some areas and thickened and more independent in others. At the arched lower border of the transversus muscle, the

transversalis fascia is thought to fuse with the fascia on the external surface of the transversus and to form a sheet extending to the inguinal ligament. This fascia extends under the inguinal ligament to form the anterior wall of the femoral sheath (see page 19). Lateral to this, in the area where the transversus abdominis arises from the turned-under edge of the external oblique aponeurosis and the related iliac fascia, the transversalis fascia fuses with the iliac fascia.

The extraperitoneal tissue (subserous fascia) is thin and comparatively free from fat on the roof and anterolateral abdominal wall, except in the lowest portion where it is loose and fatty to allow for the expansion of the bladder. In contrast to the situation on the roof and most of the anterolateral abdominal wall, the extraperitoneal tissue on the posterior wall of the abdominal cavity is large in amount and quite fatty, particularly around the great vessels and kidneys.

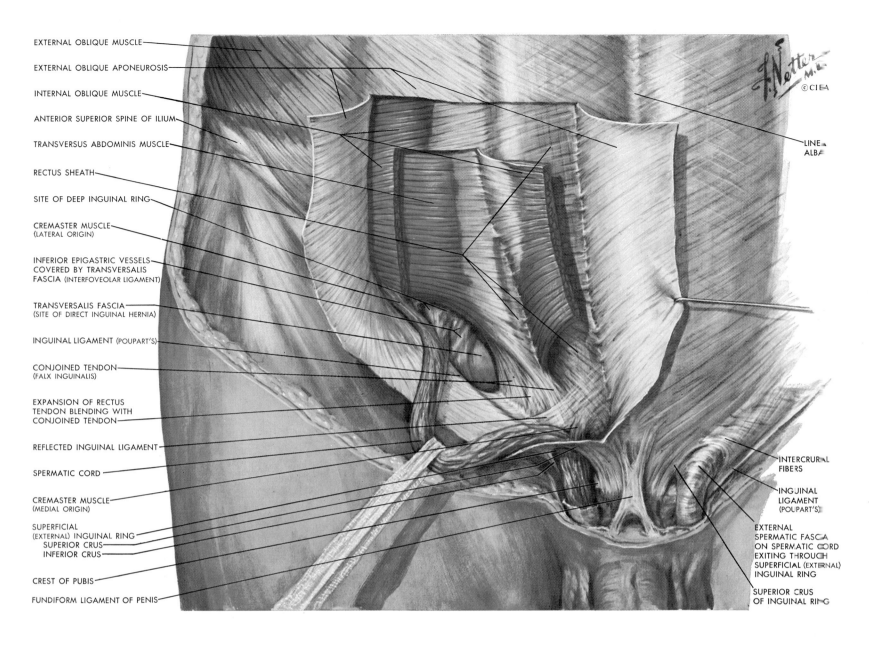

EXTERNAL OBLIQUE MUSCLE

EXTERNAL OBLIQUE APONEUROSIS

INTERNAL OBLIQUE MUSCLE

ANTERIOR SUPERIOR SPINE OF ILIUM

TRANSVERSUS ABDOMINIS MUSCLE

RECTUS SHEATH

SITE OF DEEP INGUINAL RING

CREMASTER MUSCLE
(LATERAL ORIGIN)

INFERIOR EPIGASTRIC VESSELS
COVERED BY TRANSVERSALIS
FASCIA (INTERFOVEOLAR LIGAMENT)

TRANSVERSALIS FASCIA
(SITE OF DIRECT INGUINAL HERNIA)

INGUINAL LIGAMENT (POUPART'S)

CONJOINED TENDON
(FALX INGUINALIS)

EXPANSION OF RECTUS
TENDON BLENDING WITH
CONJOINED TENDON

REFLECTED INGUINAL LIGAMENT

SPERMATIC CORD

CREMASTER MUSCLE
(MEDIAL ORIGIN)

SUPERFICIAL
(EXTERNAL) INGUINAL RING
SUPERIOR CRUS
INFERIOR CRUS

CREST OF PUBIS

FUNDIFORM LIGAMENT OF PENIS

LINEA ALBA

INTERCRURAL FIBERS

INGUINAL LIGAMENT (POUPART'S)

EXTERNAL SPERMATIC FASCIA ON SPERMATIC CORD EXITING THROUGH SUPERFICIAL (EXTERNAL) INGUINAL RING

SUPERIOR CRUS OF INGUINAL RING

INGUINAL CANAL

The space occupied by the spermatic cord and its coverings, as it passes obliquely through the anterolateral abdominal wall in the male, is called the inguinal canal. A similar inguinal canal is present in the female, which transmits the round ligament of the uterus toward its termination in the labium majus. For the sake of convenience, the description given here will be based on the male. In general, it can be said that the canal and the structures described in relation to it are much the same in the female, although somewhat less well developed.

The inguinal canal is an oblique tunnel, 3 to 5 cm. long, through the muscular and deep fascial layers of the anterior abdominal wall, which lie parallel to and just above the *inguinal ligament*. The canal extends between the *deep inguinal ring,* located in the *transversalis fascia* approximately halfway between the *anterior superior spine of the ilium* and the pubic symphysis, and the *superficial inguinal ring,* located in the *aponeurosis of the external abdominal oblique muscle* just superior and lateral to the pubic tubercle. The deep (abdominal or internal) inguinal ring can be described as a funnel-shaped opening in the transversalis fascia, as it is the site at which this fascia is continued onto the spermatic cord to become the innermost covering of the cord,

the internal spermatic or infundibuliform fascia. The *inferior epigastric vessels* (see page 16) are just inferomedial to the deep inguinal ring and the most lateral part of the inferior border of the transversus muscle is just superolateral to this ring. The superficial (subcutaneous or external) inguinal ring is formed by a splitting apart of the fibers of the external abdominal oblique aponeurosis, with those fibers which pass superomedial to the ring going to intermingle with similar ones of the opposite side and attach to the anteroinferior surface of the symphysis pubis. This portion of the external oblique aponeurosis is called the *superior* (medial) *crus of the superficial ring.* The fibers of the external oblique aponeurosis, which pass inferolateral to the superficial inguinal ring, are called the *inferior* (lateral) *crus of the ring* which, in a sense, is the medial end of the inguinal ligament.

The lower border of the external oblique aponeurosis (see page 13) is folded under upon itself, with the edge of the fold (and variable added fibrous strands) forming the inguinal ligament. The fascia lata on the anterior aspect of the thigh is closely blended to the full length of the inguinal ligament, and its approximately lateral half, folded under the aponeurosis, is firmly fused with the iliac fascia as the iliacus muscle passes into the thigh. As to the approximately medial half of the inguinal ligament, the folded edge is actually formed by the fibers of the aponeurosis rolling under in such a way that the fibers forming the inferolateral margin of the

superficial inguinal ring become the most inferior fibers at the attachment to the pubic bone and thus attach most inferiorly on the pubic tubercle, while the fibers which were originally more inferior attach higher up on the tubercle and in sequence along the medial part of the pecten pubis for a variable distance, with the lowest fibers in the aponeurosis attaching farthest laterally on the pecten. The portion of the aponeurosis which runs posteriorly and superiorly from the folded edge to the pecten pubis can be called the pectineal part of the inguinal ligament or the *lacunar (Gimbernat's) ligament* (see Plate 10). The fibers of the external oblique aponeurosis, described above, are attached to the pubic tubercle and the pecten pubis and continue, to a varying extent, beyond these points of attachment. Those which continue from the pecten pubis superiorly and medially superficial to the *conjoined tendon* reach the midline and blend to some extent with the external oblique aponeurosis of the opposite side. They are called the *reflected inguinal ligament.*

Lateral to the superficial inguinal ring, variable fibrous strands course roughly perpendicular to the fibers of the external oblique aponeurosis and are blended with the fibers of the superficial surface of this aponeurosis. These fibers, called the *intercrural fibers* (see also page 12), can be thought of as helping to prevent the split between the fibers of the external oblique aponeurosis (the superficial

(Continued on page 18)

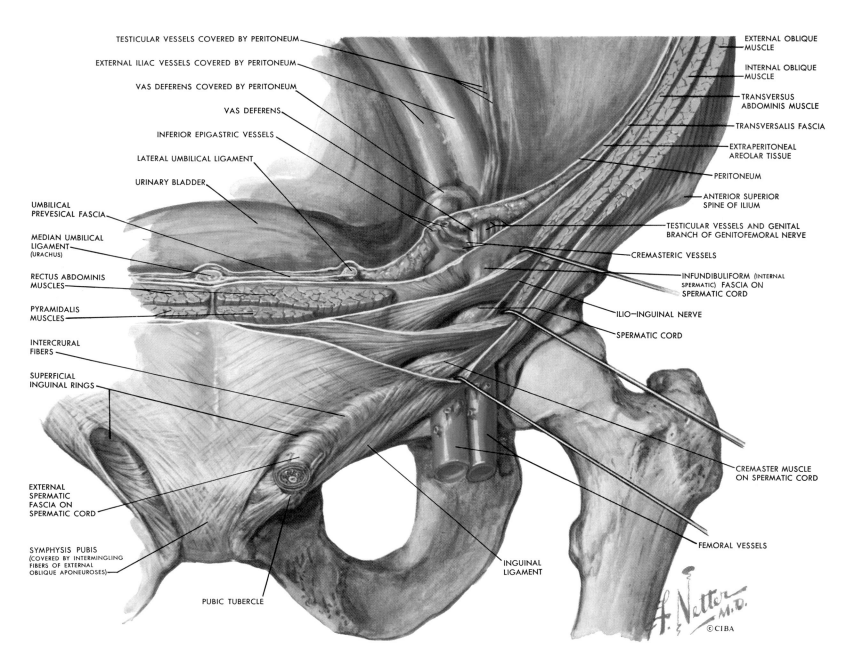

TESTICULAR VESSELS COVERED BY PERITONEUM

EXTERNAL ILIAC VESSELS COVERED BY PERITONEUM

VAS DEFERENS COVERED BY PERITONEUM

VAS DEFERENS

INFERIOR EPIGASTRIC VESSELS

LATERAL UMBILICAL LIGAMENT

URINARY BLADDER

UMBILICAL PREVESICAL FASCIA

MEDIAN UMBILICAL LIGAMENT (URACHUS)

RECTUS ABDOMINIS MUSCLES

PYRAMIDALIS MUSCLES

INTERCRURAL FIBERS

SUPERFICIAL INGUINAL RINGS

EXTERNAL SPERMATIC FASCIA ON SPERMATIC CORD

SYMPHYSIS PUBIS (COVERED BY INTERMINGLING FIBERS OF EXTERNAL OBLIQUE APONEUROSES)

PUBIC TUBERCLE

EXTERNAL OBLIQUE MUSCLE

INTERNAL OBLIQUE MUSCLE

TRANSVERSUS ABDOMINIS MUSCLE

TRANSVERSALIS FASCIA

EXTRAPERITONEAL AREOLAR TISSUE

PERITONEUM

ANTERIOR SUPERIOR SPINE OF ILIUM

TESTICULAR VESSELS AND GENITAL BRANCH OF GENITOFEMORAL NERVE

CREMASTERIC VESSELS

INFUNDIBULIFORM (INTERNAL SPERMATIC) FASCIA ON SPERMATIC CORD

ILIO-INGUINAL NERVE

SPERMATIC CORD

CREMASTER MUSCLE ON SPERMATIC CORD

FEMORAL VESSELS

INGUINAL LIGAMENT

SECTION IX—PLATE 9

INGUINAL CANAL

(Continued from page 17)

inguinal ring) from extending farther laterally.

Another structure which is frequently described as being formed by fibers from the external abdominal oblique aponeurosis, and which has considerable clinical significance as a firm structure to which sutures can be anchored in the surgical repair of hernia, is the *pectineal ligament* or *Cooper's ligament* (see Plate 10 and pages 20, 208, 210 and 211). This ligament runs along the sharp edge of the pecten pubis and has the effect of heightening this ridge. It is often described and pictured as being formed by fibers of the lateral part of the pectineal portion of the inguinal ligament (lacunar ligament) which, as they approach the pecten, turn sharply supero-laterally to run along it. The pectineal ligament can also be interpreted as a building up of the periosteum along the pecten pubis, which is more in keeping with what appears to be the situation in many cadavers.

The origins and insertions of the internal abdominal oblique muscle and the transversus abdominis muscle have been described previously (see page 14), but certain details in regard to the portions of these muscles related to the inguinal canal merit emphasis or added

description. The exact amount of the turned-under edge of the external abdominal oblique aponeurosis (and the adjacent iliac fascia to which this edge of the aponeurosis is closely related) from which these two muscles take origin is quite variable, and it may be difficult to separate these muscles in this area. The origin of the internal oblique muscle, more times than not, extends far enough medially so that some fasciculi of the muscle are anterior to the spermatic cord as its constituent structures come together at the deep inguinal ring, thus reinforcing this area to a certain extent. The origin of the transversus abdominis muscle (if it can be adequately separated) usually does not extend medially beyond the lateral border of the abdominal inguinal ring, if it extends that far. Since the conjoined tendon inserts on the pecten pubis and the crest of the pubis and thus along a line which angles from the pecten onto the crest, the part of this tendon inserting on the pecten is in one plane and that inserting on the crest is in a somewhat different plane. The part of the conjoined tendon inserting on the pecten pubis is partially fitted to the contour of the spermatic cord, and it approaches the pecten from behind the spermatic cord to meet the lacunar ligament (pectineal part of the inguinal ligament) which approaches the pecten from below the spermatic cord.

The inguinal canal and the structures in rela-

tion to it can be further elucidated by thinking of this tubular tunnel as having a roof, a floor and anterior and posterior walls, although, of course, since the tunnel is tubular, being shaped to accommodate a cylindrical structure (the spermatic cord), no sharp boundary between any of the four walls can be established. It should be further remembered that the openings at the ends of the tunnel are not in planes perpendicular to the long axis of the tunnel but are in planes which form an acute angle with the long axis of the tunnel, so that the posterior wall of the canal extends farther medially than does the anterior wall and the anterior wall extends farther laterally than does the posterior wall. The two openings, of course, are the deep inguinal ring in the transversalis fascia at the internal (lateral) end of the canal and the superficial inguinal ring in the aponeurosis of the external abdominal oblique muscle at the external (medial) end of the canal. The external abdominal oblique aponeurosis, strengthened by the *intercrural fibers,* is present in the entire length of the anterior wall of the canal. For approximately the lateral one quarter to one third of the canal, fibers of the internal oblique muscle, which arise from the inguinal ligament and related iliac fascia, form the anterior wall of the canal deep to the external oblique aponeurosis. Superficial to the external oblique aponeurosis lie the superficial fascia and the skin

(Continued on page 19)

INGUINAL CANAL

(Continued from page 18)

which, of course, continue medially beyond the anterior wall of the canal above the superficial inguinal ring. The *floor (inferior boundary) of the canal* is formed in its medial two thirds to three quarters by the rolled-under portion of the external oblique aponeurosis together with the lacunar ligament (pectineal portion of the inguinal ligament), forming a shelf upon which the spermatic cord rests. The transversalis fascia is present for the entire length of the *posterior wall of the canal.* Toward the medial end of the canal, and thus reinforcing the part of this wall posterior to the superficial inguinal ring, is the reflected inguinal ligament to the extent present just anterior to the conjoined tendon of the transversus and internal oblique muscles (see page 14). A quite variable expansion from the tendon of the rectus abdominis muscle (called by some authors the inguinal falx) fuses, to a variable extent, with the posterior aspect of the conjoined tendon. All of the reinforcing structures just described are, of course, anterior to the transversalis fascia. Posterior or deep to the transversalis fascia are the subserous fascia and *peritoneum* which continue across behind the deep inguinal ring. At the lateral end of the canal, the *inferior epigastric artery* and *vein* are posterior to the canal in the subperitoneal fascia as they are in relation to the medial (inferomedial) margin of the deep inguinal ring. Overlying these vessels, a thickening in the transversalis fascia is variably present, which has been called the *interfoveolar ligament* (see also page 16). A slight depression in the parietal peritoneum, as seen from within, is apt to be present at the site of the deep inguinal ring. The *roof of the inguinal canal* can be said to be formed by the most inferior fasciculi of the internal oblique muscle as they gradually pass in a slightly arched fashion, from a position at their origin anterior to the canal to a position at their insertion (by way of the conjoined tendon) posterior to the canal. At the lateral end of the canal, the lower fasciculi of the transversus abdominis arch similarly over the canal. It should be pointed out that, although the description above of a roof and a floor of the canal can serve a useful purpose in talking about the canal, the anterior and the posterior walls of the canal, in a sense, come together superior and inferior to the canal, and the roof and much of the floor are, perhaps, manufactured for descriptive purposes.

The weakest area in the anterolateral wall in relation to the inguinal canal is the area of the superficial inguinal ring, which, to a varying extent, is reinforced by the reflected inguinal ligament, the conjoined tendon and the expansion laterally and inferiorly from the tendon of the rectus muscle to the pecten pubis. This generally weakened area, through which direct inguinal herniae pass, is often described as a triangle bounded

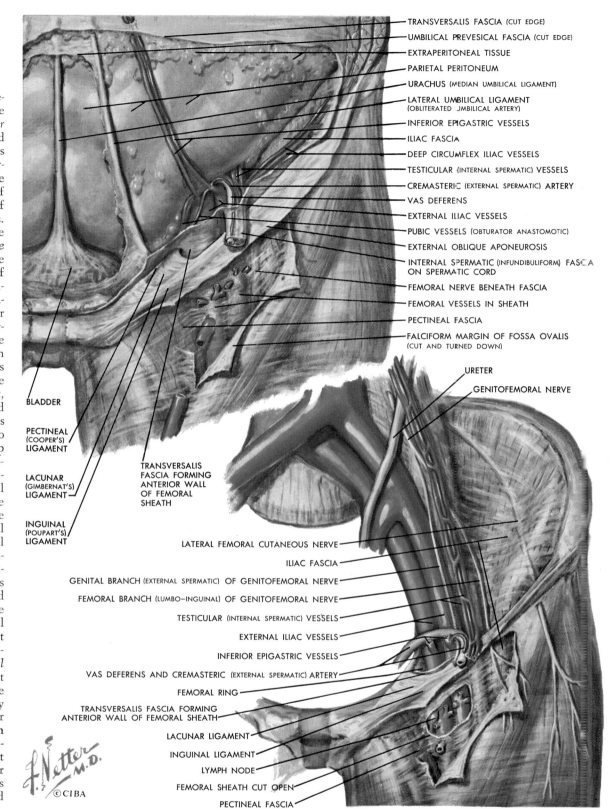

TRANSVERSALIS FASCIA (CUT EDGE)
UMBILICAL PREVESICAL FASCIA (CUT EDGE)
EXTRAPERITONEAL TISSUE
PARIETAL PERITONEUM
URACHUS (MEDIAN UMBILICAL LIGAMENT)
LATERAL UMBILICAL LIGAMENT (OBLITERATED UMBILICAL ARTERY)
INFERIOR EPIGASTRIC VESSELS
ILIAC FASCIA
DEEP CIRCUMFLEX ILIAC VESSELS
TESTICULAR (INTERNAL SPERMATIC) VESSELS
CREMASTERIC (EXTERNAL SPERMATIC) ARTERY
VAS DEFERENS
EXTERNAL ILIAC VESSELS
PUBIC VESSELS (OBTURATOR ANASTOMOTIC)
EXTERNAL OBLIQUE APONEUROSIS
INTERNAL SPERMATIC (INFUNDIBULIFORM) FASCIA ON SPERMATIC CORD
FEMORAL NERVE BENEATH FASCIA
FEMORAL VESSELS IN SHEATH
PECTINEAL FASCIA
FALCIFORM MARGIN OF FOSSA OVALIS (CUT AND TURNED DOWN)

BLADDER
PECTINEAL (COOPER'S) LIGAMENT
LACUNAR (GIMBERNAT'S) LIGAMENT
INGUINAL (POUPART'S) LIGAMENT
TRANSVERSALIS FASCIA FORMING ANTERIOR WALL OF FEMORAL SHEATH

URETER
GENITOFEMORAL NERVE

LATERAL FEMORAL CUTANEOUS NERVE
ILIAC FASCIA
GENITAL BRANCH (EXTERNAL SPERMATIC) OF GENITOFEMORAL NERVE
FEMORAL BRANCH (LUMBO-INGUINAL) OF GENITOFEMORAL NERVE
TESTICULAR (INTERNAL SPERMATIC) VESSELS
EXTERNAL ILIAC VESSELS
INFERIOR EPIGASTRIC VESSELS
VAS DEFERENS AND CREMASTERIC (EXTERNAL SPERMATIC) ARTERY
FEMORAL RING
TRANSVERSALIS FASCIA FORMING ANTERIOR WALL OF FEMORAL SHEATH
LACUNAR LIGAMENT
INGUINAL LIGAMENT
LYMPH NODE
FEMORAL SHEATH CUT OPEN
PECTINEAL FASCIA

F. Netter M.D.
©CIBA

superolaterally by the inferior epigastric vessels, superomedially by the lateral margin of the rectus and inferiorly by the inguinal ligament, and is called Hesselbach's triangle (see page 16).

Developmentally, the inguinal canal is established by an outpouching in the lower part of the anterior abdominal wall, comprising all of the layers from the parietal peritoneum outward, in preparation for the descent of the testis (see also CIBA COLLECTION, Vol. 2, page 26), from where it is formed on the posterior body wall down through the inguinal canal into the scrotum. Originally, the outpouching was straight dorsoventrally, but further regional development causes it to become oblique. The peritoneal outpouching (processus vaginalis) normally loses its connection with the parietal peritoneum of the abdominopelvic cavity, and all that remains of this is the double-walled serous sac (tunica vaginalis) par-

tially surrounding the testis. The outpouchings of the other layers remain as coverings of the spermatic cord and testis, which are picked up by the spermatic cord as it passes through the successive layers of the anterolateral abdominal wall. The covering acquired from the transversalis fascia is called the internal spermatic or infundibuliform fascia. Some authors consider the outpouching as having passed inferior to the lower border of the transversus abdominis, whereas others consider the transversus as combining with the internal oblique muscle in contributing a covering to the testis and spermatic cord. The covering derived from the internal abdominal oblique muscle (and perhaps the transversus) and its fascia is the *cremasteric muscle* and fascia. The covering of the spermatic cord and testis procured from the external abdominal oblique muscle and/or the deep fascia blended with it is the external spermatic or intercrural fascia.

POSTERIOR WALL OF ABDOMINAL CAVITY

The bodies of the *five lumbar vertebrae,* together with the related intervertebral disks, form a distinct longitudinally running midline elevation in the posterior wall of the abdominal cavity, which actually comes within a relatively short, but quite variable, distance (a few centimeters) of the inner surface of the anterior abdominal wall. The intervertebral disks produce bulges in this elevation, and the *anterior longitudinal ligament,* with the closely attached crura of the diaphragm, covers its anterior surface. Just lateral (on each side) to the lumbar vertebrae are the *psoas major* and *minor* (if present) *muscles.* Lateral to the psoas major muscle in the area inferior to the crest of the ilium is the *iliacus muscle,* and in the area between the twelfth rib and the crest of the ilium is the *quadratus lumborum muscle.*

The *psoas major muscle* arises from: (1) the anterior surfaces of the bases and the inferior borders of the transverse processes of all of the lumbar vertebrae; (2) the lateral aspect of the intervertebral disk above each of the lumbar vertebrae and from the adjacent parts of the vertebra above and the vertebra below each of these disks by five slips; and (3) from tendinous arches stretching across the concavity at the side of the body of each of, at least, the first four lumbar vertebrae. This muscle courses inferiorly along, slightly overhanging, the brim of the pelvis and passes beneath the inguinal ligament to enter the thigh and insert on the lesser trochanter of the femur. (For innervation, see pages 41 and 42.)

Present in 40 to 60 per cent of the cases, the *psoas minor muscle* arises from the lateral aspect of the bodies of the twelfth thoracic and first lumbar vertebrae and the intervertebral disk between them. It courses inferiorly on the anterior aspect of the psoas major, ending in a long flat tendon which inserts into the pecten pubis and the iliopectineal eminence (see page 11).

The *iliacus muscle* fills much of the iliac fossa (which actually forms the lateral wall of this part of the abdomino-

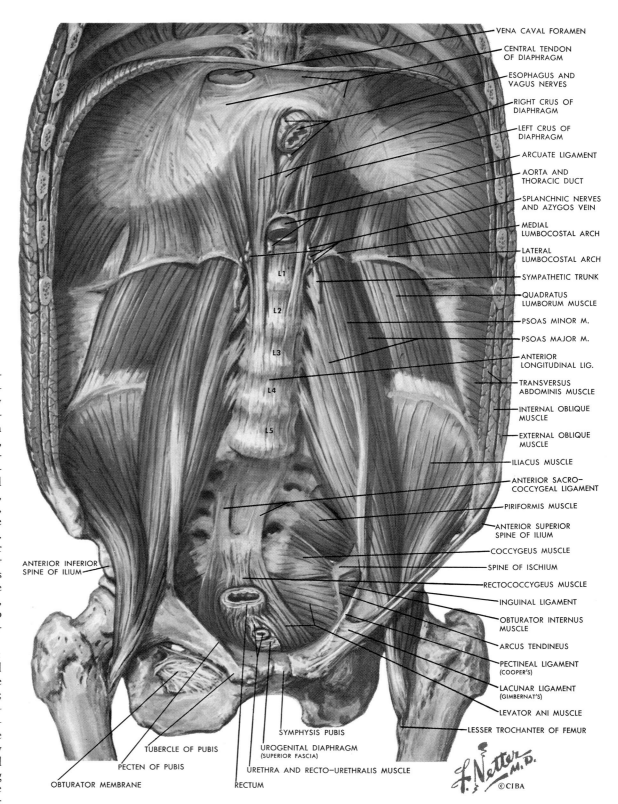

pelvic cavity) and arises from the upper two thirds of this fossa, the inner lip of the crest of the ilium, the anterior sacro-iliac and iliolumbar ligaments, and the base of the sacrum. Its fibers converge as they course inferiorly to insert, for the most part, into the lateral side of the tendon of the psoas major muscle. Some of the fibers are prolonged onto the body of the femur just below and anterior to the lesser trochanter. Since most of the iliacus muscle inserts into the tendon of the psoas major, the two muscles are often described as the "iliopsoas muscle" and, of course, have a common action.

The *quadratus lumborum muscle* arises from the posterior part of the crest of the ilium (inner lip), the iliolumbar ligament and the transverse process of the fifth (and perhaps fourth, third and second for a sometimes demonstrable anterior layer of the muscle) lumbar vertebra, and inserts into the lower border of

the medial part (half or so) of the twelfth rib, with some insertion into the transverse processes of the upper four lumbar vertebrae. It draws the last rib down and thus acts as anchorage for the diaphragm to the crest of the ilium, and it also bends the lumbar portion of the lumbar spine laterally.

The postero-inferior part of the diaphragm may be considered as part of the posterior abdominal wall. Depending on where the posterior limit of the antero-lateral abdominal wall is arbitrarily placed, the portions of the transversus abdominis muscle (overlain by the internal and external obliques) just lateral to the quadratus lumborum muscle can also be considered as helping to form the posterior abdominal wall.

The structures of the lower part of the back (see page 15) are, of course, external to what has been described here and would have to be traversed were the abdominal cavity approached from behind.

Image labels

VENA CAVAL FORAMEN
CENTRAL TENDON OF DIAPHRAGM
ESOPHAGUS AND VAGUS NERVES
RIGHT CRUS OF DIAPHRAGM
LEFT CRUS OF DIAPHRAGM
ARCUATE LIGAMENT
AORTA AND THORACIC DUCT
SPLANCHNIC NERVES AND AZYGOS VEIN
MEDIAL LUMBOCOSTAL ARCH
LATERAL LUMBOCOSTAL ARCH
SYMPATHETIC TRUNK
QUADRATUS LUMBORUM MUSCLE
PSOAS MINOR M.
PSOAS MAJOR M.
ANTERIOR LONGITUDINAL LIG.
TRANSVERSUS ABDOMINIS MUSCLE
INTERNAL OBLIQUE MUSCLE
EXTERNAL OBLIQUE MUSCLE
ILIACUS MUSCLE
ANTERIOR SACRO-COCCYGEAL LIGAMENT
PIRIFORMIS MUSCLE
ANTERIOR SUPERIOR SPINE OF ILIUM
COCCYGEUS MUSCLE
SPINE OF ISCHIUM
RECTOCOCCYGEUS MUSCLE
INGUINAL LIGAMENT
OBTURATOR INTERNUS MUSCLE
ARCUS TENDINEUS
PECTINEAL LIGAMENT (COOPER'S)
LACUNAR LIGAMENT (GIMBERNAT'S)
LEVATOR ANI MUSCLE
LESSER TROCHANTER OF FEMUR

L1 L2 L3 L4 L5

ANTERIOR INFERIOR SPINE OF ILIUM
OBTURATOR MEMBRANE
PECTEN OF PUBIS
TUBERCLE OF PUBIS
SYMPHYSIS PUBIS
UROGENITAL DIAPHRAGM (SUPERIOR FASCIA)
URETHRA AND RECTO-URETHRALIS MUSCLE
RECTUM

F. Netter M.D.
©CIBA

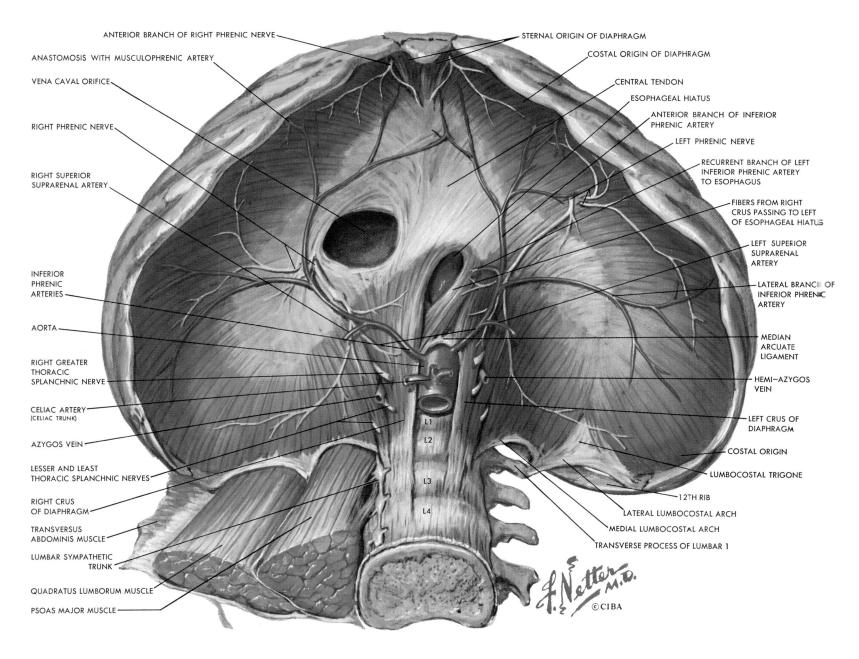

DIAPHRAGM

The dome-shaped roof of the abdominopelvic cavity is formed by a musculo-aponeurotic septum, the diaphragm, which also forms the floor of the thoracic cavity and thus is the partition between these two cavities. This unique muscular structure takes *origin* by its entire circumference from the inner aspect of, roughly, the *lower margin of the thoracic cage.* The muscular fibers course for the most part upward and inward to insert in the margins of a *central tendon.* The *sternal origin* is, by way of a fairly short, fleshy slip (a right and a left one), from the posterior aspect of the xiphoid process, which, on its way to the anterior margin of the central tendon, does not ascend nearly as much as do the fibers from the other two areas of origin. In fact, depending on the position of the individual and the degree of contraction of the diaphragm, the fibers from the sternal origin may even course downward.

The *costal origin* is, in general, the inner surfaces of the costal cartilages and the adjacent parts of the lower six ribs by a digitation (some-times more than one) from each, which interdigitates with the origin of the transversus abdominis muscle (see page 14). The *lumbar origin* consists of a crus, a *medial lumbocostal arch* and a *lateral lumbocostal arch* on each side. The crura begin as tendinous structures, which attach to the fronts and sides of the upper lumbar vertebrae (one to three or four for the right and one to two or three for the left) and related intervertebral disks, blending with the anterior longitudinal ligament. The *right crus* is stouter as well as longer than the left and, as it becomes muscular, usually splits to send *a portion* to the left of the *esophageal hiatus.* The medial margins of the two crura converge to meet in the midline to form an arch across the anterior aspect of the aorta (*median arcuate ligament*). The medial lumbocostal arch (medial arcuate ligament) is a tendinous arch, blended with or a thickening in the fascia over the upper part of the *psoas major muscle,* extending from the side of the body of the second (or first) lumbar vertebra, where it blends with the lateral margin of the corresponding crus to the end of the *transverse process* of the first (or second) *lumbar vertebra.* The lateral lumbocostal arch (lateral arcuate ligament) is a thickening in the fascia over the *quadratus lumborum muscle* and reaches from the end of the transverse process of the first (or second) lumbar vertebra to the tip and lower margin of the twelfth (or eleventh) rib.

The central tendon is a thin but strong and densely felted aponeurosis, closer to the sternal origin than the costal and lumbar origins. It is shaped somewhat like a thick and widely opened V, with slight indentations, which produce three leaflets. The fibrous pericardium is blended with its superior surface.

Several openings (hiatus) permit the passage of structures between the thoracic and abdominal cavities. The *vena caval hiatus* at the junction of the right and middle leaflets of the central tendon is the most anterior and the highest of the three large openings, being at the level of the disk between T8 and T9. It often transmits also a branch of the phrenic nerve. The esophageal hiatus is in the muscular portion just posterior to the central tendon, a little to the left of the midline and about at the level of T10, and transmits the vagus nerves (see CIBA COLLECTION, Vol. 3/1, page 44), small blood vessels and the esophagus. The *aortic hiatus* (really a notch in the posterior margin of the diaphragm) is at the level of T12 and also transmits the thoracic duct and the *azygos vein* (the latter may pierce the right crus). The *greater and lesser splanchnic nerves* pierce the crura and, in addition, the left crus is pierced by the *hemi-azygos vein.*

Intervals at the origin where muscle is replaced by areolar connective tissue occur at the sternocostal triangle and, with great variation, at the lateral lumbocostal arches.

The innervation of the diaphragm is discussed on page 44.

SYMPHYSIS PUBIS

ARCUATE LIGAMENT

CREST OF PUBIS

HIATUS FOR DORSAL VEIN OF PENIS

TUBERCLE OF PUBIS

TRANSVERSE LIGAMENT OF PELVIS
(ANTERIOR MARGIN OF UROGENITAL DIAPHRAGM)

SUPERIOR RAMUS OF PUBIS

SUPERIOR FASCIA OF UROGENITAL DIAPHRAGM

PECTEN PUBIS
(PECTINEAL LINE)

HIATUS FOR URETHRA

OBTURATOR CANAL

VISCERAL EXTENSIONS FROM LEVATOR
ANI MUSCLE TO RECTUM (TO CONJOINED
LONGITUDINAL MUSCLE)

OBTURATOR FASCIA

PUBORECTALIS
PUBOCOCCYGEUS } LEVATOR ANI
ILIOCOCCYGEUS   MUSCLE

RIM OF ACETABULUM

ARCUS TENDINEUS
OF LEVATOR ANI MUSCLE

ANTERIOR
INFERIOR
SPINE OF
ILIUM

OBTURATOR
INTERNUS
MUSCLE

FLOOR OF
ABDOMINOPELVIC CAVITY

ALA (WING) OF ILIUM

LINEA TERMINALIS

SPINE OF ISCHIUM

SACRO-ILIAC JOINT

SACRUM

ANORECTAL HIATUS

ANTERIOR SACROCOCCYGEAL LIGAMENT

ANTERIOR SACRAL FORAMINA

PIRIFORMIS MUSCLE

COCCYGEUS MUSCLE

F. Netter M.D.
©CIBA

The outlet of the pelvis (inferior aperture of the pelvis) is, for the most part, closed by the slinglike structure known as the pelvic diaphragm which, together with the urogenital diaphragm, gives the inferior and postero-inferior support to the abdominopelvic viscera. As usually described, the pelvic diaphragm consists of the right and left levator ani muscles, the right and left coccygeus muscles and the fascia on both surfaces of these muscles.

The *levator ani muscle* (described in more detail on pages 61 to 63) arises (1) from the pelvic surface of the pubis along a line from a little lateral to the lower part of the symphysis to near the *obturator foramen*, (2) from the *arcus tendineus musculi levatoris ani*, which is a thickening of the fascia on the pelvic surface of the obturator internus muscle along a line extending from the lateral end of the pubic origin of the levator ani to the ischial spine, and (3) from the pelvic surface of the *ischial spine*. In general, the fibers of the right and left levator ani muscles run backward, downward and medially, with varying degrees of obliquity, to come into relationship with each other in the midline by inserting into the anococcygeal ligament (perineal body) and the front and sides of the coccyx, or to blend closely with the midline viscera, where they are interposed between the two muscles. Approximately the anterior half (often called the *pubococcygeus muscle*) of the levator ani can be described in at least three parts—the most anterior fibers inserting into the perineal body, clasping the prostate in the male (puboprostaticus) and the vagina in the female, the intermediate fibers forming a sling around the anorectal junction (*puborectalis*) and the most posterior fibers passing in a plane above the iliococcygeus muscle

to insert into the coccyx and anococcygeal ligament (pubococcygeus proper). The remainder of the levator ani muscle is called the *iliococcygeus muscle*. The nerve supply of the levator ani muscle is from the fourth sacral nerve by way of the perineal branch of the pudendal nerve (see page 81).

The *coccygeus muscle,* which is closely applied to the deep surface of the sacrospinal ligament and is in much the same plane as the iliococcygeus muscle, is a flat triangular muscle arising from the ischial spine and inserting into the margin of the lower two sacral segments and the first two segments of the coccyx. It receives its nerve supply from the anterior primary ramus of the fourth sacral nerve.

The bony framework of the pelvis minor ("true pelvis"), supplemented by the sacrospinal and sacrotuberous ligaments, presents several openings, each of which is, to a great extent, closed by muscle. The

obturator internus, a muscle of the lower extremity, covers the obturator foramen except for the obturator canal through which the obturator vessels and nerve pass. It arises from the pelvic aspect of the *obturator fascia* and the adjacent bone and passes through the lesser sciatic foramen (mostly filling this opening) on its way to the medial side of the greater trochanter of the femur, where it inserts (see page 11). Anterosuperior to the origin of the levator ani muscle (see above), the obturator internus muscle forms a portion of the wall of the pelvic cavity. The *piriformis,* also a muscle of the lower extremity, arises from the pelvic surface of the sacrum between and lateral to the second, third and fourth anterior *sacral foramina* and mostly fills the greater sciatic foramen in traversing this foramen on its way to insert on the summit of the greater trochanter of the femur. The piriformis muscle thus also contributes to the pelvic parietes.

PERITONEUM

The peritoneum is the extensive serous membrane which, in general, lines the parietes of the abdominopelvic cavity and reflects from these parietes to cover, to a differing extent, the various viscera which are contained within the abdominopelvic cavity. A general concept which one might have of the pleura or the serous pericardium can be carried over to the peritoneum. In all of these situations, the serous membrane lining the parietes is continuous with that on the surfaces of the viscera contained within the portions of the body cavity involved, and one refers to parietal and visceral portions of the respective serous membrane. Also, under normal circumstances, the contained viscera fill the respective portion of the body cavity so completely that the visceral and parietal portions or adjacent visceral or adjacent parietal portions of the serous membrane in question are separated from each other by only a thin film of fluid, and thus a potential cavity comes into existence, which is named the cavity of the particular serous membrane. These cavities are all closed cavities, except the peritoneal cavity of the female, in which the lumen of each uterine tube is continuous with the peritoneal cavity at the abdominal ostium of the tube. From what has been stated above, it is obvious that the names peritoneal cavity and abdominal or abdominopelvic cavity should not be used synonymously.

The peritoneum is much more complicated in its arrangement than either the pleura or the serous pericardium. This is essentially due to the fact that parts of several viscera invaginate the peritoneal serous membrane to various degrees because, in the course of the fetal development, the rotations of the gut, combined with the propensity of one free peritoneal surface to fuse with another free surface (see pages 4 to 7), result in complex changes of the arrangement which, in the earliest stages of development, was as simple as in the case of the two other serous membranes. The stomach — to cite only one example of the manifold rearrangements in the visceroperitoneal relations — in its primary vertical position was attached by one double

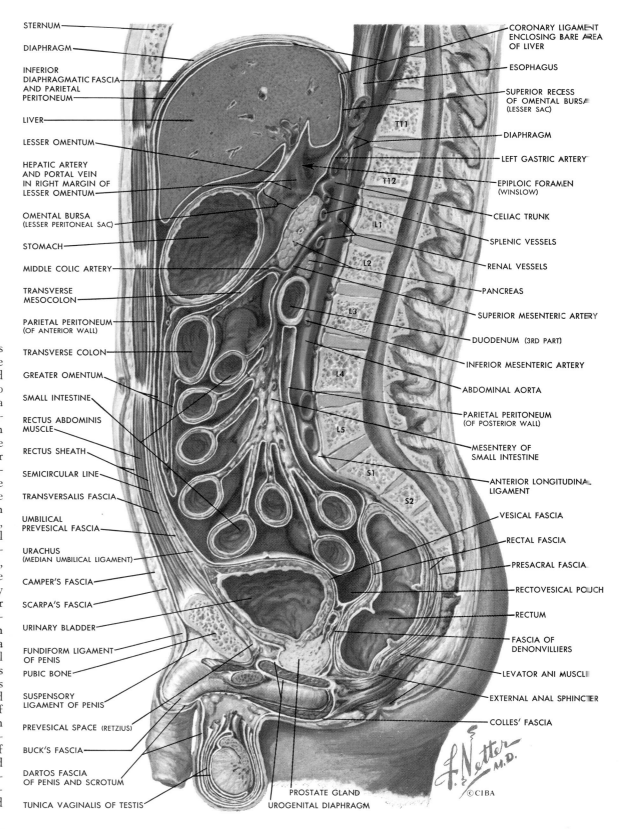

layer of peritoneum, the ventral mesogastrium, to the ventral body wall, and by another double layer, the dorsal mesogastrium, to the posterior wall. When the stomach rotates, its original left side becoming the anterosuperior surface and the original right side the postero-inferior surface, the dorsal mesogastrium is swept toward the left and forms, as a result of extensive growth and fusions of its layers, an outpouching of the peritoneal cavity, which presents itself at an early developmental stage (6 weeks) as the so-called lesser sac, or omental bursa, communicating with the general (main) cavity or greater sac by only a small opening, the epiploic foramen (of Winslow), located a little to the right of the midline postero-inferior to the liver.

The best way to obtain a general concept of the arrangement of the peritoneum is to trace it in three planes — a midsagittal plane and two horizontal

planes, one at the level of the epiploic foramen, the other at the level of the umbilicus — in a preferably fresh specimen at the autopsy table. Lacking this opportunity, the use of these three planes (see Plates 14, 15 and 16) still remains methodically the most informative approach to study the peritoneal continuity and its relationship to the abdominopelvic viscera.

In the near midsagittal plane (shown on this page somewhat schematically, simplified for didactic reasons) the greater and lesser peritoneal sacs must be pursued separately, because they are not continuous anywhere in this plane. In following the cut edge of the *greater sac*, one can start with the *parietal peritoneum* on the inner surface of the *anterior wall* at the level of the umbilicus. Progressing superiorly, the peritoneum continues onto the inferior surface of the

(Continued on page 24)

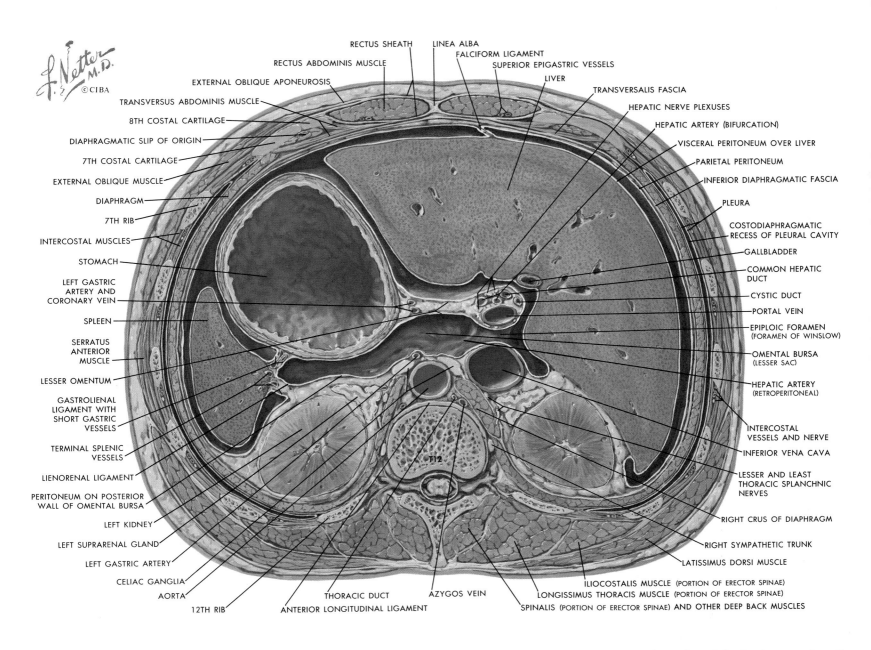

RECTUS SHEATH — LINEA ALBA
RECTUS ABDOMINIS MUSCLE — FALCIFORM LIGAMENT
SUPERIOR EPIGASTRIC VESSELS
EXTERNAL OBLIQUE APONEUROSIS — LIVER
TRANSVERSUS ABDOMINIS MUSCLE — TRANSVERSALIS FASCIA
8TH COSTAL CARTILAGE — HEPATIC NERVE PLEXUSES
DIAPHRAGMATIC SLIP OF ORIGIN — HEPATIC ARTERY (BIFURCATION)
7TH COSTAL CARTILAGE — VISCERAL PERITONEUM OVER LIVER
EXTERNAL OBLIQUE MUSCLE — PARIETAL PERITONEUM
DIAPHRAGM — INFERIOR DIAPHRAGMATIC FASCIA
7TH RIB — PLEURA
INTERCOSTAL MUSCLES — COSTODIAPHRAGMATIC RECESS OF PLEURAL CAVITY
STOMACH — GALLBLADDER
LEFT GASTRIC ARTERY AND CORONARY VEIN — COMMON HEPATIC DUCT
— CYSTIC DUCT
SPLEEN — PORTAL VEIN
— EPIPLOIC FORAMEN (FORAMEN OF WINSLOW)
SERRATUS ANTERIOR MUSCLE — OMENTAL BURSA (LESSER SAC)
LESSER OMENTUM — HEPATIC ARTERY (RETROPERITONEAL)
GASTROLIENAL LIGAMENT WITH SHORT GASTRIC VESSELS
TERMINAL SPLENIC VESSELS — INTERCOSTAL VESSELS AND NERVE
— INFERIOR VENA CAVA
LIENORENAL LIGAMENT
PERITONEUM ON POSTERIOR WALL OF OMENTAL BURSA — LESSER AND LEAST THORACIC SPLANCHNIC NERVES
LEFT KIDNEY — RIGHT CRUS OF DIAPHRAGM
LEFT SUPRARENAL GLAND — RIGHT SYMPATHETIC TRUNK
LEFT GASTRIC ARTERY — LATISSIMUS DORSI MUSCLE
CELIAC GANGLIA — ILIOCOSTALIS MUSCLE (PORTION OF ERECTOR SPINAE)
AORTA — LONGISSIMUS THORACIS MUSCLE (PORTION OF ERECTOR SPINAE)
12TH RIB — THORACIC DUCT — AZYGOS VEIN — SPINALIS (PORTION OF ERECTOR SPINAE) AND OTHER DEEP BACK MUSCLES
ANTERIOR LONGITUDINAL LIGAMENT
T12

SECTION IX—PLATE 15

PERITONEUM

(*Continued from page 23*)

diaphragm and along this until it is reflected to the liver as the superior (anterior) layer of the *coronary* (left triangular) *ligament.* From here it extends along the anterosuperior surface of the liver, around the free margin of the liver and onto its visceral surface, until it is reflected toward the lesser curvature of the stomach as the anterior layer of the *lesser omentum,* which then advances onto the anterosuperior surface of the stomach, leaving the latter as the anterior surface of the greater omentum. At the free margin of the greater omentum, this layer turns superiorly to become the posterior surface of the greater omentum, which proceeds upward to the transverse colon, where it appears to continue onto the posterior surface of the transverse colon and then as the posterior layer of the transverse mesocolon. (The development of the situation just described is shown on Plates 3, 4 and 5 of Section VIII and discussed on pages 6, 7 and 8.) From the posterior layer of the transverse mesocolon, the peritoneum turns inferiorly from the lower border of the *pancreas* across the anterior surface of the *third portion of the duodenum* and becomes the right (superior) layer of the *mesentery* (see Plate 17). At its free margin the mesentery

completely (except for the area of mesenteric attachment) surrounds the small intestine and continues to the posterior body wall as the left (inferior) layer of the mesentery. On reaching the body wall, it runs as the *parietal peritoneum of the posterior wall* inferiorly on the anterior surface of the aorta and then on the vertebral column to about the second sacral level, where it comes to lie on the anterior surface of the rectum, from which, in the male, it is reflected onto the posterosuperior surface of the bladder, bounding the *rectovesical pouch.* In the female (see Plate 20) the peritoneum passes from the anterior surface of the rectum to the posterior vaginal fornix, bounding the rectovaginal (recto-uterine) pouch (of Douglas). It then passes up the posterosuperior aspect of the uterus, over the fundus of the uterus, and down on its antero-inferior aspect to about the junction of the body and cervix, whence it reflects onto the posterosuperior aspect of the bladder, bounding the vesicouterine pouch. In both the male and the female the peritoneum passes from the superior surface of the *bladder* to the inner surface of the anterior body wall, a variable distance above the symphysis pubis, depending on the degree of distention of the bladder. From here it continues superiorly to the point at which this tracing of the peritoneum was started.

In following the cut edge of the *lesser sac* peritoneum in a near midsagittal plane, a start can be made on the anterior surface of the pancreas, and the peritoneum can be traced superiorly from

here onto the surface of the diaphragm and until it reflects from the diaphragm to the liver as the inferior (posterior) layer of the *coronary* (left triangular) *ligament.* From here it can be traced along the posterior and then the inferior surfaces of the liver to the point at which it leaves the liver to go to the lesser curvature of the stomach as the posterior layer of the lesser omentum, which continues onto the postero-inferior surface of the stomach and to the greater curvature, where it leaves the stomach to extend for a variable distance into the greater omentum. This distance depends on the degree of fusion of the peritoneum which has taken place (see Figure 20, page 7), often (in the adult) reaching not much beyond the transverse colon. The peritoneum turns upward on the anterior surface of the transverse colon, and then, in the adult, it usually forms apparently the anterior layer of the transverse mesocolon if, in development, the fusion of the primitive dorsal mesogastrium with the primitive mesentery of the transverse colon has been complete. The transverse mesocolon comes to the posterior body wall just inferior to the point at which the tracing of the lesser sac peritoneum was started.

In tracing the peritoneum in a horizontal section at the level of the epiploic foramen (see plate on this page), a start can be made with the greater sac peritoneum on the inner surface of the anterior abdominal wall in the midline. Following the cut edge of the *parietal peritoneum* to the left

(*Continued on page 25*)

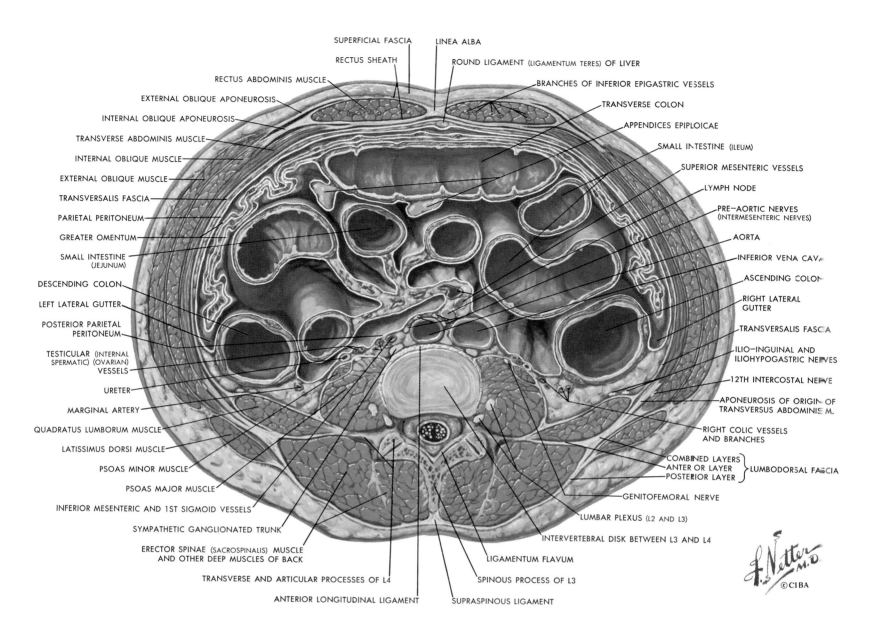

SUPERFICIAL FASCIA — LINEA ALBA
RECTUS SHEATH — ROUND LIGAMENT (LIGAMENTUM TERES) OF LIVER
RECTUS ABDOMINIS MUSCLE — BRANCHES OF INFERIOR EPIGASTRIC VESSELS
EXTERNAL OBLIQUE APONEUROSIS — TRANSVERSE COLON
INTERNAL OBLIQUE APONEUROSIS — APPENDICES EPIPLOICAE
TRANSVERSE ABDOMINIS MUSCLE — SMALL INTESTINE (ILEUM)
INTERNAL OBLIQUE MUSCLE — SUPERIOR MESENTERIC VESSELS
EXTERNAL OBLIQUE MUSCLE — LYMPH NODE
TRANSVERSALIS FASCIA — PRE-AORTIC NERVES (INTERMESENTERIC NERVES)
PARIETAL PERITONEUM — AORTA
GREATER OMENTUM — INFERIOR VENA CAVA
SMALL INTESTINE (JEJUNUM) — ASCENDING COLON
DESCENDING COLON — RIGHT LATERAL GUTTER
LEFT LATERAL GUTTER — TRANSVERSALIS FASCIA
POSTERIOR PARIETAL PERITONEUM — ILIO-INGUINAL AND ILIOHYPOGASTRIC NERVES
TESTICULAR (INTERNAL SPERMATIC) (OVARIAN) VESSELS — 12TH INTERCOSTAL NERVE
URETER — APONEUROSIS OF ORIGIN OF TRANSVERSUS ABDOMINIS M.
MARGINAL ARTERY — RIGHT COLIC VESSELS AND BRANCHES
QUADRATUS LUMBORUM MUSCLE — COMBINED LAYERS ANTERIOR LAYER POSTERIOR LAYER } LUMBODORSAL FASCIA
LATISSIMUS DORSI MUSCLE — GENITOFEMORAL NERVE
PSOAS MINOR MUSCLE — LUMBAR PLEXUS (L2 AND L3)
PSOAS MAJOR MUSCLE — INTERVERTEBRAL DISK BETWEEN L3 AND L4
INFERIOR MESENTERIC AND 1ST SIGMOID VESSELS
SYMPATHETIC GANGLIONATED TRUNK — LIGAMENTUM FLAVUM
ERECTOR SPINAE (SACROSPINALIS) MUSCLE AND OTHER DEEP MUSCLES OF BACK — SPINOUS PROCESS OF L3
TRANSVERSE AND ARTICULAR PROCESSES OF L4 — ANTERIOR LONGITUDINAL LIGAMENT — SUPRASPINOUS LIGAMENT

SECTION IX—PLATE 16

PERITONEUM

(Continued from page 24)

along the inner surface of the anterolateral wall to the region of the posterior wall, it will be found to pass onto the anterolateral surface of the left *kidney,* from where it reflects to the hilar area of the spleen, forming the external (greater sac) layer of the *lienorenal ligament,* and then completely surrounds the spleen except at the hilar area. From the anterior margin of the hilum of the spleen, the peritoneum passes to the stomach as the external (greater sac) layer of the *gastrolienal ligament.* The peritoneum can then be followed along the anterosuperior surface of the stomach to the lesser curvature, where it leaves the stomach as the anterior (greater sac) layer of the *lesser omentum,* which can be followed to the right until the free margin is reached a short distance to the right of the midline. Here the peritoneum passes around the free margin of the lesser omentum (anterior boundary of the epiploic foramen) to become the lesser sac peritoneum, which continues to the left, as the posterior layer of the lesser omentum, to the lesser curvature of the stomach, where it continues onto the postero-inferior surface of the stomach, which it follows until it leaves the stomach to form the internal (lesser sac) layer of the gastrolienal

ligament. From the spleen the peritoneum goes to form the internal (lesser sac) layer of the lienorenal ligament and then travels to the right in front of the *aorta* and the *inferior vena cava.* At the right margin of the inferior vena cava, the peritoneum again becomes greater sac peritoneum and continues to the right onto the anterior aspect of the right kidney. From here the tracing of the peritoneum could differ, depending on whether the bare area of the liver were to extend down just far enough to be encountered in the plane of the tracing, as is the case in the schematic section shown in Plate 15, or whether the plane of tracing passes just inferior to the bare area of the liver, as is often shown in text figures. In the former case the peritoneum would pass from the kidney as the inferior layer of the coronary ligament to the liver, and would follow around the liver to its anterosuperior surface, where it would leave the liver as the left layer of the *falciform ligament* of the liver, to go to the inner surface of the anterior body wall and to the left to the point from which the tracing started. To complete the tracing in this plane, one must follow the peritoneum from the right layer of the falciform ligament onto the anterosuperior surface of the liver, and to the right along this surface to the superior layer of the coronary ligament, along this to the diaphragm and then anteriorly on the inner surface of the parietes to the right layer of the falciform ligament. If the plane of section passes just inferior to the bare area of the liver as the peritoneum

leaves the anterior surface of the inferior vena cava (the posterior boundary of the epiploic foramen), it passes across the anterior surface of the right kidney, then to the diaphragm and forward on the inner surface of the parietes to the falciform ligament. The picture would be the same as in Plate 15, except that no connection would be seen between the peritoneum crossing the right kidney and the peritoneum encircling the portion of the liver cut in the section.

In tracing peritoneum in a horizontal section at about the level of the umbilicus (see plate on this page), one can start at the midline of the inner surface of the anterior abdominal wall and follow from this point the parietal peritoneum to the left along the inner surface of the wall to the posterior wall, where it reflects onto the left side of the *descending colon* to cover also the anterior surface and right side of this structure, from which it passes to the posterior body wall. [In early development the descending colon was suspended by the primitive dorsal mesentery, but, by peritoneal fusion during embryologic development [see Section VIII, Plate 4 and page 6], it comes to have the adult relationship to the peritoneum just described.] The peritoneum continues to the right on the posterior body wall to about the midline, where it reflects forward to form the left (inferior) layer of the mesentery (see Plate 17). The small intestine is completely surrounded (except at its mesenteric attachment) in the free margin of the mesentery; from

(Continued on page 26)

INFERIOR VENA CAVA
HEPATIC VEINS
CORONARY LIGAMENT OF LIVER
EPIPLOIC FORAMEN (WINSLOW) BEHIND RIGHT FREE MARGIN OF LESSER OMENTUM
RIGHT TRIANGULAR LIGAMENT OF LIVER
FALCIFORM LIGAMENT OF LIVER
SUPERIOR RECESS OF LESSER SAC
ATTACHMENT OF LESSER OMENTUM; LEFT GASTRIC ARTERY
ESOPHAGUS
LEFT TRIANGULAR LIGAMENT OF LIVER
GASTROPHRENIC LIGAMENT; LEFT INFERIOR PHRENIC ARTERY
GASTROLIENAL LIGAMENT; SHORT GASTRIC VESSELS
LIENORENAL (PHRENICOLIENAL) LIGAMENT; SPLENIC VESSELS
DIAPHRAGMATIC FASCIA
SUPRARENAL GLANDS
HEPATIC AND SPLENIC ARTERIES (RETROPERITONEAL)
PHRENICOCOLIC LIG.
ATTACHMENT OF GREATER OMENTUM (RIGHT GASTRO-EPIPLOIC VESSELS)
ATTACHMENT OF TRANSVERSE MESOCOLON
ROOT OF MESENTERY; SUPERIOR MESENTERIC VESSELS
SITE OF DESCENDING COLON
TRANSVERSALIS FASCIA
SITE OF ASCENDING COLON
ATTACHMENT OF SIGMOID MESOCOLON; SIGMOID VESSELS
SUPERIOR RECTAL (HEMORRHOIDAL) VESSELS
PARIETAL PERITONEUM
URETERS (RETROPERITONEAL)
SACROGENITAL FOLD
TESTICULAR VESSELS (RETROPERITONEAL)
SITE OF DEEP INGUINAL RING
INFERIOR EPIGASTRIC VESSELS (RETROPERITONEAL)
MEDIAN UMBILICAL FOLD (CONTAINING URACHUS)
LATERAL UMBILICAL FOLDS
RECTUM
BLADDER

PERITONEUM

(Continued from page 25)

here the peritoneum is traced posteriorly to the posterior body wall as the right (superior) layer of the mesentery. Next, the peritoneum can be followed to the right onto the posterior body wall, until it reflects from here to cover the left, anterior and right surfaces of the *ascending colon*. (This structure was also suspended originally by the primitive dorsal mesentery; see Section VIII.) From the right side of the ascending colon, the peritoneum passes to the posterior body wall and then forward on the inner surface of the parietes until it reaches the midline in front, where the tracing was started. Also in a section at about the level of the umbilicus, one would expect to find the greater omentum cut, which is present as an island of peritoneum not connected in this section to the rest of the peritoneum. If the transverse colon is hanging low enough, it too would be cut as an island with its peritoneum continuous with that of the greater omentum (as shown in Plate 16).

Worth-while additions to the general concept of the distribution of the peritoneum, gained by tracing it in several planes as done above, can be obtained by careful study of a view of the posterior half of the abdominopelvic cavity (shown on this page), in which all of the viscera (except the bladder and rectum) which invaginate the peritoneum to any degree have been removed, cutting the peritoneum along its lines of reflection from the posterior body wall or the anterior surfaces of the viscera and vessels which do not invaginate the peritoneum to any degree. The *right* and *left kidneys*, the *pancreas* (except for the tip of its tail), the *second, third* and most of the *fourth parts of the duodenum* and the *aorta* and *inferior vena cava* do not invaginate the peritoneum to any degree. The peritoneum covers the inner surface of the abdominopelvic parietes as parietal peritoneum, except where it is lifted away from them by the structures just listed, the bare area of the liver against the diaphragm (see Plate 14), the ascending and descending colon, the roots of the mesentery, the transverse mesocolon and sigmoid mesocolon, the ureters and inferior mesenteric vessels, the rectum and bladder and, in

the female, also the uterus and broad ligaments, other folds in the pelvis and folds on the inner surface of the anterior abdominal wall. The folds on the inner surface of the anterior abdominal wall (see page 16) are: the *falciform ligament* of the liver (a remnant of the ventral mesogastrium, ventral to where the liver grew into it), running superiorly and a little to the right from the umbilicus, with the ligamentum teres (obliterated umbilical vein) of the liver in its free margin; the *median umbilical fold* (containing the urachus), running from the bladder up the midline to the umbilicus; and the right and left *lateral umbilical folds* (medial umbilical folds of P.N.A.), containing the obliterated umbilical arteries and also running up toward the umbilicus. The *inferior epigastric artery* and *vein* on each side may produce a slight elevation remindful of a fold by pulling the peritoneum a little away from the body wall, but

definite folds are seldom formed in this manner. The depression between the *median* and *lateral umbilical folds* is called the supravesical fossa, the one between the lateral umbilical and "epigastric fold" is named the medial inguinal fossa and the one lateral to the "epigastric fold" is the lateral inguinal fossa. Parietal peritoneum is thus seen to be applied to practically the entire extent of the inner surface of the anterolateral abdominal wall, and virtually any incision through this wall including the parietal peritoneum will open into the peritoneal cavity.

Much of the diaphragm has parietal peritoneum on its abdominal surface, but much less of the posterior abdominal wall is directly lined by peritoneum on its inner surface, because it is here that several viscera and the main vessels lie behind the peritoneum and from here, for the most part, that the abdom-

(Continued on page 27)

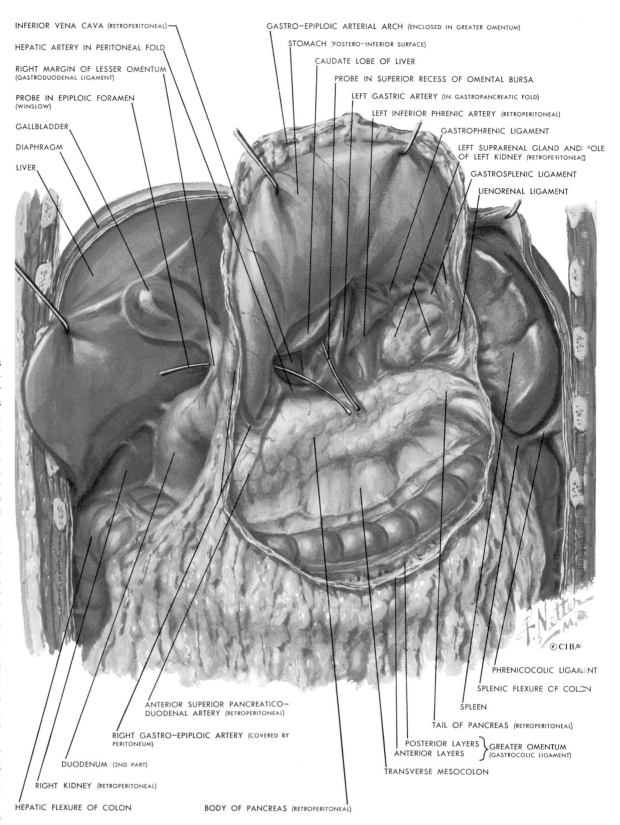

INFERIOR VENA CAVA (RETROPERITONEAL)
HEPATIC ARTERY IN PERITONEAL FOLD
RIGHT MARGIN OF LESSER OMENTUM (GASTRODUODENAL LIGAMENT)
PROBE IN EPIPLOIC FORAMEN (WINSLOW)
GALLBLADDER
DIAPHRAGM
LIVER

GASTRO-EPIPLOIC ARTERIAL ARCH (ENCLOSED IN GREATER OMENTUM)
STOMACH (POSTERO-INFERIOR SURFACE)
CAUDATE LOBE OF LIVER
PROBE IN SUPERIOR RECESS OF OMENTAL BURSA
LEFT GASTRIC ARTERY (IN GASTROPANCREATIC FOLD)
LEFT INFERIOR PHRENIC ARTERY (RETROPERITONEAL)
GASTROPHRENIC LIGAMENT
LEFT SUPRARENAL GLAND AND POLE OF LEFT KIDNEY (RETROPERITONEAL)
GASTROSPLENIC LIGAMENT
LIENORENAL LIGAMENT

PHRENICOCOLIC LIGAMENT
SPLENIC FLEXURE OF COLON
SPLEEN
TAIL OF PANCREAS (RETROPERITONEAL)
POSTERIOR LAYERS } GREATER OMENTUM
ANTERIOR LAYERS } (GASTROCOLIC LIGAMENT)
TRANSVERSE MESOCOLON

ANTERIOR SUPERIOR PANCREATICO-DUODENAL ARTERY (RETROPERITONEAL)
RIGHT GASTRO-EPIPLOIC ARTERY (COVERED BY PERITONEUM)
DUODENUM (2ND PART)
RIGHT KIDNEY (RETROPERITONEAL)
HEPATIC FLEXURE OF COLON
BODY OF PANCREAS (RETROPERITONEAL)

PERITONEUM

(*Continued from page 26*)

inal viscera invaginate the peritoneum.

From the preceding description it is obvious that the degree to which the various abdominal viscera are covered by peritoneum (visceral peritoneum) varies from the situation in which peritoneum covers just part of one surface of the viscus in question to the situation in which peritoneum covers the viscus entirely, except for the area of attachment of a suspending double-layered fold of peritoneum. Several terms are used in various ways by different authors to designate varying degrees of peritoneal covering, but, since most of these terms do not have a generally accepted connotation, it is suggested that one can be more specific in the description of peritoneal covering of a specific viscus by stating which parts of which surfaces of the viscus are covered by peritoneum, a description which is best given as part of the description of a particular organ. "Retroperitoneal" is, of course, a very commonly used descriptive term having the general meaning of "behind the peritoneum", which is well agreed upon, but some authors refer to certain organs as retroperitoneal which other authors would not designate in this fashion.

Additional detail concerning the peritoneum is given below by describing certain named parts of the peritoneum as well as some of the named fossae or recesses.

The *"mesentery"* (see Plate 14) is ordinarily taken to mean the mesentery of the small intestine, *i.e.,* the jejuno-ileal portion of the small intestine, which is the portion having a mesentery or a double-layered fold of peritoneum suspending it from the posterior abdominal wall. The *root* or attached border *of the mesentery* (see Plate 17) is about 15 cm. in length, and its line of attachment varies a bit with the shape of the duodenum, but, in general, it courses from a little to the left of the second lumbar vertebra downward and to the right, crossing the third part of the duodenum, the aorta, the inferior vena cava, the right ureter and the right psoas major muscle to reach a point near the right sacro-iliac joint. The free or unattached border which contains the jejuno-ileum is

frilled out to such an enormous degree that it may attain a length varying from 3 to sometimes more than 6 m. The distance from the attached to the free border measures 15 to 22 cm., which may definitely increase with age, probably owing to the stretching of the mesentery due to laxity of the abdominal wall. Between the two layers of peritoneum on the two surfaces of the mesentery are the *superior mesenteric artery* and its branches, the accompanying *veins,* lymphatics, 100 to 200 lymph nodes, autonomic nerve plexuses, connective tissue and varying amounts of adipose tissue, which is present in greater amounts near the root. The mesentery divides the area below the transverse mesocolon into two compartments, which are important in determining collections of fluid and the localization of infection.

The *transverse mesocolon* (see Plates 14, 16 and 18) is the broad peritoneal fold suspending the trans-

verse colon from the posterior body wall. The root *of the transverse mesocolon* (see Plate 17) crosses the anterior surface of the right kidney, the second portion of the duodenum and the head of the pancreas, and then passes along the lower border of the body and tail of the pancreas above the duodeno-jejunal flexure, to end on the anterior surface of the left kidney. It contains the middle colic artery, branches of the right and left colic arteries, accompanying veins, lymphatic structures and autonomic nerve plexuses, as well as a considerable thickness of connective tissue.

The *sigmoid mesocolon* (see page 54) is the mesentery of the sigmoid colon. When the peritoneum begins to surround the large intestine near the crest of the ilium and thus suspends what is often called the iliac colon (when it is not suspended) as well as the pelvic colon, the attachment of the sigmoid meso-

(*Continued on page 28*)

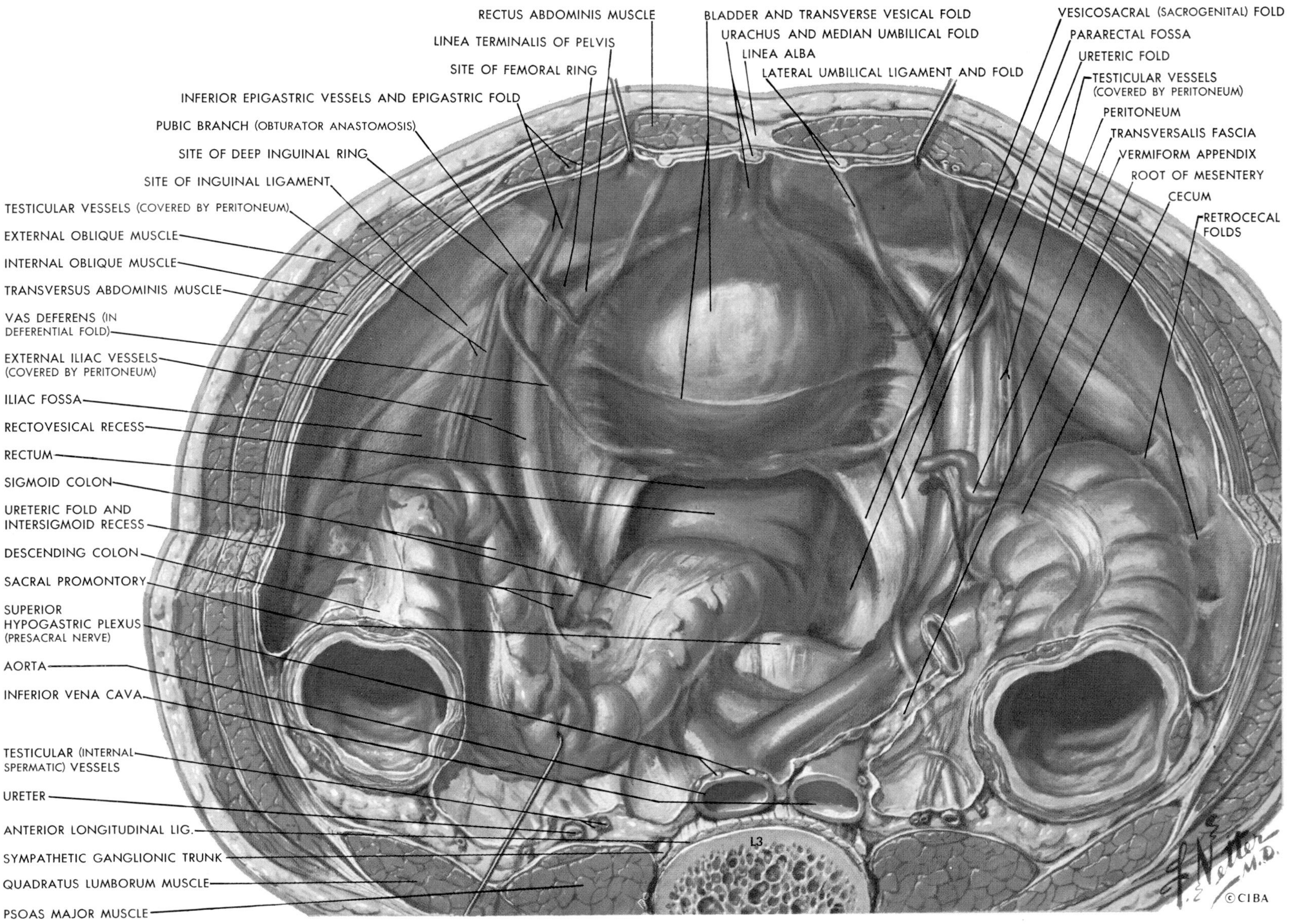
RECTUS ABDOMINIS MUSCLE
LINEA TERMINALIS OF PELVIS
SITE OF FEMORAL RING
INFERIOR EPIGASTRIC VESSELS AND EPIGASTRIC FOLD
PUBIC BRANCH (OBTURATOR ANASTOMOSIS)
SITE OF DEEP INGUINAL RING
SITE OF INGUINAL LIGAMENT
TESTICULAR VESSELS (COVERED BY PERITONEUM)
EXTERNAL OBLIQUE MUSCLE
INTERNAL OBLIQUE MUSCLE
TRANSVERSUS ABDOMINIS MUSCLE
VAS DEFERENS (IN DEFERENTIAL FOLD)
EXTERNAL ILIAC VESSELS (COVERED BY PERITONEUM)
ILIAC FOSSA
RECTOVESICAL RECESS
RECTUM
SIGMOID COLON
URETERIC FOLD AND INTERSIGMOID RECESS
DESCENDING COLON
SACRAL PROMONTORY
SUPERIOR HYPOGASTRIC PLEXUS (PRESACRAL NERVE)
AORTA
INFERIOR VENA CAVA
TESTICULAR (INTERNAL SPERMATIC) VESSELS
URETER
ANTERIOR LONGITUDINAL LIG.
SYMPATHETIC GANGLIONIC TRUNK
QUADRATUS LUMBORUM MUSCLE
PSOAS MAJOR MUSCLE
BLADDER AND TRANSVERSE VESICAL FOLD
URACHUS AND MEDIAN UMBILICAL FOLD
LINEA ALBA
LATERAL UMBILICAL LIGAMENT AND FOLD
VESICOSACRAL (SACROGENITAL) FOLD
PARARECTAL FOSSA
URETERIC FOLD
TESTICULAR VESSELS (COVERED BY PERITONEUM)
PERITONEUM
TRANSVERSALIS FASCIA
VERMIFORM APPENDIX
ROOT OF MESENTERY
CECUM
RETROCECAL FOLDS
L3
F. Netter M.D.
©CIBA

SECTION IX—PLATE 19

Peritoneum

(Continued from page 27)

colon follows a fairly straight line from the posterior part of the left iliac fossa downward and medially to reach the third sacral segment. If, as is the case in the other extreme of the range of variation (see page 56), the colon is closely bound down in the iliac fossa, the line of attachment of the sigmoid mesocolon goes posteriorly along the pelvic brim until it crosses the sacro-iliac joint, and then descends along the ventral aspect of the sacrum to the level of its second to third segment. The sigmoid colon is enwrapped by the free margin of the sigmoid mesocolon, which has its greatest width (distance from attached to free border) at its attachment to the first sacral segment. This width varies from about 5 to 18 cm., although it occasionally may be as much as 25 cm. Between the layers of the sigmoid mesocolon run the sigmoidal and superior rectal arteries, the accompanying veins, lymphatics and autonomic nerve plexus and connective tissue, which may, of course, include varying amounts of adipose tissue.

The *greater omentum,* gastrocolic omentum or ligament (see Plates 14, 16 and 18) is the largest peritoneal fold, which may hang down like a large apron from the greater curvature of the stomach in front of the other viscera as far as the brim of the pelvis or even into the pelvis, or perhaps into an inguinal hernia (more commonly on the left side). It also may be much shorter than this, even just a fringe on the greater curvature of the stomach, or it may be of some length and found folded in between coils of the small intestine, tucked into the left hypochondriac area or turned upward in front of the stomach. The upper end of the left border is continuous with the gastrolienal ligament, and the upper end of the right border extends as far as the beginning of the duodenum. The greater omentum is usually thin, with a delicate layer of fibroelastic tissue as its framework, and somewhat cribriform in appearance, although it usually contains some adipose tissue and may accumulate a large amount of fat in an obese individual. In the make-up of the greater omentum, the lesser sac peritoneum on the postero-inferior surface of the stomach and the greater sac peritoneum on the anterosuperior surface of the stomach meet at the greater curvature of the stomach and course inferiorly to the free border of the greater omentum, where they turn superiorly to the transverse colon. Early in development these two layers, which are the elongated dorsal mesogastrium, course superiorly in front of the transverse colon and transverse mesocolon to the anterior surface of the pancreas. Owing to fusions of these two layers of peritoneum to each other and to the peritoneum on the transverse colon and the anterior surface of the primitive transverse mesocolon, it appears, in the fully developed state, as though the "two layers" of peritoneum, running superiorly as the posterior layer of the greater omentum, separate from each other to surround the transverse colon and continue as the two layers of the transverse mesocolon (see Plate 14). Frequently, there is enough fusion in the four-layered primitive greater omentum inferior to the transverse mesocolon so that it is possible actually to make out no definite cavity (omental bursa, see below) in the greater omentum and little more than minimal connective tissue with an anterior and a posterior covering surface. Close to the greater curvature of the stomach, the right and left gastro-epiploic vessels course, anastomosing with each other in the greater omentum. The greater omentum, if of any length, has a great deal of mobility and can shift around to fill what would otherwise be temporary gaps between viscera or to build up a barrier against bacterial invasion of the peritoneal cavity by becoming adherent at a potential danger spot.

The *lesser omentum,* hepatogastric and hepatoduodenal ligaments (see Plates 14 and 15) extend from the postero-inferior surface of the liver to the lesser curvature of the stomach and the beginning of the duodenum (see also Ciba Collection, Vol. 3/iii, page 6). It is extremely thin, particularly the part to the left, which is sometimes fenestrated. The part to the right is thicker and ends in a free, rounded margin, which contains the common bile duct to the

(Continued on page 29)

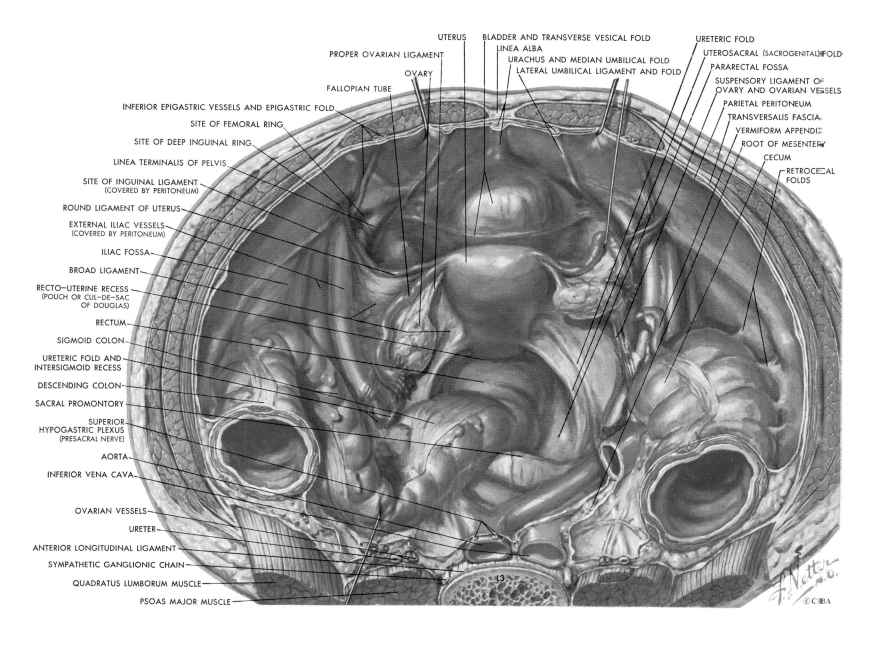

UTERUS
PROPER OVARIAN LIGAMENT
OVARY
FALLOPIAN TUBE
INFERIOR EPIGASTRIC VESSELS AND EPIGASTRIC FOLD
SITE OF FEMORAL RING
SITE OF DEEP INGUINAL RING
LINEA TERMINALIS OF PELVIS
SITE OF INGUINAL LIGAMENT (COVERED BY PERITONEUM)
ROUND LIGAMENT OF UTERUS
EXTERNAL ILIAC VESSELS (COVERED BY PERITONEUM)
ILIAC FOSSA
BROAD LIGAMENT
RECTO-UTERINE RECESS (POUCH OR CUL-DE-SAC OF DOUGLAS)
RECTUM
SIGMOID COLON
URETERIC FOLD AND INTERSIGMOID RECESS
DESCENDING COLON
SACRAL PROMONTORY
SUPERIOR HYPOGASTRIC PLEXUS (PRESACRAL NERVE)
AORTA
INFERIOR VENA CAVA
OVARIAN VESSELS
URETER
ANTERIOR LONGITUDINAL LIGAMENT
SYMPATHETIC GANGLIONIC CHAIN
QUADRATUS LUMBORUM MUSCLE
PSOAS MAJOR MUSCLE

BLADDER AND TRANSVERSE VESICAL FOLD
LINEA ALBA
URACHUS AND MEDIAN UMBILICAL FOLD
LATERAL UMBILICAL LIGAMENT AND FOLD

URETERIC FOLD
UTEROSACRAL (SACROGENITAL) FOLD
PARARECTAL FOSSA
SUSPENSORY LIGAMENT OF OVARY AND OVARIAN VESSELS
PARIETAL PERITONEUM
TRANSVERSALIS FASCIA
VERMIFORM APPENDIX
ROOT OF MESENTERY
CECUM
RETROCECAL FOLDS

L3

SECTION IX — PLATE 20

PERITONEUM

(Continued from page 28)

right, the hepatic artery to the left and the portal vein posterior to these two, and forms the anterior border of the epiploic foramen (see below). In addition to the structures just listed, the lesser omentum contains the right and left gastric arteries (close to the lesser curvature of the stomach) and the accompanying veins, lymphatics and autonomic nerve plexuses. The peritoneum forming the anterior layer of this omentum and continuing onto the anterosuperior surface of the stomach is greater sac peritoneum, and that forming the posterior layer and continuing onto the postero-inferior surface of the stomach is lesser sac peritoneum. The lesser omentum reaches the liver at the porta, and to the left of the porta it extends to the bottom of the fossa for the ligamentum venosum (obliterated ductus venosus; see CIBA COLLECTION, Vol. 3/III, page 5).

The *omental bursa,* lesser sac of the peritoneum (see Plates 14, 15, 17 and 18), is a large fossa or outpouching from the general peritoneal cavity (the development of which is described in Section VIII). It is bounded in front, from above down, by the *caudate lobe of the liver,* the *lesser omentum,* the *postero-inferior surface of the stomach* and the *anterior*

layer of the greater omentum (at least in part). Behind it, from below upward, are the posterior layer of the greater omentum (amount of this depends on the variable inferior extent of the bursa), the *transverse colon,* the anterior layer of the *transverse mesocolon,* the anterior surface of the *pancreas, left suprarenal gland,* upper end of the *left kidney* and, to the right of the esophageal opening into the stomach, that part of the diaphragm which supports the caudate lobe of the liver. The horizontal extent of the bursa reaches from the epiploic foramen (described below) at the right to the hilum of the spleen at the left, where it is limited by the *phrenicolienal* and *gastrolienal ligaments.* Inferiorly, the bursa may extend about as far as the transverse colon, its cavity having originally reached as far down as the free margin of the omentum before becoming obliterated by fusion of its layers. The portion of the bursa between the caudate lobe of the liver and the diaphragm is called the superior recess, and the narrow portion from the epiploic foramen across the head of the pancreas to the gastropancreatic fold (see Plate 18) is called the vestibule of the bursa.

The *epiploic foramen* (of Winslow) (see Plates 14, 15, 17 and 18) is the opening by which the omental bursa communicates with the general peritoneal cavity (greater sac). It is somewhat circular and usually is large enough to admit one or two fingers. Anterior to the foramen is the free margin of the lesser omentum (see above), containing the *common bile duct,*

hepatic artery and *portal vein.* Its posterior border is the peritoneum covering the inferior vena cava; superior to it is the peritoneum on the caudate process of the liver, and its inferior boundary is the peritoneum which covers the beginning of the duodenum and the hepatic artery.

Many extremely variable and inconstant fossae or recesses have been described which are of interest to the surgeon because of the possibility of herniation of a loop of intestine into any one of them (see page 218). The more common ones are located either in the region of the fourth portion of the duodenum or in the region of the cecum and ileocecal junction (see page 51). A relatively common "intersigmoid recess" is found on the left side of the line of attachment of the sigmoid mesocolon (see page 54) at the angle which is present in this line when the colon is tightly bound down in the iliac fossa.

A characteristic of the peritoneum covering the surfaces of the various parts of the colon is the presence of little outpouchings of peritoneum containing adipose tissue, which are called *appendices epiploicae* (see page 55).

The parietal peritoneum is supplied by the nerves to the adjacent body wall and is thus pain sensitive. The visceral peritoneum is insensitive to ordinary pain stimuli. The roots of the mesenteries contain receptors which give rise to pain in response to stretching of the mesentery.

When moist surfaces of peritoneum which are in contact become irritated, adhesions tend to form which often become permanent.

F. Netter M.D. ©CIBA

URACHUS (MEDIAN UMBILICAL LIGAMENT)
UMBILICAL PREVESICAL FASCIA
LATERAL UMBILICAL LIGAMENT
TRANSVERSALIS FASCIA
VESICAL FASCIA
SUPERIOR WING OF HYPOGASTRIC SHEATH
OBLITERATED UMBILICAL ARTERY
INFERIOR EPIGASTRIC VESSELS
ROUND LIGAMENT OF UTERUS

SYMPHYSIS PUBIS
DORSAL VEIN OF CLITORIS (PENIS)
TRANSVERSE LIGAMENT OF PELVIS (ANTERIOR FUSED MARGIN OF UROGENITAL DIAPHRAGM)
MEDIAL PUBOVESICAL LIGAMENT
LATERAL PUBOVESICAL LIGAMENT
PILLAR OF BLADDER
SUPRA–ANAL (SUPRALEVATOR) FASCIA
CARDINAL LIGAMENT; UTERINE ARTERY
ARCUS TENDINEUS OF PELVIC FASCIA
ARCUS TENDINEUS OF LEVATOR ANI
SUPERIOR WING (CUT) OF HYPOGASTRIC SHEATH
LINEA TERMINALIS OF PELVIS
OBTURATOR FASCIA

OVARIAN VESSELS (INFUNDIBULOPELVIC LIGAMENT)
SUPERIOR VESICAL ARTERY
URETER
UTERINE ARTERY
INFERIOR VESICAL AND VAGINAL ARTERIES
MIDDLE RECTAL ARTERY
BRANCH OF SUPERIOR RECTAL ARTERY
PRESACRAL (RETRORECTAL) SPACE
PRESACRAL FASCIA
UTEROVAGINAL FASCIA
MIDDLE SACRAL VESSELS
RECTAL FASCIA
RECTOVAGINAL SPACE

ILIOPSOAS FASCIA
UMBILICAL (SUPERIOR VESICAL) ARTERY
OBTURATOR ARTERY
INTERNAL ILIAC VESSELS
HYPOGASTRIC SHEATH
INFERIOR WING OF HYPOGASTRIC PRESACRAL WING SHEATH
PREVESICAL SPACE (RETZIUS)
WING OF VAGINA
VESICOVAGINAL AND VESICOCERVICAL SPACES

PELVIC FASCIA AND PERINEOPELVIC SPACES

The steadily changing pressure and filling conditions in the pelvis require an exquisite adaptability of those structures the essential function of which is to support the viscera within the funnellike frame of the pelvis. Part of such support derives from the anorectal musculature and the levator ani (see pages 22 and 61 to 63). But since these muscles are, to a great extent, involved in the sphincteric and emptying functions of the anorectal canal, their supporting tasks need indispensable assistance from connective tissue structures with adequate tensile strength, *i.e.*, from the pelvic fascia. With the recognition of this fact, the pelvic fascia is removed from the passive rôle of an undifferentiated "subserous tissue", which, in former times, was assigned to it. Oversimplified descriptions such as these disguise the physiologic and, particularly, the surgical significance of the pelvic fascia. Admittedly, its anatomic relation is complex, but it is now generally recognized that the fascia is best divisible into a visceral and a parietal portion. The former lies entirely above the pelvic diaphragm, forming the fascial investments of the pelvic viscera, the perivascular sheaths and the intervisceral and pelvovisceral ligaments, which are described below.

The parietal portion of the pelvic fascia may be divided into those parts which lie in the supra-anal (supralevator) and the infra-anal (infralevator) planes, the levator ani muscle demarcating the division. At the supralevator level the parietal pelvic fascia is a continuation downward of the parietal abdominal fascia (see Plate 22). The *iliopsoas fascia* and the *transversalis fascia* of the abdo-

men are attached along the iliopectineal line (*linea terminalis*) to the bony pelvis and then extend downward into the pelvis over the inner surface of the *obturator internus muscle* as the *obturator fascia* (see Plate 23). Anteriorly, the transversalis fascia is attached to the inner surface of the pubic bones and symphysis. The prevertebral fascia of the abdomen continues downward into the pelvis as the *presacral fascia*.

The supra-anal (supralevator) fascia or superior layer of the pelvic diaphragm arises from the *arcus tendineus* of the levator ani muscle (see Plate 22), which, in truth, is a line of thickening in the obturator fascia, running arcwise, convex downward from the posterior surface of the pubic ramus (1 or 2 cm. in front of the obturator foramen) to a point above the ischial spine. From this arcus the supralevator fascia spreads out to cover the superior (inner) surface of the levator ani and coccygeus muscles.

Anteriorly, the supra-anal fascia spans the infrapubic interval in front of the *transverse ligament of the pelvis* (anterior fused margin of the urogenital diaphragm; see next page and CIBA COLLECTION, Vol. 2, page 13). The fascia descends here just a few millimeters to form a small fossa, the bottom of which is pierced by the *dorsal vein of the penis or clitoris*, respectively. On each side of this small fossa, a thickening in the fascia extends backward from each side of the lower end of the symphysis pubis to the prostate in the male and to the bladder in the female. These thickened parts are the medial puboprostatic ligaments (or anterior true ligaments of the prostate) in the male, to which correspond the *medial pubovesical*, also pubo-urethral or anterior true ligaments of the bladder in the female. The lateral puboprostatic or pubovesical ligaments (or lateral true liga-

(Continued on page 31)

PERITONEUM

PRESACRAL SPACE
(RETRORECTAL SPACE)

PRESACRAL FASCIA
(PARIETAL)

RECTAL FASCIA

PRERECTAL
SPACE

DENONVILLIERS' FASCIA
(RECTOGENITAL SEPTUM)

RETROVESICAL SPACE

SEMINAL VESICLE

PERITONEUM

VESICAL FASCIA

UMBILICOVESICAL
FASCIA (URACHUS)

UMBILICAL
PREVESICAL
FASCIA

TRANSVERSALIS
FASCIA

RECTAL
FASCIA

SYMPHYSIS
PUBIS

RECTUS
SHEATH

SCARPA'S
FASCIA

CAMPER'S
FASCIA

PREVESICAL
SPACE
(RETZIUS)

ARCUATE
LIGAMENT

PELVIC FASCIA AND PERINEOPELVIC SPACES

(Continued from page 30)

ments of prostate or bladder) lie just posterior to this and consist of lateral reflections from the supra-anal fascia to the prostate or bladder, respectively.

The thickenings in the supra-anal fascia, which comprise the medial puboprostatic or pubovesical ligaments, continue backward in a slight curve, concave downward, gradually diverging to the region of the ischial spine. This constitutes on each side the *arcus tendineus of the pelvic fascia,* which lies considerably more medially and below the *arcus tendineus of the levator ani.* The supralevator pelvic fascia also continues medially and below its arcus tendineus. Anterior to the rectum, it spans the interval between the crura of the pubococcygeus muscles and, coursing around their free margins, fuses with the deep (superior) layer of the urogenital diaphragm. Here also it is reflected upon the prostate and bladder in the male and the vagina in the female as the visceral fascial sheaths of these respective organs.

Continuing posteriorly, the supra-anal fascia (see Plate 24) surrounds the rectum as that organ starts to pass through the pelvic diaphragm. It is reflected there as a sheath upon the rectum as the visceral (*rectal*) *fascia,* but it also blends with the longitudinal rectal musculature and contributes fibrous extensions to the formation of the fibromuscular, conjoined longitudinal muscle of the anal canal (see page 60). The reflection of the *supra-anal* (parietal) *fascia* (see Plate 21) upon the pelvic viscera to be converted into the visceral fascia takes place largely at the arcus tendineus of the pelvic fascia, but also more medially and more caudally in the region where

LEVATOR ANI
MUSCLE
(LEVATOR PLATE)

SUPRA–ANAL FASCIA
(SUPERIOR LEVATOR ANI
FASCIA)

INFRA–ANAL FASCIA
(INFERIOR LEVATOR ANI
FASCIA)

DEEP POSTANAL SPACE

SUPERFICIAL
EXTERNAL SPHINCTER

SUPERFICIAL POSTANAL SPACE

INTERMUSCULAR SPACE

SUBCUTANEOUS
EXTERNAL SPHINCTER

SUBMUCOUS
SPACE

INTERNAL SPHINCTER

CONJOINED LONGITUDINAL
MUSCLE

SUPERFICIAL EXTERNAL SPHINCTER

DEEP EXTERNAL SPHINCTER

RECTO–URETHRALIS MUSCLE

RETROPROSTATIC SPACE

PROSTATIC FASCIA (CAPSULE)

COLLES' FASCIA (MAJOR LEAF)

BULBOCAVERNOSUS MUSCLE

BUCK'S FASCIA

SCROTAL SEPTUM

TRANSVERSE LIGAMENT OF PELVIS

DARTOS FASCIA OF SCROTUM

UROGENITAL DIAPHRAGM

the viscera begin to penetrate the pelvic diaphragm.

At the infralevator plane the obturator fascia continues downward on the side walls of the pelvis below the arcus tendineus of the levator ani muscle. It covers the obturator internus muscle and is attached to the bony pelvis about the margins of that muscle. In its lower portion the fascia is split to form a more or less horizontal *canal* (*Alcock's*), in which course the *internal pudendal vessels* and the *pudendal* and *dorsal nerves of the penis.* The fascial layer which forms the medial wall of this canal is known as "*lunate fascia*". The *infra-anal fascia* is a comparatively thin sheet which extends from the arcus tendineus of the levator ani muscle and covers the inferior surface of this and the coccygeus muscle. As circumanal fascia it continues around the lower rectum and the anal canal. It is reflected into the anterior recess of the *ischiorectal space,* finally fusing with the

deep (superior) layer of the urogenital diaphragm.

The perineal fascia consists of a superficial subcutaneous (essentially panniculus adiposus) and a deep membranous layer. The former is unnamed but is considered to correspond to Camper's fascia of the abdominal wall; the latter is *Colles' fascia,* corresponding to Scarpa's fascia of the abdomen. (For a more detailed description of the perineal fascia, see CIBA COLLECTION, Vol. 2, pages 10, 11, 12, 13 and 89, 91 and 92, respectively.) The superficial layer varies considerably throughout the perineum. Over the anal triangle it forms the fatty layer of the *peri-anal space,* whereas laterally over the ischial tuberosities, it is made up of fibrous fascicles which connect to the underlying bone and form, directly over the ischial tuberosities, fibrous bursal sacs. The main part of the deep layer of Colles' fascia has a firm attachment

(Continued on page 32)

PELVIC FASCIA AND PERINEOPELVIC SPACES

(Continued from page 31)

PSOAS FASCIA

EXTERNAL ILIAC VESSELS

PERI-ANAL SPACE (EXTERNAL HEMORRHOIDAL PLEXUS)

ILIOPECTINEAL LINE

ISCHIAL TUBEROSITY

OBTURATOR INTERNUS MUSCLE AND FASCIA

SUBMUCOUS SPACE (INTERNAL HEMORRHOIDAL PLEXUS)

PUDENDAL CANAL (ALCOCK'S) WITH INTERNAL PUDENDAL VESSELS, PUDENDAL NERVE, DORSAL NERVE OF PENIS

INTERMUSCULAR SPACE

PERI-ANAL SPACE

ISCHIORECTAL SPACE } ISCHIORECTAL FOSSA

LUNATE FASCIA

ARCUS TENDINEUS

URETER

SUPRALEVATOR SPACE (PELVIRECTAL SPACE)

SACROGENITAL FOLD

INTERMUSCULAR GROOVE (WHITE LINE OF HILTON)

LEVATOR ANI MUSCLE WITH ITS SUPRA-ANAL AND INFRA-ANAL FASCIA

MUSCULUS SUBMUCOSAE ANI

TRANSVERSE SEPTUM OF ISCHIORECTAL FOSSA

INTERNAL ANAL SPHINCTER

CONJOINED LONGITUDINAL MUSCLE

SUPERFICIAL FASCIA (DEEP LAYER)

PERITONEUM

EXTERNAL ANAL SPHINCTER (DEEP, SUPERFICIAL AND SUBCUTANEOUS)

RECTAL FASCIA

to the pubic rami and to the posterior margin of the urogenital diaphragm. It spreads medially across the urogenital triangle, constituting the floor of the superficial perineal compartment, which lies between it and the inferior layer of the urogenital diaphragm and contains the superficial perineal musculature (see CIBA COLLECTION, Vol. 2, page 13).

As described, the visceral pelvic fascia invests, one by one, each of the pelvic viscera forming their fascial capsule (the *vesical fascia, prostatic fascia,* vaginal-uterine fascia [see CIBA COLLECTION, Vol. 2, page 95], *rectal fascia*). It also comprises the ligaments which connect these viscera with each other and with the pelvic walls and floor, as well as the perivascular sheaths. The latter consist of the *hypogastric sheath* and its several "wings". The hypogastric sheath arises on each side from the parietal pelvic fascia over a roughly triangular area (its root) in the posterolateral angle of the pelvis, encloses the hypogastric ("internal iliac", according to the 1955 P.N.A.) *vessels,* as well as the *ureter,* nerves and lymphatics, and extends downward as far as the spine of the ischium. The sheath fans out into three (superior, inferior and posterior or presacral) wings. The *superior wing* (see Plate 21) extends anteriorly to the superolateral border of the bladder, where it splits into superior and inferior layers, which blend, respectively, with the superior and lateral aspects of the vesical fascia (fascial capsule of the bladder). Laterally, the superior hypogastric wing spreads to the pelvic wall, where it blends with the parietal fascia. The superior vesical branches of the umbilical vessels course within this

wing. Posteriorly, in the female, the superior wing fuses with the *infundibulopelvic ligament* containing the *ovarian vessels* (see also CIBA COLLECTION, Vol. 2, pages 89 and 96).

The *inferior wing* springs from the caudal end of the hypogastric sheath. Laterally, it blends with the supra-anal (parietal) pelvic fascia (vide supra) and medially with the inferolateral aspects of the bladder or prostatic fascial capsule, *i.e.,* with the *vesical* or *prostatic capsule.* In a sense, it thus constitutes a reflection from the supra-anal (parietal) fascia to the vesical (visceral) fascia along the *arcus tendineus of the pelvic fascia,* its anterior portion comprising the lateral true ligaments of the bladder or prostate. Posteriorly, the transversely placed *cardinal ligament* (see Plate 21) of the uterus extends to the inferior wing, which contains the *ureter,* the *inferior vesical vessels* and autonomic nerves.

The *presacral wing* extends medially from the hypogastric sheath in front of the sacrum and *presacral fascia,* lying in a more or less vertical plane, in contrast to the superior and inferior wings, which unfold in an almost horizontal plane. Upon reaching the sides of the rectum, the presacral wing splits into two leaves which encircle the rectum as the rectal (visceral) fascia (see Plate 21). This wing contains the *superior* and *middle* hemorrhoidal (*rectal*) vessels, the inferior hypogastric or pelvic nerve plexus (see page 81) and many lymphatics.*

The origin, course and insertion of the pelvic mus-

(Continued on page 33)

---

*It should be emphasized that many of these fasciae, particularly the hypogastric sheath and its wings, are not distinct structures but are, rather, somewhat more densified or thickened extraperitoneal connective tissue.

PELVIC FASCIA AND PERINEOPELVIC SPACES

(*Continued from page 32*)

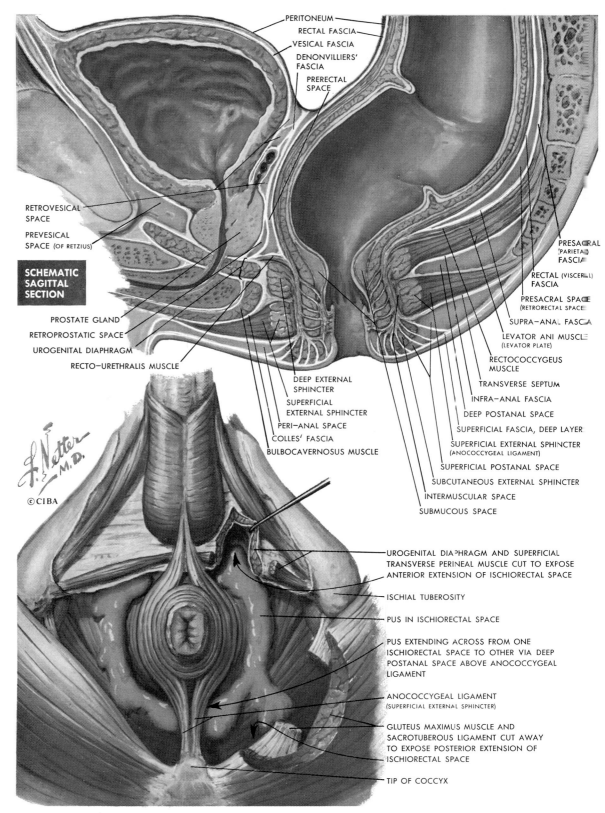

PERITONEUM
RECTAL FASCIA
VESICAL FASCIA
DENONVILLIERS' FASCIA
PRERECTAL SPACE

RETROVESICAL SPACE
PREVESICAL SPACE (OF RETZIUS)

SCHEMATIC SAGITTAL SECTION

PROSTATE GLAND
RETROPROSTATIC SPACE
UROGENITAL DIAPHRAGM
RECTO–URETHRALIS MUSCLE

DEEP EXTERNAL SPHINCTER
SUPERFICIAL EXTERNAL SPHINCTER
PERI-ANAL SPACE
COLLES' FASCIA
BULBOCAVERNOSUS MUSCLE

PRESACRAL (PARIETAL) FASCIA
RECTAL (VISCERAL) FASCIA
PRESACRAL SPACE (RETRORECTAL SPACE)
SUPRA-ANAL FASCIA
LEVATOR ANI MUSCLE (LEVATOR PLATE)
RECTOCOCCYGEUS MUSCLE
TRANSVERSE SEPTUM
INFRA-ANAL FASCIA
DEEP POSTANAL SPACE
SUPERFICIAL FASCIA, DEEP LAYER
SUPERFICIAL EXTERNAL SPHINCTER (ANOCOCCYGEAL LIGAMENT)
SUPERFICIAL POSTANAL SPACE
SUBCUTANEOUS EXTERNAL SPHINCTER
INTERMUSCULAR SPACE
SUBMUCOUS SPACE

F. Netter M.D.
©CIBA

UROGENITAL DIAPHRAGM AND SUPERFICIAL TRANSVERSE PERINEAL MUSCLE CUT TO EXPOSE ANTERIOR EXTENSION OF ISCHIORECTAL SPACE
ISCHIAL TUBEROSITY
PUS IN ISCHIORECTAL SPACE
PUS EXTENDING ACROSS FROM ONE ISCHIORECTAL SPACE TO OTHER VIA DEEP POSTANAL SPACE ABOVE ANOCOCCYGEAL LIGAMENT
ANOCOCCYGEAL LIGAMENT (SUPERFICIAL EXTERNAL SPHINCTER)
GLUTEUS MAXIMUS MUSCLE AND SACROTUBEROUS LIGAMENT CUT AWAY TO EXPOSE POSTERIOR EXTENSION OF ISCHIORECTAL SPACE
TIP OF COCCYX

cles and the figuration of the anorectal musculature (see pages 60 to 63), together with the supra- and infralevator fasciae, discussed above, give rise to a number of *perineopelvic spaces,* which require more than mere anatomic recognition, because they have a fundamental importance for an adequate concept of the pathogenesis and extensions of infectious and malignant processes of pelvis and perineum. As with the fasciae, these spaces are conveniently separated into a supra- and an infralevator group.

At the supralevator level, in the male, four main spaces can be discerned: (1) the prevesical space (Retzius), (2) the rectovesical space, (3) the bilateral pararectal spaces and (4) the retrorectal space.

The *prevesical space of Retzius* is, in both sexes, a potentially large cavity surrounding the front and lateral walls of the bladder. The main cavity in front of the bladder comprises two superimposed anteromedian recesses and two lateral compartments. The upper anteromedial recess lies behind the anterior abdominal wall (*i.e.,* behind the most medial parts of the *transversalis fascia;* see Plate 22) and is roofed by the peritoneal reflection from the dome of the bladder supported by the *umbilicovesical fascia* (*urachus*) and the *umbilical prevesical fascia.* Its lateral borders are demarcated by the *obliterated umbilical arteries* (lateral umbilical ligaments, see Plate 21). The lower recess, continuous with the above, lies behind the symphysis and pubic bones and in front of the bladder. Its floor is formed by the pubovesical (pubo-urethral) ligaments in the female or the puboprostatic ligaments in the

male (true ligaments of the bladder). The lateral recesses of the prevesical space are bounded by a lateral wall formed by the obturator and supra-anal fasciae (see above) and a median wall presented by the bladder and the inferior hypogastric fascial sheath. They contain the ureter and the main neurovascular supply to the bladder and, in the male, to the prostate. The floor of the lateral recess is the supra-anal fascia, which affords attachment to the true lateral ligaments of the bladder. Dorsally, the lateral recess of the prevesical space extends as far as the root of the hypogastric sheath in the region of the ischial spine — a point not generally appreciated. The roof is formed by the superior hypogastric fascial wing covered by the peritoneum, where these tissues are reflected from the lateral pelvic wall.

The *retrovesical compartment* in the male, divisible into three subspaces, lies between the bladder and

the prostate, covered by the vesical and prostatic fasciae anteriorly, and the rectum, covered by the rectal fascia posteriorly. Its roof is formed by the *rectovesical recess* or pouch of the peritoneum, which comes into existence by the continuity of the peritoneal reflection from the rectum to the bladder. Its floor is the posterior part of the urogenital diaphragm. Denonvilliers' fascia (rectogenital septum), originating from the undersurface of the rectovesical peritoneal pouch (see also CIBA COLLECTION, Vol. 2, page 9) and extending caudally in a coronal plane, divides into two leaves, an anterior leaf, blending with the prostatic fascia or capsule, and a posterior leaf, attaching below to the urogenital diaphragm medially and to the inferior hypogastric wing laterally. Thus the retrovesical compartment becomes partitioned into the *retrovesical space* and *retroprostatic space* arte-

(*Continued on page 34*)

PELVIC FASCIA AND
PERINEOPELVIC SPACES

(*Continued from page 33*)

riorly and the *prerectal space* posteriorly. The inferior wing of the hypogastric fascial sheath, with its contents (see above), marks the lateral boundary of the two anterior spaces and also the separation from the lateral recess of the space of Retzius. Caudally, the prerectal space terminates where the *recto-urethralis muscle,* covered by a fibrous extension of the *rectal fascia,* attaches itself to the urogenital diaphragm or its superior fascia (see CIBA COLLECTION, Vol. 2, page 11). The retroprostatic space (Proust's space) terminates caudally in the same region but varies, depending on the very variable caudal limits of Denonvilliers' fascia and its attachments to the prostatic capsule.

In the female, as in the male, the area between the bladder and the rectum is divided into three spaces (for this and the following paragraphs see Plate 22). The dominant dividing structure, however, is not the rectogenital septum (Denonvilliers' fascia) but the much more bulky vagina and cervix uteri. Anterior to these structures, two spaces come into existence: the *vesicocervical space* above and the *vesicovaginal space* below. They are separated by a fascial septum, the supravaginal septum or vesicocervical ligament, which forms the floor of the vesicocervical space and the roof of the vesicovaginal space. The vesicocervical space is roofed by the uterovesical fold of the peritoneum (see CIBA COLLECTION, Vol. 2, page 89) and extends caudally to the point where the urethra and vagina are in apposition above the superior layer of the urogenital diaphragm. In the floor of this space, the medial and lateral *pubo-urethral ligaments* surround the urethra which lies in a fused musculofascial sheath. Laterally, the vesicovaginal space is limited by the strong fascial connections between the bladder and the cervix, the uterovesical ligaments or *"pillars of the bladder".*

In the female, of course, the posterior compartment of the rectovesical space, *i.e., rectovaginal space,* is farther from the anterior compartments, because the substantial mass of the cervix uteri and the vagina provide more separation. Whether or not the small area between the rectum and the genital organs can be divided into a retrovaginal and a *prerectal space* is a controversial question of no practical significance. A separation into two spaces would be brought about by the rectovaginal septum (corresponding to Denonvilliers' septum in the male), the existence of which, in the female, still remains to be proved. Of more practical importance is the fact that the rectovaginal space is roofed by the peritoneal fold which forms the *recto-uterine pouch* of Douglas. The boundaries of this space are, anteriorly, the *vaginal fascia* and, posteriorly, the *rectal fascia* (see also Plate 21). Laterally, the space extends to the fusion of the vaginal and rectal fascial collars, which, in this region, form the wings of the vagina. The space terminates caudally at the line of fusion between the posterior vaginal wall and the anal canal. It is apparent that, in this region, numerous fascial and muscular elements fuse. This fact prompted the term "perineal body", or "central point of the perineum".

The pararectal space extends on each side from the rectogenital septum (male) and the cardinal ligament (female) to the presacral fascial wing. It lies on the supra-anal fascia covering the superior surface of the pubococcygeus mus-

cle, alongside the inferolateral parts of the rectum or its fascial enclosure. Its roof is made up, in both sexes, of the peritoneum reflected from the lateral aspects of the rectum to the pelvic parietes, forming the floor of the pararectal peritoneal fossa.

The presacral space, similar in both sexes, constitutes the interval between the parietal pelvic fascia, covering the sacrum as well as the piriformis, coccygeus and pubococcygeus muscles, and the presacral fascial wing of the hypogastric sheath, which envelops the rectum as the *rectal fascia.* Where the posterior rectal wall lies almost horizontally, the ventral lining of the presacral space is produced by the rectal fascial collar. Cranially, the space becomes continuous with the prevertebral-retroperitoneal areolar tissue. A strong lateral barrier for this space is provided by the attachment of the hypogastric sheath to the parietal fascia, a fact which explains why retrorectal abscesses are more apt to rupture into the rectum than to penetrate into the other supralevator spaces.

In the group of spaces below the levator level (infralevator spaces), the *submucous space,* encircling the sphincteric portion of the rectum and extending from the anorectal muscle ring to the dentate line, is the highest or most cranial. Its practical significance is explained by its contents: the terminal anastomotic network of the internal hemorrhoidal (rectal) plexus and a rich lymphatic plexus, both embedded in a supportive fibro-elastic connective tissue. It also contains the well-developed muscularis mucosae and the proximal portion of the musculus submucosae ani (see page 60).

A potential, not truly anatomic space, with somewhat ill-defined borders, lies within the conjoined longitudinal muscle between the internal and external anal sphincters. This *intermuscular space* surrounds the entire circumference of the anal canal, from the junction of the external sphincter with the levator ani to the intramuscular groove. Abscesses in this intermuscular space may develop as a result of infection of the peri-anal glands expanding within it (see pages 58 and 173). The submucous and intermuscular spaces are not interfascial, but, rather, intravisceral.

The peri-anal space is located between the skin and the transverse septum of the ischiorectal fossa (see Plates 21 and 23). Its boundaries, projected to the surface, correspond to the anal triangle (see CIBA COLLECTION, Vol. 2, page 13). Anteriorly, the space extends to the posterior border of the superficial transverse perineal muscle and laterally as far as the ischial tuberosities. Medially, the peri-anal space is confined by the anoderm upward as far as the latter's firm attachment to the internal sphincter and musculus submucosae ani (see page 58). Numerous fibrous extensions from the conjoined longitudinal muscle (*i.e.,* the corrugator cutis ani, see page 60), which pass through the subcutaneous external sphincter, transverse the peri-anal space. It is important to note that, circumanally, the peri-anal space reaches to the lower end of the internal sphincter, within the subcutaneous external sphincter. The space contains the external hemorrhoidal (rectal) venous plexus and superficial peri-anal lymphatics. Posteriorly, extending as far as the coccyx, the peri-anal space changes its name and becomes the *superficial postanal space,* which extends from the anal canal to the subcutaneous tissue below the extensions of the superficial external sphincter (*anococcygeal ligament*), as the latter attach to the

dorsal surface of the coccyx. It is noteworthy that the peri-anal space of each side communicates with its counterpart of the opposite side via this superficial postanal space below the anococcygeal ligament in just the same fashion as the ischiorectal spaces of each side communicate above this ligament via the deep postanal space (vide infra). Postanally, the relationships to the extensions of the conjoined longitudinal muscle and the fibers of the corrugator cutis ani are the same as described in conjunction with the peri-anal space (see above), but, in this postanal region, that arrangement has a particular significance, since it confines — as commonly observed in abscesses and fistulas complicating anal fissures — the posterior anal infections to the superficial tissues.

The largest and most important of the infralevator spaces are the paired *ischiorectal spaces* (average 6 to 8 cm. anteroposteriorly, 2 to 4 cm. wide, 6 to 8 cm. deep). Each of these is irregularly wedge-shaped, with the apex at the pubic angle and the base at the gluteus maximus muscle. Its superior medial wall is formed by the circumanal and infra-anal fasciae covering the superficial and deep portions of the external sphincter and the superimposed *puborectalis* and *pubococcygeus portions* of the levator ani muscle. The attachments of this muscle and the infra-anal fascia to the urogenital diaphragm mark the medial wall of the *anterior extension* (Waldeyer), which extends above the urogenital diaphragm. At the most cranial point of the ischiorectal fossa, the inner wall joins its outer wall, which is made up by the *obturator* and *lunate fasciae,* overlying the *obturator internus muscle,* and farther down by the *ischial tuberosity.* The infra-anal fascia covering the iliococcygeus muscle roofs the ischiorectal space. The coccyx and the sacrospinous and sacrotuberous ligaments (see page 63), overlapped by the gluteus maximus muscle, constitute the base or posterior wall of the fossa. These structures thus confine the *posterior extension* of the ischiorectal space, which has, posteriorly to the anal canal, no medial walls. The fossae of each side communicate with each other by what is known as the *deep postanal space,* which lies above the anococcygeal ligament or posterior extension of the external anal sphincter and below the levator plate. This deep postanal space is also known as the posterior communicating space, because through it communicate the right and left ischiorectal spaces. The deep postanal space is thus the usual pathway for purulent infections to spread from one ischiorectal space to the other, resulting in the semicircular or "horseshoe" posterior anal fistula (see page 173). The floor of the ischiorectal space behind the urogenital diaphragm is the transverse septum of the ischiorectal fossa (see Plate 23 and page 60). In the anterior recess the floor is formed by the urogenital diaphragm. The ischiorectal space is filled with large fat globules, lying in a matrix of thin collagenous fibrils. The inferior hemorrhoidal (rectal) vessels and nerves cross each space obliquely from its posterior-lateral angle en route from the pudendal vessels and nerves in Alcock's canal to the anal canal (see Plate 23).

The superficial and deep compartments of the *urogenital diaphragm* (see CIBA COLLECTION, Vol. 2, pages 10, 11, 12, 13 and 91, 92, 93, 94 and 95 for the male and female, respectively) occupy the space within the pubic arch and contain the urogenital musculature which is in close functional relationship to the pelvic diaphragm and the anorectal sphincters.

BLOOD SUPPLY
OF THE ABDOMEN

The aorta, after entering the abdomen at the level of T12 in midline behind the diaphragm, through a hiatus formed by the arcuate ligament (see pages 20 and 21), gives off its first parietal branches, *the inferior phrenic aa.*,* which commonly originate between the diaphragmatic crura and course to the dome of the diaphragm, where they divide into anterior and posterior branches. The latter of these anastomose with the intercostal aa. (see Plate 26), whereas the former anastomose with twigs of the contralateral a., with the *musculophrenic aa.* and the *pericardiacophrenic* and the *internal thoracic aa.* (for the last two see Plate 26), but communications also exist, through the coronary ligament and bare area of the liver (see CIBA COLLECTION, Vol. 3/III, page 5), with the hepatic arterial system. The size and origin of the inferior phrenic aa. vary greatly (caliber from 1 to 4 mm.; bilateral start [60 per cent], either both from the aorta or celiac a. or one from the former and the other from the latter; common trunk [40 per cent], either from the aorta [20 per cent], from the celiac [18 per cent] or from the left gastric [2 per cent] a., Greig *et al.*). From the trunk or the posterior branch of the inferior phrenic a., the *superior suprarenal aa.* take off, which, with the *middle* (from the aorta) and the *inferior suprarenal aa.* from the renal or accessory renal aa., will be described and specifically illustrated in the volume on the endocrine system (now in preparation). Another vessel, especially important surgically (transthoracic esophagectomy, Torek), is the *recurrent esophageal branch,* which is given off by the left inferior phrenic a. shortly after it has passed under the esophagus (see CIBA COLLECTION, Vol. 3/I, page 41). From the right inferior phrenic a. egress minute branches to the vena cava.

From the dorsal surface of the aorta, opposite the four upper lumbar vertebral bodies, arise four *lumbar aa.,* either via a common trunk or separately on each side. Since the aorta ends at L4 a *fifth pair* of *lumbar aa.* frequently originate from the middle sacral or sometimes from the internal iliac aa. The lumbar aa. curve around the vertebral bodies and pass beneath the lumbar sympathetic chain (see page 81), psoas and quadratus lumborum muscles, except for the fourth lumbar a., which often traverses in front of the latter. The right lumbar aa. lie behind the inferior vena cava, and the two upper ones lie behind the cisterna chyli (see page 39). Each lumbar a. gives

*In this and the following page, "artery" and "arteries" are abbreviated "a." and "aa.", respectively.

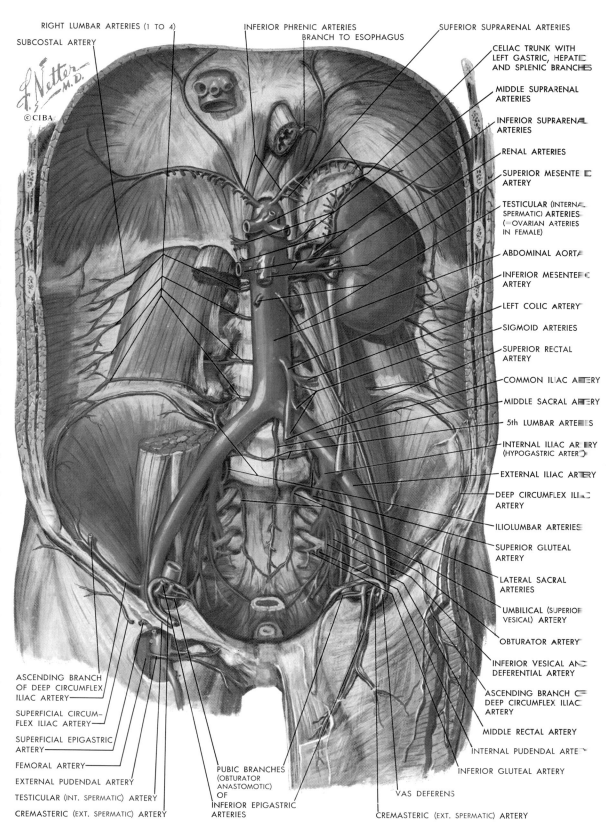

off a long dorsal branch, which, via medial, lateral and spinal rami, supplies the skin and muscles of the back, the spinal ligaments and the cord, respectively. Leaving the lateral border of the quadratus lumborum muscle, the lumbar aa. continue between the muscular layers of the abdominal wall until they reach the rectus muscle, releasing en route cutaneous branches and anastomosing with the lower *intercostal, iliolumbar, superior* and *inferior epigastric aa.* and the *ascending branch* of the *deep circumflex iliac a.* The lumbar aa. participate also in a perirenal arterial circle (Hughes, Albarran), in the subperitoneal tissue, formed by adipose capsular branches from the renal, suprarenal and gonadal aa.

The visceral branches from the abdominal aorta, feeding the entire intestines, are described on pages 64 to 70. The renal aa., taking off at the level of L1 or between L1 and L2, are scheduled to be illustrated

and discussed in a future volume that will deal with the kidney and urinary passages. An account of the gonadal (*testicular and ovarian*) aa. has been given on pages 16 and 97 of Volume 2. These aa. start predominantly from the anterior surface of the aorta below the renal aa. at a level varying from L1 to L3, but they may also arise from a suprarenal, phrenic, superior mesenteric, lumbar common or internal iliac a. In many instances (17 per cent) they appear in duplicate on one or, less frequently, on both sides. An important (because of a possible effect on the renal pedicle) abnormality concerns the arched gonadal a. (arched testicular a. of Luschka), which, after its start behind or below the renal vein, ascends first to curve over and then to descend in front of the renal vein.

After an average length of 14 cm. (12 cm in women, Taniguchi), the aorta divides at the level of

(Continued on page 36)

Labels on illustration:
RIGHT LUMBAR ARTERIES (1 TO 4)
SUBCOSTAL ARTERY
INFERIOR PHRENIC ARTERIES BRANCH TO ESOPHAGUS
SUPERIOR SUPRARENAL ARTERIES
CELIAC TRUNK WITH LEFT GASTRIC, HEPATIC AND SPLENIC BRANCHES
MIDDLE SUPRARENAL ARTERIES
INFERIOR SUPRARENAL ARTERIES
RENAL ARTERIES
SUPERIOR MESENTERIC ARTERY
TESTICULAR (INTERNAL SPERMATIC) ARTERIES (=OVARIAN ARTERIES IN FEMALE)
ABDOMINAL AORTA
INFERIOR MESENTERIC ARTERY
LEFT COLIC ARTERY
SIGMOID ARTERIES
SUPERIOR RECTAL ARTERY
COMMON ILIAC ARTERY
MIDDLE SACRAL ARTERY
5th LUMBAR ARTERIES
INTERNAL ILIAC ARTERY (HYPOGASTRIC ARTERY)
EXTERNAL ILIAC ARTERY
DEEP CIRCUMFLEX ILIAC ARTERY
ILIOLUMBAR ARTERIES
SUPERIOR GLUTEAL ARTERY
LATERAL SACRAL ARTERIES
UMBILICAL (SUPERIOR VESICAL) ARTERY
OBTURATOR ARTERY
INFERIOR VESICAL AND DEFERENTIAL ARTERY
ASCENDING BRANCH OF DEEP CIRCUMFLEX ILIAC ARTERY
MIDDLE RECTAL ARTERY
INTERNAL PUDENDAL ARTERY
INFERIOR GLUTEAL ARTERY
ASCENDING BRANCH OF DEEP CIRCUMFLEX ILIAC ARTERY
SUPERFICIAL CIRCUMFLEX ILIAC ARTERY
SUPERFICIAL EPIGASTRIC ARTERY
FEMORAL ARTERY
EXTERNAL PUDENDAL ARTERY
TESTICULAR (INT. SPERMATIC) ARTERY
CREMASTERIC (EXT. SPERMATIC) ARTERY
PUBIC BRANCHES (OBTURATOR ANASTOMOTIC) OF INFERIOR EPIGASTRIC ARTERIES
VAS DEFERENS
CREMASTERIC (EXT. SPERMATIC) ARTERY

BLOOD SUPPLY
OF THE ABDOMEN

(Continued from page 35)

the lower third of L4 into the approximately 6 mm.-wide *common iliac aa.*, the lengths of which vary from 1 to 9 cm. Up to the point at which they divide into external and internal iliac aa. (see pages 19 and 70 and CIBA COLLECTION, Vol. 2, pages 14, 97 and 98), the common iliac aa., except for a few unnamed branches to the peritoneum and subperitoneal tissue, release no branches.

The *superior epigastric* and *musculophrenic aa.* (both terminal branches of the internal thoracic [mammary] a.) supply the anterolateral wall from above. The latter vessels, in their course downward behind the lower costal cartilages, send branches to the seventh to ninth intercostal spaces, to the lower parts of the pericardium and to the upper portions of the flat abdominal muscles. Terminating at the tenth and eleventh intercostal spaces, they *anastomose* with the *intercostal aa.* of these spaces, with the *subcostal, lumbar* and the *deep circumflex iliac (ascending branch) aa.* A branch piercing the diaphragm communicates with the anterior ramus of the inferior phrenic a. (see page 21). The superior epigastric a., entering the rectus sheath behind the seventh costal cartilage and descending behind the rectus abdominis muscle, ramifies to supply this muscle and to give off a number of small cutaneous branches. It terminates by anastomosing with the inferior epigastric a. (see below).

The main vessels that feed the abdominal wall from below are the *inferior epigastric* and the *deep circumflex iliac aa.* Both arise from the *external iliac a.*, the former on its medial, the latter on its lateral side just above the inguinal ligament (see page 19). Coursing upward and obliquely toward the umbilicus (see also pages 14 and 16) between the peritoneum and the transversalis fascia, the inferior epigastric a., at the level of the semicircular line (see page 14), pierces the fascia to enter the rectus sheath, after having given off, during its course, several branches which supply the flat abdominal muscles and the overlying subcutaneous tissue and skin. Connecting terminally with the superior epigastric and the lower intercostal aa., the inferior epigastric a. releases numerous small vessels to the rectus abdominis muscle. Shortly after its origin the inferior epigastric a. releases the *cremasteric a.* and a *pubic branch* (see page 19), which latter passes below or sometimes above the femoral ring to reach the pelvic surface of the os pubis, where it anastomoses with a branch of the obturator a. The cremasteric a. accompanies the spermatic cord

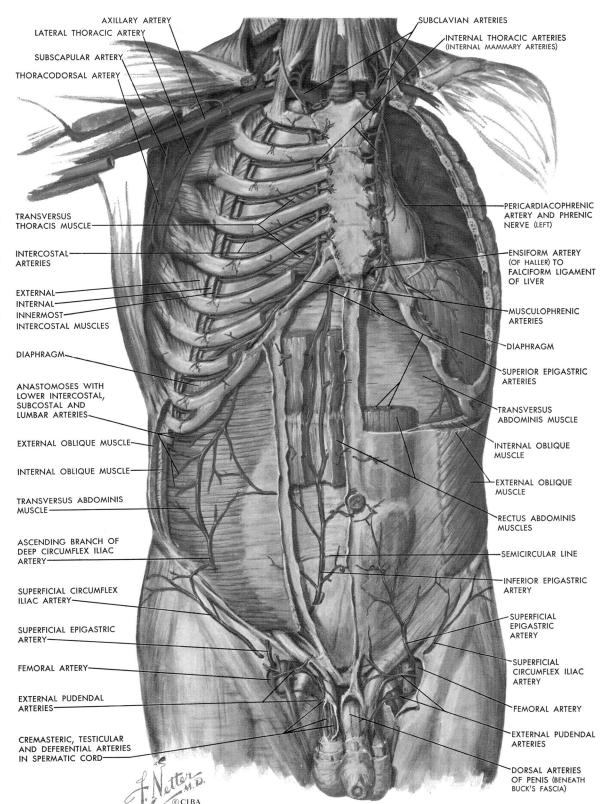

AXILLARY ARTERY
LATERAL THORACIC ARTERY
SUBSCAPULAR ARTERY
THORACODORSAL ARTERY

SUBCLAVIAN ARTERIES
INTERNAL THORACIC ARTERIES (INTERNAL MAMMARY ARTERIES)

TRANSVERSUS THORACIS MUSCLE
INTERCOSTAL ARTERIES
EXTERNAL
INTERNAL
INNERMOST
INTERCOSTAL MUSCLES
DIAPHRAGM
ANASTOMOSES WITH LOWER INTERCOSTAL, SUBCOSTAL AND LUMBAR ARTERIES
EXTERNAL OBLIQUE MUSCLE
INTERNAL OBLIQUE MUSCLE
TRANSVERSUS ABDOMINIS MUSCLE
ASCENDING BRANCH OF DEEP CIRCUMFLEX ILIAC ARTERY
SUPERFICIAL CIRCUMFLEX ILIAC ARTERY
SUPERFICIAL EPIGASTRIC ARTERY
FEMORAL ARTERY
EXTERNAL PUDENDAL ARTERIES
CREMASTERIC, TESTICULAR AND DEFERENTIAL ARTERIES IN SPERMATIC CORD

PERICARDIACOPHRENIC ARTERY AND PHRENIC NERVE (LEFT)
ENSIFORM ARTERY (OF HALLER) TO FALCIFORM LIGAMENT OF LIVER
MUSCULOPHRENIC ARTERIES
DIAPHRAGM
SUPERIOR EPIGASTRIC ARTERIES
TRANSVERSUS ABDOMINIS MUSCLE
INTERNAL OBLIQUE MUSCLE
EXTERNAL OBLIQUE MUSCLE
RECTUS ABDOMINIS MUSCLES
SEMICIRCULAR LINE
INFERIOR EPIGASTRIC ARTERY
SUPERFICIAL EPIGASTRIC ARTERY
SUPERFICIAL CIRCUMFLEX ILIAC ARTERY
FEMORAL ARTERY
EXTERNAL PUDENDAL ARTERIES
DORSAL ARTERIES OF PENIS (BENEATH BUCK'S FASCIA)

F. Netter M.D.
©CIBA

(see page 19) to supply the cremasteric muscle and coverings of the cord and ultimately anastomoses with the testicular a. (In the female the a. accompanies the round ligament.)

The deep circumflex iliac a. courses in a sheath formed by the union of the transversalis and iliac fasciae (or between the latter and the peritoneum) laterally and upward to the anterior iliac spine, continuing after piercing the transversalis fascia along the inner lip of the iliac crest. At the midpoint of the crest, it passes through the transverse abdominal muscle to pursue a backward course between this and the internal oblique muscle. An ascending branch, leaving the main a. shortly below the anterior iliac spine, *anastomoses* with the *subcostal, lumbar* and *lower intercostal aa.*, while other branches communicate with the superficial circumflex iliac, inferior epigastric, iliolumbar and superior gluteal aa.

The next three aa. participating in the blood supply of the abdominal wall stem from the *femoral a.* The *superficial epigastric*, after piercing the cribriform fascia (see page 12), passes over the inguinal ligament and courses toward the umbilicus, supplying the superficial group of inguinal lymph nodes (see page 39), the skin and the subcutaneous tissue of the medial region of the lower abdomen. The *superficial circumflex iliac a.*, coursing below and parallel with the inguinal ligament (after piercing the fascia lata), provides blood to parts of the upper thigh and also to the lateral side of the abdomen. The *external pudendal aa.* (the superficial one emerging through the fossa ovalis) cross medially the spermatic cord (or round ligament) to supply the skin and subcutaneous tissue in the suprapubic region. One branch anastomoses with the dorsal a. of the penis (or clitoris).

VENOUS DRAINAGE OF THE ABDOMEN

The main collecting vessels of the abdomen are the inferior vena cava (IVC) and the portal v.* The latter has been treated in connection with the vv. transporting blood from the intestinal viscera (see pages 71 and 72 and CIBA COLLECTION, Vol. 3/III, page 18), as well as in connection with the intrahepatic vascular system (see ibidem, pages 10 to 12). The tributaries of the IVC are taken up here, starting with the superficial vv. serving the anterolateral abdominal wall. All these vv. accompany the homonymous arteries (see page 36), mostly in duplicate (venae comitantes) on both sides of the artery, being enwrapped in the same sheath.

The *external pudendal v.*, aside from branches coming from the region above the symphysis pubis, receives the vv. draining the external genitalia (*superficial dorsal v. of the penis* [clitoris] and the subcutaneous *vv. of the scrotum* [labium majus]), and joins, in most cases, the *great saphenous v.* (in other instances, the *femoral v.*). The *superficial epigastric* and *superficial circumflex iliac vv.*, draining the medial and more lateral parts of the lower abdominal wall, respectively, pass over the inguinal ligament and, piercing the cribriform fascia, enter the femoral (in many instances, the great saphenous) v. In the lateral body line the superficial vv. of the upper and lower halves of the trunk communicate through the *thoraco-epigastric v.*, which unites in the axilla with the *lateral thoracic v.*, a branch of the *axillary v.* This system of anastomosis plays an important rôle in the event of an obstruction of the superior or inferior caval v. Some vv., emerging from the lateral aspect of the mammary gland (areolar venous plexus), also drain into the thoraco-epigastric v. (Massopust and Gardner).

Another collateral venous circulation of clinical significance comes about by the superficial supra- and infra-umbilical vv., which, by means of five or six *para-umbilical vv.* (Sappey) arising from the integument and the musculo-aponeurotic structures of the abdominal wall, course within the ligamentum teres and enter the left branch of the portal v. (see CIBA COLLECTION, Vol. 3/III, page 18). When, as in liver cirrhosis, the portal venous pressure rises (see ibidem, page 69), the para-umbilical vv. establish collaterals with the superior and inferior epigastric and other abdominal vv. and become enlarged and tortuous, assuming a radial pattern known as "caput medusae" (see ibidem, pages 70 and 71).

The two deeper vv. still serving the

<hr>

*In this and the following page, "vein" and "veins" are abbreviated "v." and "vv.", respectively.

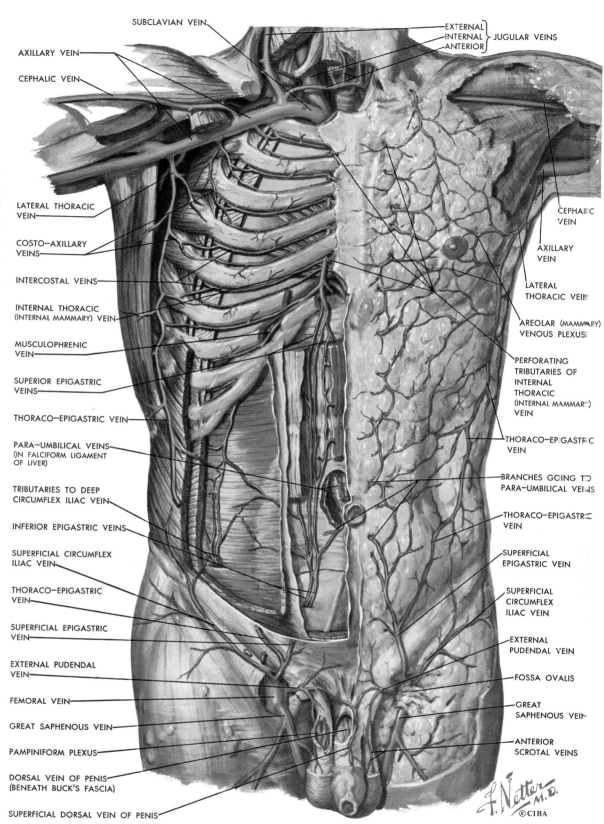

SUBCLAVIAN VEIN

AXILLARY VEIN

CEPHALIC VEIN

EXTERNAL INTERNAL ANTERIOR } JUGULAR VEINS

LATERAL THORACIC VEIN

COSTO-AXILLARY VEINS

INTERCOSTAL VEINS

INTERNAL THORACIC (INTERNAL MAMMARY) VEIN

MUSCULOPHRENIC VEIN

SUPERIOR EPIGASTRIC VEINS

THORACO-EPIGASTRIC VEIN

PARA-UMBILICAL VEINS (IN FALCIFORM LIGAMENT OF LIVER)

TRIBUTARIES TO DEEP CIRCUMFLEX ILIAC VEIN

INFERIOR EPIGASTRIC VEINS

SUPERFICIAL CIRCUMFLEX ILIAC VEIN

THORACO-EPIGASTRIC VEIN

SUPERFICIAL EPIGASTRIC VEIN

EXTERNAL PUDENDAL VEIN

FEMORAL VEIN

GREAT SAPHENOUS VEIN

PAMPINIFORM PLEXUS

DORSAL VEIN OF PENIS (BENEATH BUCK'S FASCIA)

SUPERFICIAL DORSAL VEIN OF PENIS

CEPHALIC VEIN

AXILLARY VEIN

LATERAL THORACIC VEIN

AREOLAR (MAMMARY) VENOUS PLEXUS

PERFORATING TRIBUTARIES OF INTERNAL THORACIC (INTERNAL MAMMARY) VEIN

THORACO-EPIGASTRIC VEIN

BRANCHES GOING TO PARA-UMBILICAL VEINS

THORACO-EPIGASTRIC VEIN

SUPERFICIAL EPIGASTRIC VEIN

SUPERFICIAL CIRCUMFLEX ILIAC VEIN

EXTERNAL PUDENDAL VEIN

FOSSA OVALIS

GREAT SAPHENOUS VEIN

ANTERIOR SCROTAL VEINS

f. Netter M.D.
©CIBA

anterolateral abdominal wall are the *inferior epigastric* and *deep circumflex iliac vv.*, both of which enter the external iliac v. (the continuation of the femoral v.) after having drained the same regions supplied by the corresponding arteries (see page 36). This network of anastomoses, with the musculophrenic, the superior epigastric vv. above or through their pubic branches with the obturator v. below, likewise conforms with that of the arteries. The *external iliac v.*, beginning behind the inguinal ligaments, courses with its homonymous artery upward along the brim of the lesser pelvis to unite with the internal iliac (hypogastric) v. in front of the sacro-iliac articulation to form the common iliac v.

The *internal iliac v.* collects the blood from all pelvic structures, except the upper part of the rectum and the sigmoid colon (see page 73). During its course starting near the upper part of the greater

sciatic foramen and while ascending over the piriform and psoas major muscles, it receives the *superior* and *inferior gluteal*, the *internal pudendal*, the *obturator*, the *lateral sacral*, the *middle rectal* and the *superior vesical vv.* Many of these vessels have their origins in a rich venous plexus, such as the *pudendal*, *urethrovesical* and *uterovaginal plexuses*, which do not belong within the scope of this book.

The *common iliac vv.* continue the course of the external iliac vv. in a median direction until the left meets the right v., marking the starting point of the IVC. The left common iliac v., somewhat longer than its right counterpart in many instances, receives the middle sacral when this unpaired vessel does not enter (as it does frequently) in the angle of the two iliac vv. Both common iliac vv. receive, furthermore, the *iliolumbar v.* and, in some instances, the lateral

(Continued on page 38)

VENOUS DRAINAGE
OF THE ABDOMEN

(*Continued from page* 37)

sacral v., if the latter has not entered the internal iliac v. or has not joined the fifth lumbar v. to send its blood directly into the IVC.

The *IVC* commences at the right of L5, ascends along the aorta in front of the vertebral column and continues behind the posterior surface of the liver in a groove between the bare area and the caudal lobe (see CIBA COLLECTION, Vol. 3/III, page 5). Immediately after the reception of usually three hepatic vv. (draining the segmental divisions of the liver; Healey and Schroy, see ibidem, page 13, and Part I, pages 41 and 42), the IVC leaves the abdomen at the level of T8 to the right of the right diaphragmatic crus through a hiatus in the central tendon (see page 21). As the caval hiatus lies higher than the opening for the aorta and the union of the two common iliac vv. is lower than the aortic bifurcation, the abdominal IVC is about 7 to 8 cm. longer than the abdominal aorta. The IVC's first tributaries are the *lumbar vv.* The lowest fifth of them connects with the iliolumbar v.; the upper four, lying on the bodies of the vertebrae and accompanying the arteries, drain, in most instances, into the posterior wall of the IVC but frequently also into the azygos or hemi-azygos vv. The connections which the lumbar vv. make with the renal, suprarenal, gonadal, deep circumflex, iliac and other abdominal vv. are manifold; the most important, from the physiologic and pathophysiologic viewpoints, concerns the longitudinal anastomosis effected through the *ascending lumbar vv.* These veins, beginning in the pelvis as a continuation of the lateral sacral veins, ascend deep in the sulcus between the tendinous origins of the psoas major muscle (see page 20) and the bodies and transverse processes of the vertebrae, and, after serial reception of the branches from all the lumbar vv., the right ascending lumbar v. drains into the azygos and the left into the hemi-azygos (see CIBA COLLECTION, Vol. 3/I, page 42) or sometimes into the left renal v. Posteriorly, the ascending lumbar vv. make numerous connections with the valveless plexiform network of the vertebral venous system (see CIBA COLLECTION, Vol. I, page 54) and thus bring into relation the venous drainage of the entire caval-azygos-hemi-azygos system with the vv. of the spine, the cord, the dural sinuses and the brain. These relationships, the significance of which has been recently demonstrated (Batson), provide the explanation for the spread of infectious processes, tumors (Jonassan et al.) and thrombi from their original site in the pelvis or abdomen (and also in the thorax) into the brain, the cord or bony structures of the skull and spine.

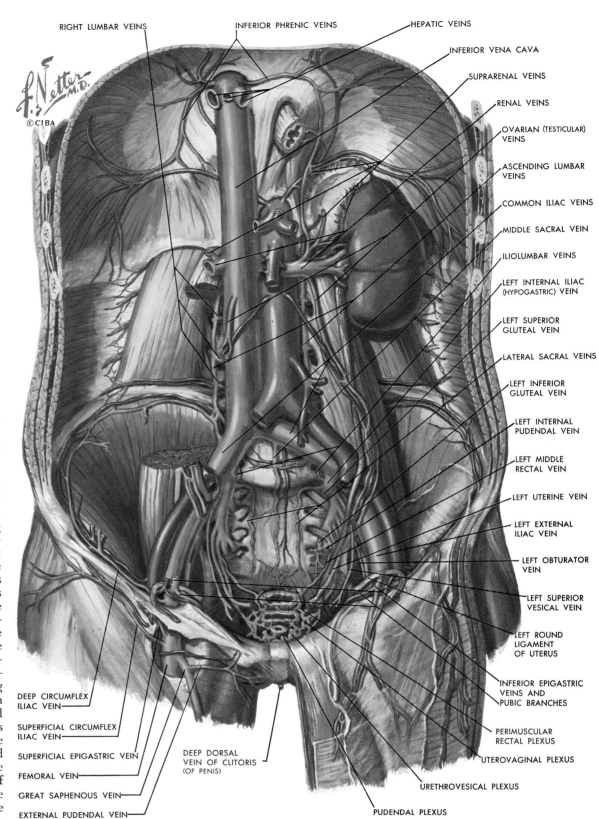

RIGHT LUMBAR VEINS — INFERIOR PHRENIC VEINS — HEPATIC VEINS — INFERIOR VENA CAVA — SUPRARENAL VEINS — RENAL VEINS — OVARIAN (TESTICULAR) VEINS — ASCENDING LUMBAR VEINS — COMMON ILIAC VEINS — MIDDLE SACRAL VEIN — ILIOLUMBAR VEINS — LEFT INTERNAL ILIAC (HYPOGASTRIC) VEIN — LEFT SUPERIOR GLUTEAL VEIN — LATERAL SACRAL VEINS — LEFT INFERIOR GLUTEAL VEIN — LEFT INTERNAL PUDENDAL VEIN — LEFT MIDDLE RECTAL VEIN — LEFT UTERINE VEIN — LEFT EXTERNAL ILIAC VEIN — LEFT OBTURATOR VEIN — LEFT SUPERIOR VESICAL VEIN — LEFT ROUND LIGAMENT OF UTERUS — INFERIOR EPIGASTRIC VEINS AND PUBIC BRANCHES — PERIMUSCULAR RECTAL PLEXUS — UTEROVAGINAL PLEXUS — URETHROVESICAL PLEXUS — PUDENDAL PLEXUS — DEEP DORSAL VEIN OF CLITORIS (OF PENIS) — EXTERNAL PUDENDAL VEIN — GREAT SAPHENOUS VEIN — FEMORAL VEIN — SUPERFICIAL EPIGASTRIC VEIN — SUPERFICIAL CIRCUMFLEX ILIAC VEIN — DEEP CIRCUMFLEX ILIAC VEIN

The right *testicular (ovarian) v.* enters the IVC above the lumbar vv., whereas the left gonadal vv. usually merge with the left renal or suprarenal or one of the lumbar vv. (Anson et al., Notkovich). The testicular vv., starting from the pampiniform plexus (see CIBA COLLECTION, Vol. 2, pages 14 and 23), ascend along the ductus deferens as major constituents of the spermatic cord, pass through the inguinal canal and, following the artery, course cranially on the psoas major muscle behind the peritoneum. The ovarian vv., deriving from the uterovaginal and ovarian plexuses (see ibidem, pages 97 and 99), take a similar course.

The *large renal vv.*, next in order of the IVC tributaries, lie in front of the corresponding arteries, are seldom multiple and show a far less remarkable variational pattern than do the arteries. The right v. rarely receives tributaries, whereas on the left side super-

numerary vv. may be present, and connections with adjacent vv. are frequent, the most important of which is the one with the lumbar (usually second) v. (see above).

The right *suprarenal v.* usually terminates either directly in the IVC, occasionally in the right renal v. The left suprarenal drains into the left renal or inferior phrenic v., with which, in any event, it is connected by several anastomoses.

The uppermost tributaries of the IVC (just above the entrance of the hepatic vv.) are the *inferior phrenic vv.*, which, in general, follow the course of the homonymous arteries. The left one may join the left renal v. separately or via a common trunk with the left suprarenal v. (25 per cent). The vv. of the left diaphragmatic dome provide a very adequate collateral circulation between the superior vena cava and the IVC (Gillot and Hureau).

LYMPH DRAINAGE OF THE ABDOMEN

The major lymphatics of the posterior abdominal wall as well as the intervening lymph nodes are essentially located along the large blood vessels. Thus the *external iliac* lymph vessels, interrupted by *nodes* of the same name, course with the external iliac arteries and veins. Entering the greater pelvis behind the inguinal ligament about midway between the anterior superior spine of the ilium and symphysis pubis, these lymphatics receive lymph from the deep (and thereby also superficial) inguinal nodes, through which passes the drainage of the lower extremities, the lower parts of the anterolateral abdominal wall and the perineum (including the external genitalia and anal region). The internal iliac lymph vessels run, interrupted by the *internal iliac (hypogastric) nodes,* with the artery and vein of identical name and drain the larger part of the organs and wall of the true pelvis, whereas the remaining part of this region releases lymph via the presacral lymphatics. The external and internal iliac lymphatics join over, or in the neighborhood of, the common iliac artery to form the common iliac lymph vessels, between which nodes carrying the same designation are inserted. They receive afferents from the presacral lymphatics with their lateral and middle sacral nodes. The latter are situated in the retrorectal connective tissue over the concavity of the os sacrum. In the region of the aortic bifurcation, the common iliac lymph vessels proceed cranially along the lateral walls of the aorta to become the right and left lumbar trunks. These trunks and the interposed lumbar (lateral aortic) nodes receive afferents from the kidney and the pre-aortic lymph nodes (see page 75). The extremely large area of drainage which the lumbar trunks serve includes thus, in particular, the walls and organs of the lower abdomen as well as of the lower extremities.

Both lumbar trunks unite in the area of the aortic hiatus in front of the vertebral column, in the majority of cases at the level of the upper third of L1 and the intervertebral disk between T12 and L1 (Jdanow), to form the beginning of the thoracic duct, which, in about 50 per cent of individuals, starts with a distinctive, elongated, saccular dilatation (approximately 1 to 1.5 cm. in diameter and 5 to 7 cm. in length), the cisterna chyli. Its three main roots are the single intestinal or gastro-intestinal trunk (see page 74) and the two lumbar trunks

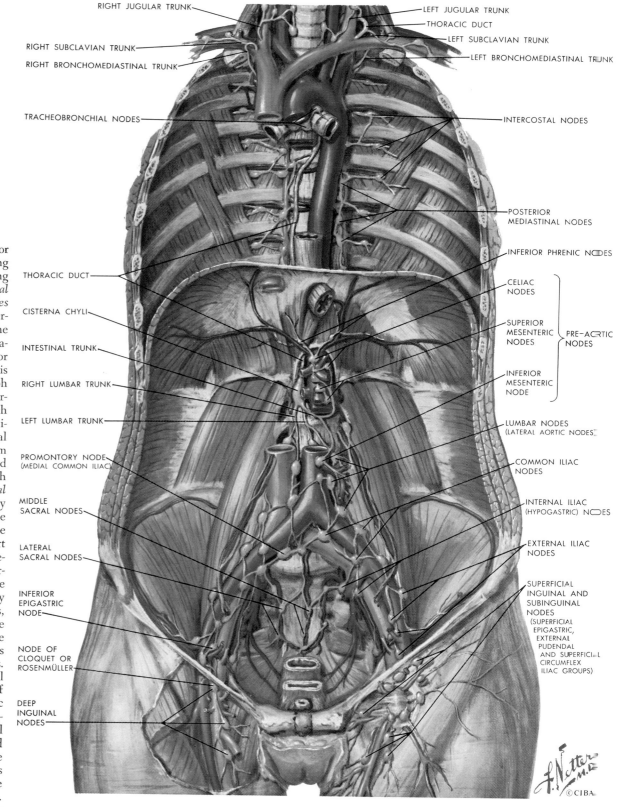

RIGHT JUGULAR TRUNK

RIGHT SUBCLAVIAN TRUNK

RIGHT BRONCHOMEDIASTINAL TRUNK

TRACHEOBRONCHIAL NODES

THORACIC DUCT

CISTERNA CHYLI

INTESTINAL TRUNK

RIGHT LUMBAR TRUNK

LEFT LUMBAR TRUNK

PROMONTORY NODE (MEDIAL COMMON ILIAC)

MIDDLE SACRAL NODES

LATERAL SACRAL NODES

INFERIOR EPIGASTRIC NODE

NODE OF CLOQUET OR ROSENMÜLLER

DEEP INGUINAL NODES

LEFT JUGULAR TRUNK

THORACIC DUCT

LEFT SUBCLAVIAN TRUNK

LEFT BRONCHOMEDIASTINAL TRUNK

INTERCOSTAL NODES

POSTERIOR MEDIASTINAL NODES

INFERIOR PHRENIC NODES

CELIAC NODES

SUPERIOR MESENTERIC NODES

PRE-AORTIC NODES

INFERIOR MESENTERIC NODE

LUMBAR NODES (LATERAL AORTIC NODES)

COMMON ILIAC NODES

INTERNAL ILIAC (HYPOGASTRIC) NODES

EXTERNAL ILIAC NODES

SUPERFICIAL INGUINAL AND SUBINGUINAL NODES (SUPERFICIAL EPIGASTRIC, EXTERNAL PUDENDAL AND SUPERFICIAL CIRCUMFLEX ILIAC GROUPS)

(see above), but two smaller tributaries (a pair of descending intercostal lymph trunks) coming from a cranial direction and descending through the aortic opening of the diaphragm into the abdominal cavity also join the cisterna chyli. The thoracic duct passes first to the right across the dorsal surface of the aorta, through the aortic hiatus of the diaphragm into the mediastinum, ascending then in front of the lower thoracic vertebrae lying between the aorta and the vena azygos ventral to the right intercostal arteries. On reaching the level of the fifth thoracic vertebra, it changes over behind the esophagus to the left side of the spinal column, where it runs for a short distance along the right of the aorta and then crosses behind the aortic arch to continue its ascent. Opposite the third thoracic vertebra, the thoracic duct draws away from the spinal column in a ventral direction and proceeds between the left common carotid artery and the left subclavian artery, through the upper thoracic aperture, into the left supraclavicular fossa. Here it describes a curve over the arch of the subclavian artery and, finally, opens either into the angle at which the left jugular and left subclavian veins join to form the left innominate vein (vena brachiocephalica sinistra) (see CIBA COLLECTION, Vol. 3/1, page 34) or, less often, into one of the two veins forming this angle. At its point of entry into the veins, the thoracic duct does not always form a single entity but sometimes divides into a deltalike structure composed of two or more branches. During its passage through the thorax, the thoracic duct is joined by vessels connecting with the retrocardiac, infracardiac, posterior parietal, tracheobronchial and posterior mediastinal nodes (see CIBA COLLECTION, Vol. 3/1, page 43) and others draining the thoracic wall and intrathoracic organs.

INNERVATION OF ABDOMEN AND OF PERINEUM

The segmentally arranged spinal nerves (see CIBA COLLECTION, Vol. 1, pages 49 to 52) are attached to the sides of the spinal cord by a series of *ventral* and *dorsal roots*. These roots from each of the spinal segments unite to form the *spinal nerve trunk*, which emerges through the corresponding intervertebral foramen (see CIBA COLLECTION, Vol. 1, page 21). The ventral roots contain the axons of the larger anterior cornual motor cells, and the dorsal roots contain the axons of the pseudo-unipolar sensory cells located in the *dorsal root ganglia*.

After emerging from the intervertebral foramen, each spinal nerve receives a branch or branches (*gray rami communicantes*) from an adjacent ganglion of the *sympathetic trunk*, and the thoracic and the first two or, occasionally, three lumbar spinal nerves each contribute a branch or branches (white rami communicantes) to the corresponding sympathetic trunk ganglia. The gray rami contain sympathetic postganglionic fibers; the white rami contain sympathetic preganglionic fibers and constitute the sympathetic component of the autonomic outflow (see CIBA COLLECTION, Vol. 1, page 82).

The spinal nerves are short. Before dividing into *ventral* and *dorsal primary rami*, each of the spinal nerves gives off a small recurrent *meningeal branch*. The primary rami contain fibers from both ventral and dorsal nerve roots and also from the gray rami communicantes, and thus are mixtures of efferent and afferent somatic, as well as efferent and afferent autonomic, fibers.

In general, the dorsal primary rami are smaller than the ventral and do not unite to form plexuses. They divide into *medial* and *lateral branches* for the supply of the muscles and skin of the back. The usually larger ventral primary rami supply the anterolateral aspects of the trunk (see also next page) and the limbs. In the cervical (see CIBA COLLECTION, Vol. 1, page 49), lumbar, sacral and coccygeal regions (see Plate 32), several of the ventral rami converge to form plexuses, but in the thoracic region they maintain their segmental character and each runs separately and independently to the site or structure it innervates.

The thoracic ventral rami (*intercostal nerves*) are distributed chiefly to the anterolateral walls of the thorax and abdomen. They are twelve in number on

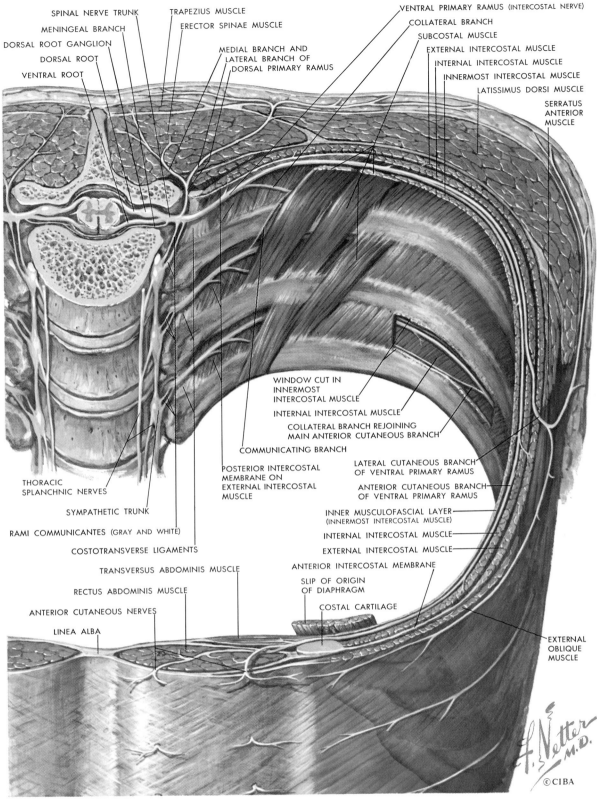

each side, but only eleven are intercostal. The twelfth pair lie below the last ribs and are termed subcostal. The upper six pairs of intercostal nerves are limited in their supply to the thoracic parietes and, in addition, a considerable number of fibers of the uppermost two pairs participate in the formation of the brachial plexus, *i.e.*, the innervation of the upper limbs. The lower five pairs of intercostal nerves and the subcostal nerves supply the parietes of the thorax and abdomen and also contribute fibers to the diaphragm.

Typically, a lower (seventh to eleventh) thoracic (intercostal) nerve courses forward along the thoracico-abdominal wall below the corresponding rib and intercostal vessels (see page 36). Posteriorly, the nerve lies between the pleura and the *posterior intercostal membrane* and then passes between the *internal* and *innermost intercostal muscles*. Each nerve gives off a *collateral branch* and a *lateral cutane-*

ous branch. The former, separating from the primary ramus only a few centimeters away from the vertebrae, inclines downward in the same intermuscular plane as the parent nerve, runs along the lower border of the intercostal space and ends anteriorly as a small cutaneous nerve or by rejoining the main ramus. The lateral cutaneous branch accompanies the main intercostal nerve as far as the midaxillary line before piercing the intercostal muscles obliquely and dividing into anterior and posterior branches, which are mainly cutaneous in distribution. The intercostal nerves supply intercostal, subcostal and transverse thoracic muscles. The lower five or six intercostal nerves also supply filaments to the peripheral parts of the diaphragm (see Plate 34).

The lower five intercostal nerves and the subcostal nerves pass behind the lower *costal cartilages* and
(Continued on page 41)

INNERVATION OF ABDOMEN AND OF PERINEUM

(Continued from page 40)

enter the abdominal wall to supply the *oblique, transverse* and *rectus abdominal muscles* and end as *anterior abdominal cutaneous branches.* The tenth nerve serves the dermatome (see CIBA COLLECTION, VOL. I, page 55) at the level of the umbilicus. The lateral cutaneous branch of the subcostal nerve (T12) pierces the internal and external oblique abdominal muscles and then descends over the iliac crest to assist in supplying the skin over the upper lateral part of the thigh (see Plates 32 and 33).

The ventral primary rami of the lower spinal nerves (five lumbar, five sacral and one coccygeal) divide and reunite in a plexiform fashion to form the *lumbar, sacral* and *coccygeal plexuses* (see next page). They are interconnected as described above (*rami communicantes*) with the *sympathetic trunks.*

The *lumbar plexus* is formed by the ventral rami of the first three lumbar nerves and the greater part of the fourth (with a contribution from the subcostal twelfth thoracic). It is situated in front of the lumbar vertebral transverse processes and is embedded in the posterior part of the psoas major muscle, which (as, *e.g.,* in picture on next page) would have to be dissected to make the plexus accessible. The most common course and distribution of the components of the plexus and its relationship to the bony structures and muscular and aponeurotic layers are demonstrated on the following two pages, but it should be kept in mind that variations in the makeup of the lumbar plexus are frequent.

The first lumbar nerve, after receiving a twig from the subcostal nerve, splits into an upper and a smaller lower branch. The former divides into the *iliohypogastric* and *ilio-inguinal nerves,* and the latter unites with a twig of the second lumbar to form the *genitofemoral nerve.* The rest of the second lumbar nerve, the third and that part of the fourth which contributes to this plexus, each divide also into anterior and posterior sections, which combine to constitute the *obturator* and *femoral nerves,* respectively. The *accessory obturator nerve,* when present, is formed by branchlets from the anterior divisions of the third and fourth nerves, whereas the *lateral femoral cutaneous nerve* evolves by the fusion of small offshoots from the posterior divisions of the

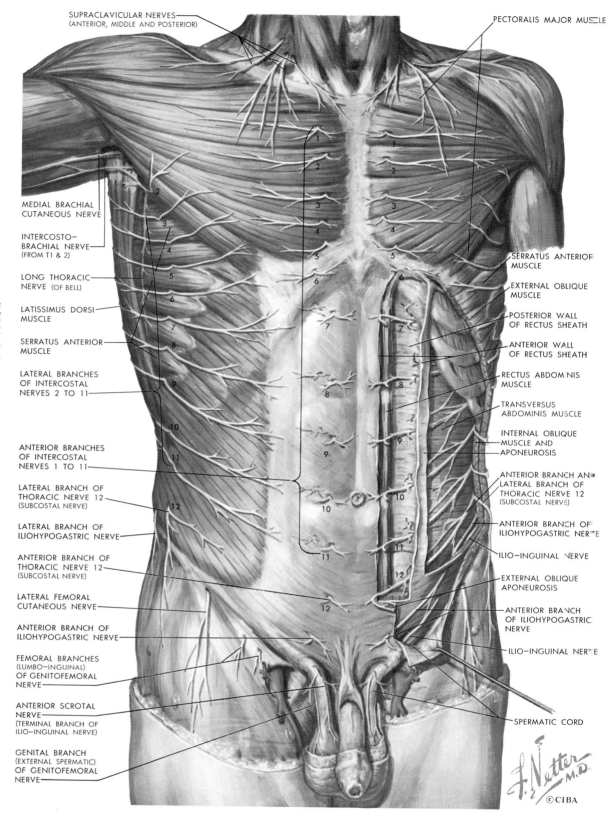

second and third lumbar nerves. *Muscular branches* from the subcostal and upper four lumbar nerves supply the *quadratus lumborum muscle* (see Plate 33), and those of the first and second reach the *major and minor psoas muscles.* The psoas major muscles are further innervated by branches from the third and, sometimes, fourth lumbar nerves, which also supply the *iliacus muscles.*

The *iliohypogastric* and *ilio-inguinal nerves* resemble the thoracic nerves in their course and distribution, being analogous, respectively, to the main trunk and the collateral branch of an intercostal nerve. The former nerve gives off a *lateral branch* which crosses the iliac crest a short distance behind the corresponding branch of the subcostal nerve (see above), both nerves then going to the skin of the upper lateral part of the thigh (see also page 15). Continuing forward, the *anterior branch of the iliohypogastric nerve* sends

filaments to the transverse and the oblique abdominal muscles, pierces the *external oblique aponeurosis* about 3 cm. above the superficial inguinal ring and terminates innervating the skin above the pubis.

The ilio-inguinal nerve supplies filaments to the adjacent muscles and, after piercing the same muscles as the iliohypogastric nerve, enters the inguinal canal, runs below the spermatic cord and emerges through the superficial inguinal ring to supply the upper inner side of the thigh, the root of the penis and the anterior part of the scrotum in the male, and the mons pubis and labium majus in the female.

The *genitofemoral nerve,* after emerging from the lumbar plexus (see above), passes through the psoas major muscle and descends on its anterior surface, behind the peritoneum, to divide, at about the level of the fifth lumbar vertebra, into the *genital* and *femoral*

(Continued on page 42)

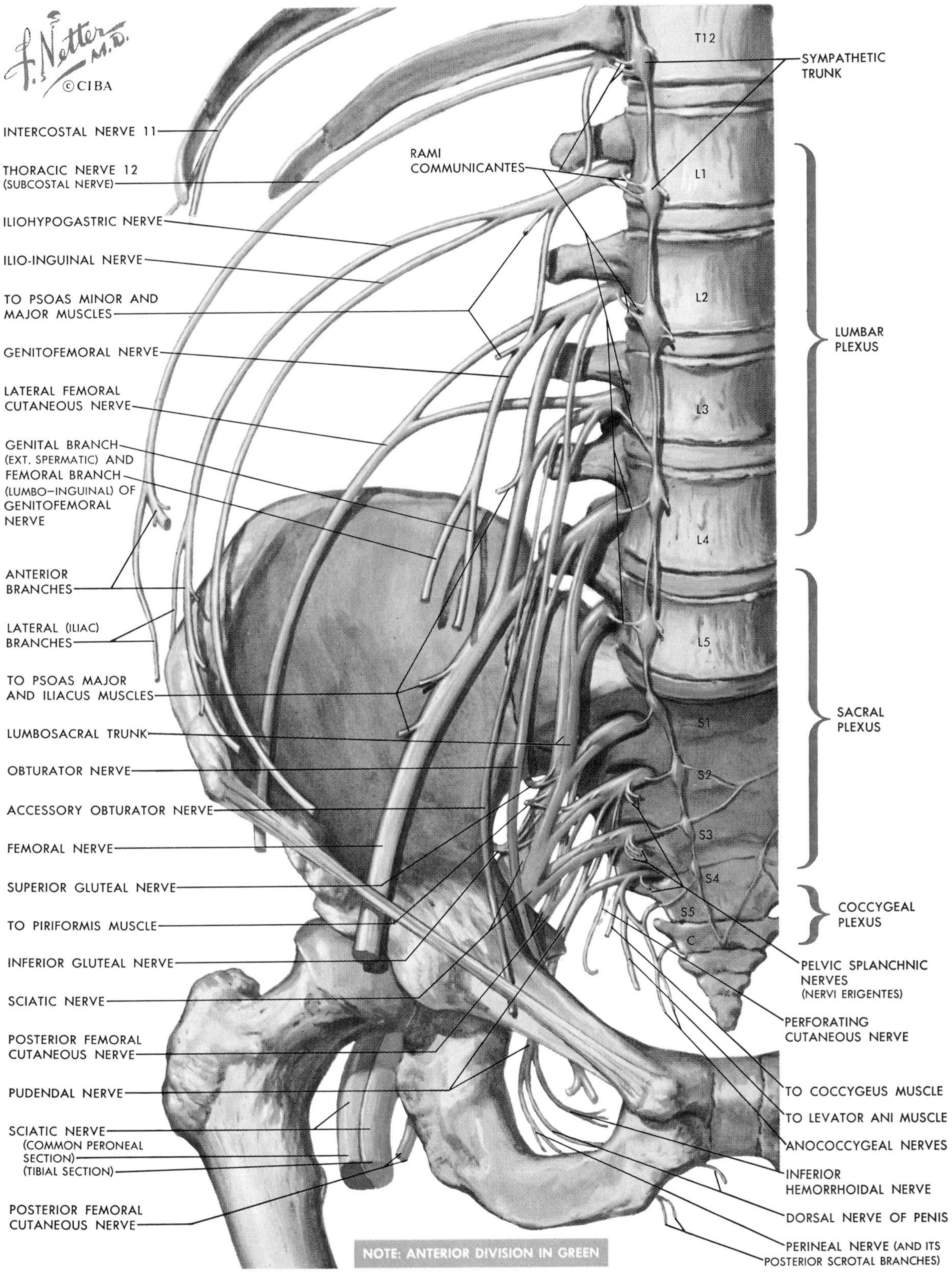

f. Netter M.D.
©CIBA

INNERVATION OF ABDOMEN AND OF PERINEUM

(Continued from page 41)

branches. The former branch enters the inguinal canal through the deep inguinal ring, supplies the cremaster muscle and contributes some twigs to the skin of the scrotum, or the labium majus of the female *(external spermatic nerve).* The femoral (lumbo-inguinal) branch runs lateral to the external iliac and femoral arteries (see also page 19), passes behind the inguinal ligament and, after piercing the anterior layer of the femoral sheath and the fascia lata, ramifies in the superficial tissues and skin over the upper part of the femoral triangle (Scarpa's). The genitofemoral nerve and its branches carry many of the efferent and afferent fibers to and from the common iliac, external iliac and femoral arteries.

Other branches of the lumbar plexus (*e.g.,* the largest, the *femoral nerve*), except for muscular rami to quadratus lumborum, psoas major and iliacus muscles, are distributed to the lower limb and, consequently, are not discussed in this volume.

The anterior (ventral) rami of the sacral and coccygeal nerves, which, in contrast to the lumbar nerves, diminish in size progressively from above down, divide and reunite to form the *sacral* and *coccygeal plexuses.* These lie on the posterior wall of the pelvis, behind the ureters, the internal iliac vessels and intestinal coils, and in front of the piriformis and coccygeus muscles. The lower and smaller part of the fourth lumbar nerve (nervus furcalis) unites with the ventral ramus of the fifth lumbar nerve to appear as the *lumbosacral trunk,* which, together with the ventral rami of the first three and the upper part of the fourth sacral nerves, constitutes the sacral plexus. The lower part of the fourth sacral joins the fifth sacral and coccygeal nerves to form the small coccygeal plexus.

Each nerve entering into the composition of these two plexuses receives postganglionic fibers by way of one or more gray rami communicantes from an adjacent ganglion of the sympathetic trunk. Parasympathetic preganglionic fibers emerge through the second, third, and fourth sacral nerves and leave them as pelvic splanchnic nerves (nervi erigentes) (see Plate 33 and page 76), constituting the sacral part of the autonomic outflow.

The *sacral plexus,* by convergence and fusion of its roots, develops into a flattened band, from which many branches arise, before its largest part passes as the *sciatic nerve* through the greater sciatic foramen below the piriformis muscle (see page 22). This large nerve consists of a *tibial* and a *common peroneal section,* which usually

(Continued on page 43)

Labels (illustration):

- INTERCOSTAL NERVE 11
- THORACIC NERVE 12 (SUBCOSTAL NERVE)
- ILIOHYPOGASTRIC NERVE
- ILIO-INGUINAL NERVE
- TO PSOAS MINOR AND MAJOR MUSCLES
- GENITOFEMORAL NERVE
- LATERAL FEMORAL CUTANEOUS NERVE
- GENITAL BRANCH (EXT. SPERMATIC) AND FEMORAL BRANCH (LUMBO-INGUINAL) OF GENITOFEMORAL NERVE
- ANTERIOR BRANCHES
- LATERAL (ILIAC) BRANCHES
- TO PSOAS MAJOR AND ILIACUS MUSCLES
- LUMBOSACRAL TRUNK
- OBTURATOR NERVE
- ACCESSORY OBTURATOR NERVE
- FEMORAL NERVE
- SUPERIOR GLUTEAL NERVE
- TO PIRIFORMIS MUSCLE
- INFERIOR GLUTEAL NERVE
- SCIATIC NERVE
- POSTERIOR FEMORAL CUTANEOUS NERVE
- PUDENDAL NERVE
- SCIATIC NERVE (COMMON PERONEAL SECTION) (TIBIAL SECTION)
- POSTERIOR FEMORAL CUTANEOUS NERVE
- T12
- RAMI COMMUNICANTES
- SYMPATHETIC TRUNK
- L1
- L2
- L3
- L4
- L5
- LUMBAR PLEXUS
- S1
- S2
- S3
- S4
- S5
- C
- SACRAL PLEXUS
- COCCYGEAL PLEXUS
- PELVIC SPLANCHNIC NERVES (NERVI ERIGENTES)
- PERFORATING CUTANEOUS NERVE
- TO COCCYGEUS MUSCLE
- TO LEVATOR ANI MUSCLE
- ANOCOCCYGEAL NERVES
- INFERIOR HEMORRHOIDAL NERVE
- DORSAL NERVE OF PENIS
- PERINEAL NERVE (AND ITS POSTERIOR SCROTAL BRANCHES)

NOTE: ANTERIOR DIVISION IN GREEN

NERVES	ANTERIOR DIVISION		POSTERIOR DIVISION	
	LUMBAR	SACRAL	LUMBAR	SACRAL
Sciatic, tibial sec.	4, 5	1, 2, 3		
common peroneal sec.			4, 5	1, 2
To m. quadr. femoris and gemellus inf.	4, 5	1		
To m. obturator int. and gem. sup.	5	1, 2		
Superior gluteal			4, 5	1
Inferior gluteal			5	1, 2
To m. piriformis				1, 2
To m. levator ani and coccygeus				(3) 4
Pudendal		2, 3, 4		
Pelvic splanchnic		2, 3, 4		
Posterior femoral cutaneous		2, 3		1, 2
Perforating cutaneous				2, 3 (4)
Perineal branch of S4				4

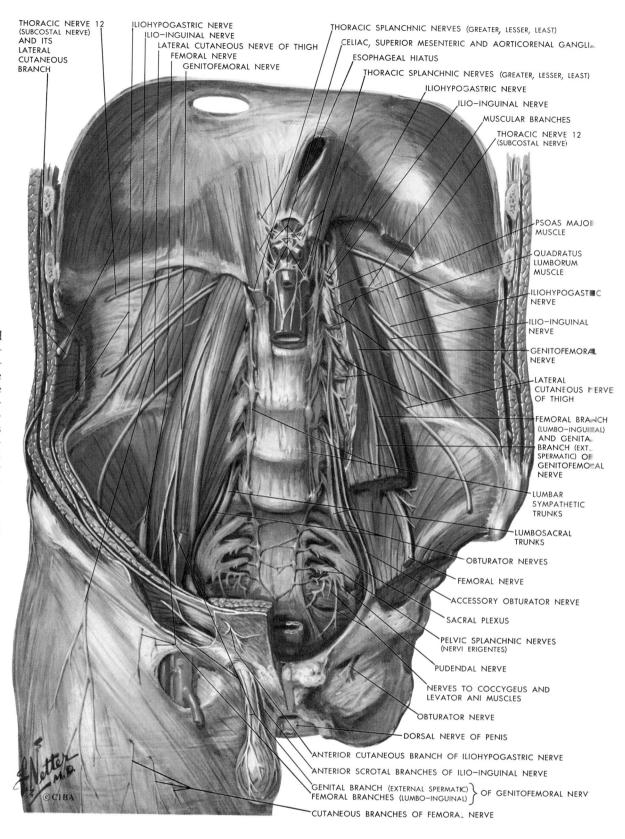

THORACIC NERVE 12 (SUBCOSTAL NERVE) AND ITS LATERAL CUTANEOUS BRANCH
ILIOHYPOGASTRIC NERVE
ILIO-INGUINAL NERVE
LATERAL CUTANEOUS NERVE OF THIGH
FEMORAL NERVE
GENITOFEMORAL NERVE

THORACIC SPLANCHNIC NERVES (GREATER, LESSER, LEAST)
CELIAC, SUPERIOR MESENTERIC AND AORTICORENAL GANGLIA
ESOPHAGEAL HIATUS
THORACIC SPLANCHNIC NERVES (GREATER, LESSER, LEAST)
ILIOHYPOGASTRIC NERVE
ILIO-INGUINAL NERVE
MUSCULAR BRANCHES
THORACIC NERVE 12 (SUBCOSTAL NERVE)

PSOAS MAJOR MUSCLE
QUADRATUS LUMBORUM MUSCLE
ILIOHYPOGASTRIC NERVE
ILIO-INGUINAL NERVE
GENITOFEMORAL NERVE
LATERAL CUTANEOUS NERVE OF THIGH
FEMORAL BRANCH (LUMBO-INGUINAL) AND GENITAL BRANCH (EXT. SPERMATIC) OF GENITOFEMORAL NERVE
LUMBAR SYMPATHETIC TRUNKS
LUMBOSACRAL TRUNKS
OBTURATOR NERVES
FEMORAL NERVE
ACCESSORY OBTURATOR NERVE
SACRAL PLEXUS
PELVIC SPLANCHNIC NERVES (NERVI ERIGENTES)
PUDENDAL NERVE
NERVES TO COCCYGEUS AND LEVATOR ANI MUSCLES
OBTURATOR NERVE
DORSAL NERVE OF PENIS
ANTERIOR CUTANEOUS BRANCH OF ILIOHYPOGASTRIC NERVE
ANTERIOR SCROTAL BRANCHES OF ILIO-INGUINAL NERVE
GENITAL BRANCH (EXTERNAL SPERMATIC) / FEMORAL BRANCHES (LUMBO-INGUINAL) } OF GENITOFEMORAL NERVE
CUTANEOUS BRANCHES OF FEMORAL NERVE

INNERVATION OF ABDOMEN AND OF PERINEUM

(Continued from page 42)

remain fused until about the lower third of the thigh, but which may occasionally be separated at their points of origin or may divide before the nerve leaves the pelvis. The nerve roots of the sacral plexus split into anterior and posterior divisions, which, in some individuals, unite again to produce the nerves as summarized in the table on the preceding page. Most branches of the sacral plexus supply structures in the lower limb and cannot be included in this discussion. Others are distributed in the pelvic and perineal regions.

The *nerves* (origin, see table) *to the piriformis muscle,* to the levator ani and to the coccygeus muscle (see pages 20 and 22) pierce the anterior or pelvic surfaces of these muscles. The nerve to the *obturator internus muscle* (not to be confused with the obturator nerve) leaves the pelvis through the greater sciatic foramen below the piriformis muscle, crosses the ischial spine lateral to the pudendal nerve and internal pudendal vessels, re-enters the pelvis through the lesser sciatic foramen and sinks into the pelvic surface of the obturator internus muscle.

The *pudendal nerve* (origin, see table), after passing between the piriformis and coccygeus muscles (see Plate 34), leaves the pelvis through the greater sciatic foramen, together with the sciatic nerve, and enters the buttock. Crossing the ischial spine medial to the internal pudendal artery (see page 70), it accompanies that vessel through the lesser sciatic foramen into the pudendal (Alcock's) canal on the obturator internus fascia (see page 30). As the nerve enters the canal, it gives off the inferior hemorrhoidal (rectal) nerve and shortly thereafter terminates by splitting into the perineal nerve and the dorsal nerve of the penis or clitoris, respectively (see CIBA COLLECTION, Vol. 2, pages 19 and 104).

The inferior rectal nerve perforates the medial wall of the pudendal canal, crosses obliquely the ischiorectal fossa with the inferior rectal vessels and divides into branches, which are the main supply of the external sphincter ani and for the lining of the lower part of the anal canal and the skin around the anus. Its branches communicate with the perineal branches of the posterior femoral

cutaneous, fourth sacral and perforating cutaneous nerves (see Plate 32) and the *perineal nerve,* which is the larger terminal branch of the pudendal nerve. This latter nerve runs forward in the pudendal canal below the internal pudendal artery toward the posterior border of the urogenital diaphragm, near which it divides into *superficial and deep rami.* The superficial one divides into medial and lateral posterior scrotal (or labial) nerves, which spread over the skin of the scrotum (or major labia), communicating with the perineal branch of the posterior femoral cutaneous nerve. The deep branches supply the anterior parts of the external sphincter ani, the superficial and deep transverse perineal, *bulbo-* and *ischiocavernosus muscles* (see Plate 34), and sphincter urethrae (and, in a subsidiary fashion, the levator ani). A twig, termed the nerve of the bulb, arises from the branch to the bulbocavernosus muscle and is distributed to

the erectile tissue of the corpus spongiosum and the mucous membrane of the urethra.

The *dorsal nerve of the penis* accompanies the internal pudendal artery in its course through the *deep transversal perineal muscle* and passes forward to the pubic arch under cover of the ischiocavernosus muscle, whence a branch goes to the corpus cavernosum penis. Passing through a gap between the inferior fascia and the apex of the urogenital diaphragm, the nerve comes to lie alongside the dorsal artery of the penis and continues as far as the glans and the prepuce. (In the female the dorsal nerve of the clitoris is smaller, but its distribution is similar.)

The *posterior femoral cutaneous nerve* (small sciatic nerve) (origin, see table), besides innervating the skin of the posterior thigh, gives off a gluteal branch, the inferior cluneal nerve, supplying the

(Continued on page 44)

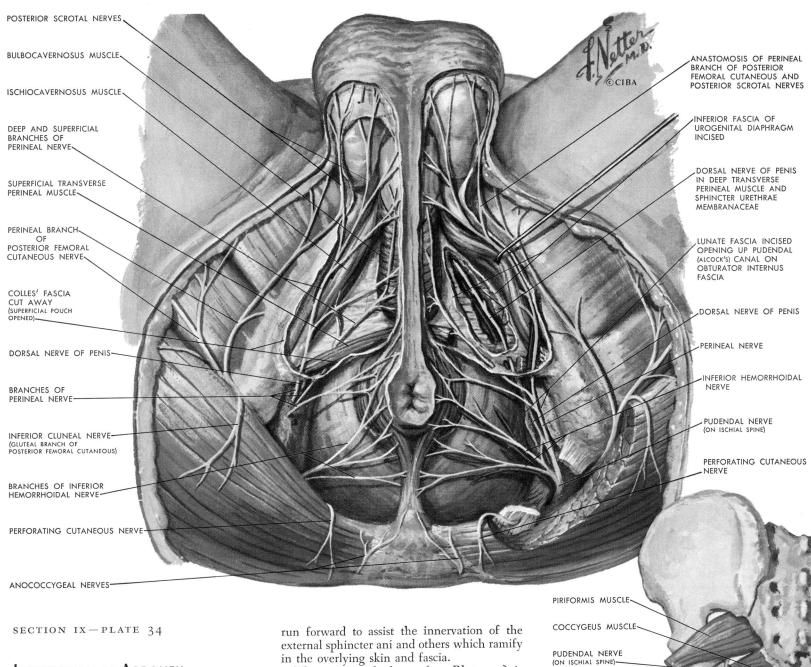

POSTERIOR SCROTAL NERVES

BULBOCAVERNOSUS MUSCLE

ISCHIOCAVERNOSUS MUSCLE

DEEP AND SUPERFICIAL
BRANCHES OF
PERINEAL NERVE

SUPERFICIAL TRANSVERSE
PERINEAL MUSCLE

PERINEAL BRANCH
OF
POSTERIOR FEMORAL
CUTANEOUS NERVE

COLLES' FASCIA
CUT AWAY
(SUPERFICIAL POUCH
OPENED)

DORSAL NERVE OF PENIS

BRANCHES OF
PERINEAL NERVE

INFERIOR CLUNEAL NERVE
(GLUTEAL BRANCH OF
POSTERIOR FEMORAL CUTANEOUS)

BRANCHES OF INFERIOR
HEMORRHOIDAL NERVE

PERFORATING CUTANEOUS NERVE

ANOCOCCYGEAL NERVES

ANASTOMOSIS OF PERINEAL
BRANCH OF POSTERIOR
FEMORAL CUTANEOUS AND
POSTERIOR SCROTAL NERVES

INFERIOR FASCIA OF
UROGENITAL DIAPHRAGM
INCISED

DORSAL NERVE OF PENIS
IN DEEP TRANSVERSE
PERINEAL MUSCLE AND
SPHINCTER URETHRAE
MEMBRANACEAE

LUNATE FASCIA INCISED
OPENING UP PUDENDAL
(ALCOCK'S) CANAL ON
OBTURATOR INTERNUS
FASCIA

DORSAL NERVE OF PENIS

PERINEAL NERVE

INFERIOR HEMORRHOIDAL
NERVE

PUDENDAL NERVE
(ON ISCHIAL SPINE)

PERFORATING CUTANEOUS
NERVE

PIRIFORMIS MUSCLE

COCCYGEUS MUSCLE

PUDENDAL NERVE
(ON ISCHIAL SPINE)

OBTURATOR INTERNUS
MUSCLE

LEVATOR ANI MUSCLE

INFERIOR HEMORRHOIDAL NERVE

EXTERNAL SPHINCTER ANI

SECTION IX—PLATE 34

INNERVATION OF ABDOMEN AND OF PERINEUM

(Continued from page 43)

skin area over the lower part of the gluteus maximus and, in the same region, a perineal branch, which curves forward and medially below the ischial tuberosity to the skin and fasciae of the perineum, scrotum and root of the penis (perineum, labium majus and root of the clitoris in the female), where its terminal twigs communicate with the inferior rectal and perineal branches of the pudendal and terminal filaments of the ilio-inguinal nerves. The *perforating cutaneous nerve* (origin, see table) pierces the sacrotuberous ligament and turns around the lower margin of the gluteus maximus to become cutaneous a short distance lateral to the coccyx. Its origin and distribution, however, are not constant. It may be joined or replaced by branches from the pudendal or posterior femoral cutaneous nerve, or the *perineal branch of the fourth sacral nerve,* arising from a loop between the third and fourth sacral nerves, may take over its function. This branch reaches the posterior angle of the ischiorectal fossa (see page 32) by perforating the coccygeus muscle and then divides into some twigs which

run forward to assist the innervation of the external sphincter ani and others which ramify in the overlying skin and fascia.

The *coccygeal plexus* (see Plate 32) is formed by the union of the lower part of the ventral ramus of the fourth sacral nerve with those of the fifth sacral and coccygeal nerves. The plexus is small and really consists of two loops on the pelvic surface of the coccygeus and the levator ani muscles. It gives off fine twigs to the parts adjacent to both these structures, as well as the delicate anococcygeal nerves which pierce the sacrotuberous ligament and supply the skin in the vicinity of the coccyx.

Having demonstrated and discussed the nerves supplying the wall of the abdominal cavity, the formation of the lumbar and sacral plexus and the nerve branches they release to innervate part of the abdominal viscera and floor (pelvis as well as perineum) of the abdominal cavity, it remains to consider the innervation of that muscular tendinous organ, the diaphragm, which represents the roof of the abdominal cavity.

The diaphragm (see page 21 and CIBA COLLECTION, Vol. 3/1, page 39) is supplied by the phrenic and lower intercostal nerves. The phrenics contain both motor and sensory fibers. (The latter convey afferent impulses from the pleura, pericardium, peritoneum, etc.) The motor fibers are the axons of the phrenic nucleus located in the third, fourth and fifth cervical cord segments (see CIBA COLLEC-

TION, Vol. 3/1, pages 29 and 34). If one phrenic is destroyed, complete muscular atrophy occurs in the corresponding half of the diaphragm, so it is presumed the intercostal nerve supply must be sensory.

The phrenic nerves are distributed mainly on the inferior surface of the diaphragm. The right pierces the central tendon just lateral to the vena caval orifice and divides into ventral and dorsal branches which supply all the muscle fibers on the same side, including the crural fibers on the right side of the esophagus and those arising from the lumbocostal arches. The left nerve pierces the diaphragm about 3 cm. anterior to the central tendon and, thereafter, supplies the left half of the muscle, including the fibers of the right crus lying to the left of the esophageal hiatus.

The phrenic branches communicate with autonomic fibers from the celiac plexus accompanying the inferior phrenic arteries. On the right side a small ganglion marks one of these interconnections.

Section X

ANATOMY OF THE LOWER DIGESTIVE TRACT

by

FRANK H. NETTER, M.D.

in collaboration with

R. V. GORSCH, M.D., F.I.C.S., F.A.P.S., D.A.P.B.
Plates 10-17

NICHOLAS A. MICHELS, M.A., D.Sc.
Plates 18-27

PROF. G. A. G. MITCHELL, O.B.E., T.D., M.B., Ch.M., D.Sc.
Plates 30-34

PROF. GERHARD WOLF-HEIDEGGER, M.D., Ph.D.
Plates 1-9, 28 and 29

SMALL INTESTINE I

Topography and Relations

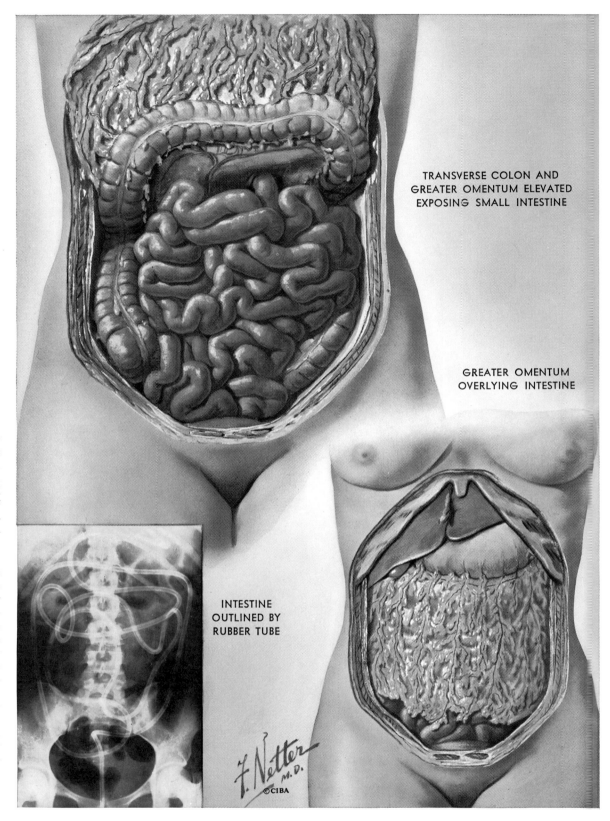

TRANSVERSE COLON AND
GREATER OMENTUM ELEVATED
EXPOSING SMALL INTESTINE

GREATER OMENTUM
OVERLYING INTESTINE

INTESTINE
OUTLINED BY
RUBBER TUBE

The small intestine consists of a retroperitoneal portion, the duodenum (see CIBA COLLECTION, Vol. 3/1, pages 50, 54 and 55), and a mesenteric portion comprising the *coils of the jejunum and ileum.* Since the mesenteric portion of the small intestine is subject to considerable individual and functional variations, its total length varies considerably, the average for adults being around 5 m., approximately two fifths of which are accounted for by the upper part (the jejunum) and three fifths by the lower part (the ileum). The jejunum commences at the duodenojejunal flexure (see CIBA COLLECTION, Vol. 3/1, page 50) on the left side of the second lumbar vertebra or, occasionally, somewhat more cranially; the ileum joins the large intestine in the region of the right iliac fossa (see page 52). The duodenojejunal flexure is situated high up in the inferior, *i.e.,* infra-mesocolic, zone of the peritoneal cavity and may sometimes be partially concealed by the parietal line of attachment of the transverse mesocolon. Between the site of the duodenojejunal flexure and that of the ileocolic junction, the parietal line of attachment of the small-intestinal mesentery (see page 26) runs obliquely from above on the left to below on the right, passing across the lumbar portion of the spine, the large prevertebral blood vessels (aorta and inferior vena cava), the right psoas major and the right ureter. As the mesentery is only about 15 to 20 cm. in length at its parietal line of attachment, as compared with several meters (corresponding to the length of the intestine) along its intestinal attachment, it splays out toward the intestine like a fan. The mesentery, consisting of two layers of peritoneum, affords the intestinal coils a wide range of movement. The space between the two layers of peritoneum is filled with connective tissue and fat tissue, the latter varying greatly from one

individual to another; embedded in this tissue are blood and lymph vessels running between the intestine and the dorsal wall of the abdomen, as well as nerves and mesenteric lymph nodes.

The various *portions of the large intestine* (see page 54), describing a horseshoe-shaped arch, form a frame enclosing the convolutions of the small intestine. This frame, however, may be overlapped ventrally by the coils of the small intestine, particularly on the side of the descending colon. Similarly, depending on their filling and on their relationship with the pelvic organs, the coils of the small intestine may either bulge downward into the true pelvis or, alternatively, if the pelvic organs are greatly distended (*e.g.,* in pregnancy), may be displaced in a cranial direction.

Greatly varying in shape and highly mobile as far as its position is concerned, the *greater omentum*

hangs down apronlike from the greater curvature of the stomach (see page 23 and CIBA COLLECTION, Vol. 3/1, page 49) and spreads between the anterior abdominal wall and the coils of the small intestine.

The greater part of the coils of the jejunum lie upward to the left, while those forming the ileum are situated lower to the right. Since, owing to its mesentery, the small intestine is capable of considerable movement, its individual coils vary greatly in position even in one and the same subject, depending, *e.g.,* on the state of intestinal filling and peristalsis and on the position of the body, as can be observed under X-ray examination after oral introduction of a rubber tube. The only portion which, in line with its progressively shortened mesentery, has a more or less constant position is the terminal ileum, which passes from the left across the right psoas major to the site of the ileocolic junction (see page 51).

SMALL INTESTINE II

Structure

The freely mobile portion of the small intestine, which is attached to the mesentery, extends from the duodenojejunal flexure (see CIBA COLLECTION, Vol. 3/1, page 50) to the ileocolic orifice (Bauhin's valve), where the small intestine joins the large intestine (see page 51). This portion of the small intestine consists of the jejunum and the ileum. Between these two parts no distinct dividing line exists. They run imperceptibly into each other, the transition being marked by a gradual change in the diameter of the lumen and by various structural alterations, as pointed out below.

The walls of the jejunum and ileum, which are virtually identical in structure, consist, like the entire gastro-intestinal tract, of five coats—the *mucosa* (M.), *submucosa* (S.M.), *circular muscularis* (C.M.), *longitudinal muscularis* (L.M.) and *serosa* (S.). The innermost layer, the mucous membrane, is thickly plicated by macroscopically visible folds, circular or convoluted in shape and known as *circular* or *Kerckring's folds*. These folds vary in height, projecting into the lumen from 3 to 10 mm. Some of these plicae extend all the way around the internal circumference, some of them make only half or two thirds of the circle and still others spiral around twice or even more times. The circular folds of Kerckring, running in a transverse direction to the longitudinal axis of the lumen, have also been named valvulae conniventes ("closing valves"), though they can scarcely act in the sense of a true valve. Projecting into the lumen, they will slow down, to a certain extent, the progression of the luminal contents, but their essential function is certainly to increase the absorptive surface area. This principle is all the more obvious since the folds' surface is, furthermore, equipped with tiny fingerlike projections, the villi, the microscopic and ultramicroscopic structures of which are discussed below.

Below the epithelial surface of the mucosa, but participating in the formation of Kerckring's folds and the villi, lies the tunica (*lamina*) *propria,* which is a loose coat of predominantly reticular connective tissue, assuming, in parts, a lymphatic character. The tunica propria also contains thin fibers of smooth muscles radiating from the muscularis mucosae and extending upward to the tips of the villi, which, when these fibers are relaxed, have an even surface, whereas they become jagged or indented when the

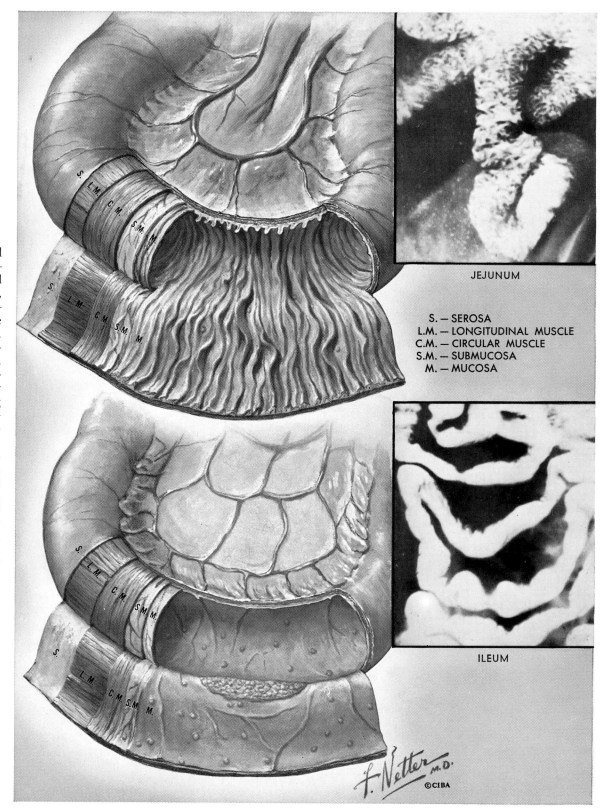

JEJUNUM

S. — SEROSA
L.M. — LONGITUDINAL MUSCLE
C.M. — CIRCULAR MUSCLE
S.M. — SUBMUCOSA
M. — MUCOSA

ILEUM

fibers contract (see upper right corner of Plate 3). The muscular fibrils are assumed to act as motors maintaining the pumping function of the villi. Situated in the tunica (*lamina*) *propria* and especially in the stroma of the villi are the terminal ramifications of the blood vessels, the *central lacteal* or chyliferous vessel of the villus (see Plate 4) and nerve fibers. Many solitary lymph nodes (see also below) are embedded in the tunica propria, which, at times, reach far into the submucosal layer.

The *muscularis mucosae,* which separates the mucous membrane from the submucosal coat, is composed of two thin nonstriated muscle layers, which keep the movable mucosal layer in place. The outer longitudinal layer is thinner than the inner circular layer, from which the muscular fibers in the core of the villi, mentioned above, emanate. The tunica submucosa is made up of collagen connective tissue, the

fibers of which form a network of lozenge-shaped meshes. By altering the angles of its meshes, this submucosal network is able to adapt itself to changes in the diameter and length of the intestinal lumen (peristalsis and pendular movements; see page 84). The submucosa contains a rich network of capillaries and larger vessels, numerous lymphatics and the submucous nerve plexus of Meissner (see page 78).

The *muscular layer* is built up of smooth muscle cells. The thick inner circular layer and the thinner outer longitudinal layer are connected by convoluted transitional fascicles in the area where they border on each other. Between the two layers is spread a network of nonmyelinated nerve fibers and ganglion cells, the myenteric plexus of Auerbach (see page 78).

The *serosa* is composed of a layer of flat, polygonal epithelia, and the subserosa of very loose connective

(Continued on page 49)

SMALL INTESTINE II
Structure

(Continued from page 48)

tissue. The serosal coat covers the entire circumference of the intestinal tube, except for a narrow strip at the posterior wall, where the visceral peritoneum connects with the two serous layers of the fan-shaped mesentery.

Though essentially built along the same principles, the jejunum and ileum differ in several respects. The lumen of the ileum is narrower and the diameter of the total wall is thinner than that of the jejunum. The average diameter of the jejunum measures 3 to 3.5 cm. and that of the ileum 2.5 cm. or less. Owing to this difference, the contents of the intestine show up more clearly through the ileum than through the jejunum, so that, when seen after opening the abdomen, the jejunum has a whitish-red hue, whereas the ileum, during life as well as after death, takes on a darker appearance. At variance, furthermore, are the frequency and height of the folds as well as of the villi. They become smaller and decrease in number as the small intestine continues. In the lower reaches of the ileum, the folds appear only here and there.

In the jejunum, lymphatic tissue is encountered only in the form of solitary nodules (*folliculi lymphatici solitarii*), which appear as pinhead-sized elevations on the surface of the mucosa. They become more numerous and more pronounced as they near the large intestine. In addition, aggregate nodules (*folliculi lymphatici aggregati* or Peyer's patches) occur, but these are exclusively confined to the ileum. They are invariably situated opposite the attachment of the mesentery and, generally, are of an elongated oval or ellipsoid shape, their longest diameter always coinciding with the longitudinal axis of the intestinal lumen. Their average width is 1 to 1½ cm., whereas they may vary in length from 2 cm. up to 10 or 12 cm. or, occasionally, even more. They differ in number from one individual to another, the average total fluctuating from 20 to 30.

Finally, another difference between the jejunum and ileum concerns the fat content of the respective mesentery. In the adult the ileac mesentery contains more fatty tissue and appears, thus, to be thicker than does that of the jejunum.

The entire mucosal surface of the small intestine, over and between the circular folds of Kerckring (see above), is covered with the *intestinal villi*, projections 0.5 to 1.5 mm. long (*i.e.*, just vis-

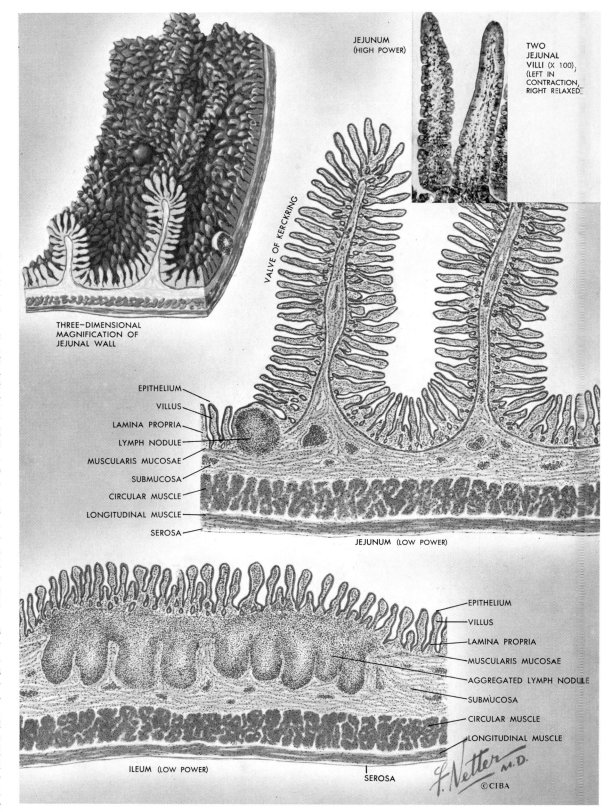

THREE–DIMENSIONAL MAGNIFICATION OF JEJUNAL WALL

JEJUNUM (HIGH POWER)

TWO JEJUNAL VILLI (X 100); (LEFT IN CONTRACTION, RIGHT RELAXED)

VALVE OF KERCKRING

EPITHELIUM
VILLUS
LAMINA PROPRIA
LYMPH NODULE
MUSCULARIS MUCOSAE
SUBMUCOSA
CIRCULAR MUSCLE
LONGITUDINAL MUSCLE
SEROSA

JEJUNUM (LOW POWER)

EPITHELIUM
VILLUS
LAMINA PROPRIA
MUSCULARIS MUCOSAE
AGGREGATED LYMPH NODULE
SUBMUCOSA
CIRCULAR MUSCLE
LONGITUDINAL MUSCLE
SEROSA

ILEUM (LOW POWER)

F. Netter M.D. ©CIBA

ible to the naked eye). The mass of these villi (estimated at 4 million altogether in the jejunum and ileum [Elze]) accounts for the velvetlike appearance of the mucosa. In the jejunum they are somewhat longer and broader than in the ileum. The valleys or indentations between the villi end up in nonramified pits, each of which harbors one or two tubular structures, the intestinal glands or *crypts of Lieberkühn*. The entire inner surface is covered by a single line of epithelial cells, the majority of which are cylindrical, *i.e.*, highly prismatic columnar cells bearing on their surface a well-developed cuticular border (see Plate 4). Between these columnar cells are interspersed three other types of cells, namely, the *goblet cells,* the *oxyphilic granular cells of Paneth* and the *argentaffine cells.* The goblet cells secrete an alkaline, mucous fluid which coats the whole mucosa. The majority of goblet cells are found in the crypts

or along the lower parts of the villi, but a considerable number of them are located also in the upper parts of the villi, where they seem to be squeezed in between the otherwise closely contiguous row of epithelial cells. The characteristic elements of the floor of the crypts are Paneth's cells, which, because of their staining qualities and the granules they contain, are also named "oxyphilic granular cells" (see upper right corner of Plate 4). They probably participate in enzyme production. A fourth type of cell is referred to as argentaffine or yellow cells (also cells of Schmidt or of Kultschitzky). They contain basal-staining granules with a high affinity for silver and chromium. Their habitat is, again, the fundi of Lieberkühn's crypts (see lower right corner of the plate on page 55).

As to the functional significance of these argentaf-
(Continued on page 50)

SMALL INTESTINE II
Structure

(Continued from page 49)

fine cells, opinions are still conflicting, but, since it has been shown that carcinoid tumors arise from them (see page 165), the evidence is strong for their having an endocrine rather than an exocrine function. They are, in all probability, the source of serotonin, the physiologic rôle of which still remains to be established.

Within the tunica propria a great variety of cells are found, most of them originating from reticular cells which have a marked capacity for differentiation. Besides the usual connective tissue cells, numerous lymphocytes and plasma cells are present. The lymphocytes show a marked tendency to migrate through the epithelium toward the lumen.

The principal task of the gastro-intestinal tract is to serve as an organ which supplies the body with substances adequate to satisfy its caloric requirements and elementary material. The tract in toto, from the mouth to the large intestine, is, therefore, equipped with a variety of structures, such as the gland and the muscular apparatus, which are specifically suitable to prepare and transform the life-sustaining matter, *i.e.*, the foodstuffs, for their admission by the organism. The structure that takes care of this admission, *i.e.*, of the absorption, is the long row of epithelial cells which coat the inner surface of the small intestine. These epithelial cells, together with the villi which they cover, should be considered THE organ of absorption. More intimate knowledge about the structure of the columnar cells investing the villi has been obtained only within the last two decades by means of ultramicroscopic studies, *i.e.*, by phase microscopy and, particularly, by electron microscopy. The latter disclosed that the long-known (Koelliker, 1885) striated or cuticular border, with which the luminal surface of the epithelial cells is equipped, consists of an exceedingly great number of extremely fine projecting rods, called *microvilli* (Granger and Baker; Dalton; Dalton *et al.*; Palay and Karlin). It has been calculated that each epithelial cell is provided with about 1000 microvilli, which increase the cellular surface approximately twenty-four times. The microvilli seem to vary only little in size (average length 1 micron, width 0.07 micron) and appear, when visualized in a transverse cross section, to be set in a hexagonal array. Covered by a continuation of the cell membrane, they contain, in the core, fine fibrils which are con-

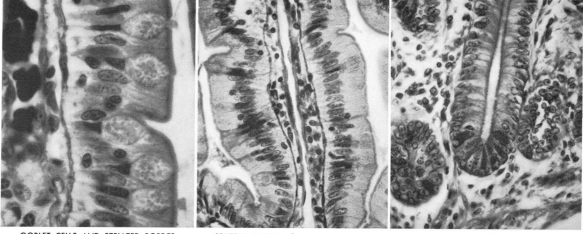

GOBLET CELLS AND STRIATED BORDER
OF HUMAN JEJUNAL VILLUS
(AZAN STAIN, X 650)

CENTRAL LACTEAL (CHYLIFEROUS VESSEL)
IN HUMAN JEJUNAL VILLUS
(AZAN STAIN, X 325)

FLOOR OF CRYPT OF LIEBERKÜHN WITH
GRANULATED, OXYPHILIC CELLS OF PANETH
(HEMATOXYLIN-EOSIN, X 325)

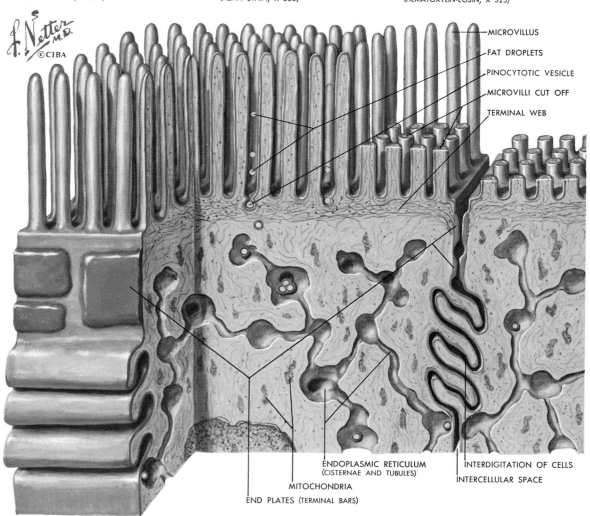

MICROVILLUS
FAT DROPLETS
PINOCYTOTIC VESICLE
MICROVILLI CUT OFF
TERMINAL WEB

ENDOPLASMIC RETICULUM
(CISTERNAE AND TUBULES)
MITOCHONDRIA
END PLATES (TERMINAL BARS)
INTERDIGITATION OF CELLS
INTERCELLULAR SPACE

THREE-DIMENSIONAL SCHEMA OF STRIATED BORDER OF INTESTINAL EPITHELIAL CELLS (BASED ON ULTRAMICROSCOPIC STUDIES)

nected with the network of fibrils, termed *"terminal web"*, just beneath the striated border.

At some time after the ingestion of a fat meal (in the mouse, about 20 minutes after administration of corn oil; Palay and Karlin), fine lipid droplets have been observed in the intermicrovillous spaces; slightly later the droplets appear in the area of the terminal web, where they accumulate in minute vesicles, which owe their existence to a *pinocytotic activity,* probably of the intermicrovillous plasma membrane. The droplets then seem to proceed and can be found in the main body of the epithelial cell, where they coalesce to larger units in vesicles or cisternae, which are connected with each other by intracellular tubules. This system of cisternae and tubules is termed the *endoplasmic reticulum.* Through this reticulum the fat droplets pass toward the lateral cell surfaces. From the intercellular spaces the droplets traverse the base-

ment membrane and the interstitial spaces of the lamina propria to enter the central lacteals (see above) of the villi.

The nucleus, the mitochondria and the other organelles of the cell body show no particular or specific features. The lateral surfaces of the epithelial cells are characterized by the fact that they are not smooth and even. In the region below the microvilli and the terminal web, the profile of the lateral surfaces is irregular, because *end plates,* the terminal bars (recognized even by light microscopy), project outward, probably as a result of variations in the thickness of the cell membrane. Farther toward the base of each cell, the membrane is plicated or undulated, by which means the adjacent cells become interdigitated, remindful in a way — transferring the ultramicroscopic aspect into macroscopic dimensions — of the sutura serrata of the bones of the skull.

ILEOCOLIC ARTERY
COLIC BRANCH
ILEAL BRANCH
SUPERIOR MESENTERIC ARTERY
POSTERIOR CECAL ARTERY
APPENDICULAR ARTERY
ANTERIOR CECAL ARTERY
ILEOCOLIC FOLD
(SUPERIOR ILEOCECAL FOLD)
ILEOCOLIC FOSSA
(SUPERIOR ILEOCECAL FOSSA)
ILEOCECAL FOLD
(INFERIOR ILEOCECAL FOLD;
BLOODLESS FOLD OF TREVES)
ILEOCECAL FOSSA
(INFERIOR ILEOCECAL FOSSA)
MESO-APPENDIX
APPENDICULAR ARTERY

RETROCECAL FOSSA
RETROCECAL FOLDS
RETROCOLIC FOLD (COLIC FOLD)
RIGHT PARACOLIC GUTTER

ANTERIOR
(FREE)
TAENIA
(TAENIA
LIBERA)
APPENDICULAR
ARTERY
DORSOMEDIAL
(MESOCOLIC)
TAENIA
DORSOLATERAL
(OMENTAL)
TAENIA
POSTERIOR CECAL ARTERY
RETROCECAL FOLDS
RETROCECAL FOSSA

SOME VARIATIONS IN POSTERIOR PERITONEAL ATTACHMENT OF CECUM

ATTACHED AREA — LINE OF POSTERIOR PERITONEAL REFLECTION
ATTACHED AREA — LINE OF POSTERIOR PERITONEAL REFLECTION
ATTACHED AREA — LINE OF POSTERIOR PERITONEAL REFLECTION
ATTACHED AREA — LINE OF POSTERIOR PERITONEAL REFLECTION

ILEOCECAL REGION

The most caudal portion of the small intestine, the terminal ileum, lying in the pelvis over the right iliac fossa, opens, coming sideways from the left, into the medial wall of the large intestine. The section of the latter, caudally or below this junction, is a blind sac and, hence, is designated as a blind gut or *cecum*. The part of the large intestine above the junction constitutes the beginning of the colon and continues upward, or in a cranial direction, as the *ascending colon*. Strictly speaking, the ileum thus opens neither into the cecum, as implied by the term "ileocecal orifice", nor into the colon, as inferred by the designation "ileocolic orifice" but between these two portions of the large intestine. Projected to the anterior abdominal wall, the orifice, *i.e.*, the entry of the ileum into the large intestine, though subject to wide variation, lies commonly at a point where the line of Monro, connecting the anterior superior iliac spine with the umbilicus, crosses the lateral edge of the rectus abdominis muscle (McBurney's point) (see also page 53). The cecum, the widest portion of the large intestine, lies in the right iliac fossa and rests on the iliac muscle. If abnormally large, it may extend downward, overlapping the psoas major and even reaching beyond the margin of the latter into the true pelvis. When empty, the cecum is usually overlapped by coils of the small intestine and, depending on its size and position, by the greater omentum, whereas when full, and especially when distended with intestinal gases, it bulges anteriorly into contact with the anterior abdominal wall, yielding a distinct tympanitic note when percussed. When the cecum is neither particularly large nor particularly full, it does not reach as far as the depression running along and posterior to the inguinal ligament, into which loops of the small intestine usually protrude. The medial circumference of the cecum is in contact

with the terminal ileum, which hangs into the pelvis.

Where the ileum joins the large intestine, a peritoneal fold extends in almost all individuals from the terminal part of the ileal mesentery across the front of the ileum to the cecum and lowermost part of the ascending colon. This fold is variously known as the *"ileocolic fold"* or as the *"superior ileocecal fold"*. It contains the anterior cecal artery (see page 67), and it forms the anterior wall of a fossa, correspondingly termed the *"ileocolic"* or *"superior ileocecal fossa"*. The posterior wall of this fossa is made up of the terminal ileum and its mesentery. Its mouth opens downward and somewhat to the left. Commonly, another fold, known as *"ileocecal"* or *"inferior ileocecal fold"*, is encountered in front of the meso-appendix, extending from the lower or right side of the terminal ileum to the cecum. Together with the meso-appendix as the posterior wall, the fold again forms

a fossa, the *ileocecal* or *inferior ileocecal fossa,* of which the fold represents the anterior wall. The ileocecal fold contains no important vessel and has, therefore, been named the *"bloodless fold of Treves"*.

The third peritoneal extension, the *meso-appendix* or appendicular mesenteriolum, serves as the mesentery of the vermiform appendix. It stretches from the posterior leaf of the mesentery of the terminal ileum and behind the latter (to which it is usually attached) to the left side of the cecum and to the entire length of the appendix, which it enwraps. It thus assumes a triangular shape, and it transmits between its two layers the appendicular artery or one of its numerous variations (see page 66).

In some individuals one or more thin peritoneal folds spread from the parietal peritoneum of the posterolateral abdominal wall to the lateral (right) side

(Continued on page 52)

LABIAL FORM OF
ILEOCECAL SPHINCTER
AS SEEN COMMONLY POST MORTEM
AND OCCASIONALLY IN VIVO

ILEOCECAL REGION

(*Continued from page 51*)

FRENULUM

PAPILLARY FORM OF
ILEOCECAL SPHINCTER
AS FOUND MOST COMMONLY
IN THE LIVING SUBJECT

of the cecum or ascending colon. They are known as *retrocecal* and *retrocolic folds,* respectively, and create, between and below them, small shallow recesses or fossae which are, only in rare instances, large enough to admit loops of the small intestine. Their apertures are normally too wide to permit the formation of an internal hernia (see page 218).

The degree of mobility of the cecum depends upon the level at which the posterior part of its visceral peritoneum is reflected to the parietal peritoneum of the posterior abdominal wall. This level and also the contour of the reflection vary considerably. Occasionally, the *peritoneum may turn so low* that the cecum, as well as the terminal ileum, is firmly fused to the posterior abdominal wall. In other instances the *reflection occurs high up* from the surface of the ascending colon, so that the entire cecum, including parts of the colon, is surrounded on all sides by visceral peritoneum. In the majority of cases, the reflection lies between these two extremes. The line of reflection may be straight, convex or concave, or it may incline downward to the right or left or may be characterized by a narrow downward prolongation forming a sort of mesocecum.

At the junction the terminal ileum, as if thrust with all its coverings (except for the serosa) into the wall, invaginates the large intestine, creating within the lumen of the latter what has been known as the *ileocolic valve* (valvula Bauhini). When this sphincter is exposed in the dead body, the ileal aperture, in some 60 per cent of the cases (Di Dio), is bounded by two approximately horizontal folds referred to as the upper and lower lips of the valve, respectively. At both ends of the lips, where they seem to coalesce, two mucosal ridges extend horizontally in the lumen of the large intestine, resembling the crescent-shaped folds of the colon (see page 55). These ridges, known

CIRCULAR MUSCLE OF COLON
DORSOMEDIAL TAENIA OF COLON
FIBERS TO PAPILLA
FIBERS TO ILEUM
FIBERS AROUND MARGINS OF
ILEOCECAL JUNCTION
FIBERS TO TAENIA } LONGITUDINAL
FIBERS TO PAPILLA } MUSCLE
                    OF ILEUM
CIRCULAR MUSCLE OF ILEUM

SCHEMA OF MUSCULATURE AT ILEOCECAL SPHINCTER (AFTER DI DIO)

as the frenula of the valve, form the dividing line between the cecum and the colon ascendens. In vivo, as recently demonstrated very impressively (Di Dio), the ileum protrudes into the large intestine in the form of a round *papilla,* the lumen of which assumes a starlike aspect when closed. The appearance of this papilla has been compared to the appearance of the cervix uteri projecting into the vagina. In view of the bilabial aspect of the orifice in the cadaver, it was thought that this structure acted as a "flap valve", but recent studies (Di Dio) indicate that it is more likely to act like a true sphincter (see also page 85) which is under neural and/or hormonal control. The arrangement of the ceco-ileal musculature supports the concept of a true sphincter. Some fibers from the mesocolic (dorsomedial) taenia, descending from the colon and cecum to the appendix, turn inward and pass into the ileocolic papilla, while others turn out-

ward to become continuous with the longitudinal muscle of the ileum. Still others pass elliptically around the margins of the papilla and continue within the taenia. The longitudinal muscle of the ileum likewise takes divergent courses, some fibers passing into the papilla, others joining fibers of the taenia. The circular muscle fibers of the ileum and large intestine circle around the papilla, the latter surrounding the former. The two circular layers enclose the longitudinal fibers deriving from the taenia, except in the region close to the ostium, where the two circular layers meet. Both circular layers are considerably thicker at the base of the papilla and somewhat thicker at its free end, so that one obtains the impression that a double sphincter exists. It is hypothesized that the circular muscle layer — much the stronger — closes the sphincter, whereas the longitudinal muscle layer opens it.

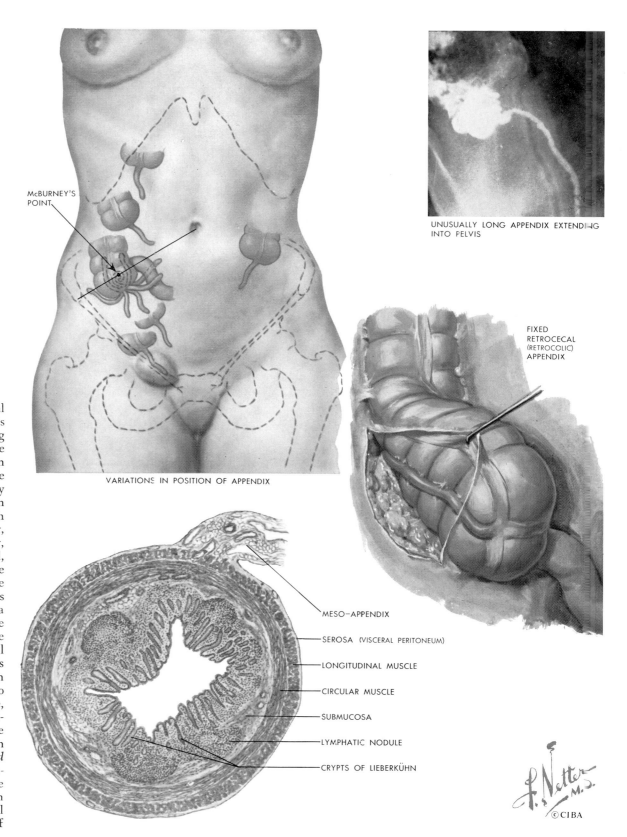

McBURNEY'S POINT

VARIATIONS IN POSITION OF APPENDIX

UNUSUALLY LONG APPENDIX EXTENDING INTO PELVIS

FIXED RETROCECAL (RETROCOLIC) APPENDIX

MESO-APPENDIX

SEROSA (VISCERAL PERITONEUM)

LONGITUDINAL MUSCLE

CIRCULAR MUSCLE

SUBMUCOSA

LYMPHATIC NODULE

CRYPTS OF LIEBERKÜHN

APPENDIX VERMIFORMIS

A structure of considerable clinical significance, the vermiform appendix is part of the cecum. Its surface marking lies on the transition of the outer to the middle third of an imaginary line drawn from the anterosuperior iliac spine to the umbilicus (*McBurney's point*). In early fetal life the cecum extends caudally in the form of a cone, the tip of which grows more in length than in diameter, thus creating a vermiform process. Later, during embryologic development and, again, as a result of a difference in the speed of growth of the cecal walls, the point where the appendix arises shifts from the distal end of the blind sac to a site on the dorsomedial wall, where the three taeniae of the large intestine merge into one uniform coat of longitudinal muscle. In man and apes the appendix is a rather rudimentary, narrow and thin (from 2.5 to 25 cm. long; average 6 to 9 cm.) offshoot of the large intestine, which has no intestinal function (in contrast to the processus vermiformis of some birds and mammals in which it may attain considerable length). The *course and position of the appendix differ* individually and change also in one and the same individual, depending essentially upon the length and width of the peritoneal fold, which represents the mesentery of the appendix.

This peritoneal fold, known as the mesenteriolum, has been described in connection with other peritoneal recesses in the same region (see page 51). The mesenteriolum permits the high degree of mobility characteristic of the appendix, which, as a rule, hangs downward for a varying distance into the true pelvis and may actually come into contact with the pelvic organs, *e.g.,* with the uterus or its adnexa or with the bladder. Sometimes the appendix can be found within the sac of an indirect inguinal hernia (see page 214) or involved in a direct inguinal hernia. The appendix may also turn upward and extend behind or in front of the cecum or ileum. The appendix may have wandered into the retro-

cecal fossa and be capable of emerging again, in contrast to a so-called *"fixed" retrocecal appendix* (see also page 148). This fixation may have taken place as a result of inflammatory adhesions, or the appendix may have been trapped in the retrocecal position during fetal life at a time when the ascending colon fuses to the posterior abdominal wall (see pages 5 and 6). Such a posteriorly fixed appendix may, in fact, extend high enough behind the gut so as to be more properly called "retrocolic" rather than retrocecal.

The layers composing the wall of the appendix are the same as those in other parts of the intestinal tract. The tube is enwrapped by *visceral peritoneum,* except for a narrow line between the attachment of the two layers of the mesenteriolum. The *longitudinal muscle* invests the entire circumference. The *circular muscle* layer is well developed along the entire length of the appendix, though it may occasionally be defi-

cient in one or two small regions, where the submucosal tissue becomes contingent with the serous coat. The *submucous layer* is endowed with masses of lympho-epithelial tissue, the abundance of which is characteristic of the appendix and explains why the appendix has been termed "the intestinal tonsil". The structure of the *mucosa* is essentially the same as in the large intestine, except for a relative paucity of glandular elements. Occasionally, Paneth's cells can be found within the epithelium of the pits. The occurrence of yellow basal granular (argentaffine) cells explains the frequency of carcinoid tumors in the appendix (see pages 148 and 165).

The appendix can be *visualized in X-ray* studies about 24 hours after the ingestion of barium. It usually fills uniformly, but the appearance of segments is not to be interpreted as an expression of a pathologic process.

COLON

Topography and Relations

The large intestine varies extraordinarily in caliber, depending on its functional state. Moreover, since the haustra form sacculations separated by constricting furrows, the lumen bulges and contracts alternately (see page 55). The caliber is greatest at the commencement of the large intestine (cecum) (see page 52) and narrows toward the rectum. Viewed as a whole, the various parts of the large intestine describe an arch in the shape of a horseshoe. The total length of the large intestine is approximately 120 to 150 cm. Of the four segments of the colon, known as the ascending, transverse, descending and sigmoid (pelvic) colon, the ascending and descending colon are situated retroperitoneally and the transverse and sigmoid colon intraperitoneally.

The *ascending colon* averages about 15 to 20 cm. in length and runs in a more or less straight course from the upper lip of the ileocolic valve to the right colic (or hepatic) flexure, where it passes into the transverse colon. Starting in the right iliac fossa and after crossing the iliac crest, it lies in the angle between the psoas major and the quadratus lumborum and transversus abdominis muscles. The right colic flexure, responsible for the so-called colic impression on the undersurface of the right lobe of the liver (see CIBA COLLECTION, Vol. 3/III, page 5), lies anterior to the caudal portion of the right kidney, the two organs being linked together by loose connective tissue. The proximal portion of the transverse colon is furthermore related to the descending part of the duodenum as it turns leftward losing its direct connection with the medial surface of the right kidney (see CIBA COLLECTION, Vol. 3/I, page 50). To what extent the ascending colon enters into contact with the anterior abdominal wall depends upon its filling or upon the degree to which it is overlapped by the convolutions of the small intestine.

The *transverse colon*, varying from 30 to 60 cm. in length, extends from the hepatic (right) flexure to the slightly more cranially situated left colic (or splenic) flexure. It lies intraperitoneally and thus is attached to the posterior abdominal wall by a peritoneal fold (mesentery), the transverse mesocolon, which is very short in the region of the flexures and longest in the middle of the transverse colon. When its longitudinal musculature is contracted, the transverse colon ascends from left to right, forming a ventrally convex arch which, when

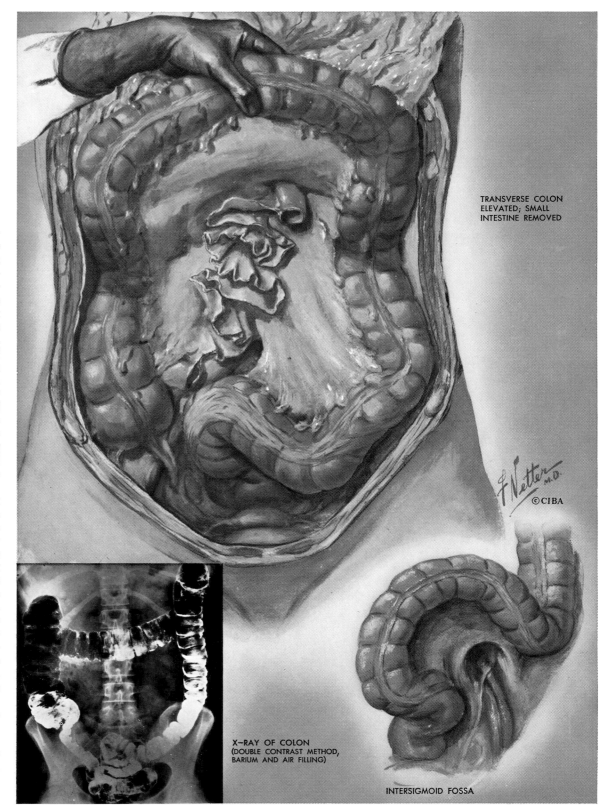

TRANSVERSE COLON
ELEVATED; SMALL
INTESTINE REMOVED

X-RAY OF COLON
(DOUBLE CONTRAST METHOD,
BARIUM AND AIR FILLING)

INTERSIGMOID FOSSA

seen in anterior-posterior projection, appears more or less straight. As its mesentery is longest in the middle, affording the colon a considerable range of movement in this area, a long transverse colon, especially when its longitudinal musculature is relaxed, may sag down some distance toward the pelvis like a U-shaped tube. Viewed from left to right, the parietal line of attachment of the transverse mesocolon crosses first the descending part of the duodenum, then the pancreas and, finally, the left kidney. At the lateral edge of the kidney near the lower pole of the spleen is situated the left (or splenic) flexure of the colon. The posterior surface of the greater omentum adheres to the upper surface of the transverse mesocolon and to the serosal coating on the anterior side of the transverse colon. Whereas in its middle part the transverse colon is covered only by the double fold of the omentum descending from the stomach and otherwise

lies directly adjacent to the anterior abdominal wall, it is overlapped to a greater or lesser degree, depending on the filling and position of the various organs, by the liver and gallbladder on the right and by the stomach and spleen on the left.

The retroperitoneal *descending colon,* some 20 to 25 cm. in length, extends downward from the left colic flexure to the iliac crest or beyond it into the left iliac fossa. After running first in the angle between the lateral edge of the kidney and the quadratus lumborum muscle and then over the iliac muscle, it finally passes in front of the psoas major, crossing the femoral and genitofemoral nerves, and continues with no sharp dividing line into the pelvic (sigmoid) colon, at which point the colon becomes intraperitoneal again. On its anterior surface the descending colon is overlapped by the greater omentum and generally by coils of the small intestine.

STRUCTURE OF COLON

Corresponding to the structure of the entire intestinal tract, the wall of the colon and cecum consists of a mucosa, a submucosa, a double-layered muscularis and—depending on its relationship with the peritoneum—a serosa and subserosa or adventitia. The external aspect of the colon, however, differs from that of the small intestine not only because of its greater caliber but also because of the appearance of three typical formations: (1) the three taeniae, (2) the haustra and (3) the appendices epiploicae.

The three *taeniae* are longitudinal bands, approximately 8 mm. in width, running along the total length of the colon, which owe their existence to the fact that the outer muscle layer, *i.e.*, the longitudinal musculature, does not constitute a uniform coat. In the region of these three bands, the longitudinal musculature is conspicuous by its thickness, whereas in the spaces between them it consists merely of a very thin coating. Each of the taeniae is named by reference to its topographical situation in relation to the transverse colon. One, the taenia mesocolica, is situated dorsal to the transverse colon at the line of attachment of the transverse mesocolon and comes to lie dorsomedially on the ascending and descending colon. The second taenia, named taenia omentalis because it is related to the line of attachment of the greater omentum on the ventrocranial surface of the transverse colon, runs along the dorsolateral aspect of the ascending and descending portions. The third taenia, called taenia libera because it is free, *i.e.*, not related to any mesenteric or omental attachment, is generally found on the caudal (inferior) surface of the transverse and on the anterior aspect of the ascending and descending colon. Where the appendix joins the cecum (see page 51) and also where the sigmoid passes into the rectum (see page 60), the three taeniae merge into one uniform muscular coat, which, however, in the proximal rectum, is more strongly developed in its anterior and posterior parts than it is laterally. Generally, the posterolateral and anterior taeniae coalesce into a broad longitudinal band in the region of the middle and lower sigmoid.

The *haustra* are more or less prominent sacculations formed in the spaces between the taeniae. They are separated from each other by constricting circular furrows of varying depth. The degree of their prominence depends on contraction

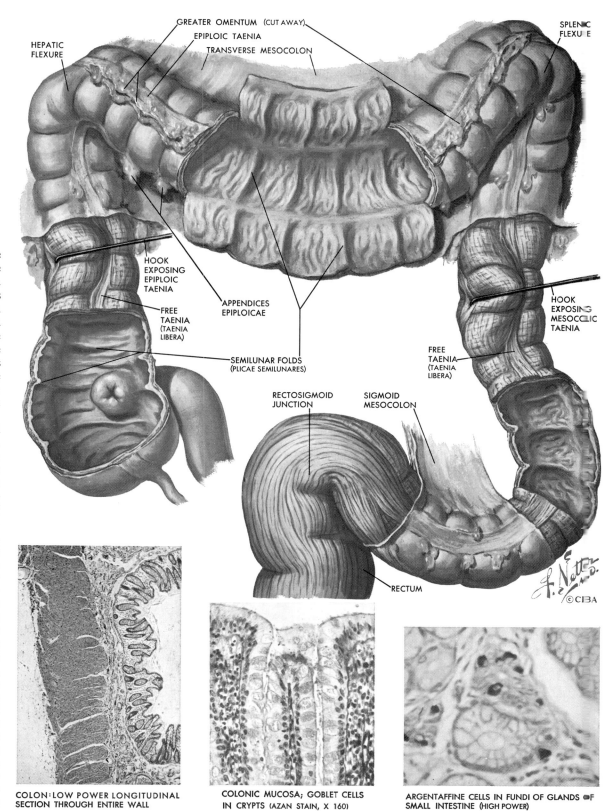

COLON: LOW POWER LONGITUDINAL SECTION THROUGH ENTIRE WALL

COLONIC MUCOSA; GOBLET CELLS IN CRYPTS (AZAN STAIN, X 160)

ARGENTAFFINE CELLS IN FUNDI OF GLANDS OF SMALL INTESTINE (HIGH POWER)

of the taeniae; the more the latter contract, the more marked the haustration of the large intestine becomes, whereas it is almost completely absent when the taeniae are totally relaxed.

The third structural characteristic, the *appendices epiploicae,* consist of subserous pockets filled with fat, shaped like grapes and varying in size according to the individual's state of nutrition. On the ascending and descending colon, they are generally distributed in two rows, whereas on the transverse colon they form only one row along the line of the taenia libera.

Corresponding to the furrows between the haustra visible on the outer surface, the mucous membrane of the large intestine forms crescent-shaped transverse folds, known as the *plicae semilunares*. As a rule, the length of these folds corresponds to the distance between two taeniae, although sometimes they may be somewhat longer. Whereas Kerckring's folds in

the small intestine (see page 49) consist merely of mucosa and submucosa, the plicae semilunares also include the circular muscle layer.

In contrast to the small intestine, the mucosa of the large intestine is not covered with villous projections but contains deep tubular pits, which increase in depth toward the rectum and extend as far as the muscularis mucosae. In the submucosa, besides the usual structures (blood vessels, lymphatics, Messner's submucosal plexus), numerous solitary lymphatic nodules are located, originating in the reticular tissue of the tunica propria and penetrating through the muscularis mucosae into the submucosa.

The mucosal epithelium of the large intestine comprises one layer built up of tall prismatic cells, which when fixed in a fresh state display a cuticular border on their surface. Goblet cells are very numerous, especially at the base of the pits.

SIGMOID COLON

The exact point of commencement of the *sigmoid colon, i.e.,* the transition from descending colon to sigmoid colon, is indefinite. The sigmoid is generally considered to be that part of the large bowel between the descending colon and the rectum, which, as a result of its attachment to a mesentery (see below), is freely movable. Since (as shown by Anson and others) this mesentery is subject to great variations, the extent of the sigmoid also becomes variable. It has been described as beginning anywhere between the left iliac crest and the margin of the left psoas muscle or brim of the pelvis minor (true pelvis). Other authorities regard the sigmoid colon as comprising the iliac colon (an iliac portion which has no mesentery) and the pelvic portion (pelvic colon) with a mesentery commencing at the brim of the pelvis minor. The "mesenteriolized" sigmoid colon assumes, as a rule, an omega-shaped flexure arching over the pelvic inlet toward the first or second sacral vertebra or toward the right side of the pelvis. It finally joins the rectum at an acute angle at the level of approximately the third sacral vertebra. This *typical shape* of the sigmoid is, however, not a constant finding. The *sigmoid* may be *short,* in which case it will run straight and *obliquely* into the pelvis, or it may be so long that the *loop extends far to the right* or, in an extreme case, *high into the abdomen.* Its average length is about 40 cm. in adults and 18 cm. in children. With the variations, as mentioned, it may reach 84 cm. (and even more). The root of its mesentery, *i.e.,* of the mesosigmoid, is variable but, characteristically, starts in the upper left iliac

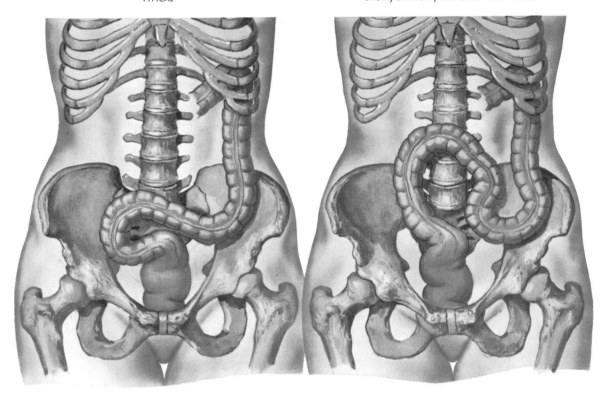

TYPICAL

SHORT, STRAIGHT, OBLIQUELY INTO PELVIS

LOOPING TO RIGHT SIDE

ASCENDING HIGH INTO ABDOMEN

fossa, proceeds downward a few inches, then mesially and again upward to a point on the psoas muscle a little to the left of the fourth lumbar vertebra, whence it turns downward into the pelvis. The line of mesenteric attachment takes the shape of an irregular and blunt inverted "V". Turning caudally after having reached its highest point, the attachment line of the mesosigmoid crosses over the left common iliac artery and vein (see page 66) just above the division of the artery. The length of the mesosigmoid, *i.e.,* the distance from its root to the bowel wall, is extremely variable. A small peritoneal fossa — the intersigmoid fossa or recess (see page 54) — is formed by the mesosigmoid while twisting around the vascular pedicle, which, however, is only very rarely the cause of a retroperitoneal hernia. It is, nevertheless, a valuable guide to the vascular stalk. The left ureter passes retroperitoneally behind the intersigmoid recess.

The mucosa and submucosa of the sigmoid colon are practically identical with the corresponding structures of other parts of the colon (see page 55). The same holds true for the arrangement of the circular and longitudinal muscle layers, except for the most distal parts of the sigmoid colon, where the three flat longitudinal muscle bands, typical of the large intestine, spread out to form a completely encircling longitudinal muscle layer at the rectosigmoid junction. In the same region the circular layer thickens, in some instances to such an extent that its prominence is alluded to as the sphincteric muscle of the junction ("third sphincter of O'Beirne"). It is questionable, however, whether this thickening has a true sphincter function.

Throughout the course of the sigmoid colon, the appendices epiploicae of the serous coat diminish gradually in number and size.

RECTUM AND ANAL CANAL

The terminal part of the intestines comprises the *rectum* and the *anal canal,* which derive embryologically from quite different anlagen (see pages 4 and 8). The rectum extends from the *recto-sigmoid junction,* at the level of the third sacral vertebra, 10 to 15 cm. downward to the anorectal line (see below). The peritoneal coat continues down from the sigmoid, but only over the anterior and lateral rectal walls, for 1 to 2 cm. A very small mesorectum may occasionally be present but only close to the rectosigmoid junction. The rectum is thus generally a truly retroperitoneal organ. From the upper anterior rectal surface, the peritoneum is reflected into the interval between the rectum and the bladder in the male, or rectum and uterus in the female, forming the *rectovesical* or *recto-uterine* recess or *pouch,* respectively. The depth to which these reflections extend varies. The average distance from the anus to these peritoneal sacs is 7 cm. in the male and 4 cm. in the female. Laterally, the peritoneum is reflected from the rectum to the sacral wall and to the pararectal fossae (see page 28).

The small segment of the rectum covered by peritoneum is sometimes referred to as part of the sigmoid or "pelvic" colon (see page 56). From the functional point of view, a division into an ampullary and a sphincteric portion of the rectum seems to be more appropriate. The former, although presenting itself, when empty, as a more or less transverse slit, varies in size and form at different times in the same individual, essentially depending on its state of fullness and on the intra-abdominal pressure. It may be pear- or balloon-shaped or tubelike. With a circumference of approximately 15 cm. at the rectosigmoid junction and of 35 cm. or more at its widest part, the rectum narrows at the level where it passes through the pelvic diaphragm, *i.e.,* at the anorectal muscle ring, roughly opposite the middle of the prostate in the male or the middle of the vagina in the female. The length of the rectum is subject, as is the diameter, to great variation. The rectum in women, *e.g.,* is, on the average, much smaller than in men. The axis of the ampullary portion of the rectum conforms, in general, to the sacral curve. Its posterior wall hugs the anterior aspect from the sacrum to the sacrococcygeal articulation, where it comes to lie more or less horizontally over the *levator shelf.* The anterior wall is comparatively straight and follows closely a line parallel to the posterocephalic axis of the vagina in the female or the rectogenital septum in the male. In any event, the rectum is anything but straight (the Latin term rectus [straight] derives from the early anatomists' experience in dissecting mammals that do not walk upright).

The rectal ampullary portion usually

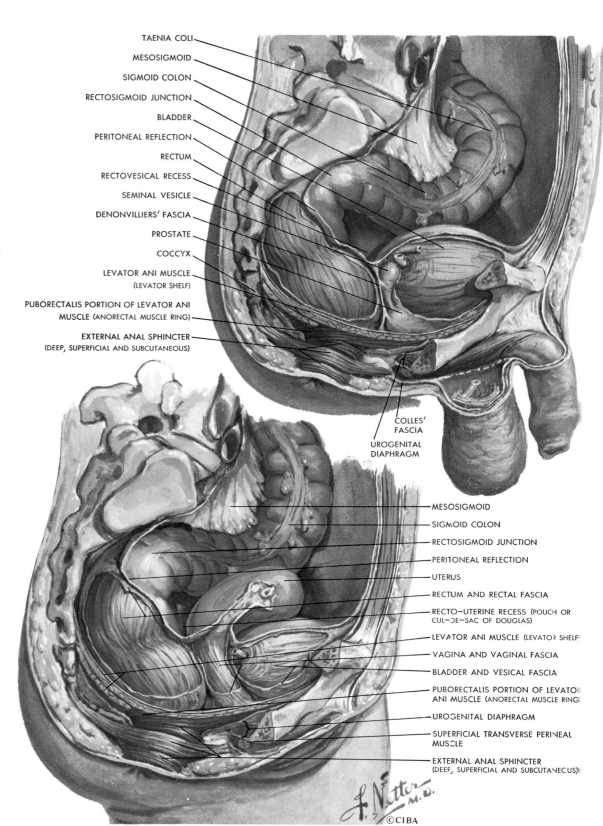

TAENIA COLI
MESOSIGMOID
SIGMOID COLON
RECTOSIGMOID JUNCTION
BLADDER
PERITONEAL REFLECTION
RECTUM
RECTOVESICAL RECESS
SEMINAL VESICLE
DENONVILLIERS' FASCIA
PROSTATE
COCCYX
LEVATOR ANI MUSCLE
(LEVATOR SHELF)
PUBORECTALIS PORTION OF LEVATOR ANI
MUSCLE (ANORECTAL MUSCLE RING)
EXTERNAL ANAL SPHINCTER
(DEEP, SUPERFICIAL AND SUBCUTANEOUS)

COLLES'
FASCIA
UROGENITAL
DIAPHRAGM

MESOSIGMOID
SIGMOID COLON
RECTOSIGMOID JUNCTION
PERITONEAL REFLECTION
UTERUS
RECTUM AND RECTAL FASCIA
RECTO-UTERINE RECESS (POUCH OR
CUL-DE-SAC OF DOUGLAS)
LEVATOR ANI MUSCLE (LEVATOR SHELF)
VAGINA AND VAGINAL FASCIA
BLADDER AND VESICAL FASCIA
PUBORECTALIS PORTION OF LEVATOR
ANI MUSCLE (ANORECTAL MUSCLE RING)
UROGENITAL DIAPHRAGM
SUPERFICIAL TRANSVERSE PERINEAL
MUSCLE
EXTERNAL ANAL SPHINCTER
(DEEP, SUPERFICIAL AND SUBCUTANEOUS)

presents three frequently quite prominent lateral curvatures or flexures. Of these, the middle one bulges to the left, the upper and lower to the right. All three bends correspond to the indentations on the opposite side of the internal rectal wall, which are produced by crescentlike plications of the mucosa and submucosa, including also the circular musculature but not the longitudinal. These more or less marked folds, known as *rectal valves,* encircle about one third to one half of the rectal circumference. The *superior* and *inferior rectal valves* are located on the left side, the former about 4 cm. below the rectosigmoid junction and the latter about 2 to 3 cm. above the dentate line (see below) at a site where the ampullary rectal portion begins to narrow. The middle rectal valve lies, usually, on the right side at or slightly above the level of the peritoneal reflection, *i.e.,* about 6 to 7 cm. above the dentate line. It is worth noting that this

distance is about the limit to which a probing finger may reach in rectal digital examination. In most instances this middle one is the largest of all three valves, but their size varies individually, as does their number. One or two additional folds or valves may be encountered, or only two may be present.

The sphincteric portion of the rectum, often considered to be the upper third of the *surgical anal canal* (Milligan, Morgan), begins at the clinically palpable upper edge of the anorectal muscle ring (see page 60), usually about 4 to 6 cm. above the anal verge, where the rectum narrows considerably. It extends down to the *anatomic anorectal line (dentate line, pectinate line,* linea sinuosa), an irregular or undulating demarcation in the rectal mucosa about 2 to 3 cm. above the anal verge. It has been assumed that this line marks the junction of the endodermal primitive

(Continued on page 58)

RECTUM AND ANAL CANAL

(Continued from page 57)

gut with the ectodermal proctodeum; histologic evidence, however, has since disclosed that this transition of the two fetal structures is not abrupt but spreads gradually over several centimeters (see below). Nevertheless, the dentate line is visually recognizable, encircling the bowel, presenting from 6 to 12 cranial extensions and an equal number of intervening caudal sinuosities. The cranial extensions of the dentate line are generally related to and overlie columnlike bulges in the rectal (anal) mucosa, known as *"rectal columns"* or *"columns of Morgagni"*. These stretch from 2 to 3 cm. upward and blend insensibly, at their most cranial point, into the level of the surrounding mucosa. They contain a richer lymphatic and vascular bed than does the intervening tissue. The valley-like depressions between the rectal columns are the *"rectal sinuses"* or *"sinuses of Morgagni"*.

At their lower extremities (*i.e.*, at the dentate line), the rectal columns are joined together by mucosal folds, the *"anal valves"*, also named *"semilunar valves"* because of the concavity of their free upper margins. (These anal valves should not be confused with the rectal valves [see above].) Most, but not all, of the rectal sinuses extend caudad, external to the anal valves to form pockets, designated as *"anal crypts"* or referred to as "anal pockets", "anal sinuses", "crypts of Morgagni" and "saccules of Horner", which may be 1 cm. or more deep. Their mouths open cranially into the rectal sinuses, and their luminal walls are formed by the anal valves. In the depths of the anal crypts, the ducts of *peri-anal glands* (see below) may open.

The dentate line projects cranially a variable distance correlative to the rectal columns. These projections may be 1 to 1.5 cm. long, and the peninsulas of anoderm enclosed by them are designated *anal columns*. It is apparent that the anal columns are aligned with the rectal columns which lie cranial to them. Occasionally, the anal columns form papillary projections into the rectal lumen, and the name "anal papillae" has been applied to these teatlike processes. In most instances, however, the anal papillae are absent, but they may, when present and exposed to chronic infection, hypertrophy and become so prominent as to appear like fibrous polyps (see page 172), which may even prolapse through the anal canal. Between the rectal columns, the dentate line corresponds to the upper free margin of the anal valves.

The lower two thirds of the surgical anal canal is identical with the *anatomic anal canal*, which starts at the dentate line and extends to the anal verge, *i.e.*, to the margin where the anal tube opens outward or to the circumference, somewhat difficult to define, but roughly iden-

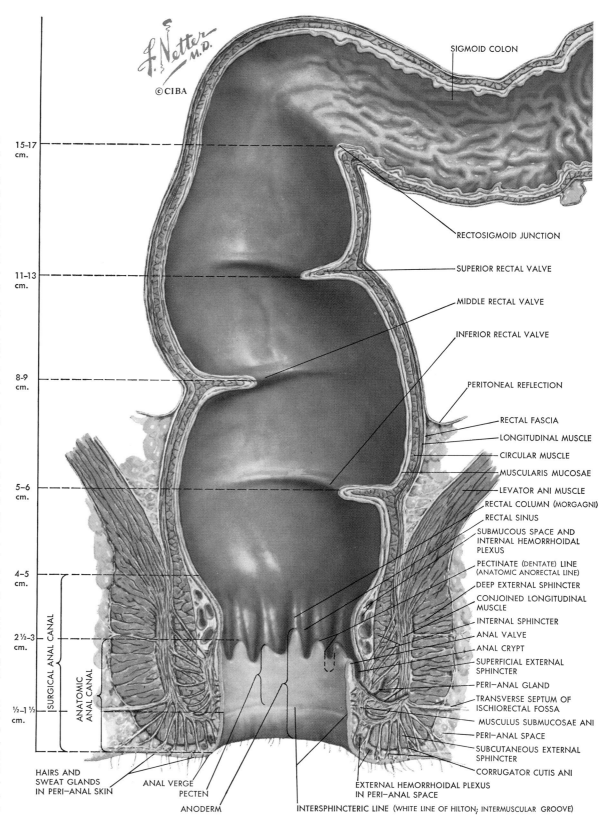

tical with the margin of the anal skin where hair stops growing. The comblike upper border, *i.e.*, the dentate line, gave rise to the designation of the upper part of the anatomic anal canal as pecten (comb), which comprises not only the mucocutaneous cover, called *anoderm* (Gorsch), but also its subepithelial, areolar and connective tissue and structures, such as the anastomoses between the *internal* and *external hemorrhoidal* (rectal) *plexuses* (see page 73), the connections between the autonomic innervation of the rectum and the peripheral nerve supply of the anal canal (see page 81), and the lymphatics (see page 75). The pecten, surrounded by all muscles which constitute the anal muscular ring (see pages 60 to 63), extends downward a varying length of 1 to 1½ cm.; namely, to the *intersphincteric line* (also named *white line of Hilton* or *intermuscular groove*), which is a readily palpable landmark created by the

attachment of the *conjoined longitudinal muscle* to the anoderm and its fusion with the *musculus submucosae ani* (see also page 60), the level of which corresponds to the narrow gap between the blunt lower margin of the internal anal sphincter and the subcutaneous portion of the external sphincter. The clinical significance of the pecten is indicated by its being the predilection zone for anal fissures, fibrosis (pectenosis) and inflammatory processes. (The pecten should not be confused with the controversial and now obsolete term: "pecten band".)

The 1-cm.-broad ring of cutaneous tissue, starting at the intermuscular groove, where it joins the pecten, is also covered by the anoderm and terminates the anal canal at the anal verge. The anoderm superposes here the peri-anal space (see page 33), part of the anorectal musculature (see pages 60 to 63)

(Continued on page 59)

RECTUM AND ANAL CANAL

(Continued from page 58)

and the external hemorrhoidal (rectal) plexus (see page 73).

The axis of the anal canal (anatomic as well as surgical) is, in adults, directed upward and anteriorly toward the umbilicus (in contrast to that of the rectum, see above). In infants both axes, that of the rectum and that of the anal canal, take the same direction, because the child still lacks the adult rectal curves. This fact predisposes anal and rectal prolapse in childhood.

The inner *circular* and outer *longitudinal muscular* coats and the particularly well-developed muscularis mucosae of the rectum are discussed in context with the anorectal musculature (see pages 60 to 63).

Within the submucosa of the sphincteric rectal portion lies the *internal hemorrhoidal (rectal) venous plexus* in the submucous space (see page 33). The submucosa is also particularly rich in lymphatics and terminal nerve fibers (see pages 75 to 81).

As compared with the sigmoid colon, the *mucous membrane of the rectum* is thicker. It also becomes increasingly redder and more richly vascularized as it reaches the surgical anal canal, until its lowermost portion assumes an almost plum color. The extreme vascularity predisposes to hemorrhagic disorders. The mobility of the rectal mucosa is also greater, and large rugous folds, sometimes referred to as pseudopolyps, may form. The simple, true columnar mucosal epithelium of the rectum is similar to that of the colon, though it tends to become somewhat more cuboidal toward the lower end. Like the remainder of the colon, the rectum also contains mucigenous tubular glands (of Lieberkühn), which here, in line with the increased vascularity, are particularly well developed and contain an abundance of goblet cells. The cuboidal or columnar epithelium of the rectum extends downward into the upper third of the surgical anal canal, where it changes irregularly *above* the *dentate line* (see below) into a stratified squamocuboidal type, which directly covers the internal hemorrhoidal plexus as well as the *rectal columns* and *sinuses of Morgagni* (see above). This epithelial transition zone, which is sometimes referred to as the "anal mucosa", does not (in contrast to previous concepts) start abruptly but is arranged in a rather disorderly fashion, in that the squamous epithelium, overriding adjacent cuboidal columnar zones, may extend, in some places, far above the dentate line up to the region of the anorectal muscle ring (see page 60). It is, therefore, wrong to refer to the dentate line as being the "mucocutaneous junction".

The stratified squamous epithelium, which covers the rectal columns and sinuses, thickens as it reaches the ano-

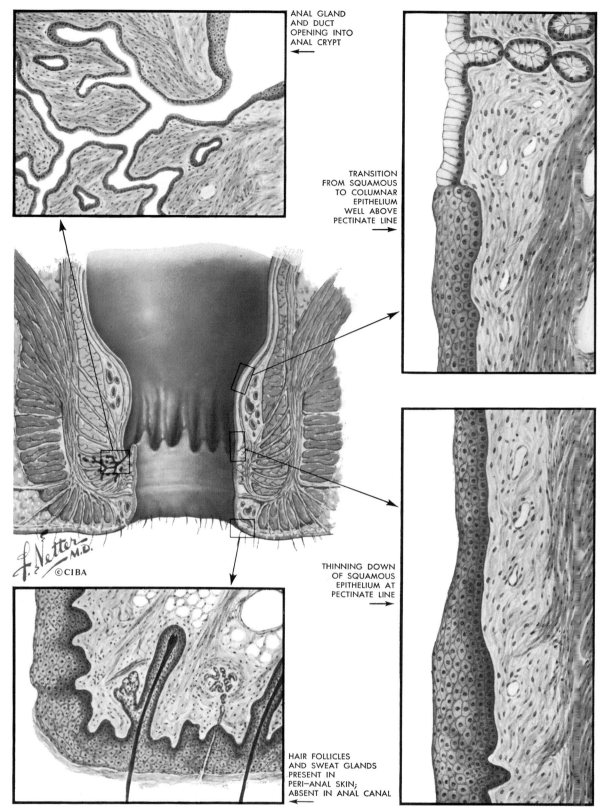

ANAL GLAND
AND DUCT
OPENING INTO
ANAL CRYPT
←

TRANSITION
FROM SQUAMOUS
TO COLUMNAR
EPITHELIUM
WELL ABOVE
PECTINATE LINE
→

THINNING DOWN
OF SQUAMOUS
EPITHELIUM AT
PECTINATE LINE

HAIR FOLLICLES
AND SWEAT GLANDS
PRESENT IN
PERI-ANAL SKIN;
ABSENT IN ANAL CANAL
←

derm lining the pecten area of the anal canal between the dentate line and the intermuscular groove. The anoderm, smooth, shiny and grayish in appearance, is devoid of mucous, sebaceous and sweat glands and is firmly attached to the subjacent muscular and fibrous tissues of the pecten, thus separating the submucous space above from the peri-anal space below (see page 33). Below the intermuscular groove the anoderm further thickens and passes insensibly into the peri-anal skin with its usual cutaneous glandular and follicular elements, which include also the special circumanal glands of Gay, the apocrine and excretory glands in which peri-anal hydradenoma may occasionally be diagnosed.

In the subepithelial and muscular strata of the anal canal, as well as of the lower rectum, simple tubular and racemose glands can be found with fair to varying regularity. They have been described as *peri-anal*

glands, intramuscular glands, anal ducts, etc. Unfortunately, knowledge about their embryologic origin and of their true anatomic site, as well as of their functional significance, is still very incomplete and confusing. The mouths of the ducts open usually into the bottom of the anal crypts, but the ducts and glands may extend for a variable distance into the adjacent tissues, even into or through the sphincteric muscles, which is the reason they are sometimes referred to as "intramuscular glands". The significance of these glandular structures as sites of anorectal infections cannot be denied. Fistulous termination of peri-anal abscesses (see page 173) arising from an anorectal nidus, despite adequate drainage, results primarily from the persistence of an "epithelial" focus in the peri-anal glands, ducts or surrounding connective tissue, and not from the crypts. Persistence of such a focus may likewise be the cause of fistula recurrence.

ANORECTAL MUSCULATURE

As do all other parts of the digestive tube, the rectum has an inner circular and an outer longitudinal muscular coat, but the arrangement of its muscular layers is different and quite peculiar in its integration with the striated anorectal musculature. The *longitudinal rectal muscle* (see also page 58) is formed by an expansion of the colonic taeniae which spread out in the region of the rectosigmoid junction to create a diffuse tunic. Similarly, the inner circular muscle of the rectum is a continuation of the circular muscle of the sigmoid colon. The ampullary section of the rectum is characterized by frequent connections of longitudinal and circular fibers. Fanlike muscular bundles of the longitudinal musculature insert into the circular layer, particularly at the site of those indentations which correspond to the rectal valves (see page 58). Inversely, fibers of the circular layer join those that are longitudinal. At the lower extremity of the rectum, the longitudinal rectal muscle fibers fuse with striated fibers from the levator ani muscle and fibro-elastic tissue from the supra-anal fascia to form the *conjoined longitudinal muscle* of the anal canal (see below), and the inner circular muscle becomes increasingly thicker, to constitute the nonstriated *internal anal sphincter muscle.*

Thus the internal anal sphincter muscle, representing a gradual enlargement of the inner circular muscle sheet of the rectum, is composed of smooth muscle fibers which are innervated by autonomic nerves via the intrinsic nerve plexuses (myenteric and submucous) (see pages 77 and 81). At the level of the intermuscular depression (½ to 1 cm. above the anal verge), the internal anal sphincter, having a thickness of 0.6 to 0.8 cm. and a length of 3 to 5 cm., ends with a sharply defined and readily palpable rounded lower margin, resulting from its strong fascial encuffment and from the recurrentlike arrangement of its more caudal muscle bundles.

The outer longitudinal muscle layer of the rectum continues on downward and, at the level where the sphincteric portion of the rectum (upper part of surgical anal canal, see page 58) passes through the pelvic diaphragm, is joined by fibromuscular extensions from the *pubococcygeus and puborectalis portions* (see Plate 15) of the levator ani muscle as well as by fibers from the supra-anal fascia to become the conjoined longitudinal muscle (see also page 22). This fibromuscular structure extends caudally, surrounding the internal anal sphincter, and is itself surrounded by the external anal sphincter. While continuing its downward course, the muscle gives off, successively, bundles of fibro-elastic tissue interwoven with muscular fibrils, which penetrate the internal sphincter. These fascicles decrease successively in their

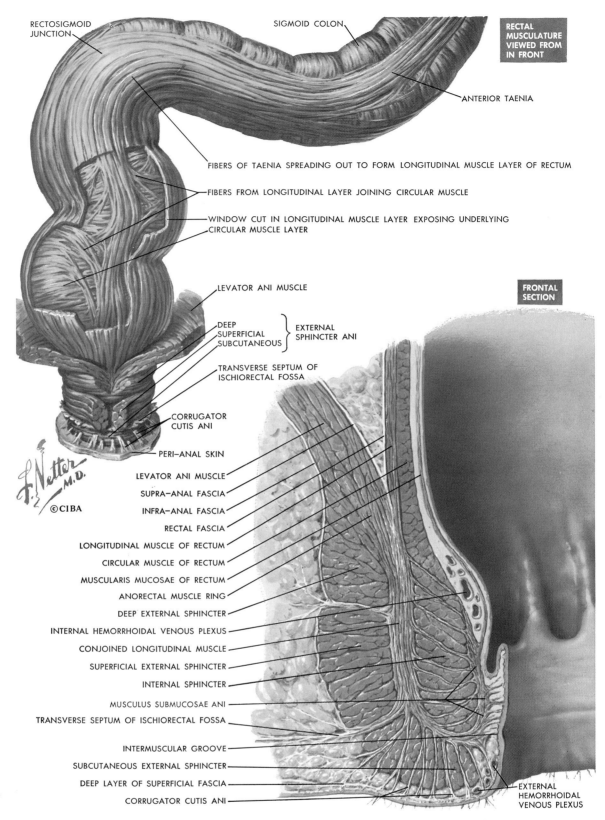

RECTAL MUSCULATURE VIEWED FROM IN FRONT

FRONTAL SECTION

obliquity as they pass through the internal sphincter, until the lowermost fascicles actually ascend. Some of these penetrating fascicles fuse with the well-developed muscularis mucosae of the anal canal and were formerly designated as "sustentator mucosae of Kohlrausch". The result of this fusion is now referred to as *musculus submucosae ani,* fibers of which anchor the anoderm of the pecten to the underlying tissue and to the lower third of the internal anal sphincter. Fixed in this fashion, the pecten prevents eversion of the anal canal and supports the superjacent *internal hemorrhoidal (rectal) venous plexus* during defecation. In total prolapse or procidentia (see page 171), it is also this fixation of the pecten which is responsible for the formation of the *intermuscular depression or groove.*

In its most caudal part the conjoined longitudinal muscle, while bending around the lower border of

the internal sphincter and before its remaining, truly terminal fibers amalgamate with the *musculus submucosae ani,* gives off in fanlike fashion a series of fibromuscular septa, which pass through the circular fibers of the subcutaneous portion of the external sphincter ani to attach themselves to the peri-anal skin. Here, the muscular elements of these septa form (together with some extended fibers of the musculus submucosae ani) the *corrugator cutis ani.*

Extensions from the outer side of the conjoined longitudinal muscle pass through the external anal sphincter. The most important of these extensions is the one which separates the subcutaneous and superficial portions of the sphincter and continues as the *transverse septum of the ischiorectal fossae* (see also page 32). Anteriorly, extensions are also reflected to the urethra above the external sphincter, forming part

(*Continued on page 61*)

ANORECTAL MUSCULATURE

(Continued from page 60)

of the recto-urethralis muscle and, posteriorly, to the coccyx as the rectococcygeus muscle (see page 33).

The significance of the conjoined longitudinal muscle for the physiology, pathology and surgery of the anorectum cannot be overemphasized. Together with the levator ani muscle, it exercises its levator and sphincteric action on the anal canal by fibers taking their course through the entire length of the conjoined longitudinal muscle. By its extensions at the level of the intermuscular groove and by its fascial frame in the upper third of the surgical anal canal, the muscle influences the spread of anorectal infections as well as the sites of the openings and main tracts of fistulas. From the surgeon's point of view, the terminal conjoined longitudinal muscle fibers are important because they permit the recognition of the lower border of the internal sphincter, which is the essential landmark in modern techniques of internal hemorrhoidectomy. Thus, ligature with the hemorrhoidal stump and conservation of the extensions into the peri-anal skin prevent retraction and denudation of the anoderm (Milligan and Morgan, Blaisdell, Gorsch). Complete annular division of the conjoined longitudinal muscle may result in the undesirable sequelae of the so-called proctoplastic hemorrhoid operations and other amputative techniques.

The outermost and also most caudal muscular elements of the anal canal belong to the *external anal sphincter,* which is a trilaminar striated muscle. Its three parts, the *subcutaneous,* the *superficial* and the *deep* (see Plate 14), are easily recognized. The subcutaneous portion, about 3 to 5 mm. in diameter, surrounds the anal orifice directly above the anal margin and is readily palpable and often discernible as a distinct annular ridge. Separated from the internal anal sphincter by fibers of the conjoined longitudinal muscle (previously erroneously called a "septum") at the level of the intermuscular groove, the subcutaneous portion is situated below and slightly lateral to the internal sphincter. Seen from below, the subcutaneous portion usually has an annular form, though its fibers may cross and branch in all directions and may extend posteriorly with the next higher, *i.e.,* the superficial portion. In the male, *anterior muscular extensions to the median raphé* are not uncommon, and it may also be found that uncrossed posterior extensions of the subcutaneous external sphincter connect with the coccyx. In the female, the subcutaneous portion is much more strongly developed, particularly anteriorly, where it forms a prominent annular band, frequently incised at episiotomy. The subcutaneous muscle is functionally integrated with the levator ani muscle through *exten-*

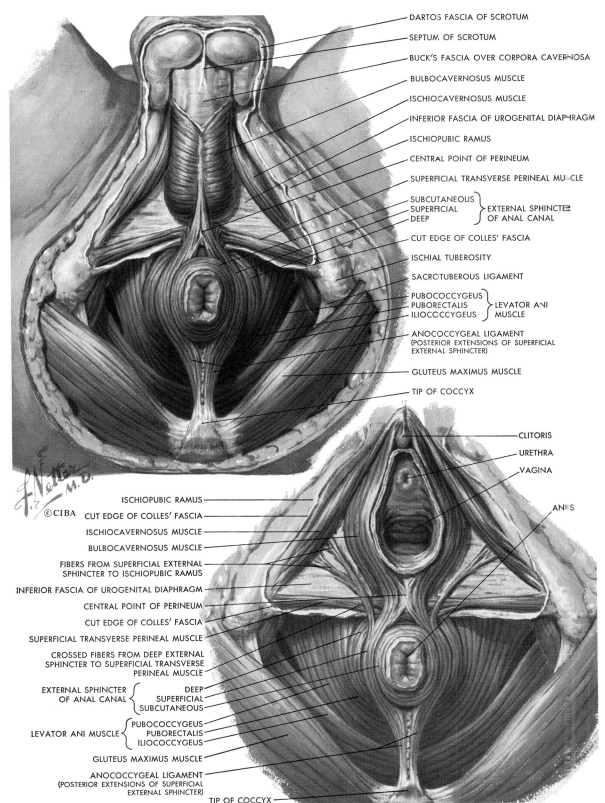

DARTOS FASCIA OF SCROTUM
SEPTUM OF SCROTUM
BUCK'S FASCIA OVER CORPORA CAVERNOSA
BULBOCAVERNOSUS MUSCLE
ISCHIOCAVERNOSUS MUSCLE
INFERIOR FASCIA OF UROGENITAL DIAPHRAGM
ISCHIOPUBIC RAMUS
CENTRAL POINT OF PERINEUM
SUPERFICIAL TRANSVERSE PERINEAL MUSCLE
SUBCUTANEOUS
SUPERFICIAL } EXTERNAL SPHINCTER
DEEP } OF ANAL CANAL
CUT EDGE OF COLLES' FASCIA
ISCHIAL TUBEROSITY
SACROTUBEROUS LIGAMENT
PUBOCOCCYGEUS
PUBORECTALIS } LEVATOR ANI
ILIOCOCCYGEUS } MUSCLE
ANOCOCCYGEAL LIGAMENT
(POSTERIOR EXTENSIONS OF SUPERFICIAL EXTERNAL SPHINCTER)
GLUTEUS MAXIMUS MUSCLE
TIP OF COCCYX

CLITORIS
URETHRA
VAGINA
ANUS

ISCHIOPUBIC RAMUS
CUT EDGE OF COLLES' FASCIA
ISCHIOCAVERNOSUS MUSCLE
BULBOCAVERNOSUS MUSCLE
FIBERS FROM SUPERFICIAL EXTERNAL SPHINCTER TO ISCHIOPUBIC RAMUS
INFERIOR FASCIA OF UROGENITAL DIAPHRAGM
CENTRAL POINT OF PERINEUM
CUT EDGE OF COLLES' FASCIA
SUPERFICIAL TRANSVERSE PERINEAL MUSCLE
CROSSED FIBERS FROM DEEP EXTERNAL SPHINCTER TO SUPERFICIAL TRANSVERSE PERINEAL MUSCLE
EXTERNAL SPHINCTER { DEEP
OF ANAL CANAL { SUPERFICIAL
{ SUBCUTANEOUS
LEVATOR ANI MUSCLE { PUBOCOCCYGEUS
{ PUBORECTALIS
{ ILIOCOCCYGEUS
GLUTEUS MAXIMUS MUSCLE
ANOCOCCYGEAL LIGAMENT
(POSTERIOR EXTENSIONS OF SUPERFICIAL EXTERNAL SPHINCTER)
TIP OF COCCYX

sions of the conjoined longitudinal muscle which pass fanlike through it, to terminate as fibers of the corrugator cutis ani.

The elliptically shaped *superficial portion,* the next deeper layer, is the largest and strongest of the three laminae of the external anal sphincter. It is situated somewhat laterally to the subcutaneous portion and arises independently from the posterior aspect and *tip of the coccyx* — a fact which explains why it is sometimes referred to as the "coccygeal portion". The fibers enclose, in a crescentlike fashion, the lower third or half of the internal sphincter and insert, in the male, at or around the *central point of the perineum* and the median fascial raphé of the bulbocavernosus muscle. In the female, however, only a few fibers of the superficial portion insert at the central point of the perineum; the majority of them merge with the bulbocavernosus muscle, and

some may extend laterally as far as the *ischiopubic rami* and the *ischial tuberosities* in conjunction with, or independent of, the thin *superficial transverse perineal muscles.* It is not uncommon that *fibers,* which pass around the anal canal on the left side, *cross over* to insert anteriorly or laterally on the right side, and vice versa. Posteriorly, the superficial muscle forms the right and left muscular components of the *anococcygeal ligament.* The right and left ischiorectal spaces are continuous above this ligament through the deep postanal spaces (see also page 33), whereas the right and left peri-anal spaces communicate with each other through the superficial postanal space below the anococcygeal ligament.

The *deep* (profundus) *external anal sphincter* is, for the most part, an annular muscle bundle, usually without attachment to the coccyx. Posteriorly, as a

(Continued on page 62)

ANORECTAL MUSCULATURE

(Continued from page 61)

part of the composite anorectal muscle ring, it is intimately blended with the puborectalis muscle as the fibers of that muscle pass, slinglike, around the terminal rectum. This deep portion of the external sphincter surrounds the upper third of the surgical anal canal and, with the *prerectal muscle bundles of the levator ani,* forms part of the anterior half of the anorectal muscle ring (see below). Occasionally, some fibers may attach themselves to the *central point of the perineum* or, after crossing sides, may join the *superficial transverse perineal muscle* to extend as far as the ischium.

The essential forces which keep the recto-anal canal in position derive from muscles forming the pelvic floor, *i.e.,* the *levator ani muscle,* which is assumed to be composed of three individual components; namely, the pubococcygeus, the puborectalis and the iliococcygeus muscles. It is useful, for a proper concept of the anatomic relations of these three separate components, to consider them as enclosing the pelvic outlets in two planes — a diaphragmatic and a subdiaphragmatic plane. The former is created by a broad, sweeping, muscular sheet, for the most part by the pubococcygeus and iliococcygeus muscles, which represent the pelvic diaphragm. The puborectalis muscles contribute but a very small ventral muscle bundle to it. The subdiaphragmatic plane is formed by the caudal fasciomuscular extensions of the pubococcygeus into the musculature of the visceral outlets, particularly of the anal canal, and by the puborectalis muscle. The diaphragmatic plane lies practically horizontal, but the subdiaphragmatic plane assumes a more or less vertical axis as its caudal sections funnel around the anorectal canal and urogenital outlets.

The *pubococcygeus muscle* arises from the posterior aspect of the pubic bone and superior pubic ramus along a line extending from just lateral to the symphysis to a site in front of the obturator foramen and also from the anterior extremity of the arcus tendineus of the levator ani muscle (see below). From this origin the muscle fibers stretch medially and posteriorly along the inner boundaries of the pelvic aperture, looping around the rectum above the puborectalis muscle. The fibers of both sides join in the midline, forming a muscular raphé or plate, which inserts into the anterior aspect of the coccyx and *sacrum.* Aponeurotic extensions from this raphé continue along the sacrum as *anterior sacrococcygeal ligaments.* The described muscular sheet, together with the supra-anal fascia which covers it, presents the main component of the pelvic diaphragm and the major muscular structure in the diaphragmatic plane. That part of the pubococcygeus muscle which lies in the subdiaphragmatic plane consists of *fibromuscular extensions to the prostate gland,* the *urethra,* vagina and also the *rectum*

and anal canal. These extensions fuse with the longitudinal muscles and fascial collars of the visceral outlets or bridge the interval between them. Anterior to the rectum, the medial borders of the pubococcygeus constitute the *"pillars of the levator ani muscle",* although fibers from each side do interdigitate with those of the opposite side, and some cross from side to side as the *"prerectal bundle"* (see below).

The *puborectalis muscle,* contributing by only a small part to the pelvic diaphragm, lies almost entirely in the subdiaphragmatic plane. It is the most medial portion of the levator ani, taking its origin at the os pubis (medially to the origin of the pubococcygeus muscle) and from the *superior fascia of the urogenital diaphragm* (see page 22), to which it is firmly attached. Not readily recognizable as a separate muscular structure in its region of origin, its fibers pass backward horizontally on either side of the pelvic

aperture and gradually come to lie caudally and somewhat medially to the anal extensions of the pubococcygeus muscle. In its course the originally horizontal surface of the muscle becomes its inner surface, and its originally medial edge its inferior margin. When this twist or rotation is complete behind the anorectal junction and caudal to the looping fibers of the pubococcygeus, the puborectalis muscle forms a distinct slinglike muscle band. In conjunction with the deep portion of the external sphincter (see above), to which it adheres or is attached, this slinglike muscle band forms the posterior half of the proctologically important anorectal muscle ring. Similarly to the pubococcygeus, the puborectalis gains a bony insertion through fibrous bands or plates extending to the coccyx as part of the levator plate. The muscle also gives off, in its backward course, fibromuscular extensions

(Continued on page 63)

BULBOCAVERNOSUS MUSCLE
ISCHIOCAVERNOSUS MUSCLE
ISCHIOPUBIC RAMUS
INFERIOR FASCIA OF UROGENITAL DIAPHRAGM
CENTRAL POINT OF PERINEUM
SUPERFICIAL TRANSVERSE PERINEAL MUSCLE
VISCERAL EXTENSIONS FROM LEVATOR ANI TO CONJOINED LONGITUDINAL MUSCLE OF ANAL CANAL
PRERECTAL BUNDLE OF LEVATOR ANI
COLLES' FASCIA (CUT AWAY)
POSTERIOR PORTION OF DEEP EXTERNAL SPHINCTER FUSED WITH PUBORECTALIS (LEVATOR ANI)
CONJOINED LONGITUDINAL MUSCLE OF ANAL CANAL
ISCHIAL TUBEROSITY
INTERNAL ANAL SPHINCTER
PUBOCOCCYGEUS
PUBORECTALIS } LEVATOR ANI MUSCLE
ILIOCOCCYGEUS
ANTERIOR PORTION OF DEEP
SUPERFICIAL
SUBCUTANEOUS } EXTERNAL ANAL SPHINCTER (REFLECTED)

GLUTEUS MAXIMUS MUSCLE
TIP OF COCCYX

COMMON VARIATIONS IN EXTERNAL SPHINCTER →

CROSSED BAND FROM DEEP SPHINCTER JOINING SUPERFICIAL TRANSVERSE PERINEAL MUSCLE
CROSSED ANTERIOR EXTENSION OF SUPERFICIAL EXTERNAL SPHINCTER
CROSSED ANTERIOR EXTENSION OF SUBCUTANEOUS EXTERNAL SPHINCTER
UNCROSSED POSTERIOR EXTENSIONS OF SUBCUTANEOUS EXTERNAL SPHINCTER
UNCROSSED POSTERIOR EXTENSION OF DEEP EXTERNAL SPHINCTER

ATTACHMENT OF DEEP AND SUPERFICIAL EXTERNAL SPHINCTERS TO CENTRAL POINT OF PERINEUM

ANORECTAL MUSCULATURE

(Continued from page 62)

to the prostate or vagina and to the con-joined longitudinal muscle. It is better developed in the female.

The *iliococcygeus muscle,* or iliac portion of the levator ani, arises from the *fascia of the obturator internus muscle* along a convex downward line, a tendinous thickening, known as *"arcus tendineus of the levator ani",* which begins in front of the obturator foramen (see page 22) and extends backward to a bony attachment in the region just above the ischial spine. The muscle's fibers, directed medially, downward and slightly backward, converge and insert into the levator plate below the pubococcygeus muscle, forming, together with the *coccygeus muscle,* the posterior component of the pelvic diaphragm and the inferior muscular lamina of the levator plate.

Combined, the three individual muscular constituents of the levator ani muscle, arranged, as described, in two planes at a diaphragmatic and a subdiaphragmatic level (see above), are shaped, if observed from above (see page 22), like a cupola, the lowest point of which is marked by the hiatus for the anorectal canal. The side walls of this cupola touch upon the obturator internus muscle and the fat pads in the ischiorectal spaces (see page 32). The levator ani thus fixes the pelvic floor and acts as a sort of fulcrum against which increased abdominal pressure, as occurs in lifting, coughing, defecation, etc., may be exerted. Its pubococcygeal portion and the sling muscle of the puborectalis muscle have additional functions, in so far as they become integral parts of the anorectal muscle ring surrounding part of the rectal ampulla and the upper end of the surgical anal canal. The posterior half of this ring consists mainly of the puborectalis sling fibers, which also serve as a prominent, readily definable, proctologic landmark. The less brawny anterior half of the ring is composed of the internal sphincter, thin muscular extensions from the pubococcygeus (the *prerectal bundle* [Luschka's fibers]) and the conjoined longitudinal muscle surrounded by the deep portion of the external sphincter, which presents its main muscular component. In view of such integration between the striated, *i.e.,* voluntary musculature of the pelvic floor, and the smooth, *i.e.,* involuntary or partly mixed muscles intrinsic to the terminal structures of the intestines, the rôle of the levator ani as supplement and synergist for the contraction and relaxation of the anorectal sphincter mechanism is evident. The posterior half of the anorectal muscle ring, in conjunction with the puborectalis muscle sling, when contracted, approximates the rectum toward the os pubis and increases thereby the anorectal kink, shortens and narrows the pelvic aperture, elevates the anus and thus collaborates in closing the anal canal.

Posterior to the levator ani muscle, the

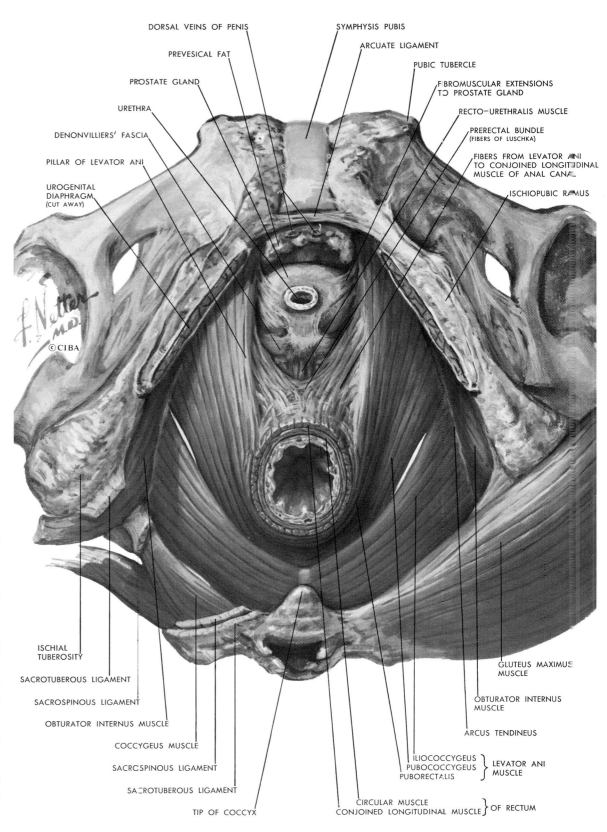

DORSAL VEINS OF PENIS
SYMPHYSIS PUBIS
ARCUATE LIGAMENT
PREVESICAL FAT
PUBIC TUBERCLE
PROSTATE GLAND
FIBROMUSCULAR EXTENSIONS TO PROSTATE GLAND
URETHRA
RECTO-URETHRALIS MUSCLE
DENONVILLIERS' FASCIA
PRERECTAL BUNDLE (FIBERS OF LUSCHKA)
PILLAR OF LEVATOR ANI
FIBERS FROM LEVATOR ANI TO CONJOINED LONGITUDINAL MUSCLE OF ANAL CANAL
UROGENITAL DIAPHRAGM (CUT AWAY)
ISCHIOPUBIC RAMUS
ISCHIAL TUBEROSITY
SACROTUBEROUS LIGAMENT
SACROSPINOUS LIGAMENT
OBTURATOR INTERNUS MUSCLE
COCCYGEUS MUSCLE
SACROSPINOUS LIGAMENT
SACROTUBEROUS LIGAMENT
TIP OF COCCYX
GLUTEUS MAXIMUS MUSCLE
OBTURATOR INTERNUS MUSCLE
ARCUS TENDINEUS
ILIOCOCCYGEUS PUBOCOCCYGEUS PUBORECTALIS } LEVATOR ANI MUSCLE
CIRCULAR MUSCLE CONJOINED LONGITUDINAL MUSCLE } OF RECTUM

pelvic floor is formed by the *coccygeus muscle* (see page 22). The levator ani and coccygeus muscles are innervated by special nerves derived from the ventral ramus of the fourth (sometimes also third) sacral nerve. These nerves course on the superior surface of the muscles until they penetrate them (see page 43 and also 44 and 31). The three laminae of the external sphincter muscle are supplied by the inferior rectal (hemorrhoidal) nerves from the internal pudendal and also, to some extent, by the perineal branch of the fourth sacral nerve.

Clinical experience, especially in surgery of anterior anal fistulas, has proved that the greater portion of the anal musculature may be severed without materially interfering with anal continence, but some degree of incontinence is apt to follow, as a result of a relatively greater retraction of the musculature, when the anorectal ring is divided, particularly in its

anterior and lateral aspects. The anorectal ring also marks the upper limit of the internal hemorrhoidal (rectal) venous plexus and presents therewith a useful guide for the so-called "high injections" of internal hemorrhoids.

A change in the anatomic relations of the anorectal musculature occurs under anesthesia, especially spinal anesthesia, a fact which is significant in anorectal surgery. All the somatic components of the musculature relax, while the visceral components tend to retain or even increase their tonus. As a result the anal canal becomes foreshortened, and the internal sphincter is displaced to a relatively lower level, becoming the principal presenting muscle surrounding the anal orifice. The subcutaneous portion of the sphincter flattens out and recedes laterally, so that the intermuscular depression may disappear and become less readily palpable.

Blood Supply of Small and Large Intestine

The blood supply to the small and large intestine is extremely variable and, in many instances, uncertain and unpredictable. The variations concerning the origin, course, anastomoses and distribution of the intestinal vessels are so frequent and so significant that the conventional textbook descriptions are inadequate and, in many respects, even misleading, a situation much the same as in the case of the blood supply of the upper abdominal organs (see Ciba Collection, Vol. 3/1, pages 56 to 61). An intimate acquaintance with the prevalent variational pattern of the gut's arterial supply is necessary to avoid, during abdominal operations, the devascularization of intestinal sections which, according to plan, should be saved, or to circumvent inadvertently induced necrosis leading to peritonitis, still a major cause of death after abdominal operations (Robillard and Shapiro; Mayo).

The *superior mesenteric a.** arises from the front of the aorta, as a rule at the vertebral level of mid L1, but in many instances as far down as the upper third of L2 (Anson and McVay). The aortic distance between the origin of the celiac and the superior mesenteric aa. — nowadays an important anatomic expediency in view of the arteriographic visualization of both arteries and the use of T12 as an earmark for the aortic puncture — varies from 1 to 23 mm., being preponderantly 1 to 6 mm. (Michels). Thus rather contiguous origins of the two vessels will be found very often, whereas a common origin from a *celiacomesenteric trunk* (see next page) is a rare occurrence (observed 3 times in over 1,500 bodies; Michels). In contrast to the frequency (17 per cent; Michels) of a *hepatomesenteric trunk,* when a replaced or an accessory right hepatic a., or even the entire hepatic trunk (see also Ciba Collection, Vol. 3/III, page 16), takes origin from the superior mesenteric a., a *lienomesenteric,* as well as a *hepatolienomesenteric,* trunk is seldom encountered. Occasionally, the right *gastro-epiploic,* the gastroduodenal, the splenic and, in rare instances, even the cystic aa. may arise from the superior mesenteric a. Aside from these variational patterns, the superior mesenteric a. is involved with the blood supply of the upper abdominal organs by its first branch, the *inferior pancreaticoduodenal a.,* which is typically the feeder line for the third portion of the duodenum and the head of the pancreas. If, as happens in 14 per cent of the cases, the dorsal pancreatic and transverse pancreatic aa. branch off from the superior mesenteric, the major por-

tions of the neck and body of the pancreas also become part of the maintenance territory of the latter vessel.

The superior mesenteric a., passing downward and forward and swinging, particularly in its lower third, to the left, gives off a variable number (13 to 21) of *intestinal aa. from its convex (left) side;* from 3 to 7 (average 5) above and from 8 to 17 (average 11) below the origin of the ileocolic a. The first of these two groups supplies the jejunum, and the second supplies part of the jejunum and the entire ileum (Kornblith). The intestinal aa., those providing the jejunum and ileum, running between the layers of the mesentery, follow prevalently the pattern shown on the accompanying plate. Each vessel courses fairly straight, for a varying distance, before it divides into branches which unite with branches from adjacent primary stem vessels to form arcades. From these pri-

mary arcades, the secondary intestinal aa., essentially shorter than the primary ones, are given off, which, in turn, form secondary arcades. Further arcades, though smaller ones, are fashioned by the same constructive principle, essentially by the more distal (ileal) aa. From the terminal arcade small straight vessels (arteriae rectae, see below) arise. Except for the blood supply of the first part of the duodenum, where, besides numerous other distinctions (see below), the first arcade is small with short arteriae rectae, the jejunal aa. are long, have a large caliber and establish primary and secondary arcades, from which multiple long arteriae rectae are given off. The stem aa. for the ileum become progressively shorter, the arcades smaller and the arteriae less elongated. The vascularization pattern of the jejunum is so characteristically different compared with that of the

(Continued on page 65)

---

*In the following, "artery" and "arteries" are abbreviated "a." and "aa.", respectively.

BLOOD SUPPLY OF SMALL AND LARGE INTESTINE

(Continued from page 64)

ileum that, by simple inspection of the gut, one can usually tell whether it is jejunum or ileum. The jejunum, with a much thicker wall and furnished with a greater digestive surface than is the ileum, receives the larger intestinal branches.

The first jejunal branch of superior mesenteric origin may be very large (6 mm. in diameter) and may have four large arcades forming branches, the length of which varies from 6 to 8 cm. and their diameter from 3 to 4 mm. In many instances, however, the first jejunal branch is very small (1 to 2 mm.) and is anastomosed with the inferior pancreaticoduodenal a. or has a common origin with it. A large primary jejunal a. may be followed by a slender second jejunal a. The distribution, as well as the caliber, of all the following intestinal branches of the superior mesenteric a. varies individually, and in one and the same individual larger and smaller branches alternate without any general rule or order. The first and second jejunal aa. are commonly stated to communicate by an arcade, but such an arcade is missing in many instances, the first jejunal a. having no connection whatsoever with the second. In a study concerned alone with the blood supply of the first 60 cm. of the jejunum, five different patterns were observed. A single jejunal branch was involved in 33 per cent (of forty specimens), three branches in 27 per cent, four branches in 20 per cent and five and six branches each in 10 per cent (Quénu *et al.*). In many instances the first (1 to 3) jejunal branches derive from the anterior or posterior pancreaticoduodenal arcades, which connect with the superior mesenteric a. either via one common pancreaticoduodenal a. (40 per cent) or via two separate vessels of this name (60 per cent; Michels). Predominantly, the first jejunal branch arises from a pancreaticoduodenal arcade (or inferior pancreaticoduodenal a.) to the right of the superior mesenteric a., coursing behind the latter to reach the jejunum. In other, by no means rare, instances the anterior or posterior (or both) pancreaticoduodenal arcade does not join the superior mesenteric a. but anastomoses with its first jejunal branch as it derives from the left side of the superior mesenteric a. Also, the anterior pancreaticoduodenal arcade may join the superior mesenteric a., while the posterior arcade joins the first jejunal branch. In strikingly aberrant cases the first jejunal branch arises from an inferior pancreaticoduodenal a., which, in turn, had taken off from an aberrant right hepatic a. of superior mesenteric origin behind the pancreas, thus bringing the jejunal blood supply in direct relation with that of the liver. This also happens when the

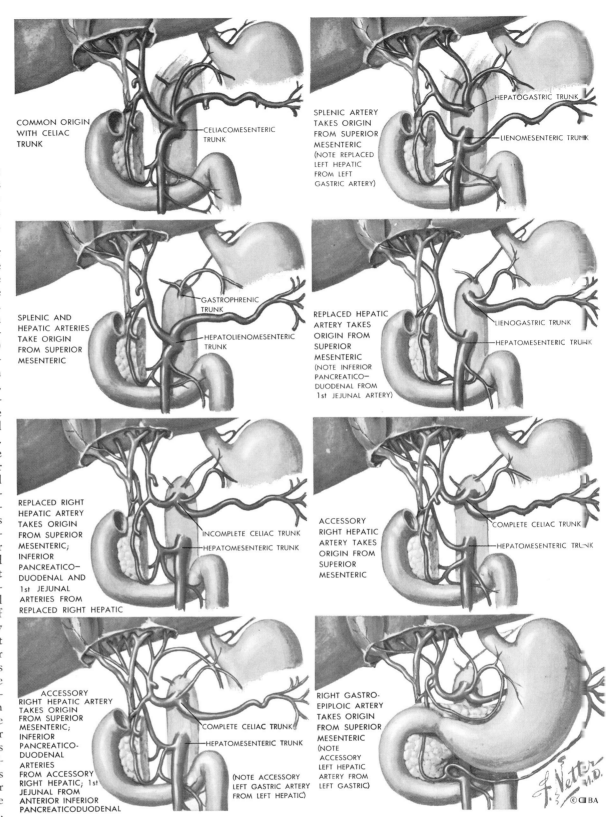

COMMON ORIGIN WITH CELIAC TRUNK — CELIACOMESENTERIC TRUNK

SPLENIC ARTERY TAKES ORIGIN FROM SUPERIOR MESENTERIC (NOTE REPLACED LEFT HEPATIC FROM LEFT GASTRIC ARTERY) — HEPATOGASTRIC TRUNK — LIENOMESENTERIC TRUNK

SPLENIC AND HEPATIC ARTERIES TAKE ORIGIN FROM SUPERIOR MESENTERIC — GASTROPHRENIC TRUNK — HEPATOLIENOMESENTERIC TRUNK

REPLACED HEPATIC ARTERY TAKES ORIGIN FROM SUPERIOR MESENTERIC (NOTE INFERIOR PANCREATICODUODENAL FROM 1st JEJUNAL ARTERY) — LIENOGASTRIC TRUNK — HEPATOMESENTERIC TRUNK

REPLACED RIGHT HEPATIC ARTERY TAKES ORIGIN FROM SUPERIOR MESENTERIC; INFERIOR PANCREATICODUODENAL AND 1st JEJUNAL ARTERIES FROM REPLACED RIGHT HEPATIC — INCOMPLETE CELIAC TRUNK — HEPATOMESENTERIC TRUNK

ACCESSORY RIGHT HEPATIC ARTERY TAKES ORIGIN FROM SUPERIOR MESENTERIC — COMPLETE CELIAC TRUNK — HEPATOMESENTERIC TRUNK

ACCESSORY RIGHT HEPATIC ARTERY TAKES ORIGIN FROM SUPERIOR MESENTERIC; INFERIOR PANCREATICODUODENAL ARTERIES FROM ACCESSORY RIGHT HEPATIC; 1st JEJUNAL FROM ANTERIOR INFERIOR PANCREATICODUODENAL — COMPLETE CELIAC TRUNK — HEPATOMESENTERIC TRUNK (NOTE ACCESSORY LEFT GASTRIC ARTERY FROM LEFT HEPATIC)

RIGHT GASTRO-EPIPLOIC ARTERY TAKES ORIGIN FROM SUPERIOR MESENTERIC (NOTE ACCESSORY LEFT HEPATIC ARTERY FROM LEFT GASTRIC)

first jejunal branch is anastomosing to the hepatic, celiac or transverse pancreatic a. via a dorsal pancreatic a. When the latter springs from the superior mesenteric below the pancreas, it may give off the first jejunal branch. A middle colic a. of celiac origin may emit the dorsal pancreatic a. to the pancreas, which, after leaving the lower border of this organ, releases the first jejunal branch. A rather odd situation may be faced during gastric resection, when the right gastro-epiploic a. and, in addition, the first jejunal branch arise from a common pancreaticoduodenal trunk, which originates from the superior mesenteric a. Variants of this situation are cases in which the superior mesenteric a. releases on its left side the gastroduodenal a. and, at about the same level, the first jejunal branch, the latter anastomosing with the common inferior pancreaticoduodenal a., while the former gives origin to the right gastro-

epiploic, the superior pancreaticoduodenal aa. and a pyloric branch (Siddharth). In one of the most bizarre patterns encountered, the first jejunal branch of superior mesenteric origin received afflux from the anterior and posterior pancreaticoduodenal arcades, while the second jejunal branch anastomosed with the anterior arcade, which, in turn, joined the transverse pancreatic a. Though numerous other examples of variations concerning the origin and communication of the first jejunal branches could be enumerated, those cited seem sufficient to justify the requirement of a careful inspection of these vessels while operating in this region.

From the wide net of communicating arcades the blood reaches the jejunal and ileal walls through straight vessels of varying lengths, the *arterial vasa rectae*. The majority of these arteriae rectae arise from the

(Continued on page 66)

BLOOD SUPPLY OF SMALL AND LARGE INTESTINE

(Continued from page 65)

most distal (ultimate) arcade formed by neighboring intestinal arteries, but quite a number of them may take origin from the primary overriding the secondary arcade. Long arteriae rectae, upon reaching the gut, predominantly proceed to the antimesenteric border to form anastomotic plexuses spreading over the wall, while the shorter arteriae rectae, stemming either from an arcade or from a long straight vessel, end at the mesenteric border of the gut. Some arteriae rectae may crisscross each other before reaching the gut, or they may divide into two branches, which proceed to the anterior and posterior surfaces. Occasionally — contrary to common opinion — the arteriae rectae form definite intermesenteric anastomoses. Most peculiar (and unrecorded; Kornblith) is the fact that often small (4 to 6 cm.) segments of the small intestine are vascularized by arteriae rectae deriving from two ultimate arcades, a more anterior one serving the anterior surface of the gut and a posterior one for the posterior surface, in a manner comparable to the arrangement of the two pancreaticoduodenal arcades serving parts of the duodenum (see CIBA COLLECTION, Vol. 3/I, page 59). As mural trunks, the arteriae rectae communicate with one another, forming a continuous network of arterial anastomoses. Proximally, the network unites with the branches of the inferior pancreaticoduodenal; distally, with the ileal branch of the ileocolic a.

From its concave, *i.e.*, right side, the superior mesenteric a., according to textbook description, releases four major branches — the *inferior pancreaticoduodenal,* middle colic, right colic and ileocolic aa. Because of the numerous variations in the origin and connections of these vessels, however, the situation is by no means as simple as such textbook description implies. The first of these aa., the inferior pancreaticoduodenal, may have a common origin with the first intestinal branch, and communicates with this in its own dangerously irregular vessel (see above) and with the anterior and/or posterior pancreaticoduodenal aa. in a great variety of ways (see above and CIBA COLLECTION, Vol. 3/I, pages 60 and 61).

The *middle colic a.,* again according to conventional descriptions, arises at the lower border of the pancreas and passes into the right half of the transverse mesocolon, where, at a variable distance from the colonic wall (5 to 7 cm.), it typically divides into two branches, one of which courses to the right to anastomose with the ascending branch of the right colic a. (see below), while the other turns to the left to anastomose with the ascending branch of the left colic a., deriving from the inferior mesenteric a. Both divisions

ANTERIOR CECAL AND POSTERIOR CECAL ARTERIES ORIGINATE FROM ARCADE BETWEEN COLIC AND ILEAL BRANCHES OF ILEOCOLIC APPENDICULAR ARTERY FROM ILEAL BRANCH

ANTERIOR CECAL AND POSTERIOR CECAL ARTERIES ORIGINATE FROM COLIC BRANCH; APPENDICULAR ARTERY FROM ILEAL BRANCH OF ILEOCOLIC ARTERY

ANTERIOR CECAL AND POSTERIOR CECAL ARTERIES HAVE COMMON ORIGIN FROM ARCADE; APPENDICULAR ARTERY FROM ILEOCOLIC ARTERY PROPER

ANTERIOR CECAL AND POSTERIOR CECAL ARTERIES ORIGINATE FROM ARCADE BETWEEN COLIC AND ILEAL BRANCHES OF ILEOCOLIC ARTERY; APPENDICULAR ARTERY FROM COLIC BRANCH BIFURCATES HIGH

ANTERIOR CECAL AND POSTERIOR CECAL ARTERIES ORIGINATE FROM ILEAL BRANCH OF ILEOCOLIC ARTERY; APPENDICULAR ARTERY FROM POSTERIOR CECAL

ANTERIOR CECAL AND TWO POSTERIOR CECAL ARTERIES ORIGINATE FROM ARCADE; APPENDICULAR ARTERY FROM ILEAL BRANCH OF ILEOCOLIC ARTERY

MULTIPLE ARCADES BETWEEN ILEAL BRANCH AND COLIC BRANCH OF ILEOCOLIC ARTERY. ANTERIOR CECAL AND POSTERIOR CECAL ORIGINATE FROM THESE ARCADES; APPENDICULAR ARTERY FROM ILEAL BRANCH

ANTERIOR CECAL AND POSTERIOR CECAL ARTERIES ORIGINATE FROM ARCADE BETWEEN COLIC AND ILEAL BRANCHES OF ILEOCOLIC ARTERY; TWO APPENDICULAR ARTERIES, ONE DERIVING FROM ARCADE, THE OTHER FROM ILEAL BRANCH, ARE PRESENT

ANTERIOR CECAL AND POSTERIOR CECAL ARTERIES ORIGINATE FROM ARCADE; TWO APPENDICULAR ARTERIES, ONE DERIVING FROM ANTERIOR CECAL, THE OTHER FROM POSTERIOR CECAL, ARE PRESENT

of the middle colic undergo subsequent variant branchings, forming primary and secondary arcades from which arteriae rectae are given off to the transverse colon. This description, however, does not fit all individuals. As a separate branch of the superior mesenteric a., the middle colic a. is frequently absent (recorded percentages vary from 5 to 22 and even to 99; Steward and Rankin; Robillard and Shapiro; Quénu *et al.*; Morgan and Griffiths; Sonneland *et al.*). In such instances the artery is usually (54 per cent; Kornblith and Siddharth) replaced by a common right middle colic trunk and, occasionally, by a branch of the left colic, the latter at times reaching the hepatic flexure. An *accessory middle colic a.* may be present (10 per cent), arising, as a rule, from the aorta somewhat above the chief middle colic. It usually anastomoses with branches from the left colic a., forming, in the left transverse meso-

colon, a secondary arc of Riolan. But such an *accessory vessel* may also *arise,* as a branch, *from the trunk of the middle colic to serve the splenic flexure.* The middle colic, furthermore, may have a *common origin* with the *right and the ileocolic aa.,* or it may arise within the pancreas from the transverse pancreatic a. and leave this organ, entering the transverse mesocolon to supply the distal third of the transverse colon. Less frequently (1.5 per cent in 200 bodies; Michels), the *middle colic a.* may *stem* directly from the *celiac trunk* or *splenic a.* via the dorsal pancreatic a., or, if of such origin, it may serve, before bifurcating, in lieu of the latter, giving off the transverse pancreatic a. and thus communicating directly with the blood supply of the pancreas. Occasionally, the middle colic a. originates behind the head of the pancreas from an accessory right hepatic

(Continued on page 67)

Blood Supply of Small and Large Intestine

(Continued from page 66)

of superior mesenteric origin or from a common trunk of the same origin which releases also the *right gastro-epiploic aa.* A pancreaticocolic trunk may come into existence when the middle colic a., arising either from the superior mesenteric a. or directly from the aorta, may release the dorsal pancreatic (and transverse pancreatic) a. It is important, furthermore, that in many instances the anastomotic connection between the superior mesenteric a. and its middle colic or accessory middle colic be established behind the pancreas and portal vein with one or more branches of celiac origin, either by one single large vessel (ramus anastomoticus of Bühler) or by a ramifying branch of the dorsal pancreatic a. The anastomosing aa. are predominantly small (1 mm. in diameter) but may, especially when connecting the superior mesenteric with the hepatic or right gastro-epiploic a., reach a diameter of 2 to 3 mm. (These celiacomesenteric anastomoses result from the persistence of a direct, primitive longitudinal anastomosis between the roots of the embryonic celiac and superior mesenteric aa. [Tandler].)

Conventionally, the *right colic a.* is described as arising from the superior mesenteric, dividing, halfway between its origin and the ascending colon, into a descending and an ascending branch, the former uniting with the ileocolic, the latter with a left branch of the middle colic a. The variability of the site, where the right colic a. takes off from the superior mesenteric, is generally admitted. It may be found to arise frequently at far higher levels, so that it may cross the descending part of the duodenum and the lower end of the right kidney. What is generally not adequately emphasized is the fact that, in about one fifth (18 per cent; Steward and Rankin) of the population, the right colic a. is entirely absent and that, in one third of the subjects studied, it arises from a common trunk with the ileocolic a. Often it constitutes but a descending part of the right branch of the middle colic a., or it may arise separately from the latter before this a. bifurcates near the lower border of the transverse colon. With the right colic a. absent in one group, the middle colic missing in another group and in view of the irregularities of their connections, the blood supply of the ascending and transverse colon becomes one of the most variable, unpredictable anatomic arrangements. Taking into account only the number of aa. that leave the superior mesenteric on its concave side above the origin of the ileocolic, three different types could be separated (dissection of 100 bodies; Quénu *et al.*). One single a. was found in 65 per cent, the territory of which covered the hepatic flexure and the trans-

verse colon, in some instances extending to the beginning of the left colon. Coursing to the right half of the transverse colon, this single a. bifurcated in one third of the cases, the left branch forming a large arcade of Riolan near the colon, which united with a branch of the left colic. In other instances the a. divided into three or four branches serving the entire transverse colon, the arc of Riolan being considerably smaller. In 33 per cent, two aa. were present, but in only one of these cases did one a. course to the transverse colon, the other to the ascending colon. In most individuals both aa. supplied the transverse colon, reaching, at times, the splenic flexure. The two aa. anastomosed, forming a variety of loops. Three aa. were existent in 2 per cent. They covered only the transverse colon but included, in one instance, the splenic flexure. These findings are, essentially, in accord with those of other authors,

since, obviously, in view of this diversity, it becomes more or less a question of terminology whether one assumes the absence of the right or the middle colic a.

The *ileocolic a.*, the last branch of the superior mesenteric on its right side, is always present, and so, as a rule, are the two chief branches — the ascending *colic* and a *descending ileal branch.* The end of the former, typically, constitutes the start of the marginal a. (of Drummond) and anastomoses with the descending branch of the right colic a. In the absence of the latter, it substitutes for it, taking over the functions of both aa. A common origin of the right colic and ileocolic has been observed in many cases (3 per cent, Robillard and Shapiro; 23 per cent, Sonneland et al.). The descending branch divides into the *anterior cecal*, the *posterior cecal* and the *appendicular aa.* A few *short colic branches* may be present. The ante-

(Continued on page 68)

67

BLOOD SUPPLY OF SMALL AND LARGE INTESTINE

(Continued from page 67)

rior cecal a. courses through the vascular superior ileocecal fold (see page 51) to reach the anterior surface of the cecum at the upper border of the ileocecal junction. The posterior cecal, sometimes double, passes behind this junction to the posterior surface of the cecum and often arises in a common trunk with the anterior cecal a.

The *appendicular a.*, although fairly uniform in its course in the mesenteriolum, varies considerably in its site of origin (see Plate 20), ten different types having been established (Anson). It may *arise* from the left or the right side of the ileal branch (35 per cent); directly *from the ileocolic a.* before it branches or at its branching point (30 per cent); *from the colic branch of the ileocolic a.*, bifurcating before passing under the terminal ileum; *from the posterior cecal*, likewise bifurcating above the ileum; or *from one* of the multiple *arcades* formed by the colic or ileal end branches of the ileocolic a. When double appendicular aa. are present (as is the case in 30 per cent; Shah and Shah), one may arise from an arcade between the colic and ileal branches of the ileocolic a., the other from its ileal branch; or one from the anterior and the other from the posterior cecal branch, or both from either one of these rami. With double appendicular aa., both may provide the entire appendix, or one may take care of the base, the other of the tip.

The ends of both the superior mesenteric and the ileocecal aa. are difficult to determine, because they unite predominantly in a circle or loop, the proximal part of which releases intestinal aa. of superior mesenteric origin, whereas those from the distal half of the loop, varying from three to six in number, are intestinal aa. from the ileal branch of the ileocolic a. Anastomoses between these intestinal aa. may form a single or double tier of arches, feeding the arteriae rectae, by which the last 3 to 6 in. of the ileum are supplied. Sometimes, however, the very last intestinal branch from the superior mesenteric a. may have failed to form an arcade. Other arcade variations in this region concern the connections between the ileal and cecal branches of the ileocolic a. (Kornblith).

The *inferior mesenteric* (see Plate 21) arises typically from the anterior aspect or left side of the aorta, 3 to 5 cm. above its bifurcation, which is situated at the level of the lower third of L4. The level at which the inferior mesenteric a. takes off varies within the distance between the middle of L2 and the disk between L3 and L4, but it is most commonly that of the middle of L3 (Taniguchi). The origin of the vessel (3 to 5 mm. in caliber, average 4 mm.) may, at times, be over-

KEY

AR — ARC OF RIOLAN
C — CELIAC TRUNK
D — DUODENUM
DP — DORSAL PANCREATIC ARTERY
H — HEPATIC ARTERY
IC — ILEOCOLIC ARTERY
IM — INFERIOR MESENTERIC ARTERY
LC — LEFT COLIC ARTERY
M — MARGINAL ARTERY
MC — MIDDLE COLIC ARTERY
RC — RIGHT COLIC ARTERY
RGE — RIGHT GASTRO-EPIPLOIC ARTERY
RRH — REPLACED RIGHT HEPATIC ARTERY
RS — RECTOSIGMOID ARTERIES
S — SIGMOID ARTERIES
SM — SUPERIOR MESENTERIC ARTERY
Sp — SPLENIC ARTERY
SR — SUPERIOR RECTAL ARTERY
TP — TRANSVERSE PANCREATIC ARTERY

ARC OF RIOLAN

DISCONTINUITY OF MARGINAL ARTERY (BETWEEN RIGHT COLIC AND ILEOCOLIC ARTERIES)

MIDDLE COLIC ARTERY ORIGINATES FROM CELIAC TRUNK VIA DORSAL PANCREATIC ARTERY

MIDDLE COLIC ARTERY GIVES ORIGIN TO DORSAL PANCREATIC ARTERY

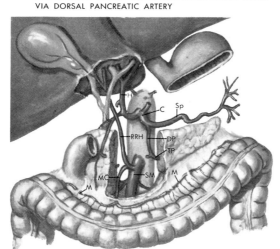

MIDDLE COLIC ARTERY ORIGINATES FROM OR WITH REPLACED RIGHT HEPATIC ARTERY (FROM SUP. MESENTERIC A.)

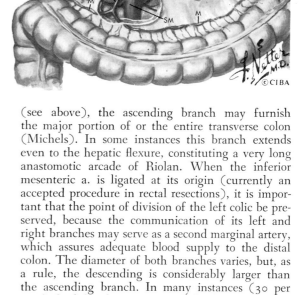

MIDDLE COLIC ARTERY HAS COMMON ORIGIN WITH RIGHT GASTRO-EPIPLOIC FROM SUPERIOR MESENTERIC ARTERY

lain by the third portion of the duodenum. Proceeding posteriorly through the mesentery to the left iliac fossa at an angle of 30 degrees with the aorta and crossing the left common iliac a., the inferior mesenteric a. gives off, at its left side, the left colic and several sigmoid aa., to continue into the lesser pelvis as the superior rectal (hemorrhoidal) a. The distributional pattern, with five to six branches, varies far less than does that of the superior mesenteric a.

The *left colic a.* takes off from 4 to 6 cm. below the origin of the inferior mesenteric and divides, after a short, fairly horizontal course, at a variable distance (3 to 10 cm.) from the gut wall, into an ascending and a descending branch. The ascending branch courses directly upward toward the splenic flexure but splits into a left and a right branch, which, respectively, join the marginal a. of the descending and transverse colon. In the absence of a middle colic a.

(see above), the ascending branch may furnish the major portion of or the entire transverse colon (Michels). In some instances this branch extends even to the hepatic flexure, constituting a very long anastomotic arcade of Riolan. When the inferior mesenteric a. is ligated at its origin (currently an accepted procedure in rectal resections), it is important that the point of division of the left colic be preserved, because the communication of its left and right branches may serve as a second marginal artery, which assures adequate blood supply to the distal colon. The diameter of both branches varies, but, as a rule, the descending is considerably larger than the ascending branch. In many instances (30 per cent) the left colic may give off the first sigmoid a., which, otherwise, emanates directly from the mesenteric inferior.

(Continued on page 69)

BLOOD SUPPLY OF SMALL AND LARGE INTESTINE

(Continued from page 68)

The inferior mesenteric a., below the origin of the left colic, proceeds downward retroperitoneally, crossing the left common iliac a. and vein to fork into the last of the sigmoid aa. and the superior rectal a. From *two to three sigmoid aa.* leave the inferior mesenteric a. to form, within the mesosigmoid, a network of arcades, from which straight vessels arise to proceed to the wall of the lower part of the descending and the sigmoid colon. The arcades anastomose similarly to those providing the small intestine, but they are less numerous, although composed of vessels with a larger caliber. The arteriae rectae to the sigmoid are longer and larger than elsewhere and generally approach and enter the gut wall in the same fashion as do the arteriae rectae of the small intestine. According to recent studies (Noer), the vessels cross the wall directly from the serosal aspect to the mucosa, as a rule in the vicinity of the lateral taenia. (For the possible relationship between the passage of small vessels and the development of colonic diverticula, see page 130.)

Proximally, the arcades emanating from the sigmoid aa. communicate with the descending branch of the left colic and, distally, at least in the majority of the cases, with the rectosigmoid branches deriving from the *superior rectal a.* This latter a., which may be considered the continuation of the inferior mesenteric a., after releasing several rectosigmoid branches providing the rectosigmoid junction, *bifurcates on the posterior surface of the rectum* (see Plate 24) into two lateral branches, which descend on either side of the rectum, to divide into smaller rami caudal to the peritoneal reflection. These secondary branches pierce the muscular coat at various sites over the entire length of the rectum and enter, finally, the submucosa, where, as straight vessels, they descend to the rectal columns of the anal canal, terminating above the anal valves in a capillary plexus. Along their course the branches of the rectal superior a. anastomose with branches of the middle and inferior rectal and middle sacral aa., which participate in the supply of the two lowest segments of the intestinal tract — the rectum and anus.

While the *internal pudendal aa.* pass through Alcock's canal, they give off, in the posterior part of the ischiorectal fossa, the inferior rectal aa., which pierce the obturator fascia and then break up into several (two to four) branches. These course medially to reach the external and internal anal sphincter muscles, which they supply and penetrate. The final offshoots provide the submucosal and subcutaneous tissue of the anal canal. Aside from the anastomoses just mentioned, they also communicate with branches of

KEY

AMC — ACCESSORY MIDDLE COLIC ARTERY

B — BIFURCATION OF SUPERIOR RECTAL ARTERY

D — DUODENUM

HF — HEPATIC FLEXURE OF COLON

IC — ILEOCOLIC ARTERY

IM — INFERIOR MESENTERIC ARTERY

LC — LEFT COLIC ARTERY

M — MARGINAL ARTERY

MC — MIDDLE COLIC ARTERY

RC — RIGHT COLIC ARTERY

RS — RECTOSIGMOID ARTERIES

S — SIGMOID ARTERIES

SF — SPLENIC FLEXURE OF COLON

SM — SUPERIOR MESENTERIC ARTERY

SR — SUPERIOR RECTAL ARTERY

COMMON ORIGIN OF RIGHT COLIC AND MIDDLE COLIC ARTERIES

COMMON ORIGIN OF RIGHT COLIC AND ILEOCOLIC ARTERIES

ABSENCE OF MIDDLE COLIC ARTERY (REPLACED BY LARGE BRANCH FROM LEFT COLIC)

ABSENCE OF RIGHT COLIC ARTERY

BRANCH OF MIDDLE COLIC ARTERY TO SPLENIC FLEXURE

ACCESSORY MIDDLE COLIC ARTERY TO SPLENIC FLEXURE

the gluteal and perineal aa. The internal pudendal aa. send also a few branches to the lower rectum that ramify in the levator ani muscle.

The *middle rectal aa.* have a varied origin and may be present in double or triple form. Most commonly, they arise from the anterior division of the *internal iliac (hypogastric) aa.;* occasionally, from the *inferior vesical a.* Below the pelvic peritoneum they transverse the connective tissue of the pelvis, spreading their branches over the anterolateral aspects of the middle of the rectum and anastomosing above with the superior rectal and below with the inferior rectal aa.

The *middle sacral a.,* which, in contrast to the above-discussed right and left rectal aa., is a single vessel, originates from the posterior surface of the aorta, a little more than 1 cm. above the aortic bifurcation, and extends to the tip of the coccyx. In addition to the lowest lumbar and the right and left lateral

sacral aa., it gives rise to a variable number of rectal branches that pass forward beneath the peritoneum or sigmoid mesocolon to the rectum, where they anastomose with other rectal aa. The significance of the blood supply to the rectum via the middle sacral is somewhat controversial, since some authors consider it negligible, whereas others have found that the bleeding from this artery in rectal excision may be very troublesome when the rectum is lifted off from the front of the sacrum (Turell).

Comparing the over-all scheme by which the small and large intestine receives arterial blood, the most striking difference will be found in the fact that the former is fed by numerous branches of one main aortic branch, the superior mesenteric a., whereas for the provision of the large intestine two main aortic branches, the superior and inferior mesenteric aa.

(Continued on page 70)

VENOUS DRAINAGE OF SMALL AND LARGE INTESTINE

(Continued from page 71)

All these tributaries follow closely the corresponding arteries, lying mostly to their left. Their anastomosing and arcade formation are the same as described for the respective arteries (see pages 67 to 69). In the region where the left colic and the upper sigmoid arteries take their origin from the inferior mesenteric artery, the corresponding vein follows a course of its own, separating from the respective artery. The vein takes a straight upward course, ascending behind the peritoneum, over the psoas muscles to the left of the fourth portion of the duodenum. It continues behind the body of the pancreas to enter most frequently (38 per cent of the observed cases) the *splenic vein,* at times 3 to 3½ cm. from the latter's union with the superior mesenteric vein, *i.e.,* the origin of the portal vein. In 29 per cent of individuals, the inferior mesenteric enters the superior mesenteric vein, and in 32 per cent it joins the latter and the splenic vein at their junction. In a few instances a second inferior mesenteric vein has been found (Douglass *et al.*).

The *portal vein* and especially the variations of its tributaries (see CIBA COLLECTION, Vol. 3/III, pages 18 and 19) are extremely important for the operative procedures recommended to produce a shunt of the portal blood flow (see ibidem, page 73) in order to relieve or ameliorate the consequences of portal hypertension (see ibidem, pages 68 and 69). It seems, therefore, appropriate to discuss in this volume those variations which particularly involve, in one way or the other, the venous drainage of the intestine, *i.e.,* those variations in which the superior or inferior mesenteric veins participate. Of the veins which in textbooks are considered portal vein feeders, the *superior pancreaticoduodenal vein* is in only 38 per cent* a single vessel but appears in 50 per cent in duplicate, one terminating in the portal, the other in the superior mesenteric vein. The gastroepiploic veins (see CIBA COLLECTION, Vol. 3/I, page 42) terminate, in 83 per cent of the cases, in the superior mesenteric vein but will, in some instances, join either the end of the splenic or the first part of the portal vein. The *coronary* (left gastric) *vein* ends mostly (58 per cent) at the superior aspect of the union of the splenic and superior mesenteric veins but has been found to join the portal vein in 24 per cent and the splenic vein distal to the just-mentioned junction in 16 per

---

*This and the following figures are from Douglass *et al.*

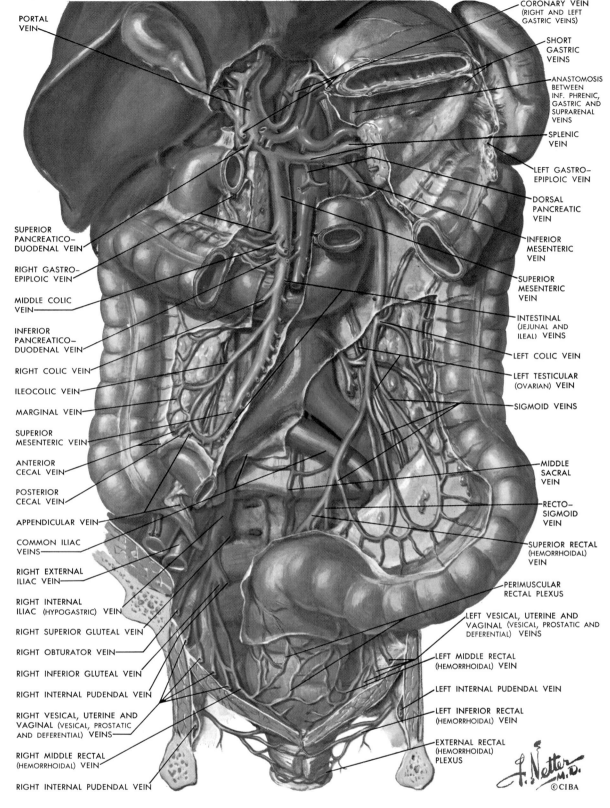

cent. More recently, it was found (Di Dio) to enter the portal vein in 66.8 per cent and the splenic vein in 33.2 per cent. The usually small pyloric (right gastric) vein (see CIBA COLLECTION, Vol. 3/III, page 18) terminates (75 per cent) in the portal vein within 3 cm. of its division into right and left branches, but in 22 per cent of instances it enters the base of the superior mesenteric or (2 per cent) the proximal segment of the right gastro-epiploic and, occasionally, the inferior pancreaticoduodenal vein.

The splenic vein, with an average length of 15 cm., is never, in contrast to the corresponding artery, tortuous or coiled. It emerges by the convergence of several trunks, arranged in fanlike fashion, from the hilus of the spleen. It demonstrates at its commencement a great number of different divisional patterns, which may include the short gastric veins and a superior polar splenic vein (Michels).

Essential to an understanding of the venous drainage of the rectum and anal canal is a basic knowledge of the regional anatomy (see pages 31 to 34 and 57 to 63). The veins serving these structures are the unpaired *superior rectal (hemorrhoidal)*, the *right* and *left middle rectal (hemorrhoidal)* and the *right* and *left inferior rectal (hemorrhoidal) veins*. These vessels follow the same course as their homonymous arteries (see page 70), but they return the blood into two different systems, *viz.,* the superior rectal into the portal system via the inferior mesenteric vein (see page 71), whereas the middle and inferior rectal veins drain into the vena cava inferior, the former directly via the internal iliac and the latter into the internal pudendal vein, which is a tributary to the internal iliac vein.

Radicals of the rectal veins begin in three venous

(Continued on page 73)

VENOUS DRAINAGE OF SMALL AND LARGE INTESTINE

(Continued from page 72)

plexuses situated in the walls of the recto-anal canal. The lowest of these plexuses, the *external rectal (hemorrhoidal) plexus,* lies in the peri-anal space (see pages 32 and 60), *i.e.,* in the subcutaneous tissue surrounding the lower anal canal below the intermuscular groove (white line of Hilton; see page 58). The *internal rectal (hemorrhoidal) plexus* is located in the submucous space of the rectum (see page 32), *i.e.,* in the loose submucosal tissue above the dentate (pectinate) line (see page 58). These two plexuses are sometimes collectively referred to as the submucous plexus or as the superior and inferior submucous plexuses. The third most proximal venous plexus surrounds the muscular wall of the rectum below its peritoneal reflection and is called the *perimuscular rectal plexus,* though some authors refer to it as the external rectal plexus, a term which leads to confusion with the first of the three plexuses described above. The perimuscular plexus, the component vessels of which are fairly large, withdraws blood chiefly from the muscular wall of the rectum and evacuates the upper portion into the superior rectal vein, but the chief route of drainage of the perimuscular plexus is to the middle rectal veins.

The internal and external rectal plexuses serve essentially the mucosal, submucosal and peri-anal tissues. The former encompasses the rectal circumference completely, but the greatest aggregation of small and large veins takes place in the rectal columns (Morgagni's) (see pages 58 and 60). The vessels returning the blood from this plexus course generally some 10 cm. upward in the submucosa. Branches deriving from these veins pierce the muscular layer of the rectum and communicate with the perimuscular plexus and directly with the superior rectal vein. Since these piercings of the musculature take place mostly above the level at which the perimuscular plexus connects with the middle rectal veins, it is apparent that the latter are to only a small degree engaged in draining the internal rectal plexus, and that the blood in this plexus returns mostly via the superior rectal vein.

Dilatation of the internal rectal plexus results in internal hemorrhoids (see page 170). Dilatation of the external rectal plexus or thrombosis of its vessels constitutes the external hemorrhoids. The two plexuses — the internal and external rectal — are separated by the musculus submucosae ani (see pages 58 and 60) and by the dense tissue of the pecten, but

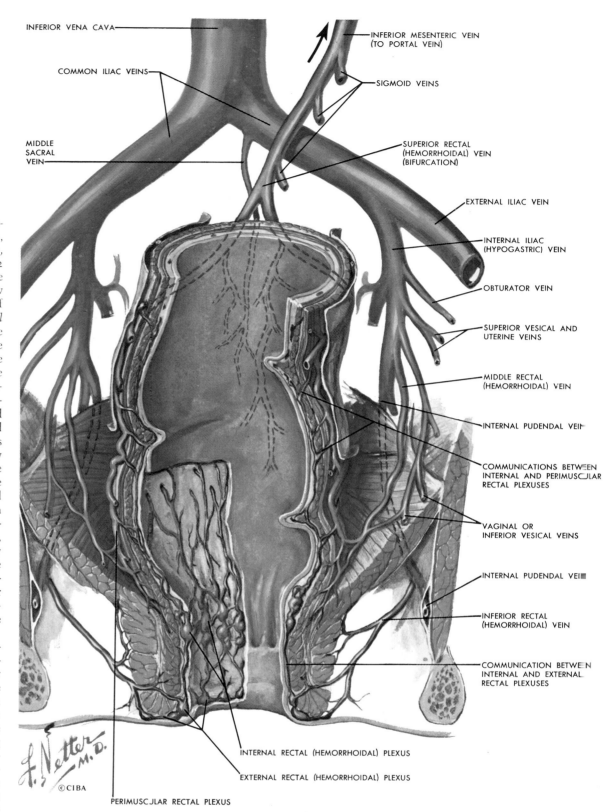

INFERIOR VENA CAVA

COMMON ILIAC VEINS

MIDDLE SACRAL VEIN

INFERIOR MESENTERIC VEIN (TO PORTAL VEIN)

SIGMOID VEINS

SUPERIOR RECTAL (HEMORRHOIDAL) VEIN (BIFURCATION)

EXTERNAL ILIAC VEIN

INTERNAL ILIAC (HYPOGASTRIC) VEIN

OBTURATOR VEIN

SUPERIOR VESICAL AND UTERINE VEINS

MIDDLE RECTAL (HEMORRHOIDAL) VEIN

INTERNAL PUDENDAL VEIN

COMMUNICATIONS BETWEEN INTERNAL AND PERIMUSCULAR RECTAL PLEXUSES

VAGINAL OR INFERIOR VESICAL VEINS

INTERNAL PUDENDAL VEIN

INFERIOR RECTAL (HEMORRHOIDAL) VEIN

COMMUNICATION BETWEEN INTERNAL AND EXTERNAL RECTAL PLEXUSES

INTERNAL RECTAL (HEMORRHOIDAL) PLEXUS

EXTERNAL RECTAL (HEMORRHOIDAL) PLEXUS

PERIMUSCULAR RECTAL PLEXUS

they communicate with each other through these tissues by slender vessels, which, however, increase in size and number with age and are also more voluminous in the presence of hemorrhoids (Reuther).

These connections between the external and internal, between the latter and the perimuscular plexuses constitute anastomoses between the inferior and superior veins and between the caval and portal venous systems. The significance of this situation is enhanced by the fact that the inferior and middle rectal veins and their collecting vessels, the internal pudendal veins, have valves, whereas the superior rectal vein is devoid of such valves, so that when the pressure in the portal vein rises, as in liver cirrhosis or other causes of portal hypertension (see CIBA COLLECTION, Vol. 3/III, page 72), the circulation in the superior rectal vein may be reversed, and portal blood may flow down through the latter vein to traverse the rectal plexuses

and be carried away by the inferior rectal vein, to be shunted via the internal iliac vein to the caval system. When this collateral venous circulation develops, the above-mentioned link between the perimuscular plexus and the middle rectal veins seems to play a less important rôle than does the route via the submucosal plexuses, which, owing to the increased blood volume and pressure, dilate to the extent that internal and external hemorrhoids are created.

In the absence of portal hypertension, spasms of the anal sphincter are said (Hiller) to be a frequent cause of external hemorrhoids, because they may shut off the outflow of blood to the inferior rectal veins. Internal hemorrhoids, on the other hand, may develop when alterations (dilatation as well as constriction) occur within the apertures of the rectal wall through which branches of the internal rectal plexus pass (see above).

LYMPH DRAINAGE OF SMALL INTESTINE

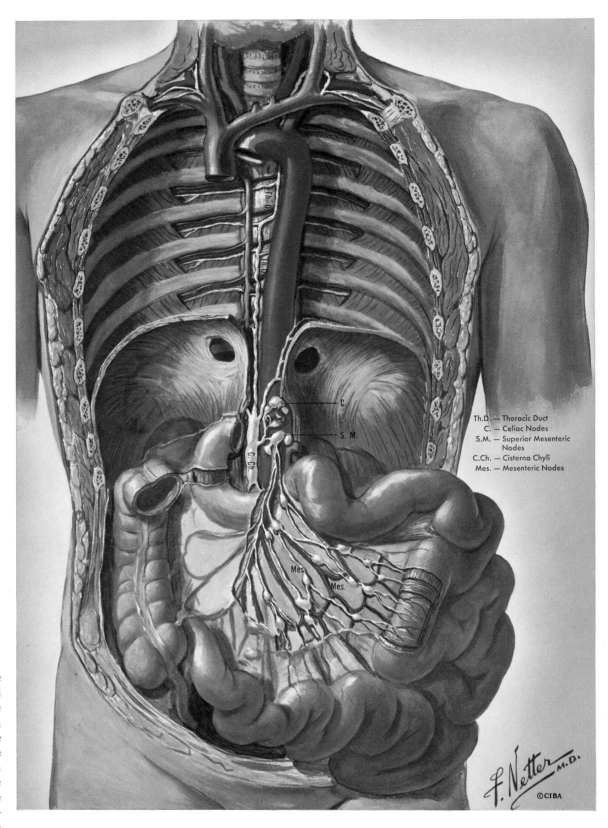

Th.D. — Thoracic Duct
C. — Celiac Nodes
S.M. — Superior Mesenteric Nodes
C.Ch. — Cisterna Chyli
Mes. — Mesenteric Nodes

The intramural lymph vessels of the small intestine begin with the central lacteals of the villi (see page 50). At the base of the villi, the central lacteals join with the lymph capillaries, draining the region of the crypts, thus forming a fine network within the tunica propria, in which the first lymphatic valves are already encountered. Many minute branches emerge from this network, penetrating through the muscularis mucosae into the submucosa, where a further network of lymphatics spreads. From this network, in which valves are a conspicuous feature, larger lymph vessels, receiving also lymph from the muscle layers and from the serosa and subserosa, pass to the line of attachment of the mesentery, where, together with the arteries and veins, they leave the intestinal wall to enter the mesentery. The lymph vessels of the small intestine have long been referred to as lacteals or chyliferous vessels, because they transport absorbed fat in emulsified form and appear, therefore, as milky-white threads after the ingestion of fat-containing food. The lymph vessels

of the mesentery drain through masses of mesenteric lymph nodes, which number some 100 to 200 and constitute the largest aggregate of lymph nodes in the whole body. They increase in number and size toward the root of the mesentery. In the root of the mesentery, larger lymphatic branches are situated, which lead into the *superior mesenteric nodes* (or mesenteric root nodes) in the area where the superior mesenteric artery arises from the aorta.

From the duodenum, lymph vessels — some of which run through the pancreatic tissue (see CIBA COLLECTION, Vol. 3/III, page 30) — pass to lymph nodes lying cranial, caudal and dorsal to the head of the pancreas; of these the upper are known as the subpyloric and right suprapancreatic nodes, the lower as the mesenteric root nodes (see CIBA COLLECTION,

Vol. 3/I, page 63) and the dorsal as the retropancreatic nodes (see CIBA COLLECTION, Vol. 3/III, page 30). Lymph flows from these various nodes into the group of celiac lymph nodes.

From the superior mesenteric nodes and the celiac nodes, the lymph passes through the short intestinal or gastro-intestinal lymph trunk, which is sometimes divided, like a deltoid mouth of a river, into several smaller parallel trunks, and enters the so-called *cisterna chyli,* a saclike expansion at the beginning of the thoracic duct (see page 39). The intestinal trunk drains not only the whole of the small intestine but also all organs whose lymph is collected in the celiac and superior mesenteric lymph nodes (especially the stomach, liver, pancreas and extensive portions of the large intestine).

LYMPH DRAINAGE OF LARGE INTESTINE

The first chain of lymph nodes encountered along the lymphatic ducts draining the large intestine consists of the not-very-numerous *epicolic nodes,* situated immediately beneath the serous membrane on the intestinal wall. (By no means do all the lymphatics draining the large intestine pass via these nodes.) The first important regional lymph nodes are the *ileocolic, right colic, middle colic* and *left colic lymph nodes,* appertaining to the respective regions of the large intestine. They start with a chain of nodes, collectively called paracolic nodes, which lie along the medial margin of the ascending transverse and descending colon and dorsal to these portions of the gut in the retroperitoneal tissue and, to a lesser extent, in the mesosigmoid, respectively. Each of these groups of lymph nodes pours its lymph into lymph ducts which run side by side with the respective blood vessels in a median direction toward the large prevertebral vessels. The majority of the lymph nodes along the course of the ileocolic artery receive their lymph from the ileocecal region, including the appendix (prececal, retrocecal, ileocecal and appendicular nodes). The fact that interconnections exist between the ileocecal and retroperitoneal lymphatics — including especially those which run near the spermatic vessels — accounts for the occasional migration of bacteria from the ileocecal zone into the superficial lymph nodes of the inguinal region. Similar interconnections also occur on the left side of the body. The larger ileocolic, right colic and middle colic lymphatics run, with the blood vessels, to the *superior mesenteric nodes.* The lymph ducts from the descending and sigmoid colon follow the branches of the inferior mesenteric vessels and lead to the *inferior mesenteric nodes.* The lymph from the region of the splenic flexure flows partly into the superior and partly into the inferior mesenteric nodes.

Some of the lymphatics emanating from the group of inferior mesenteric nodes follow the uppermost branches of the inferior mesenteric vessels (see page 67), pass from left to right in a craniomedial direction around the duodenojejunal flexure and lead to the region of the superior mesenteric nodes. In con-

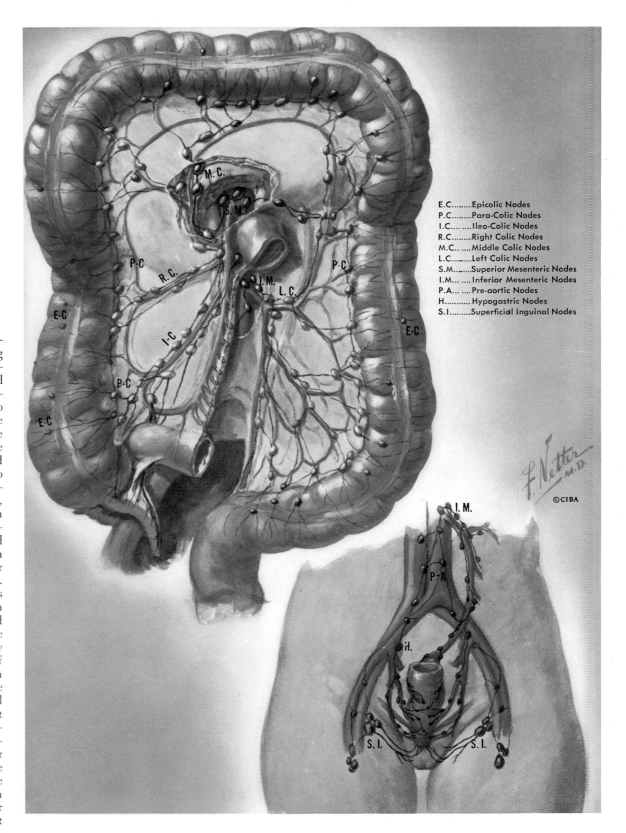

E.C.........Epicolic Nodes
P.C.........Para-Colic Nodes
I.C.........Ileo-Colic Nodes
R.C.........Right Colic Nodes
M.C.........Middle Colic Nodes
L.C.........Left Colic Nodes
S.M.........Superior Mesenteric Nodes
I.M.........Inferior Mesenteric Nodes
P.A.........Pre-aortic Nodes
H............Hypogastric Nodes
S.I..........Superficial Inguinal Nodes

trast, the lymph ducts draining the lower parts of the colon on the left run to the *pre-aortic lymph nodes* lying caudal to the inferior mesenteric nodes, and thence into the left lumbar lymphatic trunk.

The *lymphatics* emanating from the *rectum and anal canal* run in two main directions. From the lower part of the anal canal, they pass over the perineum, alongside the scrotum or labia majora and inner margin of the thigh, to the *superficial inguinal nodes.* The upper part of the anal canal is drained cranially via various intermediary nodes to the *pre-aortic lumbar lymph nodes,* which merge with the *inferior mesenteric nodes.*

From the region of the surgical anal canal (see page 58) of the rectum, the lymph passes first into the anorectal nodes lying immediately dorsal to the lower portion of the ampulla and from there to the sacral nodes situated behind and adjacent to the rec-

tum in the concavity of the sacrum. From the area of the rectal ampulla and above, lymphatics run direct to the sacral nodes, while from the lateral parts of the caudal region of the rectum, including the hemorrhoidal zone of the anal canal, lymphatics extend to the pararectal nodes lying in the paraproctium. From here the lymph flows through the lymphatics alongside the three hemorrhoidal (rectal) arteries (see page 70) in a cranial direction, i.e., (1) along the inferior hemorrhoidal (rectal) artery across the ischiorectal fossa to the *hypogastric nodes* (or internal iliac lymph nodes) and thence via the common iliac nodes to the pre-aortic nodes; (2) along the middle hemorrhoidal (rectal) artery direct to the hypogastric nodes and from there onward as in (1); and (3) along the superior hemorrhoidal (rectal) artery, then along the inferior mesenteric artery, to the inferior mesenteric nodes.

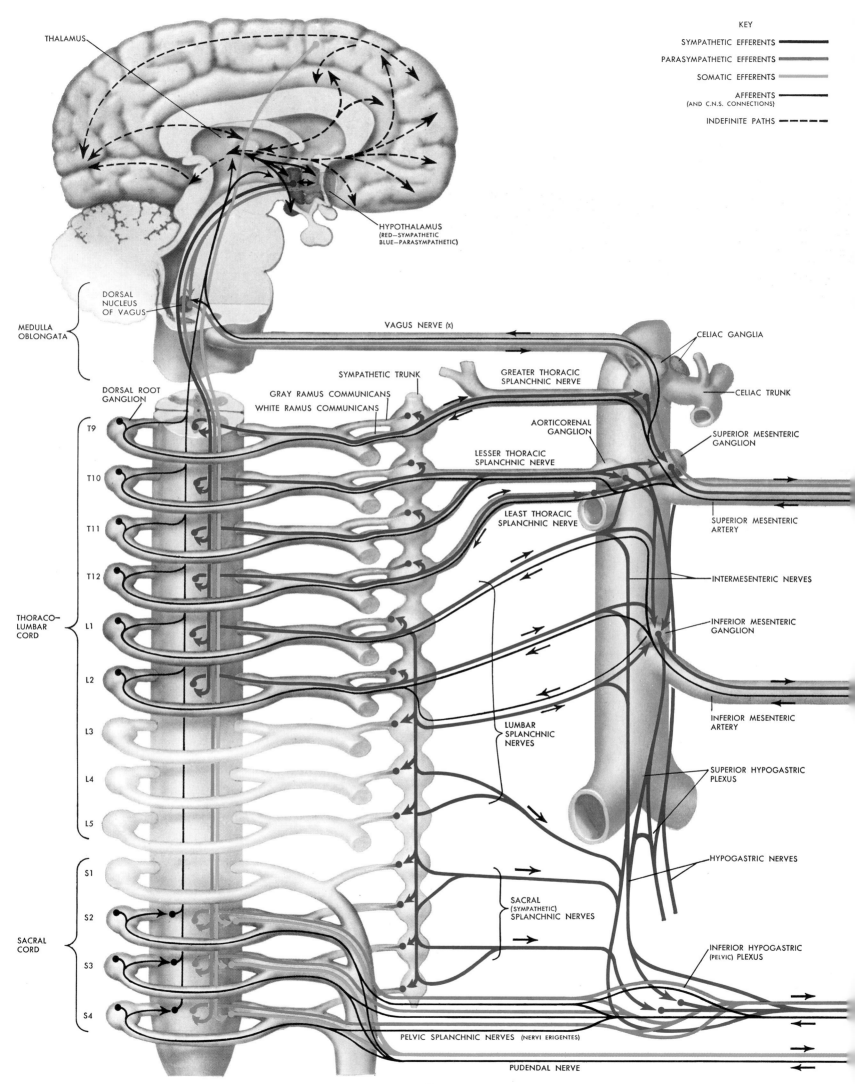

KEY
SYMPATHETIC EFFERENTS
PARASYMPATHETIC EFFERENTS
SOMATIC EFFERENTS
AFFERENTS
(AND C.N.S. CONNECTIONS)
INDEFINITE PATHS ----

THALAMUS

HYPOTHALAMUS
(RED—SYMPATHETIC
BLUE—PARASYMPATHETIC)

DORSAL
NUCLEUS
OF VAGUS

MEDULLA
OBLONGATA

VAGUS NERVE (X)

CELIAC GANGLIA

CELIAC TRUNK

DORSAL ROOT
GANGLION

SYMPATHETIC TRUNK

GREATER THORACIC
SPLANCHNIC NERVE

GRAY RAMUS COMMUNICANS
WHITE RAMUS COMMUNICANS

AORTICORENAL
GANGLION

SUPERIOR MESENTERIC
GANGLION

T9

LESSER THORACIC
SPLANCHNIC NERVE

T10

SUPERIOR MESENTERIC
ARTERY

T11

LEAST THORACIC
SPLANCHNIC NERVE

T12

INTERMESENTERIC NERVES

THORACO-
LUMBAR
CORD

L1

INFERIOR MESENTERIC
GANGLION

L2

INFERIOR MESENTERIC
ARTERY

L3

LUMBAR
SPLANCHNIC
NERVES

L4

SUPERIOR HYPOGASTRIC
PLEXUS

L5

HYPOGASTRIC NERVES

S1

SACRAL
CORD

S2

SACRAL
(SYMPATHETIC)
SPLANCHNIC NERVES

INFERIOR HYPOGASTRIC
(PELVIC) PLEXUS

S3

S4

PELVIC SPLANCHNIC NERVES (NERVI ERIGENTES)

PUDENDAL NERVE

76

INNERVATION OF SMALL AND LARGE INTESTINE

The nerves supplying the small and large intestine (and its vessels) contain both sympathetic and parasympathetic efferent and afferent fibers. They are branches of the *celiac, superior* and *inferior mesenteric* and *superior* and *inferior hypogastric plexuses* (see below). Good evidence has accumulated with regard to the importance of the *hypothalamus* as a source and terminus of pathways concerned with visceral activities, and it has *extensive cortical connections* with the premotor areas of the frontal cortex, the cingulate gyrus and the orbital surfaces of the frontal lobes. Descending fibers, germane to parasympathetic functions, arise mainly from the anterior region of the hypothalamus (preoptic and supra-optic nuclei, see CIBA COLLECTION, Vol. 1, pages 76 and 151) and form synapses with cells in the *dorsal vagal nuclei* and with cells in the *second to the fourth sacral segments* of the spinal cord. The axons of these cells constitute the *preganglionic (efferent) fibers* in the

vagal and *pelvic splanchnic nerves,* which are distributed to a large number of viscera (see CIBA COLLECTION, Vol. 1, page 81). As to the alimentary tract, the vagus nerves supply those parts derived from the fore- and midguts and the pelvic splanchnic nerves (nervi erigentes) innervate the parts derived from the hindgut. The intestinal preganglionic fibers carried in the vagal and pelvic splanchnic nerves terminate by relaying around the ganglion cells in the enteric plexuses (see below), and the axons of these ganglionic cells become the *postganglionic parasympathetic fibers,* which, together with the corresponding sympathetic fibers, serve the smooth muscle of the intestinal wall, the intramural vessels and the intestinal glands.

Fibers descending from the central nervous system, carrying sympathetic impulses concerned with intestinal activities (see also CIBA COLLECTION, Vol. 1, pages 81, 94 and 95), relay around lateral cornual cells in the four or five lowest thoracic and two or three upper lumbar segments of the spinal cord. The axons of these cells, representing the preganglionic sympathetic fibers, emerge with the ventral nerve roots of the corresponding segments (see CIBA COLLECTION, Vol. 1, pages 82 and 83) and pass in *white*

rami communicantes to the adjacent ganglia of the *sympathetic trunks.* Some of the fibers relay within these ganglia; other fibers traverse the trunk uninterruptedly, leaving it in medially directed branches as *thoracic, lumbar* or *sacral splanchnic* (pelvic sympathetic) *nerves,* which end in the above-mentioned plexuses to enter synapses with ganglionic cells. The axons of these cells, the postganglionic fibers, accompany the branches of the various arteries supplying the intestine. The chief *segmental sources of the sympathetic fibers* innervating different regions of the intestinal tract are indicated in the schematic drawing, but it should be kept in mind that, owing to overlapping, minor contributions may derive from adjacent segments.

Certain alimentary functions are probably controlled by simple reflex arcs located in the intestinal wall, but other reactions are mediated through more elaborate reflex arcs involving the central nervous system and consisting of the usual afferent, internuncial and efferent neurons. Numerous afferent fibers of relatively large caliber traverse the enteric plexuses without relaying and are carried centripetally through approximately the same sympathetic splanchnic and parasympathetic (vagal and pelvic splanchnic) nerves which transmit the preganglionic or efferent fibers (see also CIBA COLLECTION, Vol. 1, page 82). The afferent fibers are the peripheral processes of pseudo-unipolar cells in the inferior (nodose) vagal ganglia or in the *dorsal root ganglia* of those spinal ganglia which carry preganglionic intestinal fibers. The central processes enter the brain stem or the cord.

The intestines are insensitive to ordinary tactile, painful and thermal stimuli, although they respond to tension, anoxia, chemicals and so on. Specialized types of cutaneous nerve endings in the intestine are absent, except for the Vater-Pacinian corpuscles in the adjacent mesentery. The exact mode of termination of the visceral afferent fibers is, like those of the efferents, still problematic, but whorl, skein, grape, looplike and free endings have been described in the mucosal, muscular and serosal coats.

The "intrinsic innervation" is effected through the enteric plexus in the alimentary tract from the esophagus to the rectum. This plexus consists of small groups of nerve cells interconnected by networks of fibers, and it is subdivided into the myenteric (Auerbach) and the submucosal (Meissner) plexuses. The former is relatively coarse, with thicker meshes and larger ganglia at the intersections, whereas the latter is composed of finer meshes with smaller ganglia. The *myenteric plexus* lies in the interval between the circular and longitudinal muscular coats, and the main or primary meshes give off fascicles of fibers which form finer secondary and yet finer tertiary plexuses and which ramify both within and between the adjacent layers of muscle. Some fibers from the longitudinal intramuscular plexus enter the subserous tissue and constitute a rarefied *subserous plexus.* The network within the circular

(Continued on page 78)

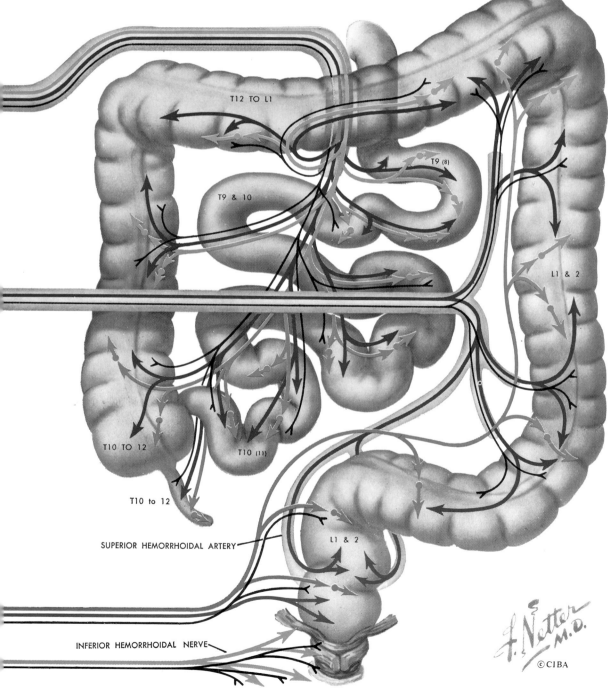

T12 TO L1

T9 (8)

T9 & 10

L1 & 2

T10 TO 12

T10 (11)

T10 to 12

L1 & 2

SUPERIOR HEMORRHOIDAL ARTERY

INFERIOR HEMORRHOIDAL NERVE

F. Netter M.D.

©CIBA

INNERVATION OF SMALL AND LARGE INTESTINE

(Continued from page 77)

muscle coat is sometimes termed the plexus muscularis profundus. The *submucosal plexus* is also subdivided into more superficial and deeper parts. Fibers from the latter enter the mucosa, where they form delicate periglandular plexuses. All these subdivisions are rather artificial, since all parts are interconnected, though the extrinsic nerves reaching the intestines along their arteries end mainly in the myenteric part of the enteric plexus.

The nerve bundles contain postganglionic sympathetic, preganglionic and postganglionic parasympathetic and afferent fibers, besides the elongated dendrites of Type II cells. The neurons are of two main types (Dogiel) — I with short dendrites, II with long dendrites; a subsidiary Type III possesses both. In general, these are multipolar cells, but some of them are pseudo-unipolar and bipolar neurons. The functions subserved by these cells are not clearly established, but the Type I may be connector, the Type II effector (motor, vasomotor and secretomotor) and the pseudo-unipolar and bipolar may be afferent and concerned in local reflex arcs, which are said to exist (Kuntz) in the intestines.

The exact course followed by the visceral afferent pathways within the central nervous system is not determined, though some evidence suggests that they behave in a fashion similar to that of the somatic pathways (see CIBA COLLECTION, Vol. 1, page 58). Some of the visceral fibers, entering the cord through the dorsal nerve roots, form synapses with posterior cornual cells near their level of entry, and the impulses are conveyed upward through tracts which lie near, or are commingled with, the anterior and lateral spinothalamic tracts. Other fibers ascend in the posterior white columns and may relay at higher levels in the brain stem. In the *medulla oblongata* these ascending fibers are joined by others from the afferent component of the *dorsal vagal nuclei,* and all continue cranialward in or near the medial and spinal lemnisci. Some of the afferent visceral fibers may pass with somatic fibers to the *thalamus,* and, like them, be relayed onward to the postcentral gyrus. Other fibers form synapses in the hypothalamus, whence fibers project to the premotor areas of the frontal cortex, the orbital surfaces and the cingulate gyri; actually, many of these hypothalamo-cortical connections are via relays in the anterior and medial nuclei of the thalamus (see also CIBA COLLECTION, Vol. 1, page 152). Possibly, the hypothalamus plays the same rôle in visceral afferent pathways as does the thalamus in their somatic counterparts (see CIBA COLLECTION, Vol. 1, page 72). (To indicate the fact that the hypothalamo-cortical as well as the cortico-hypothalamic connections follow similar routes, the lines rep-

SUBSEROUS PLEXUS

LONGITUDINAL INTRAMUSCULAR PLEXUS

MYENTERIC (AUERBACH'S) PLEXUS

CIRCULAR INTRAMUSCULAR PLEXUS

SUBMUCOSAL (MEISSNER'S) PLEXUS

PERIGLANDULAR PLEXUS

MYENTERIC PLEXUS (CROSS SECTION; HEMATOXYLIN–EOSIN, X 200)

MYENTERIC PLEXUS (PARALLEL SECTION; METHYLENE BLUE, X 200)

SUBMUCOSAL PLEXUS (LONGITUDINAL SECTION; HEMATOXYLIN–EOSIN, X 200)

LUMEN
MUCOSA AND MUCOSAL GLANDS
MUSCULARIS MUCOSAE
BRUNNER'S GLANDS
SUBMUCOSA
CIRCULAR MUSCLE
INTERMUSCULAR STROMA
LONGITUDINAL MUSCLE
SUBSEROUS CONNECTIVE TISSUE
VISCERAL PERITONEUM

Modification of a schematic drawing prepared and placed at our disposal by Mr. M. D. Thomas, B.Sc. (Hons.), Anatomy Department, University of Manchester, England

resenting these pathways have arrows on both ends.)

The *superior mesenteric plexus* is a continuation of the lowest part of the celiac plexus (see CIBA COLLECTION, Vol. 3/1, page 64) and surrounds the origin of the *superior mesenteric artery*. It is interconnected by stoutish filaments to the *celiac* and *aorticorenal ganglia*. A sizable, unpaired *superior mesenteric ganglion*, which is located usually just above the root of the artery, is incorporated in the commencement of the *superior mesenteric plexus*. The main plexus divides into subsidiary plexuses corresponding to all the branches of the artery (*inferior pancreaticoduodenal, jejunal, ileal, ileocolic, right* and *middle colic*) and innervates those parts of the intestine as indicated by their names, which, together, represent the lengthy portion of the intestine derived from the fetal midgut, extending from about the middle of the duodenum to near the end of the transverse colon. The nerves

and arteries follow the same route except for the patterns in which they approach the gut wall. The vessels advancing toward the wall form characteristic arcades (see pages 64 and 66), but the nerves pass straight outward without arcade formation, though small offshoots do accompany all the vessels and form their perivascular plexuses.

From four to twelve *intermesenteric nerves,* lying on the anterior and anterolateral aspects of the abdominal aorta between the superior and inferior mesenteric arteries and interconnected by oblique branches, form an open network, or plexus. The outermost of these nerves are lateral to the aorta and on the left side, and this may be of practical importance during sympathectomies because of the possible confusion between them and the nearby lumbar sympathetic trunk. Superiorly, the intermesenteric nerves

(Continued on page 79)

INNERVATION OF SMALL AND LARGE INTESTINE

(Continued from page 78)

are continuous with the celiac plexus, the outer ones being united to the lower parts of the celiac and aorticorenal ganglia and the intermediate ones being joined to the superior mesenteric plexus. Inferiorly, the outer fibers of the intermesenteric nerves pass down into the *superior hypogastric plexus.* The *first and second lumbar splanchnic nerves* (see Plate 30) usually end in the intermesenteric nerve plexus which gives off duodenal, pancreatic, renal, gonadal and vascular branches.

The *inferior mesenteric plexus* surrounds the origin of the *inferior mesenteric artery* and is composed mainly of the intermediate group of intermesenteric nerve fibers and smaller contributions from the outer intermesenteric nerves, as well as adjacent lumbar splanchnic nerves. One or two *ganglia,* lying contiguous to the artery, exist within the plexus. Continuations of the main inferior mesenteric plexus surround and accompany the left colic, *sigmoid* and *superior hemorrhoidal* (rectal) branches of the *inferior mesenteric artery.* The nerves, like the vessels, are distributed to the gut from the distal part of the transverse colon to the anorectal region. Their ascending branches communicate with nerves coursing alongside branches of the *middle colic artery,* and the lower branches communicate with hemorrhoidal twigs from the *inferior hypogastric plexuses.*

The *superior hypogastric plexus* (presacral nerves), situated in front of the dichotomizing aorta and between the diverging common iliac arteries, is a flattened band of intercommunicating nerves extending from the level of the lower border of the third lumbar vertebra to the upper part of the sacrum, where it ends by dividing into the right and left groups of *hypogastric nerves.* The upper and central parts of this plexus are continuous with the lower part of the inferior mesenteric plexus, and oblique *communications,* assumably conveying parasympathetic fibers to the distal colon, sometimes connect the latter plexus with the left side of the superior hypogastric plexus. The outermost intermesenteric nerves, passing down on each side of the *inferior mesenteric artery,* also join this plexus, as do the *third* and, usually, the *fourth lumbar splanchnic nerves,* which, via the hypogastric nerves, supply most of the sympathetic fibers for pelvic structures.

The *inferior hypogastric (pelvic) plexuses* are situated on each side of the rectum, prostate, seminal vesicles and posterior parts of the inferolateral surfaces and base of the bladder. In the female the cervix uteri and lateral vaginal surfaces replace the prostate and vesicles as medial relations. The inferior hypogastric plexus can be divided into *rectal* and *vesical parts,* or rectal, uterovaginal and vesical parts in the female.

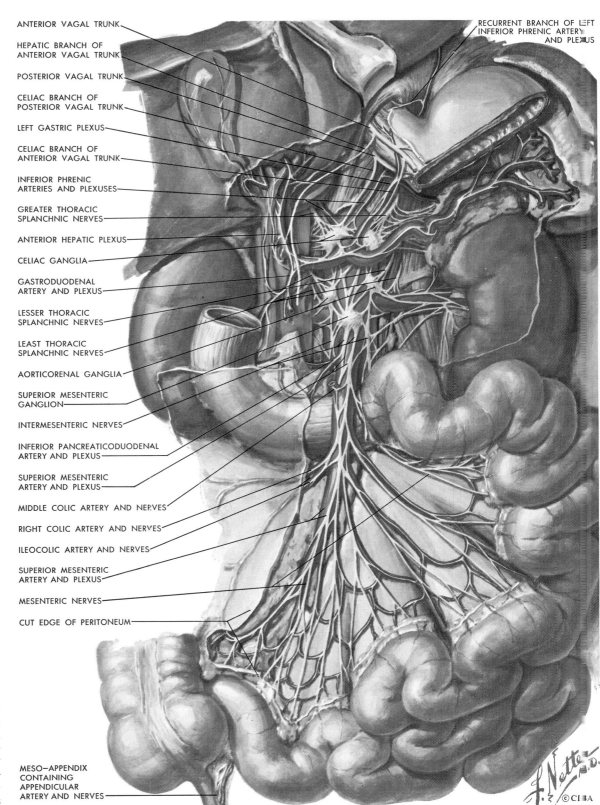

ANTERIOR VAGAL TRUNK
HEPATIC BRANCH OF ANTERIOR VAGAL TRUNK
POSTERIOR VAGAL TRUNK
CELIAC BRANCH OF POSTERIOR VAGAL TRUNK
LEFT GASTRIC PLEXUS
CELIAC BRANCH OF ANTERIOR VAGAL TRUNK
INFERIOR PHRENIC ARTERIES AND PLEXUSES
GREATER THORACIC SPLANCHNIC NERVES
ANTERIOR HEPATIC PLEXUS
CELIAC GANGLIA
GASTRODUODENAL ARTERY AND PLEXUS
LESSER THORACIC SPLANCHNIC NERVES
LEAST THORACIC SPLANCHNIC NERVES
AORTICORENAL GANGLIA
SUPERIOR MESENTERIC GANGLION
INTERMESENTERIC NERVES
INFERIOR PANCREATICODUODENAL ARTERY AND PLEXUS
SUPERIOR MESENTERIC ARTERY AND PLEXUS
MIDDLE COLIC ARTERY AND NERVES
RIGHT COLIC ARTERY AND NERVES
ILEOCOLIC ARTERY AND NERVES
SUPERIOR MESENTERIC ARTERY AND PLEXUS
MESENTERIC NERVES
CUT EDGE OF PERITONEUM
MESO—APPENDIX CONTAINING APPENDICULAR ARTERY AND NERVES

RECURRENT BRANCH OF LEFT INFERIOR PHRENIC ARTERY AND PLEXUS

These subdivisions abut upon the organs named. Each plexus is a thin, curved, fenestrated sheet of nerve bundles and ganglia, and each is connected to the superior hypogastric plexus by the corresponding group of *hypogastric nerves.* The upper parts of the plexus are applied to the lateral pelvic walls and the structures lining them. The lower parts are related to structures forming the pelvic floor, such as *levator ani* and *coccygeus muscles.* The sacral and coccygeal plexuses lie posteriorly (see pages 42 and 43).

The hypogastric nerves carry the majority of the sympathetic fibers for the pelvic plexuses, but other sympathetic fibers are conveyed through sacral splanchnic filaments from the *sacral* portion of the ipsilateral *sympathetic* trunk (see Plate 30). Parasympathetic (preganglionic) fibers, as well as afferent visceral and vascular fibers, enter the plexus as *pelvic splanchnic nerves* emanating from the sec-

ond to the fourth sacral nerves (see pages 42, 43 and 80). Some of these fibers end around ganglion cells in the pelvic plexus or plexuses; others pass through it to form synapses in minute ganglia located near, or in the wall of, the pelvic structures (distal colon, rectum, bladder, external and internal genital organs), to which they carry the impulses for vasodilator, viscero- and secretomotor functions. The old name for the pelvic splanchnic nerves, "nervi erigentes", indicates their effect in producing vasodilatation and congestion of the erectile tissue of the genitalia of both sexes.

The course of the parasympathetic fibers supplying the distal colon is peculiar. Arising on each side by several *rootlets from the inferior hypogastric plexus and hypogastric nerves,* they ascend along the sigmoid, crossing the superior hemorrhoidal and sigmoid arter-

(Continued on page 80)

INNERVATION OF SMALL AND LARGE INTESTINE

(Continued from page 79)

ies (see also page 70), and can usually be traced as far as the splenic flexure and distal parts of the transverse colon. These filaments supply delicate offshoots to the adjacent parts of the colon and communicate with branches of the inferior mesenteric plexus (see above). Evidence is available that these filaments convey the parasympathetic supply to the distal colon. Such an arrangement would explain why resection of the inferior mesenteric plexus (Rankin-Learmonth operation) spares the parasympathetic fibers to the distal colon but destroys the sympathetic supply. In a minority of individuals, most of the parasympathetic fibers to the distal colon follow an alternative route and may be carried from the inferior hypogastric plexus via hypogastric nerves to the superior hypogastric plexus and thence to the inferior mesenteric plexus *(communicating branches)*. Ablation of the latter plexus would, in such cases, destroy both the sympathetic and parasympathetic supply for the distal colon, and that explains why the Rankin-Learmonth operation does not redress the autonomic imbalances in all cases of megacolon. In some individuals the parasympathetic fibers may reach the distal colon by both of the routes described.

From the posterior part of the inferior hypogastric plexus, a series of twigs, often accompanying branches of the middle hemorrhoidal artery, detach themselves and enter the wall of the rectum. Occasionally, filaments pass to the rectum directly from the pelvic splanchnic nerves or the sacral parts of the sympathetic trunks. The rectum is also reached by terminal branches of the inferior mesenteric plexus, which follow the *superior hemorrhoidal* (rectal) *vessels* and communicate with the rectal branches of the inferior hypogastric plexus. In conformity with the general organizational arrangement in viscera which develop from midline structures, the rectum is bilaterally innervated, but the nerves from opposite sides communicate through the enteric plexus in the wall.

The subserous plexus exists naturally on those parts of the rectum which are covered by peritoneum. The myenteric (Auerbach's) and submucosal (Meissner's) elements of the enteric plexus are present in the rectum and anal canal as in other parts of the alimentary tract and extend as far as the zone of transition from columnar to squamous epithelium (see page 59). Above the pectinate line (see page 58) the ganglion cells in myenteric and submucous plexuses are almost as numerous as they are in the pyloric region (see CIBA COLLECTION, Vol. 3/1, page 46), but they rapidly fade out in the pecten and are entirely absent below the white line of Hilton. The myenteric plexus supplies the involuntary muscles in the rectum and anal canal

(Continued on page 81)

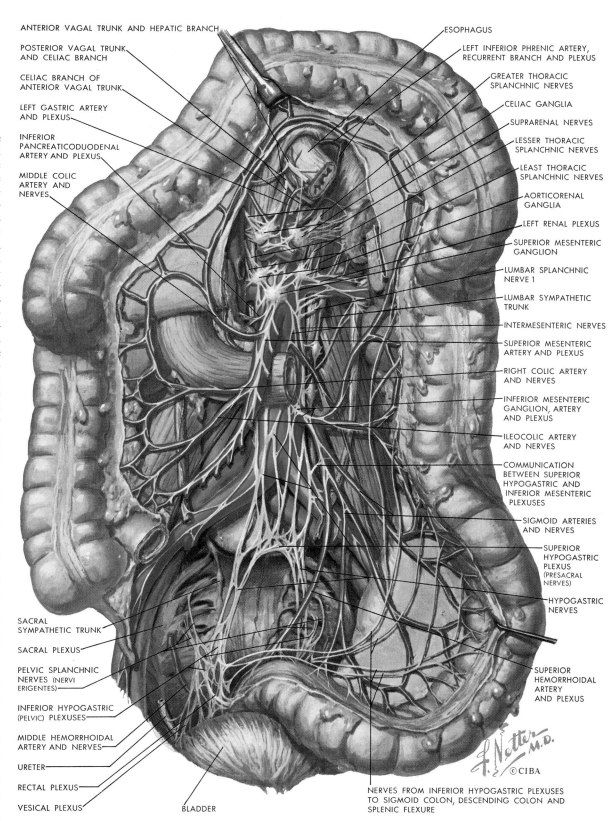

ANTERIOR VAGAL TRUNK AND HEPATIC BRANCH
POSTERIOR VAGAL TRUNK AND CELIAC BRANCH
CELIAC BRANCH OF ANTERIOR VAGAL TRUNK
LEFT GASTRIC ARTERY AND PLEXUS
INFERIOR PANCREATICODUODENAL ARTERY AND PLEXUS
MIDDLE COLIC ARTERY AND NERVES

ESOPHAGUS
LEFT INFERIOR PHRENIC ARTERY, RECURRENT BRANCH AND PLEXUS
GREATER THORACIC SPLANCHNIC NERVES
CELIAC GANGLIA
SUPRARENAL NERVES
LESSER THORACIC SPLANCHNIC NERVES
LEAST THORACIC SPLANCHNIC NERVES
AORTICORENAL GANGLIA
LEFT RENAL PLEXUS
SUPERIOR MESENTERIC GANGLION
LUMBAR SPLANCHNIC NERVE 1
LUMBAR SYMPATHETIC TRUNK
INTERMESENTERIC NERVES
SUPERIOR MESENTERIC ARTERY AND PLEXUS
RIGHT COLIC ARTERY AND NERVES
INFERIOR MESENTERIC GANGLION, ARTERY AND PLEXUS
ILEOCOLIC ARTERY AND NERVES
COMMUNICATION BETWEEN SUPERIOR HYPOGASTRIC AND INFERIOR MESENTERIC PLEXUSES
SIGMOID ARTERIES AND NERVES
SUPERIOR HYPOGASTRIC PLEXUS (PRESACRAL NERVES)
HYPOGASTRIC NERVES
SUPERIOR HEMORRHOIDAL ARTERY AND PLEXUS

SACRAL SYMPATHETIC TRUNK
SACRAL PLEXUS
PELVIC SPLANCHNIC NERVES (NERVI ERIGENTES)
INFERIOR HYPOGASTRIC (PELVIC) PLEXUSES
MIDDLE HEMORRHOIDAL ARTERY AND NERVES
URETER
RECTAL PLEXUS
VESICAL PLEXUS
BLADDER

NERVES FROM INFERIOR HYPOGASTRIC PLEXUSES TO SIGMOID COLON, DESCENDING COLON AND SPLENIC FLEXURE

	SYMPATHETIC INNERVATION		
Chief Visceral Afferent Pathways	Location of Cells		Chief Visceral Efferent Pathways
	Preganglionic	Postganglionic	
Branches from cervical and thoracic sympathetic trunks	T4-6	Cervical and thoracic ganglia of sympathetic trunks	Branches from cervical and thoracic sympathetic trunks
Gastric nerves → celiac plexus → superior thoracic splanchnic nerves; ?phrenic nerves	T6-9 (10)	Celiac plexus	Superior thoracic splanchnic nerves → celiac plexus → right and left gastric and gastro-epiploic plexuses
Ultimately aggregated in superior and middle thoracic splanchnic nerves	T9 (8)-10 (11)	Celiac and superior mesenteric ganglia	Superior and middle thoracic splanchnic nerves → superior mesenteric plexus → nerves along jejunal and ileal arteries
As above	T10-12	As above	Superior and middle thoracic splanchnic nerves → celiac and superior mesenteric plexuses → nerves along ileocolic artery
Ultimately aggregated in middle and inferior thoracic and upper lumbar splanchnic nerves	T12 (11)-L1	Superior and ? inferior mesenteric ganglia	Middle and inferior thoracic and upper lumbar splanchnic nerves → superior mesenteric plexuses → nerves along right, middle and superior left colic arteries
Lumbar splanchnic nerves and branches from sacral sympathetic trunks	L1 and 2	Inferior mesenteric and superior and inferior hypogastric plexuses	Lumbar and sacral branches of sympathetic trunks → inferior mesenteric and hypogastric plexuses → nerves along inferior left colic and rectal arteries

INNERVATION OF SMALL AND LARGE INTESTINE

(Continued from page 80)

(see pages 61 and 62). The voluntary external sphincter ani (in contrast to the involuntary internal sphincter whose function is regulated by the lower part of the intrinsic autonomic plexuses of the gut) is innervated mainly by branches of the *inferior hemorrhoidal* (rectal) *nerve* (see Plate 30) assisted by twigs from the perineal branch of the fourth sacral nerve and from the *perineal nerve.* This muscle's innervation is particularly rich, and it contains a profusion of motor end plates.

Specialized sensory endings exist in that part of the anal canal which develops from the proctodeum (see pages 3 and 4) and which is supplied by the inferior hemorrhoidal (rectal) nerve. These endings are absent in the region above Hilton's white line, where the afferent fibers end by breaking up to form fibrils or delicate plexuses between the epithelial cells. Thus, below the pecten this innervation resembles that of the skin, whereas above it the mucosa is supplied by sympathetic nerves deriving from the inferior mesenteric and inferior hypogastric plexuses and following the paths of the hemorrhoidal (rectal) arteries, and by parasympathetic fibers from the pelvic splanchnic nerves. All these nerves convey both efferent and afferent fibers to and from the terminal part of the gut. In accord with this difference in nerve supply of the anoderm (see page 58) are the differing sensory responses. The lower part, supplied by somatic nerves, is very sensitive to tactile, painful and thermal stimuli, whereas the upper part of the anal canal is almost insensitive to such stimuli but responds readily to alterations in tension. From the practical point of view, this neuro-anatomic situation explains why an anal fissure is so painful and why, in injections for piles, the puncture is scarcely .felt if the needle is inserted through the mucosa.

The table below is taken, in slightly condensed form, from Mitchell: *Anatomy of the Autonomic Nervous System,* with permission of the author and the publisher, E. and S. Livingstone, Ltd., Edinburgh, 1956.

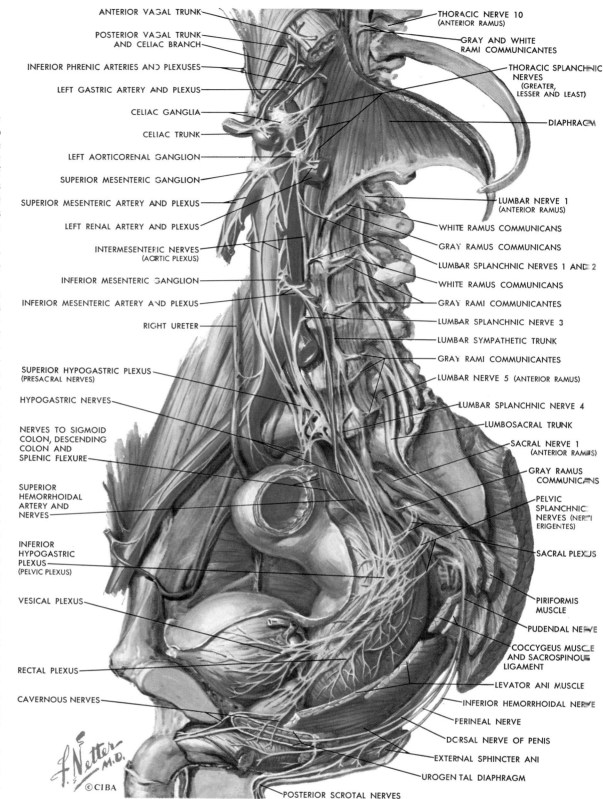

Main Functions	Structures	P A R A S Y M P A T H E T I C I N N E R V A T I O N			
		Main Functions	Chief Visceral Afferent Pathways	Location of Cells		Chief Visceral Efferent Pathways
				Preganglionic	Postganglionic	
Peristalsis diminution; ? pain transmission	Esophagus	Peristalsis increase; secretomotor; afferent transmission	Vagus nerves	Dorsal vagal nuclei	Enteric plexuses	Vagus nerves – directly and through esophageal plexus
Peristalsis and secretion diminution; pyloric contraction; vasoconstriction; pain conduction	Stomach	Peristalsis and secretion increase; pylorus relax; impulse conduction for hunger and nausea	Vagus nerves	Dorsal vagal nuclei	Enteric plexuses	Vagus nerves, gastric and pyloric branches
Peristalsis and secretion diminution; pain conduction; ? vasoconstriction	Small Intestine	Peristalsis and secretion increase; ? afferent transmission	Vagus nerves	Dorsal vagal nuclei	Enteric plexuses	Vagus nerves through celiac and superior mesenteric plexuses → jejunal and ileal nerves
Peristalsis and secretion diminution; pain conduction	Cecum and Appendix	As above	Vagus nerves	Dorsal vagal nuclei	Enteric plexuses	Vagus nerves through celiac and superior mesenteric plexuses → ileocolic nerves
As above	Colon to Splenic Flexure	As above	Vagus nerves	Dorsal vagal nuclei	Enteric plexuses	Vagus nerves through celiac and superior mesenteric plexuses → nerves along right and middle colic arteries
As above and contraction of internal anal sphincter	Splenic Flexure to Rectum	Peristalsis and secretion increase; relaxation of internal sphincter; conduction pain afferents	Nerves to distal colon and rectum → hypogastric plexuses → pelvic splanchnic nerves	In dorsolateral parts of ventral horn in mid-sacral cord	Enteric plexuses	Pelvic splanchnic nerves → hypogastric plexuses → nerves to distal colon and rectum

Section XI

FUNCTIONAL AND DIAGNOSTIC ASPECTS OF THE LOWER DIGESTIVE TRACT

by

FRANK H. NETTER, M.D.

in collaboration with

WILLIAM H. BACHRACH, M.D., Ph.D.
Plates 1-25

MITJA POLAK, M.D.
Plate 26

MOTILITY OF SMALL INTESTINE

The chyme, after its evacuation from the stomach, is propelled rather rapidly through the first and second portions of the duodenum (see CIBA COLLECTION, Vol. 3/1, page 81). The rate of progression diminishes thereafter, as the intestinal contents are moved forward and are continuously mixed by an intricate combination of various types of muscular contractions. The complexity of the intestinal motility may be appreciated by watching a motion picture of the exposed intestine in an appropriately anesthetized, recently fed animal, or by observing the intestine covered only by skin in patients with a large ventral hernia. Kymographic tracings of intraluminal pressures confirm what is observed directly or by radioscopy, permitting the separation of three principal configurations. First can be recognized periods of simple low spikes occurring at a rate of up to 14 per minute in the jejunum and 8 to 10 per minute in the terminal ileum. These spikes are the expression of the continuously shifting annular constrictions of the lumen, by which intestinal segments are formed, divided, re-formed, redivided, etc. This type of activity, the *rhythmic segmentation* (or the "pendular movements", as some authors prefer to call them), serves to mix the chyme with the jejuno-ileal secretions and to expose and re-expose it to various areas of the mucosal surface for maximal absorption. These movements also exert a pumping action on the mucosal and submucosal blood and lymph vessels, thereby enhancing the transport of absorbed material into the circulation. The rhythmic segmentations give way to periods of higher and longer-lasting contractions, corresponding to the second type of intestinal movements, the *peristaltic waves,* which (similar to the peristaltic waves of the esophagus, stomach and duodenum [see CIBA COLLECTION, Vol. 3/1, pages 76, 80 and 81]) move the intestinal contents along to more distal parts of the gut, where the rhythmic segmentation is resumed. They are slower and more sluggish than the rhythmic segmentations and move the intraluminal food masses at a rate of 1 to 2 cm. per minute, as observed directly or by X-ray studies. A third type of movement, detected kymographically by a progression of waves in multiple intraluminal pressure recordings, is characterized by the more rapid passage of a contraction wave over a long segment of intestine. It is described as *"peristaltic rush"* because, with such a contraction, the intraluminal contents move at speeds of from 2 to 25 cm. per second. The forward movements are, to some extent, and particularly in the lower ileum, counteracted by *reverse peristalsis* — antiperistaltic waves which cause a movement proximalward and serve to

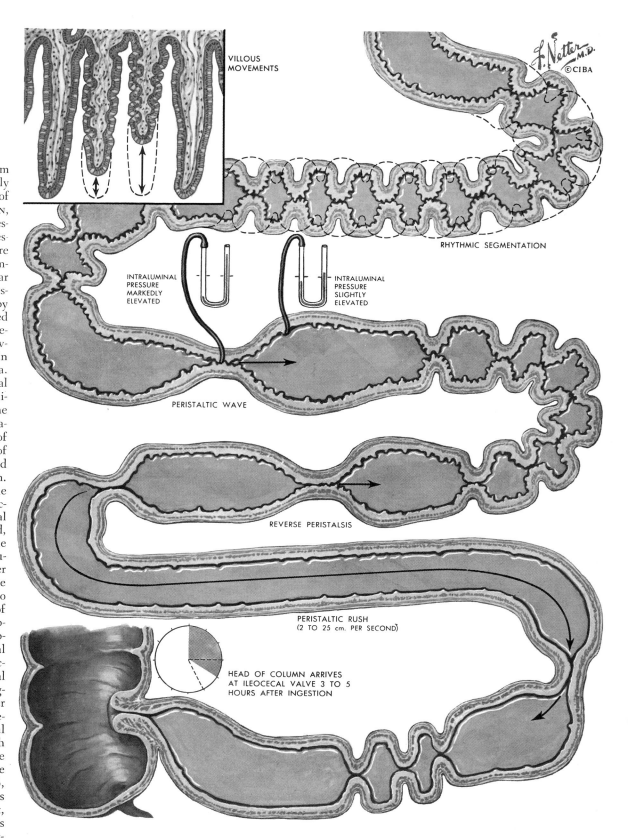

VILLOUS MOVEMENTS

RHYTHMIC SEGMENTATION

INTRALUMINAL PRESSURE MARKEDLY ELEVATED

INTRALUMINAL PRESSURE SLIGHTLY ELEVATED

PERISTALTIC WAVE

REVERSE PERISTALSIS

PERISTALTIC RUSH (2 TO 25 cm. PER SECOND)

HEAD OF COLUMN ARRIVES AT ILEOCECAL VALVE 3 TO 5 HOURS AFTER INGESTION

prolong the exposure of the contents to rhythmic segmentation. To these exteriorly visible movements must be added, finally, the *villous movements,* which shorten the villi without changing the external diameter of the wall and are thought to aid absorption by expressing the contents of the epithelial cells into the veins and lacteals.

Intestinal peristalsis is brought about by the contraction of the muscularis propria, comprising the outer longitudinal and inner circular layers, forming a continuous tube which lengthens, shortens, twists and constricts so that the enclosed contents are constantly agitated and propelled for shorter or longer distances until the remnants are driven out completely. It takes from 3 to 5 hours after ingestion of a mixed meal for the "head" of the intestinal column to reach the cecum, by which time the stomach is usually empty. The entire meal traverses the small intestine in 5 hours, a period which is shortened by the intake of another meal. Progress of the intestinal contents, owing to a more active peristalsis in the proximal parts, is more rapid through the jejunum than through the ileum. The function of the muscularis mucosae, a second muscular tube within the muscularis propria tube, remains unexplained thus far. The anatomic arrangement of this muscular layer renders it unlikely that it is engaged in the contractions of the villi, though a few of the muscle fibers within the villi (see page 49) are connected with the muscularis mucosae. The villous movements are probably initiated by stimuli furnished by components of the chyme acting upon the mucosal surface, or by a postulated, but not yet established, hormone called villikinin (see page 94).

The mechanism of peristalsis has been the subject

(Continued on page 85)

MOTILITY OF SMALL INTESTINE

(Continued from page 84)

of considerable investigation and speculation. From early experiments (Bayliss and Starling, 1899) it was concluded that the propagation of the peristaltic wave along the gut depends upon a contraction above and a relaxation below any point of excitation. This is known as the "law of the intestine" or the "myenteric reflex", but more recent evidence casts doubt on its validity. Thus it has been demonstrated that the segment immediately caudad to the point or zone of contraction is not "relaxing" but that distad to the segment in which both the longitudinal and the circular muscle layers contract, the longitudinal fibers alone contract, effecting a shortening and enlarging of the lumen. This would mean that the myenteric reflex involves differential contractile phases of the respective muscular components rather than a contraction-relaxation cycle, as the "law of the intestine" has postulated.

Another theory (Alvarez, 1928) ascribed the orderly progression of peristalsis to a number of gradients, which are defined as gradations in certain attributes, properties or biologic characteristics of the gut from the duodenum downward. The rate of rhythmic contractions, the propulsive force, tonus, resistance to distention and to the digestive action of gastric juice, secretory activity, oxygen consumption, carbon dioxide production, lactic acid, acetylcholine and catalase content, responsiveness to histamine — all these and many other indices of biologic activity, diminishing from above downward, comprise the *"gradients"* which, according to this theory, govern the transfer of material from the stomach to the colon. The integrated actions of the muscular apparatus of the intestines must derive from a fundamental and inherent property of the muscle cells, as may be concluded from the fact that evidence of polarization has been detected in mesenchymal tissue, from which the embryonic musculature of the gut develops, and in the catalase content of fetal intestines. Further proof is seen in the behavior of a loop of intestine which has been isolated, turned on its mesentery, and re-anastomosed in reverse, as indicated in the illustration. The peristalsis, under such conditions, persists in the original direction; *i.e.*, the peristaltic waves in the "turned" loop are opposite to the main peristaltic stream.

Neither the "gradient theory" nor the "law of the intestine", though both are concerned with the progression of peristalsis, explains how the intestine, when isolated as a small strip, is able to exhibit its coordinated contractile activity even when treated with cocaine, nicotine or atropine in doses sufficient to paralyze the nerve endings or to block nervous transmission to the muscle cell, or why

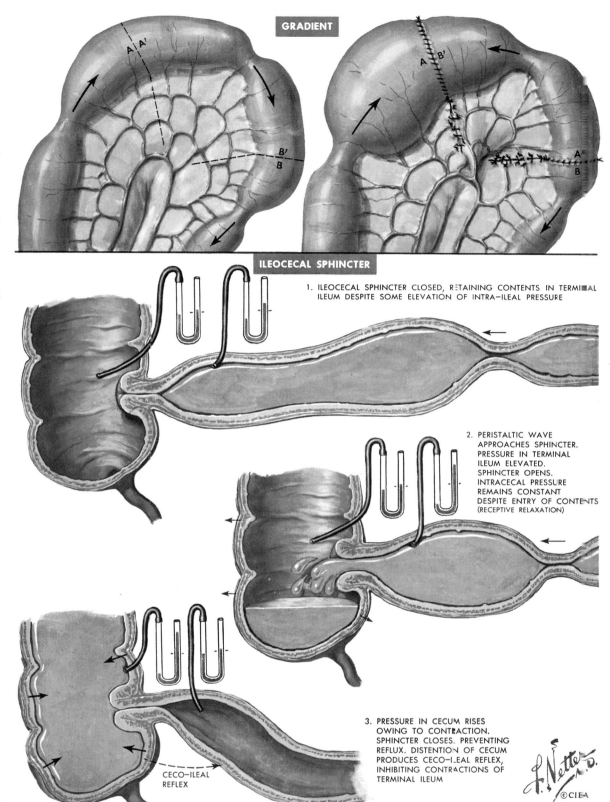

GRADIENT

ILEOCECAL SPHINCTER

1. ILEOCECAL SPHINCTER CLOSED, RETAINING CONTENTS IN TERMINAL ILEUM DESPITE SOME ELEVATION OF INTRA-ILEAL PRESSURE

2. PERISTALTIC WAVE APPROACHES SPHINCTER. PRESSURE IN TERMINAL ILEUM ELEVATED. SPHINCTER OPENS. INTRACECAL PRESSURE REMAINS CONSTANT DESPITE ENTRY OF CONTENTS (RECEPTIVE RELAXATION)

3. PRESSURE IN CECUM RISES OWING TO CONTRACTION. SPHINCTER CLOSES. PREVENTING REFLUX. DISTENTION OF CECUM PRODUCES CECO-ILEAL REFLEX, INHIBITING CONTRACTIONS OF TERMINAL ILEUM

CECO-ILEAL REFLEX

strips from which the intrinsic network has been removed are still able to contract.

Ileocecal Sphincter

The junction of the small intestine with the colon is sometimes referred to as the ileocecal valve (see page 52), partly because of its structural appearance in some anatomic specimens and partly because the end of the ileum, being wedged into the wall of the colon, seems to function, in some individuals, in the manner of a flutter valve. Observations on the living individual (Di Dio; see also page 52) indicate, however, that the ileocecal junction functions as a true sphincter, meaning that it regulates the flow of material from the ileum to the cecum, as well as preventing its retrograde passage. Thus the contact of the intestinal contents with the terminal ileal mucosa is prolonged, favoring maximal intestinal absorption. The

sphincter opens when a peristaltic wave, passing along the terminal ileum, builds up enough pressure to overcome the resistance of the sphincter. The cecum at first manifests receptive relaxation. Increasing pressure in the cecum, either by overdistention or by a peristaltic contraction, causes a reflex contraction of the sphincter, preventing overfilling of the cecum and ceco-ileal reflux. Frequently, material introduced by enema is observed to pass into the small intestine, probably owing to a functional incompetence of the sphincter or its reflex regulation. The significance of this sphincter mechanism in protecting the ileum from the reflux of cecal contents is conjectural. The hypothesis that the entry of the contents of the proximal colon into the ileum should result in absorption of toxic substances or in contamination by bacteria not ordinarily present in the small intestine, is not tenable and is not supported by good evidence.

MOTILITY OF LARGE INTESTINE

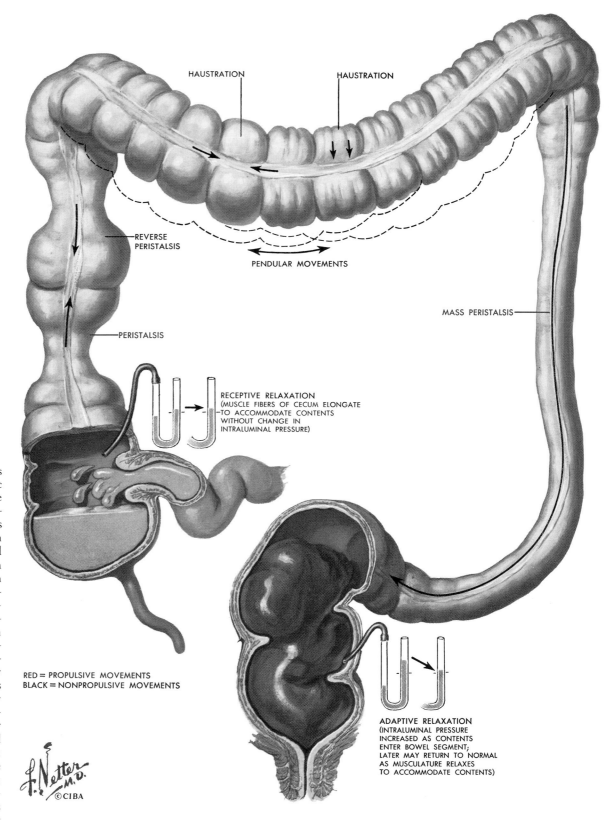

HAUSTRATION

HAUSTRATION

REVERSE PERISTALSIS

PENDULAR MOVEMENTS

MASS PERISTALSIS

PERISTALSIS

RECEPTIVE RELAXATION
(MUSCLE FIBERS OF CECUM ELONGATE TO ACCOMMODATE CONTENTS WITHOUT CHANGE IN INTRALUMINAL PRESSURE)

RED = PROPULSIVE MOVEMENTS
BLACK = NONPROPULSIVE MOVEMENTS

ADAPTIVE RELAXATION
(INTRALUMINAL PRESSURE INCREASED AS CONTENTS ENTER BOWEL SEGMENT; LATER MAY RETURN TO NORMAL AS MUSCULATURE RELAXES TO ACCOMMODATE CONTENTS)

As with the small intestine (see pages 84 and 85), various types of colonic movements can be differentiated. The *receptive relaxation* of the cecal musculature, as the terminal ileum evacuates its content, permits the accommodation of adequate quantities of the intestinal chyme before the activation of stretch receptors. The *adaptive relaxation* in other parts of the colon provides, similarly, accommodation of the fecal content without distress and without premature propulsion, as, *e.g.,* in the rectum when, for one reason or another, defecation is deferred. Such a "reservoir continence" function is a property particularly of the descending colon, and it is this feature which renders a colostomy a fairly tolerable and practical condition. *Contraction of the longitudinal muscular bands (taeniae)* shortens the bowel and forms pleats or sacculations (haustra) in which the residues of the chyme are retained to allow time for the absorption of water and a number of digestion products (see page 93). This function is abetted by *contractions of the circular muscle,* which may create small indentations within the haustra. These contractions of the longitudinal and circular musculature may be considered processes analogous to the rhythmic segmentations of the small bowel. *Pendular movements* — a slow swinging motion of the transverse colon — are probably brought about by changes in the tonus of the longitudinal muscles, and antiperistalsis, or retrograde movements, occur, to some extent, particularly in the right colon, but they are less typical there than in other parts of the intestinal tract. To these *nonpropulsive movements* must be added the *propulsive peristalsis,* which consists of (1) slow irregular contractions, which arise in a proximal segment and pass in a caudad direction for a short distance, obliterating a few haustra, and (2) the *mass peristalsis,* an analogue to the peristaltic rush of the jejunum or ileum (see page 84). The mass peristalsis, occurring only two to three times in 24 hours, initiated principally by the gastrocolic reflex (see page 95), propels the colonic contents toward the rectosigmoid by contractions which involve a broad segment of the colon.

The innervation of both the small and the large intestine has been described on pages 76 to 81. In studying the complex distribution of the autonomic innervation of the colon, it should be kept in mind that in the colon the distribution is extremely variable, particularly in the vicinity of the splenic flexure. The extrinsic nerves exert only a regulating effect on the intrinsic nerve network of the colon (see page 78), which functions autonomously and is capable of coordinating movements of adjacent segments necessary for peristaltic progression, except in a variety of pathologic conditions (see page 97).

The concept that the parasympathetics (cholinergic nerves) generally augment and the sympathetics (adrenergics) inhibit muscular contraction is acceptable as a convenient working hypothesis to formulate roughly the nature of the functional disturbances of the large bowel, provided it is understood that the net effect of stimuli reaching the colon from either component of the autonomic system is a resultant not only of the extrinsic stimuli but also of the reactivity of the intrinsic nerves, the degree of muscular excitation and other local conditions of the colon. Thus, depending upon the given situation, either cholinergic or adrenergic impulses may stimulate, on other occasions they may inhibit, and on still others they may mediate opposite effects simultaneously on different parts of the colon.

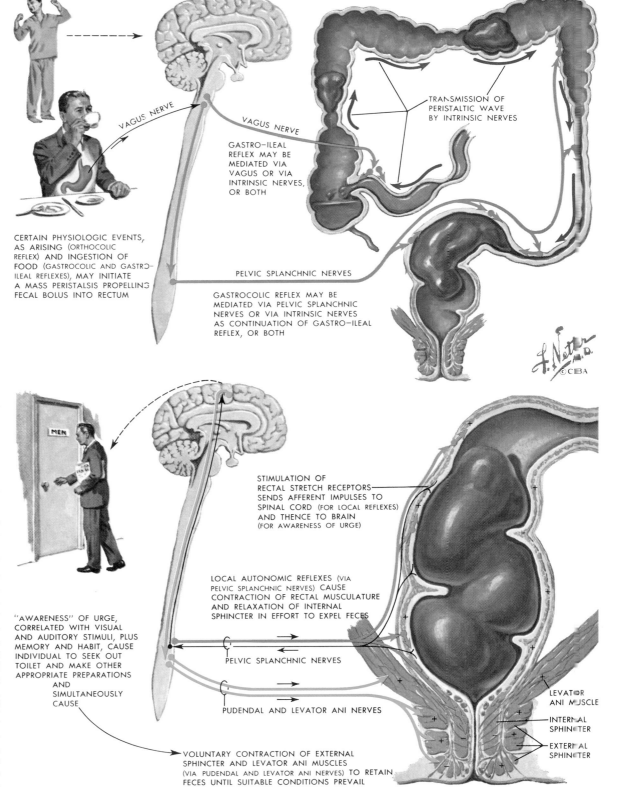

TRANSMISSION OF PERISTALTIC WAVE BY INTRINSIC NERVES

VAGUS NERVE

VAGUS NERVE

GASTRO-ILEAL REFLEX MAY BE MEDIATED VIA VAGUS OR VIA INTRINSIC NERVES, OR BOTH

CERTAIN PHYSIOLOGIC EVENTS, AS ARISING (ORTHOCOLIC REFLEX) AND INGESTION OF FOOD (GASTROCOLIC AND GASTRO-ILEAL REFLEXES), MAY INITIATE A MASS PERISTALSIS PROPELLING FECAL BOLUS INTO RECTUM

PELVIC SPLANCHNIC NERVES

GASTROCOLIC REFLEX MAY BE MEDIATED VIA PELVIC SPLANCHNIC NERVES OR VIA INTRINSIC NERVES AS CONTINUATION OF GASTRO-ILEAL REFLEX, OR BOTH

STIMULATION OF RECTAL STRETCH RECEPTORS SENDS AFFERENT IMPULSES TO SPINAL CORD (FOR LOCAL REFLEXES) AND THENCE TO BRAIN (FOR AWARENESS OF URGE)

"AWARENESS" OF URGE, CORRELATED WITH VISUAL AND AUDITORY STIMULI, PLUS MEMORY AND HABIT, CAUSE INDIVIDUAL TO SEEK OUT TOILET AND MAKE OTHER APPROPRIATE PREPARATIONS AND SIMULTANEOUSLY CAUSE

LOCAL AUTONOMIC REFLEXES (VIA PELVIC SPLANCHNIC NERVES) CAUSE CONTRACTION OF RECTAL MUSCULATURE AND RELAXATION OF INTERNAL SPHINCTER IN EFFORT TO EXPEL FECES

PELVIC SPLANCHNIC NERVES

PUDENDAL AND LEVATOR ANI NERVES

VOLUNTARY CONTRACTION OF EXTERNAL SPHINCTER AND LEVATOR ANI MUSCLES (VIA PUDENDAL AND LEVATOR ANI NERVES) TO RETAIN FECES UNTIL SUITABLE CONDITIONS PREVAIL

LEVATOR ANI MUSCLE

INTERNAL SPHINCTER

EXTERNAL SPHINCTER

DEFECATION

The mechanisms operating in the process of egestion of the alimentary residues are, in several respects, counterparts of those governing ingestion, particularly deglutition (see CIBA COLLECTION, Vol. 3/1, pages 74 to 79). Both functions involve simultaneous actions of voluntary and involuntary muscles, both are highly susceptible to derangement by emotional stimuli and both, though to a degree capable of autonomous regulation by intrinsic nerves, are seriously impaired by complete extrinsic denervation. Cerebral influences on defecation are exerted by neurons of the motor cortex, which permit the voluntary contraction of the external anal sphincter, the levator ani muscle and the musculature of the abdominal wall. A center in the midbrain has been shown to affect the tonus of the muscles of the rectum, and a medullary center in the floor of the fourth ventricle, after appropriate stimulation, appears to give rise to straining and the evacuation of stool. This center presumably involves autonomic fibers en route from the hypothalamus to the spinal cord to reach the distal third of the colon and the anorectal structures via the autonomic outflow, schematically shown on pages 76 and 77. Sympathetic impulses (via inferior mesenteric ganglia, hypogastric nerves and inferior hypogastric [pelvic] plexus) tend to exert an inhibitory effect on the rectal muscles and a variable one on the internal anal sphincter. Primarily responsible for the contraction of the rectum and the relaxation of the sphincter — and thus for the coordinated act of defecation — is the parasympathetic nerve center in the sacral segments of the spinal cord (a counterpart of the cranial centers regulating deglutition). The intrinsic nerve network, well developed in the anorectal region (see pages 77 and 81), coordinates the movements of adjacent parts of the anorectal segment and confers some degree of autonomy of action, independent of the extrinsic innervation. It is, moreover, significant that the voluntary nerve supply to the external sphincter and the levator ani (pudendal nerve) originates from the same spinal segments from which the pelvic splanchnics derive; this arrangement facilitates the reflex integration of the action of the sphincter and rectal muscles.

Of the many reflex mechanisms involved in the complex act of defecation, the following are manifestly of practical importance. Visual, auditory or olfactory receptors may inhibit or stimulate the rectum via the cerebral cortex, spinal autonomic pathways and lumbar or sacral autonomic nerves. Stretch receptors in the rectal mucosa may, via afferents to the spinal cord, influence the external sphincter and muscles concerned in squatting, bearing down, straining and supporting the pelvic floor. Receptors in the anal canal and external sphincter send stimuli via somatic afferents, to sacral segments of the spinal cord to increase, via autonomic outflow, the contraction of the rectal muscles when fecal masses are passing through the canal. Another reflex from rectum and sphincters through afferents to the sacral centers acts, via the autonomic outflow, to arrest micturition when defecation occurs. From receptors in the peri-anal skin, a reflex stimulates rectal contraction and transient contraction of the external sphincter and levator muscles via the sacral center. When the nerve terminals of the rectal mucosa are stimulated by distention, sensory impulses pass, via visceral afferents, through the dorsal root ganglia to the respective spinal segments, whence they are distributed by at least three

(Continued on page 88)

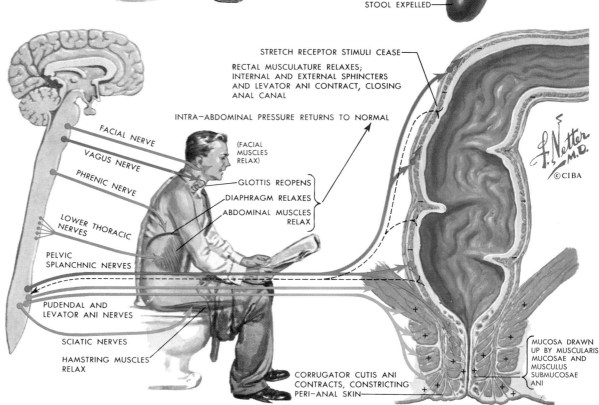

WHEN APPROPRIATE CONDITIONS PREVAIL
INHIBITORY INFLUENCE OF CORTEX CEASES

IN RESPONSE TO CONTINUING
STRETCH RECEPTOR STIMULI

RECTAL MUSCULATURE CONTRACTS,
INTERNAL AND EXTERNAL SPHINCTERS
AND MEDIAL (SPHINCTERIC) PORTION
OF LEVATOR ANI RELAX

INTRA-ABDOMINAL PRESSURE ELEVATED +

(LATERAL PORTIONS OF LEVATOR ANI CONTRACT TO MAINTAIN INTRA-ABDOMINAL PRESSURE AND SUPPORT PELVIC FLOOR)

FACIAL NERVE

VAGUS NERVE

PHRENIC NERVE

(FACIAL MUSCLES TENSE)

LOWER THORACIC NERVES

GLOTTIS CLOSED
DIAPHRAGM FIXED
ABDOMINAL MUSCLES CONTRACTED

PELVIC SPLANCHNIC NERVES

PUDENDAL AND LEVATOR ANI NERVES

SCIATIC NERVE

HAMSTRING MUSCLES CONTRACT TO INDUCE SQUATTING POSTURE

STOOL EXPELLED

STRETCH RECEPTOR STIMULI CEASE

RECTAL MUSCULATURE RELAXES;
INTERNAL AND EXTERNAL SPHINCTERS
AND LEVATOR ANI CONTRACT, CLOSING
ANAL CANAL

INTRA-ABDOMINAL PRESSURE RETURNS TO NORMAL

FACIAL NERVE

VAGUS NERVE

PHRENIC NERVE

(FACIAL MUSCLES RELAX)

GLOTTIS REOPENS
DIAPHRAGM RELAXES
ABDOMINAL MUSCLES RELAX

LOWER THORACIC NERVES

PELVIC SPLANCHNIC NERVES

PUDENDAL AND LEVATOR ANI NERVES

SCIATIC NERVES

HAMSTRING MUSCLES RELAX

CORRUGATOR CUTIS ANI CONTRACTS, CONSTRICTING PERI-ANAL SKIN

MUCOSA DRAWN UP BY MUSCULARIS MUCOSAE AND MUSCULUS SUBMUCOSAE ANI

DEFECATION

(*Continued from page 87*)

routes. The first goes via *ascending tracts to the sensory cortex* to engender awareness of the urge to defecate and to bring forth all the necessary voluntary actions connected with the discharge of fecal matter. The second impulse passes via connector neurons from dorsal to ventral horn cells to mediate reflex relaxation of the external sphincter and reflex contractions of the abdominal, perineal and hamstring muscles. The third reaches the lateral column cells, synapsing with neurons of the pelvic autonomous nerves, stimulating the longitudinal and circular rectal musculature for the coordinated action which drives the fecal mass toward and through the anus.

A mass peristalsis (see page 86), moving the content of the left colon into the rectum, may be considered to constitute the initial phenomenon of the sequence of events in defecation. The urge to defecate ordinarily occurs when the residues accumulate in the rectum; this happens at intervals varying from several times in one day to every fourth or fifth day. The majority of people feel this urge once daily, usually in the morning after breakfast, when awakening from sleep, assuming the erect position (*orthocolic reflex*), moving about and, particularly, the ingestion of food and liquids (*gastrocolic reflex*) favors the initiation of a mass peristalsis. Increased intrarectal pressure brings about a reciprocal relaxation of the anal sphincters, which, however, is counteracted by *voluntary contraction of the external sphincter,* which permits delay of defecation until circumstances permit the act to proceed. If the delay is prolonged, a temporary reduction in the intensity of the urge may ensue. These adjustments are a manifestation of the property of adaptive relaxation, *i.e.,* the ability of the rectal musculature

to adapt itself to continued distention by a reduction in the force of its contraction. It has been stated that the voluntary suppression of the defecation urge by contraction of the sphincter and levator muscles causes a diminution of the intrarectal pressure by forcing the fecal mass back into the sigmoid or even into the descending colon. Although this may be the case with fluid material, no evidence is available that it occurs with formed stool.

The urge, *i.e.,* the awareness of the need to evacuate the rectum, is responded to, under natural conditions, with a minimum of delay. The individual assumes a *squatting position,* which is facilitated by a reflex *contraction of the hamstrings,* one of those reflex mechanisms not yet developed in the newborn but acquired within the first 24 months of life. The squatting position supports the increase in the intraabdominal pressure, which is accomplished by con-

traction and *fixation of the diaphragm, closure of the glottis* and *contraction of the muscles of the abdominal wall.* The voluntary controlled contraction of the external sphincter is released, and the fecal mass is expelled by the increasing rectal contraction, which leads to intrarectal pressure of 100 to 200 mm. Hg (Hurst). Simultaneously, the muscles of the pelvic floor (see pages 22 and 63) contract, contributing to the forces that increase the intra-abdominal pressure but also acting to prevent the anus from being forced too far downward with the emerging fecal bolus. The content of the left colon, or part of it, may be emptied in a single, continuous peristaltic progression, or the anorectal structures may return to the resting state after the first bolus has been evacuated, until another contraction of the colon delivers more material into the rectum to set the sequence of events into action again.

SECRETORY, DIGESTIVE AND ABSORPTIVE FUNCTIONS OF SMALL AND LARGE INTESTINE

Secretion

The mucosa of the gut throughout its entire length is equipped with secretory cells (see pages 49 and 50 and CIBA COLLECTION, Vol. 3/I, page 55). The secretory product of the duodenal glands is an alkaline, pale-yellow, viscous fluid, consisting essentially of mucus, the primary function of which appears to be the protection of the proximal duodenum against the corrosive action of the gastric chyme. The glandular apparatus of the jejunum and ileum produces the succus entericus, the importance of which, in the normal digestive process, is difficult to assess in view of its being constantly mixed with bile and pancreatic juice. The intestinal secretion contains mucus as well as enzymes, namely, *peptidases*, nucleases, nucleosidases, phosphatase, *lipase, maltase, sucrase, lactase* and the coenzyme enterokinase, which activates trypsinogen and chymotrypsinogen of pancreatic origin to trypsin and chymotrypsin, respectively. From the fact that digestion may be only slightly disturbed in patients with a marked reduction of pancreatic secretion, it may be concluded that the intestinal enzymes may function efficiently enough to compensate for the loss of pancreatic enzymes. Under normal conditions, however, the succus entericus has a protective, diluting and lubricating function rather than a digestive one. Its flow is stimulated by the presence of an acid reaction in the upper intestine, by local mechanical and chemical stimuli, by administration of secretin, enterocrinin and pilocarpine; and by sympathectomy.

The mucous membrane of the colon, when stimulated mechanically or chemically, secretes an opalescent, alkaline fluid, composed of water, mucus and, possibly, some enzymes.

Digestion

The *intestinal digestion of proteins* is carried out by an array of enzymes, deriving partly from the intestinal glandular apparatus but primarily from the pancreas. The proteolytic action of the succus entericus, previously ascribed to a single entity called erepsin, depends upon a number of protein-splitting enzymes, each with a highly specific effect. Each one attacks only certain linkages of the protein molecule or of the degradation products resulting from the preceding effects of one or more catalytically active compounds. Similar to the specific activities of *trypsin, chymotrypsin* and carboxypeptidase (see CIBA COLLECTION, Vol. 3/III, page 55), the

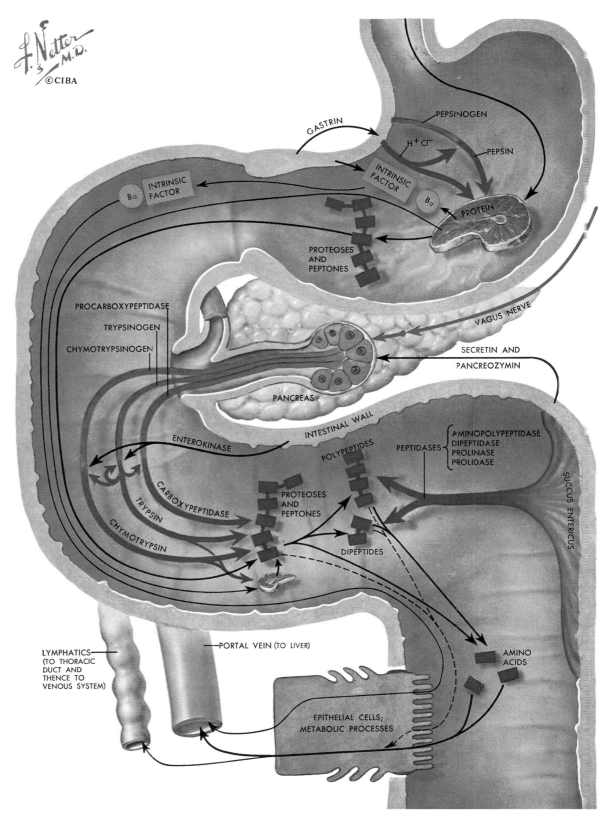

intestinal *aminopeptidase* acts only upon *polypeptides* or *peptides* containing a free amino group, liberating amino acids by scission; the *dipeptidase* acts only upon dipeptides, etc., until the original protein has been completely fragmented to its elementary components, the twenty-odd *amino acids*.

For the *digestion of nucleoproteins,* the pancreas supplies nucleases, ribonuclease, desoxyribonuclease and others which specifically hydrolyze nucleosides (pentose or desoxypentose conjugated to bases such as purines and pyrimidines). The intestinal secretion also provides nucleases and, particularly, phosphatases, which split nucleotides (phosphoric esters of nucleosides) into their components.

The processes involved in the *digestion of carbohydrates* consist generally of an enzymatic cleavage of poly- and oligosaccharides into monosaccharides. In human nutrition the most important carbohydrate

is *starch*, which is a polysaccharide occurring as an energy reservoir in plants particularly cereals, grains, roots, tubers, etc. The counterpart in animals is glycogen, another polysaccharide ingested with meat and liver. In both starch and glycogen, a large number of hexoses (monosaccharides) are linked together, forming either a straight or a branched chain of molecules. The linkage between these molecules varies, and, to open them, the organism is equipped with a variety of specifically active enzymes. The starch-splitting enzymes, called amylases, are secreted by the salivary glands (see CIBA COLLECTION, Vol. 3/I, page 71) and the pancreas (see ibidem, Vol. 3/III, page 55). The action of the amylases yields the disaccharide *maltose* and a polysaccharide fragment called *dextrin,* which is not attacked by amylase. The activity of the salivary amylase, known as ptyalin, is

(Continued on page 90)

(*Continued from page 89*)

exerted mainly in the inner portions of the food mass in the stomach before the gastric juice has sufficiently penetrated it but fails to penetrate the granules of uncooked starch. The more effective enzymes are the pancreatic amylases (two distinct types, the α- and β-amylase, have been recognized). Thus, except during the period of infancy, when the secretory activity of the pancreas has not yet fully developed, the degradation of starch into the disaccharide maltose and the monosaccharide *glucose* is completed in the lower part of the duodenum and in the jejunum and ileum. The splitting of maltose into two molecules of glucose is catalyzed by *maltase,* an enzyme formed by the intestinal glands. Other intestinal enzymes are *sucrase* (invertase) and *lactase,* which convert sucrose (our common kitchen sugar) into a molecule of glucose and *fructose,* or lactose (milk sugar) into glucose and *galactose,* respectively. The end products, thus, are simple hexose units, which the intestinal epithelial cell is prepared to absorb (see below). In the human, cellulose is indigestible, because man, in contrast to some animals, lacks enzymes capable of attacking the specific bonds of cellulose. Some exo-enzymes deriving from the bacterial flora of the human colon may act upon cellulose and upon the small amount of undigested starch reaching the distal gut.

The normal diet of humans contains a considerable amount of substances which, in contrast to carbohydrates and proteins, are not soluble in water but only in the so-called "fat solvents" (ether, chloroform, benzene and many others). This group of compounds, which includes entities of quite heterogeneous structure, is classified as *"lipids".* The term includes neutral fat, phosphatides, cerebrosides, steroids and fat-soluble vitamins. From the dietary point of view, the neutral fats are of major importance, mostly on account of their high energy value. Neutral fats, whether of plant or of animal origin, are esters of glycerol and fatty acids. These esters are called *triglycerides,* because the three alcoholic hydroxyl groups of glycerol are bound in an ester linkage to the carboxyl group (the group which determines the acid character) of either saturated or unsaturated organic acids, such as palmitic, stearic, oleic or linoleic. The *neutral fat* (neutral because no acidic group is free) is *digested* by hydrolyzation of the ester linkage, yielding the components of the esters, namely, *glycerol* and the various *fatty acids.* Evidence has been offered in recent decades that some fat molecules may escape digestion and be absorbed unchanged (see below) and that the splitting of fat occurs in stages, meaning that the *triglycerides* lose first one of the three acid molecules, leaving a *diglyceride, i.e.,* a glycerol ester containing only two acids, and this, in turn, is hydrolyzed to a *monoglyceride,* which possesses only one acid molecule. Thus, the digestion of fat furnishes a multiplicity of split products, the ratio of which, in the intestinal lumen, varies to a great extent.

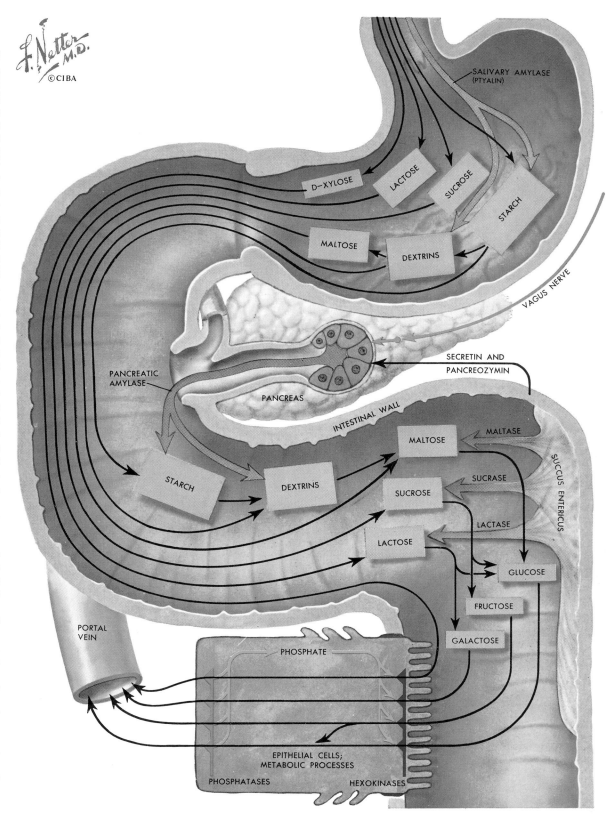

The hydrolysis of fat is accomplished by active substances called *lipases,* which are secreted by the pancreas and to a much lesser extent by the intestinal glands. A negligible amount of fat may be digested in the stomach by a lipase of gastric origin, which, in contrast to other lipases, acts in a nearly neutral environment. In adult life this gastric lipase is of no practical significance, but it may play a rôle in infancy and may be capable of hydrolyzing the highly emulsified fat of the milk. The bulk of fat in the adult diet is digested by the pancreatic lipase. In the lower duodenum the fat is mixed with bile and dispersed into a fine emulsion. The components of bile responsible for this action are the bile acids, mostly glycocholic and taurocholic acid, which are most powerful detergents. The result of the emulsification of fat in the aqueous medium of the intestinal chyme is an enormous increase of the surface of the fat particles,

facilitating the hydrolytic action of the pancreatic and intestinal lipases. As is the case with the majority of biologically active catalysts, the chemical structure of the lipolytic enzymes is unknown, nor is it known whether one lipase or several of them are produced by the cells from which they originate. In contrast to the enzymes involved in protein and carbohydrate digestion, which act with a high degree of specificity upon certain compounds or chemically well-defined groups or bonds, the action of lipases of animal or plant origin is far less specific. Being esterases, they act exclusively upon esters. It is, however, characteristic of the lipases (as of all esterases) that they not only catalyze the hydrolysis of esters but also the opposite reaction, namely, the synthesis of esters. In other words, the splitting of an ester by lipase is an easily reversible action. Hydrolysis and esterification can

(*Continued on page 92*)

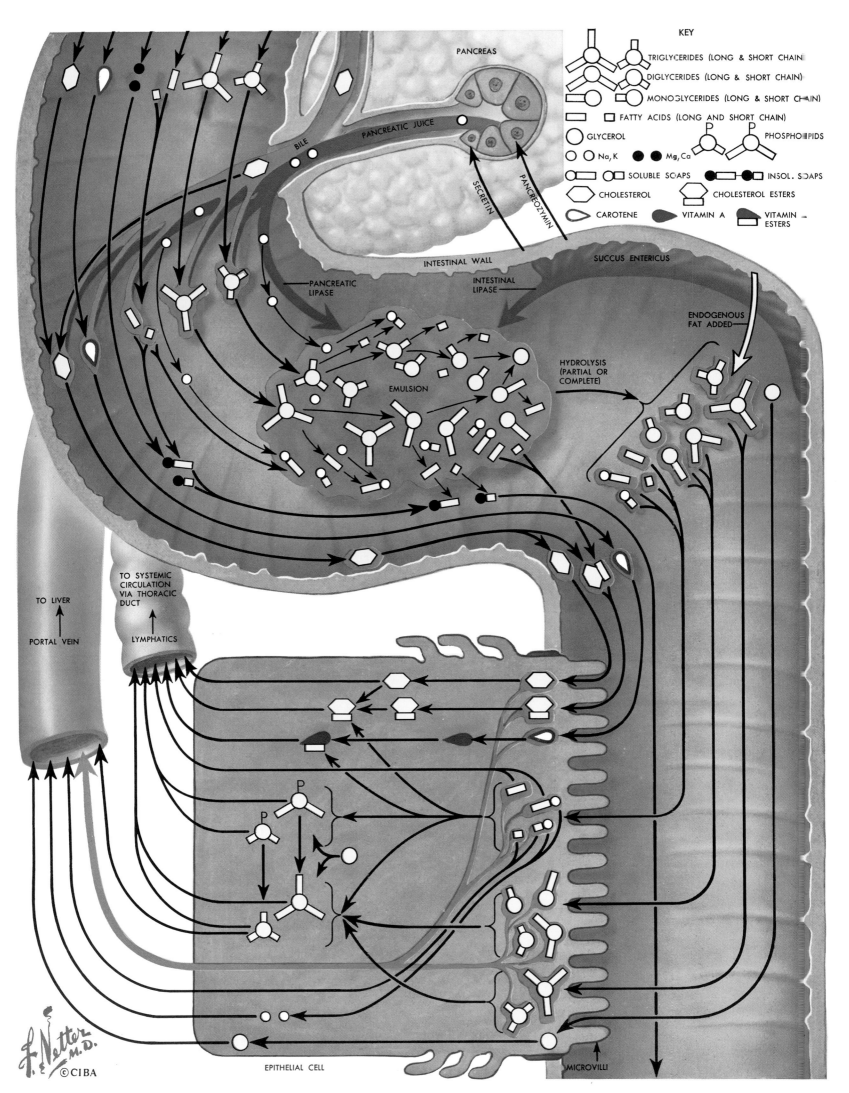

(Continued from page 90)

proceed simultaneously, the rate of the two reactions depending on an equilibrium (between substrate, enzyme, the substrate-enzyme complex and the reaction products), which has been well studied in vitro but, owing to its complexity, not in vivo. At any rate, this feature of lipase activity obviously contributes to the constant presence of tri-, di- and monoglycerides, glycerol and fatty acids in the intestinal chyme.

The fatty acids, whether ingested with the food or arising as split products of fat hydrolysis, combine in the intestine with cations, forming soluble soaps with Na and K and insoluble soaps with Ca and Mg. The soluble alkali soaps aid in the emulsification of fat and the stabilization of emulsified lipids by the same principle which makes soap useful in the household for cleansing and detergent effects. The formation of insoluble soaps represents also a sort of regulating mechanism in so far as it withdraws the fatty acids from the reaction mixture of enzymes, fat and its split products.

Other lipids, such as vitamin A (and its provitamin carotene), vitamins E and K_1, the steroids, including cholesterol and vitamin D, are not broken down within the intestine. The phospholipids (phosphatides) may remain in part unchanged, and in part are hydrolyzed into their components, viz., glycerol, fatty acids, phosphate and the special compound characteristic of the particular phospholipid (choline, serine, inositol or ethanolamine). The pancreatic juice contains a specific lecithinase which liberates isolecithin, a compound said to aid in the emulsification of dietary fat.

Absorption

The purpose of the complex enzymatic reactions to which foodstuffs are exposed within the intestinal lumen is to prepare the nutrients for transfer into and assimilation within the organism. The lumen, i.e., the space encompassed by the wall of the digestive tube, belongs, fundamentally speaking, to the outside world, and the process, or processes, by which the products of digestion enter and pass through the intestinal wall into the circulation is called absorption. The site of absorption is almost exclusively the duodenal, jejunal and ileal surface epithelium, although it is known that some absorption may take place in the colon (see below) and that both the oral and gastric mucosae are able to absorb some material. The epithelial lining of the small intestine (see pages 49 and 50) is pre-eminently and specifically equipped for its function by its length and its large surface area. The mechanisms involved in the absorptive process, though they have been studied during many past decades, have by no means been completely elucidated. The simple concept, held for some time, that this transport of nutritive split products into and out of the intestinal cells rests solely upon a few physicochemical phenomena, such as filtration, diffusion and osmosis, has been expanded by more recent studies indicating that the complexity of factors involved in the process of absorption includes, besides filtration, diffusion and osmosis, such phenomena as pinocytosis, electromotion, participation of carriers and a number of "active" energy-consuming mechanisms. The sole fact that several substances are absorbed against a concentration gradient is proof that specific cellular activities are necessary to make absorption possible, so to speak, against the physical rules that govern diffusion and osmosis. It is impossible to describe absorption in general

terms, not only because our knowledge of it is fragmentary, and to a great extent still controversial, but also because, for almost every single substance offered for absorption, a different mechanism or a different pathway is employed.

Water crosses the intestinal wall in both directions, depending essentially upon the concentration of solutes in the chyme. If the aqueous phase of the intestinal contents is hypotonic, water moves from the lumen through the cells or, possibly, between the cells through pericellular spaces into the blood (Visscher). Vice versa, if the chyme is hypertonic, water will be transferred from the blood into the lumen. As crystalloid solutes enter the wall, an obligatory transport of water from the lumen occurs to keep the solution within the tube from becoming too hypotonic. It has been suggested that the movements of water to and from the intestinal wall are regulated by osmotic forces.

A great part of the minerals, such as the salts composed of sodium, potassium and chloride ions, move with the water, but, in addition, some specific processes must be inferred to explain the selective absorption of chlorides in the presence of sulfates or the absorption of NaCl against a steep concentration gradient (Jacobs). The optimal absorption of calcium ensues under conditions of proper pH, adequate supply of bile, in the presence of a favorable ratio of digestible fat, and in the absence of those substances which, like oxalic or phytic acid, form insoluble calcium salts. The fact that diversion of bile from the intestine diminishes and stimulation of bile flow increases the absorption of calcium suggests that calcium may be transferred into and through the cells in a combination with bile acids. Large amounts of lactose (or galactose) improve the conditions for calcium absorption, especially in children, owing to the presence of lactobacilli in the gut, which ferment lactose to lactic acid, which, in turn, acidifying the intestinal contents, increases the solubility of calcium phosphate. Strong evidence is available to indicate that vitamin D, by means of a completely unknown mechanism, mediates calcium absorption. Little is known about the conditions and processes involved in the absorption of magnesium, which probably follows much the same lines as calcium. Phosphorus in the intestine, predominantly present in the form of orthophosphate, is presumably transported after esterification at the cell surface. (Iron absorption is discussed on page 88, Ciba Collection, Vol. 3/III.)

The products of protein digestion, the amino acids, are apparently absorbed (see Plate 6) as promptly as they are split off from the proteins. The mechanism by which the transfer is accomplished is obscure, but it clearly involves more than simple diffusion or osmotic movement through the cell. The rate of absorption for various amino acids is different. With the exception of tryptophan, leucine, isoleucine, valine and alanine, the L-isomers are more readily transferred than are the D-isomers. By far the greater part of the amino acids enter the circulation via the portal vein; only a small amount may leave the intestine by way of the lymphatics. Significant quantities of peptides, either entering the cells or synthesized within them, reach the circulation, as indicated by a rise of peptide nitrogen in the blood. Under special circumstances, e.g., when proteolytic enzymes are inadequately secreted or when, for unknown reasons, as in many allergic conditions, the barrier function of the epithelial lining is disturbed, intact protein molecules may be absorbed.

Carbohydrates are absorbed (see Plate 7)

almost exclusively in the form of monosaccharides, i.e., as hexoses (glucose, fructose and galactose) or pentoses (ribose, arabinose). The absorption of small amounts of disaccharides (sucrose and lactose) has been demonstrated but is of no practical significance. Galactose is more rapidly absorbed than is glucose, and the latter more rapidly than is fructose. Within fairly wide limits, the rate of hexose transfer is independent of the concentration in the chyme. From the differences in the rate of absorption of the hexoses, which should diffuse with the same speed; from the fact that one and the same hexose is more readily absorbed in the form of its dextrorotatory stereoisomer than it is absorbed as a levorotatory stereoisomer; and from the fact that pentoses, in spite of their smaller molecular structure, actually need more time to pass through the wall, it must be concluded that the transport of these simple sugars involves more than diffusion. The active, selective processes which are involved await clarification. The presence of enzymes (hexokinases) catalyzing the conversion of hexoses to hexose phosphates in the intestinal mucosa and the reduction of glucose and galactose absorption when the hexokinases are inhibited by phlorizin suggest the possibility that a phosphorylation mechanism is the active process in sugar absorption. Other evidences, however, are not in harmony with such an assumption. The picture of the absorption of pentoses is still less clear. The transfer of xylose, used now as an indicator of the efficiency of intestinal absorption (see page 107), may involve diffusion or phosphorylation, or both.

The mechanisms of absorption of fat are also still controversial. Present evidence suggests that every single component of the digestion mixture — the partially hydrolyzed products (di- and monoglycerides), the completely hydrolyzed fat components (glycerol and fatty acids), as well as undigested fat molecules — can enter the intestinal cells, and that the split products are resynthesized within the cell to fat, which leaves the cell via the lymphatics. Furthermore, it seems that glycerol and the alkali salts of long- and short-chained fatty acids (soaps), being watersoluble compounds, can enter the epithelial cell by diffusion and that the mono- and diesters of glycerol may cross the intestinal barrier without further cleavage, either in combination with bile components or on their own. All these split products are apparently re-esterified within the intestinal lining to triglycerides and, as such, they leave the cell through the lacteals (see also page 50). Esterifying enzymes are present in the cells, but it is an open question whether the cell produces them or whether they derive from the esterases in the intestinal chyme. It is possible that the pumping action of the villi plays a significant rôle in the transfer of the fat from the cells to the lacteals. In view of the prompt intracellular esterification of the split products, it is difficult to decide whether or not unhydrolyzed fat particles pass through the cell membranes from the lumen, as has been concluded from recent studies with radioactive carbon (C^{14}) incorporated into fat or its split products. Bile is important not only for the emulsification of ingested fat (see above), but it serves also as the carrier for the water-insoluble or less soluble components in the digestion mixture. Insoluble soaps, the monoglycerides, are probably "ferried" through the cellular barrier by bile acids in the form of chemical complexes, which separate in the cell spontaneously or by some unknown cellular activity. Some of the bile-salt-bound fatty

(Continued on page 93)

(Continued from page 92)

acids may pass through the cell unchanged and continue to the portal vein. This route may also be used by some of the triglycerides from short-chain fatty acids, by glycerol which has not been employed in cellular resynthesis of fat and by the bile salts split off in the cell from fatty acids, soaps and monoglycerides. By far the greater part of the fat or fat components proceed in the form of chylomicra into the lymphatics.

The absorption of other lipids, cholesterol, phosphatides and fat-soluble vitamins is intimately related to the mechanisms of fat absorption. *Cholesterol* may be esterified in the lumen and may enter the cells in a bile-ester combination, or it may enter the cell as a bile complex and be partly esterified there. Free cholesterol and the cholesterol esters leave the intestinal cells by way of the lymph stream.

The absorption of the hydrolytic products of phospholipid digestion (see above) follows the line indicated for fat absorption. The evidence relating to the *absorption of vitamin A* suggests that, within the intestinal cell, carotene, the provitamin, may form a protein complex which passes into the blood or may be converted to the free vitamin, which is then esterified and passed on to the lymphatics. As to the absorption of vitamin D, little is known except that it requires the presence of bile and pancreatic juice. The same holds true for the absorption of vitamin E (tocopherol) and vitamin K (K_1 and K_2). Most vitamin K deficiencies are conditioned by the lack of bile salts (see Ciba Collection, Vol. 3/III, page 40).

The mechanisms involved in the absorption of the water-soluble vitamins (thiamine, riboflavin, nicotinic acid, pyridoxine, pantothenic acid, ascorbic acid and cyanocobalamine [B_{12}]) are not known, except for the fact that an intrinsic factor secreted by the gastric mucosa is necessary for the absorption of B_{12} (see Ciba Collection, Vol. 3/I, page 84).

Nonmotoric Functions of the Colon

The mucous membrane of the large intestine secretes an opalescent mucoid, *alkaline fluid* composed essentially of water, mucus and, possibly, some enzymes. Secretion of this fluid is enhanced by chemical and mechanical irritation. The colonic epithelium also has an excretory function in so far as it is used by the organism as an *elimination route for metals* (lead, mercury, bismuth and, possibly, silver and calcium). The *digestive functions of the colon* are, under normal circumstances, of little practical significance but may become extremely significant as a compensatory mechanism when absorption in the small intestine is reduced by disease or surgical excision. Small amounts of starch, fat and proteins, proteoses, peptones and peptides, escaping digestion in the jejunum and ileum, may be digested in the colon, essentially by bacterial enzymes, which are capable

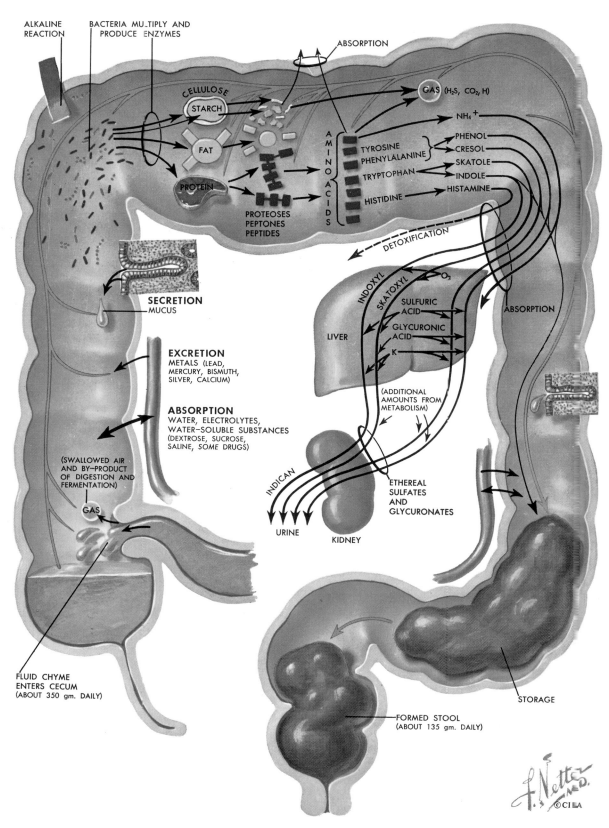

of breaking down cellulose and other food components. The ability of E. coli to split triglycerides is particularly noteworthy, because it makes the ratio of fat to fatty acids in the feces a rather unreliable index of pancreatic insufficiency. Certain amino acids, essentially *tryptophan,* but also *tyrosine, phenylalanine* and *histidine,* yield, under the influence of bacterial enzymes, such compounds as *skatole, indole, phenol, cresol* and *histamine,* respectively. These products of "putrefaction" may be absorbed in relatively small quantities by the mucosa and transported to the *liver,* where they are *detoxified* (see Ciba Collection, Vol. 3/III, pages 35 and 37), to be excreted by the *kidney* in the form of *sulfates* and *glucuronides.* The bulk of the material which remains in the colonic lumen and leaves the intestine with the feces contains indole and skatole, together with mercaptan and hydrogen sulfide, and bacterial decomposition

products of cystine, which give the feces an unpleasant odor. The color of the feces derives chiefly from stercobilin, a bacterial reduction product of bile pigment. The important *absorptive faculty* of the large intestine, especially of the ascending colon, is concerned with the uptake of water, electrolytes and a variety of water-soluble substances reaching the colon. These water-soluble substances also include some drugs (chloral hydrate, anticholinergics, xanthines, digitalis glucosides, etc.), which can, therefore, be administered rectally (by enema or suppositories). The water content of the fluid leaving the small intestine through the ileocecal valve is reduced about three- to fourfold as it passes through the ascending, transverse and descending colon, leaving, under normal conditions, a rather concentrated mixture of mucus, solids deriving from indigestible food residues and a great amount of bacteria.

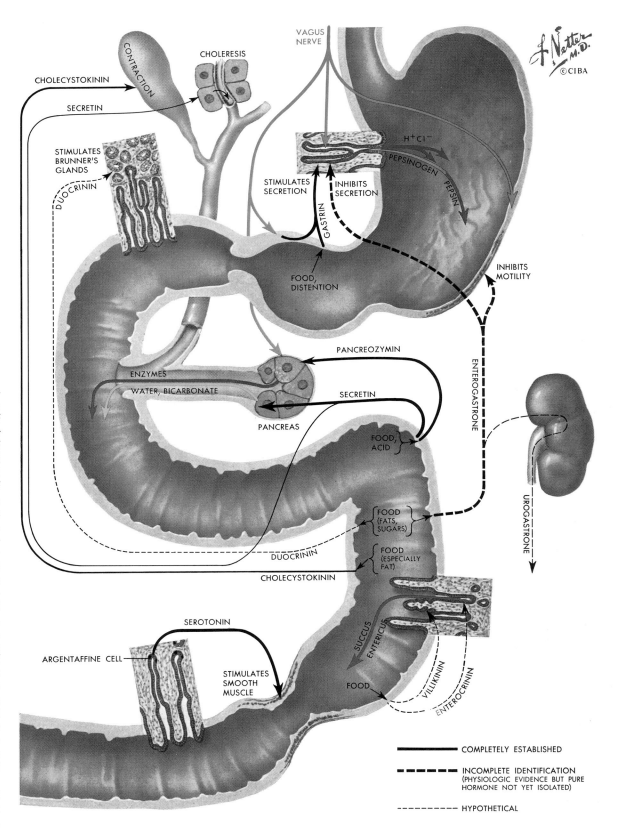

GASTRO-INTESTINAL HORMONES

Gastro-intestinal hormones are substances released by the effect of specific stimuli to the mucosa at various levels of the alimentary tract to influence other parts or functions of the tract. None of these substances has as yet been isolated in a form sufficiently pure for chemical identification. The existence of some of them has been established by physiologic evidence, whereas acceptable evidence for the existence of others is still lacking.

Gastrin, a principle released essentially from the mucosa of the pyloric portion of the stomach (Edkins) as a result of stimuli induced by distention and the contact of food with the mucosa (Grossman *et al.*), increases the secretion of hydrochloric acid and, to a lesser extent, of pepsinogen (see CIBA COLLECTION, Vol. 3/1, pages 83 and 84). Excitation of the vagus augments the liberation of gastrin, and vagotomy diminishes the responsivity of the parietal cells to the effect of gastrin. These observations provide the rationale for the surgical attempts to minimize acid secretion in ulcer patients by combining vagotomy and resection of the antral mucosa (see ibidem, page 186). The mechanism of the release of gastrin is not known.

Secretin (Bayliss and Starling, 1902) is released primarily from the duodenum and jejunum in the presence of HCl, hydrolyzed proteins, fatty acids, certain amino acids and, to a lesser extent, by other ingredients of the gastric chyme, and it stimulates the secretion of water and bicarbonates by the pancreas (see CIBA COLLECTION, Vol. 3/III, page 55). The practical application of these findings is the secretin test (see ibidem, page 58), the value of which, owing to a significant choleretic action of secretin, may be expanded to include deductions regarding the condition of the extrahepatic biliary tract (Dreiling). *Pancreozymin,* released from the same sites and as a result of the same stimuli responsible for the release of secretin, promotes the secretion of all pancreatic enzymes (see CIBA COLLECTION, Vol. 3/III, page 55). A third principle originating in the upper

intestine, *cholecystokinin* (Ivy and Oldberg), stimulates contraction and evacuation of the gallbladder (see CIBA COLLECTION, Vol. 3/III, page 52). The release of a fourth principle, *enterogastrone* (Ivy and Farrell, Lim), is evoked by fat reaching the intestine in a concentration somewhere between 10 and 15 per cent, and by sugars, also in relatively high concentrations. Enterogastrone inhibits gastric secretion and motility (see CIBA COLLECTION, Vol. 3/1, page 83), the latter, however, only if the vagus innervation is intact. The effects of this hormone are a delay in the gastric emptying time and a reduction in the acid contraction of the gastric juice.

Among the less well-established hormones is *villikinin,* which has been postulated to be responsible for the contraction of the villi during digestion (Kokas and Ludány). Another is *duocrinin* (Grossman, 1950), presumably stimulating Brunner's glands, as

suggested by animal experimentation. Based on experiments on autotransplanted loops of jejunum and ileum, *enterocrinin* (Nasset) is thought to stimulate the secretion of succus entericus.

Urogastrone is an agent extractable from urine and, when injected, causes inhibition of gastric secretions. Its status as a gastro-intestinal hormone revolves about the undecided question whether it is an excretory product of enterogastrone. Anthelone (Sandweiss), said to be present in certain extracts of small-intestinal mucosa, has been reported to prevent the development of peptic ulcers in animals (not in human beings) under conditions known to induce ulcers.

Over the years, observations have been reported suggesting the existence of a humoral mechanism for motility of the intestine. It may be that serotonin, secreted by the argentaffine cells (see pages 49, 55 and 165) of the gut, functions significantly in this capacity.

VISCERAL REFLEXES

Visceral reflexes explain a number of clinical signs, *e.g.*, much of the bizarre picture of the irritable colon syndrome (see pages 139 to 141). Afferent impulses from the hypertonic sigmoid initiate reflexes to cranial structures (headache, strange feeling in the head), to the bronchial tree (difficulty in breathing), to the stomach (epigastric distress, indigestion) and to the abdominal skin (intolerance of constricting garments).

The afferent limb of *viscerosomatic reflexes,* originating from viscera and affecting somatic structures, may be by way of sympathetic or parasympathetic nerves. The efferent limb is usually via somatic nerves or autonomic paths. In *viscerovisceral reflexes* the afferent and efferent limbs may both be over sympathetic or parasympathetic nerves, but they may be mediated by the intrinsic nerve plexuses only. *Somatovisceral reflexes* involve somatic afferents and sympathetic or parasympathetic efferents to the viscus. The so-called *"viscerosensory reflexes",* which, lacking a true efferent limb to the arc, are not true reflexes, are believed to result from a shunt or transfer of sensory impulses from autonomic (sympathetic or parasympathetic) afferents to somatic afferents. Just where this shunt or transfer takes place (dorsal root ganglion [?], spinal cord [?], nerve trunk [?]) is conjectural (Lennander, Livingston, Pottenger). The viscerosensory reflexes explain the phenomena of "referred pain" and of "skin hyperalgesia" which, in case of sympathetic reflexes, occurs in skin areas (dermatomes) innervated by the same spinal segment from which the nerve supply of the diseased viscus derives and which, in case of parasympathetic reflexes, may express itself in more remote areas (toothache or earache from gastric disease; Livingston). Of the endless number of visceral reflexes, only some are illustrated and tabulated below.

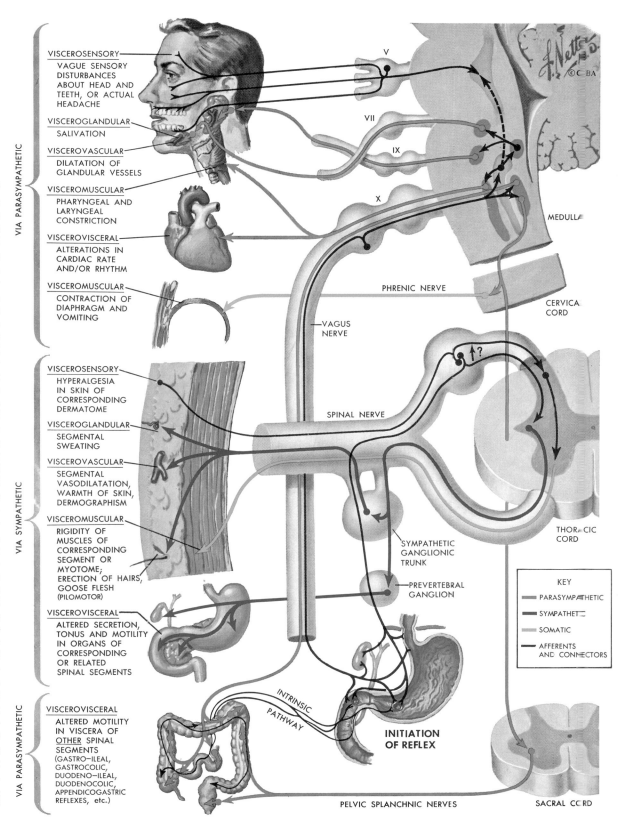

	REFLEXES	ORIGIN	EFFECT	CLINICAL SIGNIFICANCE
VISCEROSOMATIC	Visceromuscular	Diseased abdominal organ	Contraction of voluntary muscles and erectores pili muscles innervated by corresponding spinal segment; also neck and laryngeal muscles	Involuntary guarding suggests underlying visceral irritative process
	Visceroglandular	Same	Sweating in area of corresponding dermatomes	Aids in identification of level of visceral involvement
	Viscerovascular	Same	Dilatation of blood vessels, dermographia, sense of warmth in corresponding dermatome	Aids in identification of level of visceral involvement
	Viscerosensory	Same	Hyperalgesia in corresponding dermatomes	Explains, in the absence of distention, tenderness and intolerance of tight garments
VISCEROVISCERAL	Gastro-ileocolic / Duodeno-ileocolic	Food entering stomach and duodenum	Stimulation of ileac and colic motility	Accounts for "post-coffee" defecation reflex; postprandial distress in "irritable colon syndrome"
	Esophagosalivary / Gastrosalivary	Esophagus and stomach	Paroxysmal sialorrhea	Clue to neoplasm of esophagus
	Enterogastric	Distention or irritation of enteric canal	Inhibition of stomach, antral spasm	One of the mechanisms of indigestion; "biliousness", nausea
	Cologastric	Distention or irritation of colon	Same	Instigating epigastric distress in irritable colon syndrome; vomiting in appendicitis
	Urinary tract-gut	Disease of urinary tract	Inhibition, distention of gut	Acute abdominal symptoms may be of genito-urinary origin
	Viscerocardiac	Disease of gastro-intestinal organs	Diminution of coronary flow, changes in heart rhythm and rate	Myocardial disturbances (tachycardia, bradycardia, arrhythmia) may occur in G-I disorders
	Visceropulmonary	Same	Spasm of bronchioles	Accounts for sense of difficult breathing in irritable colon syndrome

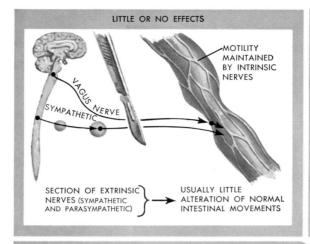

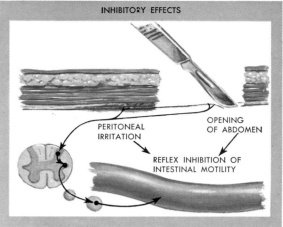

PATHOPHYSIOLOGY OF SMALL INTESTINE

The clinically recognizable disturbances of small-bowel function arise mainly from alterations in the motor activities. Distention or irritation of the small bowel tends to provoke nausea and vomiting. The second portion of the duodenum is so sensitive in this respect that it has been termed the "organ of nausea". That the duodenum may be the site of origin of the intractable nausea which sometimes occurs in patients with acute myocardial infarction is suggested by the finding of acute hemorrhagic duodenopathy in occasional patients with this disease.

Organic or functional disturbances of the jejuno-ileum evoke *pain referred to the peri-umbilical region.* From observations of this kind, it is inferred that *pain in the midabdomen* is suggestive of a *lesion of the small intestine.*

The motility of the small intestine is intensified in conditions of irritation of the mucosa, as by bacterial toxin or chemical irritant, in which case the accelerated motility is an expression of the attempt of the organism to rid itself of the irritant. The hypermotility of *mechanical obstruction* to the intestine represents the attempt of the musculature to force its contents past the obstacle.

Contraction of the intestine, in the absence of sufficient blood supply to meet the needs of the contracting musculature, results in a *relative ischemia,* with the production of abdominal pain. Thus the syndrome of abdominal pain following the ingestion of food must include, in the differential diagnosis, the possibility of occlusion of the superior mesenteric artery, or one of its main branches, by atheromatous deposits.

The grossly disordered motility which results in delayed passage of intestinal contents and the accumulation of those contents in dilated segments is seen primarily in the sprue syndrome (see page 135); the mechanism of the disturbance of the intestinal movement in this condition is not known. It is possible that the increased formation of serotonin, which has been shown to exert a disruptive effect on normal intestinal propulsion, may be a factor, inasmuch as an elevation of serotonin excretion is often demonstrable in sprue syndromes.

Disturbance of intestinal function, based on alteration in its secretory activities, has not been shown to occur. The mucoid consistency of the secretion of the glands of Brunner has led to speculations that deficiency of this secretion

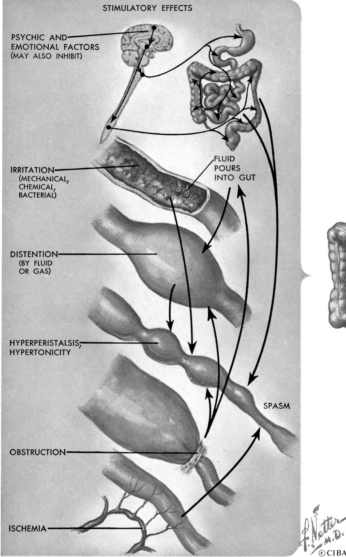

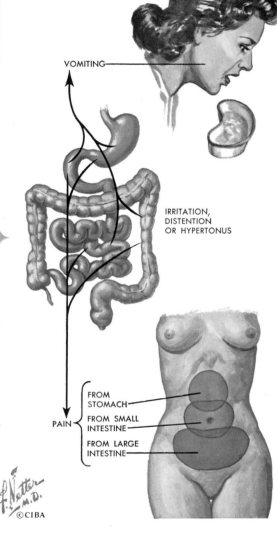

may be a factor in diminishing the susceptibility of the duodenum to the acid gastric juice in patients with peptic ulcer, but no evidence has been adduced in the human to support this theory. Likewise, no evidence of diminished secretion or action of the enzymes of the succus entericus has been forthcoming. The same situation prevails with regard to the question of alterations in the formation of the gastrointestinal hormones in the upper intestine.

Disturbances in digestion in the intestine by virtue of absence or decrease of bile and pancreatic juice, as well as disturbances of absorption in consequence of abnormalities of the intestinal mucosa, lead to motility disturbances.

Inhibition of motility of the intestine is usually of *reflex origin,* the reflex being initiated by peritoneal irritation or trauma to skeletal parts. Thus the inhibition of intestinal motility which ensues for a variable

period of time following laparotomy is assumed to be a result of the intra-abdominal irritation attendant upon the surgical manipulations. The situation is a temporary one unless further irritation is superimposed by attempts to hasten resumption of normal activity. The prevailing practice is to withhold feeding after abdominal surgery until peristaltic sounds return.

The normal stimulus for intestinal contraction is distention; therefore, distention of the walls by an inpouring of secretions into the lumen, whether for the purpose of diluting an irritant or of diluting normal intestinal content to render it of better consistency for passage through a narrowed aperture, may be expected to increase peristalsis.

Finally, peristalsis is accelerated by excessive discharge of impulses down the autonomic nervous pathways in emotional states.

PATHOPHYSIOLOGY OF THE COLON

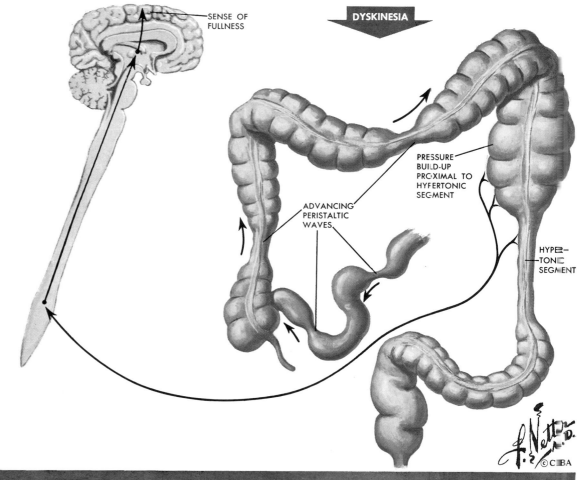

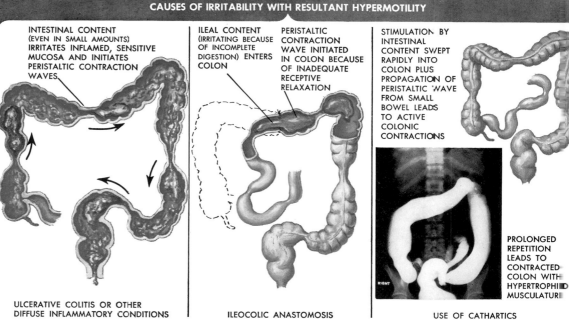

CAUSES OF IRRITABILITY WITH RESULTANT HYPERMOTILITY

INTESTINAL CONTENT (EVEN IN SMALL AMOUNTS) IRRITATES INFLAMED, SENSITIVE MUCOSA AND INITIATES PERISTALTIC CONTRACTION WAVES

ULCERATIVE COLITIS OR OTHER DIFFUSE INFLAMMATORY CONDITIONS

ILEAL CONTENT (IRRITATING BECAUSE OF INCOMPLETE DIGESTION) ENTERS COLON

PERISTALTIC CONTRACTION WAVE INITIATED IN COLON BECAUSE OF INADEQUATE RECEPTIVE RELAXATION

ILEOCOLIC ANASTOMOSIS

STIMULATION BY INTESTINAL CONTENT SWEPT RAPIDLY INTO COLON PLUS PROPAGATION OF PERISTALTIC WAVE FROM SMALL BOWEL LEADS TO ACTIVE COLONIC CONTRACTIONS

PROLONGED REPETITION LEADS TO CONTRACTED COLON WITH HYPERTROPHIED MUSCULATURE

USE OF CATHARTICS

Disturbances in motility of the large bowel are responsible for the symptoms in a high percentage of patients who complain of abdominal distress and irregularity of bowel movements. The most frequent of these disturbances consists of a dyskinesia or dyssynergia of the colon, which may be defined as an incoordination of the contractions of adjacent segments of the bowel. The motor activity of the colon is normally sluggish throughout most of the day; at intervals, a peristaltic wave, originating in the colon itself or transmitted from more proximal intestinal segments, moves the content along for a variable distance. If the content is moved forward as far as the rectum, an urge to defecate occurs, with the result that a portion of it is evacuated. If, however, the advancing wave meets an unyielding, contracted ("spastic") segment, the pressure proximal to the hypertonic segment increases and stimulates the nerve endings of the wall; this results in a feeling of fullness which may be quite distressing. In some individuals the afferent impulses arising in the hypertonic segment, especially in the distal colon, are sufficient to generate this sense of fullness. The "resting" hypertonus may dissipate if a peristaltic wave is able to pass onto and over the contracted segment; this probably explains why some patients with an irritable colon feel better for a period of time after eating. Often, however, food intake has just the opposite effect. Just how the colon motility becomes incoordinated is not known; emotional factors are frequently incriminated, but it is not clear how their effects on the colon are mediated.

A not definitely localized *hypermotility* of the large bowel is observed in three conditions. In *ulcerative colitis* (see also pages 144 to 147) or in other diffuse inflammatory diseases of the colon, any material passing down from the proximal intestine may be sufficiently irritating to initiate propulsive contractions resulting in complete evacuation of the colon in the form of a watery diarrhea which may

be so severe as to be practically continuous. A similar situation may arise after the construction of an *ileocolic anastomosis* (see also page 104).

With the chronic *misuse of cathartics*, a mechanism comes into operation which is comparable to the one just mentioned. The intestinal content is swept rapidly into the colon, where it has an irritating effect, prompting active colonic contractions which ultimately, over a period of years, may result in a diffusely contracted colon with hypertrophic musculature and a radiologic appearance indistinguishable from that of long-standing ulcerative colitis.

An extreme example of the inability of a localized colonic segment to accept an oncoming peristaltic wave is the aganglionic megacolon (see pages 118 to 120). The enormously dilated colon frequently seen in patients with malabsorption syndrome (see pages 135 to 137) is the result of several factors; it may be

the expression of an adaptation to the large volume of material arriving from the intestine, or a nutritional deficiency affecting the intrinsic nerves or a spread of the intestinal mucosal abnormality to the colonic mucosa with resulting diminution of the absorptive capacity.

The only significant disturbance of the secretory function of the colon is an excessive secretion of mucus which, as a rule, can be interpreted as a response to either mechanical, chemical or bacterial irritation, and it is this hyperirritability that must be treated.

Impairment of the absorptive function is sometimes seen in extensive ulcerative colitis (see pages 144 to 147).

A number of disorders of colon function are attributable to alteration in the nature and activities of the bacterial flora, but these are as yet too little understood to permit a rational discussion.

PATHOPHYSIOLOGY OF DEFECATION

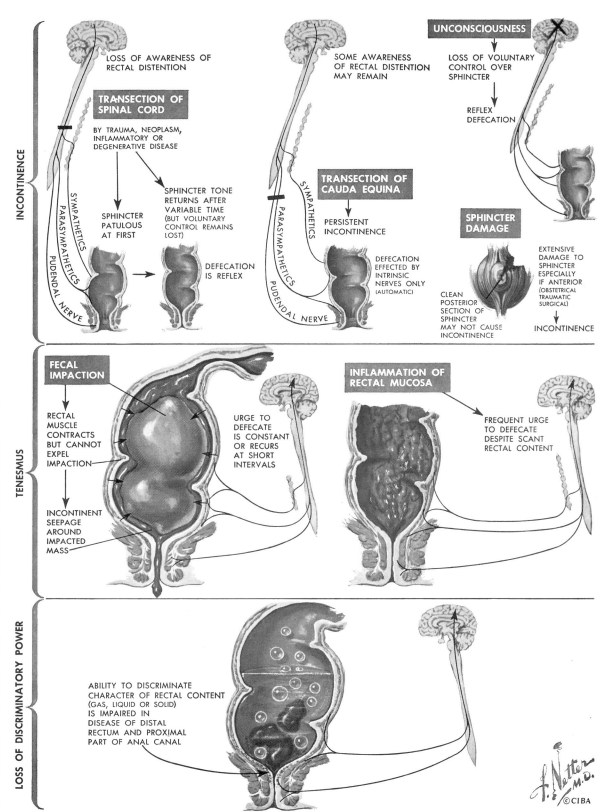

During the period of "spinal shock", which supervenes for some weeks immediately following *transection of the spinal cord* above the origin of the lumbar sympathetic nerves, the rectum and sphincters are completely paralyzed and the patient is incontinent. Thereafter, the tonus of the sphincters returns, and defecation occurs reflexly by way of the lumbosacral center. Since voluntary contraction of the external sphincter is no longer possible and since distention of the rectum is no longer perceived, the patient has no control over the act of defecation. In paraplegics this poses a difficult problem, which is managed generally by the regular use of enemas and digital evacuation of the rectum.

When the cord lesion involves the *cauda equina,* with destruction of the sacral innervation, the reflexes are abolished and defecation then becomes automatic, *i.e.,* dependent entirely on intrinsic nervous mechanisms. In these circumstances the rectum still responds, though with limited force, to distention, and the reciprocal relaxation of the already patulous sphincters enables feces to be extruded. Some awareness of rectal distention may be present if the transection is below the lumbar sympathetic outflow, and it is possible that the persistence of sympathetic connections in the absence of the sacral outflow may contribute to the sluggishness of rectal contractions.

The presence of excretory material in the rectum is not in itself sufficient to excite the urge to defecate. The content must be sufficiently large to exceed the threshold of the distention stimulus characteristic of the individual. In many patients with regular bowel habits, digital examination may reveal a considerable mass of varying consistency. However, the accumulation of a large mass in a greatly dilated rectum, occurring especially in the older age group, is suggestive of the abnormal condition known as rectal dyschezia, which results from a loss of tonicity of the rectal musculature; it

may be due to a long-standing habit of ignoring or suppressing the urge to defecate, or to degeneration of nerve pathways concerned with the defecation reflexes. When further complicated by weakness of the abdominal muscles, defecation becomes a chronic problem. In these cases evacuation may be obtained only by a mechanical washing out of the mass with enemas or by administration of cathartics which keep the stool semiliquid.

Painful *lesions of the anal canal,* such as ulcers, fissures and thrombosed hemorrhoidal veins, impede defecation by exciting a spasm of the sphincters and by voluntary suppression to avoid the resulting pain.

A rather common disturbance of defecation occurs in all age groups as a consequence of excessive *hardening of the feces,* as a result either of dietary errors or of therapeutic agents. The condition is frequently seen in patients receiving large amounts of aluminum

hydroxide or calcium carbonate. The distention of the rectum provokes a repeated, sometimes almost continuous, urge to defecate (tenesmus), but the rocklike character of the boli prevents their being molded for passage through the sphincters. If the condition cannot be dealt with by rectal infusions of oil, to render the boli more slippery, or of surface-acting agents, such as dioctyl sodium sulfosuccinate, to disintegrate the hardened masses, digital evacuation under anesthesia may become necessary.

Constant urge to defecate in the absence of appreciable content in the rectum may be caused by external compression of the rectum, by intrinsic neoplasms and, particularly, by *inflammation of the rectal mucosa.* This mucosa, normally insensitive to cutting or burning, when inflamed becomes highly sensitive to all stimuli, including those acting on the receptors mediating the stretch reflex.

DIARRHEA

Since the time of Hippocrates, the term diarrhea has been used to designate the abnormally frequent passage of loose stools. Strictly speaking, diarrhea is present only if all of the requirements of this definition are fulfilled. Frequent discharges of small amounts of mucosanguinopurulent material, but not of actual feces, as in proctosigmoiditis, is not diarrhea. The passage of an increased number of well-formed stools or the daily evacuation of a single loose stool would not constitute diarrhea. Furthermore, since the individual serves as his own "control" in regard to what is considered abnormal, a person in good health who has had a semiliquid movement after meals all his life may be said to have a hyperactive gastrocolic reflex but not diarrhea.

Nervous pathways from the cerebral cortex (see page 76) provide the route by which emotions provoke diarrhea. Depending upon the intensity and duration of the emotional disturbance, peristalsis may be accelerated throughout the small and large intestine; the effect may be transient or may persist for years. Emotogenic diarrhea may be continuous or may alternate with constipation, *e.g.*, in the irritable colon syndrome (see pages 140 and 141). The relatively infrequent diarrhea after *vagotomy* is a consequence of some autonomic imbalance, but its true mechanism has not as yet been clarified.

Endocrine disorders, affecting as they do the metabolic processes, including those of the smooth muscle of the alimentary tube, may cause diarrhea as, *e.g.*, in hyperthyroidism or adrenocortical insufficiency. In the Ellison-Zollinger syndrome (see CIBA COLLECTION, Vol. 3/1, page 88) the diarrhea has been attributed to the endocrinopathy, to the enormous volume of gastric juice pouring into the intestine and to the inactivation of pancreatic enzymes by the low pH in the upper intestine. The diarrhea in patients with a secreting carcinoid tumor (see page 165) may be a manifestation of a stimulating effect of serotonin on motility.

Physical (osmolarity, cold, liquids), *mechanical* (distention from excess intraluminal volume or from foreign bodies),

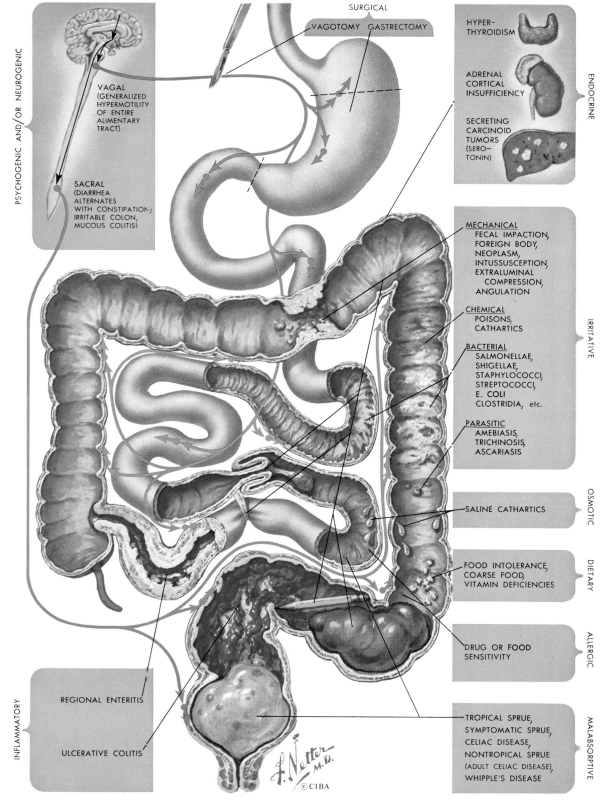

chemical or *bacterial factors*, or *food intolerance* initiate the stimulation of mucosal afferent fibers, which, in turn, evoke the response of intrinsic nervous reflexes, resulting in increased motility. A similar mechanism, by which the body is protected from noxious influences, comes into play in the regulation of the amount of nutrients absorbed (motility-stimulating action of, *e.g.*, a certain level of fat and fatty acids). In pyloric obstruction (see CIBA COLLECTION, Vol. 3/1, pages 89 and 174) diarrhea may occur because the gastric stasis gives rise to the formation of substances irritating the intestinal mucosa or because the powerful gastric contractions sweeping over onto the intestine initiate peristaltic rushes. The physiologic basis of "gastrogenous diarrhea", the term applied when achlorhydria is encountered in a patient with chronic diarrhea, has not been clarified. Possibly, the absence of HCl permits the entry of irri-

tating bacteria into intestinal segments which do not harbor them normally, or the impaired gastric digestion diminishes the concentration of proteoses or other protein-split products needed for the physiologic formation of gastro-intestinal hormones (see page 94). Likewise, it has so far not been possible to identify the precise mechanism of the diarrhea that is a presenting symptom in vitamin deficiencies.

Diarrhea may or may not be accompanied by abdominal pain, depending upon the type of motor disorder. In general, the purely hyperperistaltic diarrheas are not likely to be painful. When pain occurs with diarrhea, it suggests peristaltic waves advancing toward an obstructed or hypertonic segment, *i.e.*, a dyskinesia; in such instances nausea and anorexia may be present, and borborygmi may result from the forcing of intestinal gases through constricted segments of the gut.

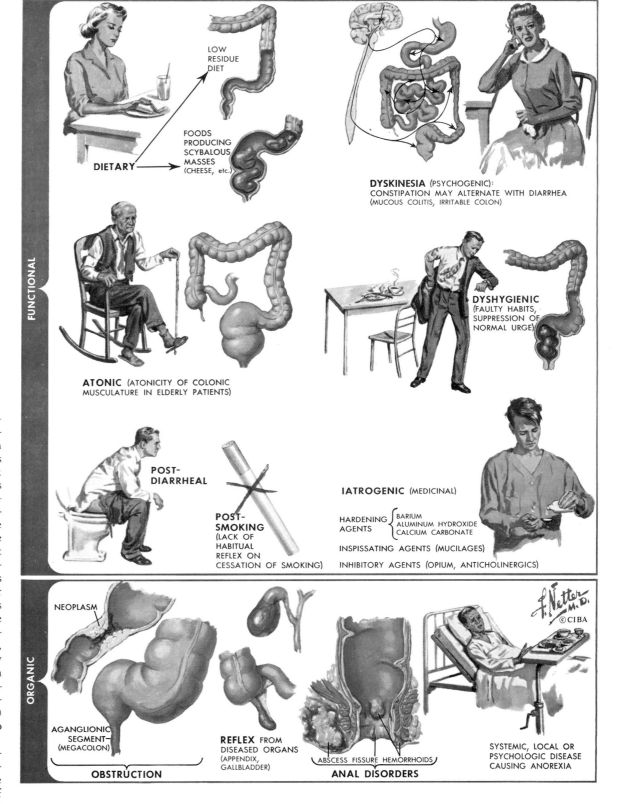

Constipation

In view of the wide individual variation in the frequency of bowel evacuations, constipation cannot be defined in terms of the number of bowel movements in any period of time. Some people think they are constipated if their evacuations do not correspond in frequency, consistency and quantity with what they consider normal. But these considerations are influenced by emotional factors, because for most individuals a bowel movement is a pleasant experience. "Subjective constipation", *i.e.*, constipation which exists only in the mind of the patient, is rather frequent and constitutes the chief basis for the enormous consumption and abuse of laxatives. Infrequency of bowel evacuation is, however, in many instances real, and a great number of conditions may cause it. Constipation may result from inadequate intake of residue- and bulk-producing foods or from excessive ingestion of foods (*e.g.*, processed cheese) which harden the stools sufficiently to render them difficult to evacuate.

Probably the most frequent and certainly the most refractory type of constipation is that associated with the condition known (among a number of other names) as "spastic colitis" (see page 141) and attributed to a motor incoordination of the distal colon. Such *dyskinesia* is usually characterized by a hypertonic or "spastic" segment in the descending portion, proximal to which pressure builds up to give rise to a feeling of abdominal fullness, discomfort, or even pain. The period of constipation is often followed by a watery stool, owing to increased fluid secretion proximal to the "spastic" segment.

Diminished tonicity of the colon and/or rectum accounts for an appreciable number of cases with constipation, particularly in elderly patients. Roentgenographic progress studies after a barium meal identify the region of the *atonicity*. Faulty habits, such as suppressing the

normal urge or the omission of an integral part of the toilet ritual, such as smoking, may lead to constipation by the disturbance of a well-balanced and elaborate reflex mechanism. *After* a period of *diarrheic stools*, constipation must be expected for several days until enough residue has accumulated in the colon. A series of therapeutic agents (aluminum hydroxide, calcium carbonate, mucilages, opiates, anticholinergics and barium given for X-ray examination) may be the cause of an *iatrogenic constipation*.

Aside from this array of *functional causes*, constipation is a frequent symptom of *organic diseases*, including those clinical or pathologic entities which manifest themselves by an obstruction somewhere in the alimentary tube. *Inflammations* of the alimentary canal or adjacent organs, such as *gallbladder* and *appendix*, or even painful injuries of skeletal structures, may disturb the normal enterocolic reflex mechanisms. *Anal irritation* (hemorrhoids, fissure, abscess) causes constipation on the basis of reflex spasm of the sphincters.

Local effects of the inability to empty the accumulating intestinal content, such as distention of the left colon, abdominal discomfort, tenderness and pain, are easily understood. More difficult to explain, however, are a great number of remote manifestations frequently observed in constipated patients, *e.g.*, hyporexia, coated tongue, halitosis, headache, dyspnea and fatigue. The concept that they are due to "toxic absorption" has been abandoned because of insufficient evidence. On the other hand, they are features of the clinical picture that are present too regularly to deny their existence as sequelae of constipation, particularly in view of the fact that they usually subside rapidly after a spontaneous or induced evacuation.

INTESTINAL OBSTRUCTION, ADYNAMIC ILEUS

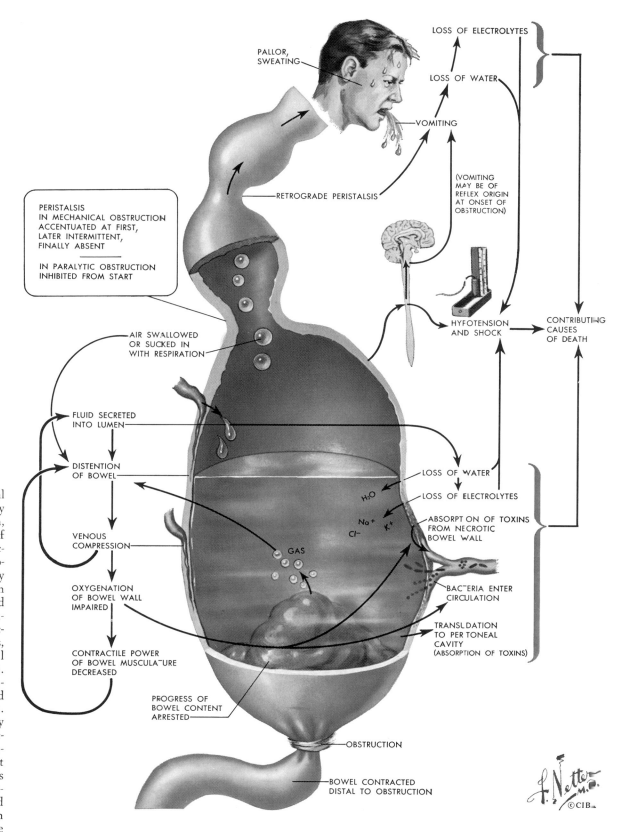

PERISTALSIS IN MECHANICAL OBSTRUCTION ACCENTUATED AT FIRST, LATER INTERMITTENT, FINALLY ABSENT

IN PARALYTIC OBSTRUCTION INHIBITED FROM START

PALLOR, SWEATING

LOSS OF ELECTROLYTES

LOSS OF WATER

VOMITING

RETROGRADE PERISTALSIS

(VOMITING MAY BE OF REFLEX ORIGIN AT ONSET OF OBSTRUCTION)

AIR SWALLOWED OR SUCKED IN WITH RESPIRATION

HYPOTENSION AND SHOCK

CONTRIBUTING CAUSES OF DEATH

FLUID SECRETED INTO LUMEN

LOSS OF WATER

LOSS OF ELECTROLYTES

H_2O

Na^+ K^+

Cl^-

DISTENTION OF BOWEL

VENOUS COMPRESSION

GAS

ABSORPTION OF TOXINS FROM NECROTIC BOWEL WALL

OXYGENATION OF BOWEL WALL IMPAIRED

BACTERIA ENTER CIRCULATION

TRANSUDATION TO PERITONEAL CAVITY (ABSORPTION OF TOXINS)

CONTRACTILE POWER OF BOWEL MUSCULATURE DECREASED

PROGRESS OF BOWEL CONTENT ARRESTED

OBSTRUCTION

BOWEL CONTRACTED DISTAL TO OBSTRUCTION

The onward passage of the intestinal content is hindered mechanically by abnormalities which occlude the lumen, partially or completely, at any level of the gastro-intestinal tract. Such obstructions may be caused by tumors; by stenoses from inflammation or scarring; by gallstones, foreign bodies or parasites in the small intestine; by adhesions and fibrous bands; by impacted feces; by compression from diseased contiguous structures; or by strangulated hernia, volvulus, intussusception or narrowed surgical stomas (see also pages 190 and 191). The progress of the intestinal content may also be diminished or arrested because of functional disturbances. Peristaltic activity may be abolished by reflexes originating from diseased structures within or remote from the abdominal cavity. Perhaps the most frequent cause of reflex inhibition of the gut is operative handling. Reflex ileus is frequently, though inappropriately, called "paralytic ileus", but it can be shown (spinal anesthesia, splanchnic nerve block) that this condition does not involve actual paralysis of the bowel. Other functional obstructions include the "metabolic ileus" encountered in cases of acute porphyria, uremia and severe electrolyte loss. Recognition of the etiology of all these forms of intestinal obstruction is important for the choice of adequate therapy, but pathophysiologic events in the wake of any obstruction, be it mechanical or functional, are very much alike, although they differ primarily in mode of onset and rate of progression.

Acute closure of the bowel may, depending on the cause, be ushered in by abdominal pain, nausea and vomiting of reflex origin; examination of the abdomen at this time discloses hyperperistalsis, which subsequently gives way to periods of alternating hyperactivity and quiescence until the latter predominates. In adynamic ileus, peristalsis ceases from the very start. As a result of loss of tonus, increased fluid secretion into the gut, and accumulation of gas (mostly air, swallowed or sucked in with respiratory movements), the intestine becomes more and more distended. In the case of a mechanical ileus, the distention is proximal to the point of obstruction, whereas in a reflex ileus the distention is more generalized. The continued stretching of the wall impairs oxygenation and occludes the venous return. Peristalsis is further weakened; the absorptive functions fail; permeability is altered so that intestinal bacteria and toxic substances pass into the peritoneal cavity. More water and electrolytes (chlorides, sodium and potassium) from the blood enter the lumen, further aggravating the distention. Vomiting ensues. The over-all effect of this chain of events is a demineralization and dehydration of blood and body tissue, leading to circulatory failure. In an effort to ascribe death from intestinal obstruction to a single cause, an endless number of experiments have been performed and several theories have been advanced. This problem is still controversial, but it may be assumed that the fatal outcome is attributable to a combination of several factors, the most important of which are indicated in the accompanying plate.

Surgical correction of mechanical obstruction should be undertaken as soon as it becomes apparent that it cannot be managed by other measures. Correction of the underlying cause of functional ileus may also require surgery. While the diagnosis is being sought, management is instituted to correct the pathologic physiology outlined above.

GASTRO-INTESTINAL HEMORRHAGE

Many gastro-intestinal disorders manifest themselves by bleeding. The loss of blood from small lesions may be so minimal that, in the absence of other symptoms, it may escape attention and, when prolonged, may lead to microcytic anemia as the first sign of a gastro-intestinal disorder. Since blood extravasating anywhere within the digestive tube, independent of the intensity of the bleeding, must be eliminated with the feces, it is important to examine for "occult" blood (see page 108) at the slightest suspicion of a lesion in the gut. More severe hemorrhages reveal themselves by the appearance of visible blood in the stool, where it may be either intermingled with the fecal material as bright-red blood (hematochezia) or cause a black discoloration, known as melena. The black color, indicating that blood has been exposed to the digestive activity of the intestinal secretions, is, as a rule, a sign that the bleeding stems from a lesion in the gut above the cecum, although, on some occasions, melena may occur with lesions located as low as the left colon. By the same token, hematochezia may derive from upper gastro-intestinal hemorrhage, in which case it signifies massive bleeding. To avoid pitfalls, it should be kept in mind that the stool may be discolored for reasons other than the presence of blood. Patients taking iron or bismuth preparations pass dark stools, and a reddish stool appears after the injection of Bromsulphalein® or when the patient has eaten beets.

The other and, as a rule, more serious signs of gastro-intestinal hemorrhage are hematemesis, *i.e.*, the vomiting of bright-red blood, or melenemesis, *i.e.*, the vomiting of dark blood or "coffee grounds" material. Here, the difference in the color of ejected blood does not permit any definite conclusions concerning the origin of the bleeding. Sanguinous vomiting depends on the accumulation of blood in the stomach or duodenum at the time the necessary conditions for vomiting (see CIBA COLLECTION, Vol. 3/1, pages 90 and 91) are fulfilled. In the majority of cases, both hematemesis

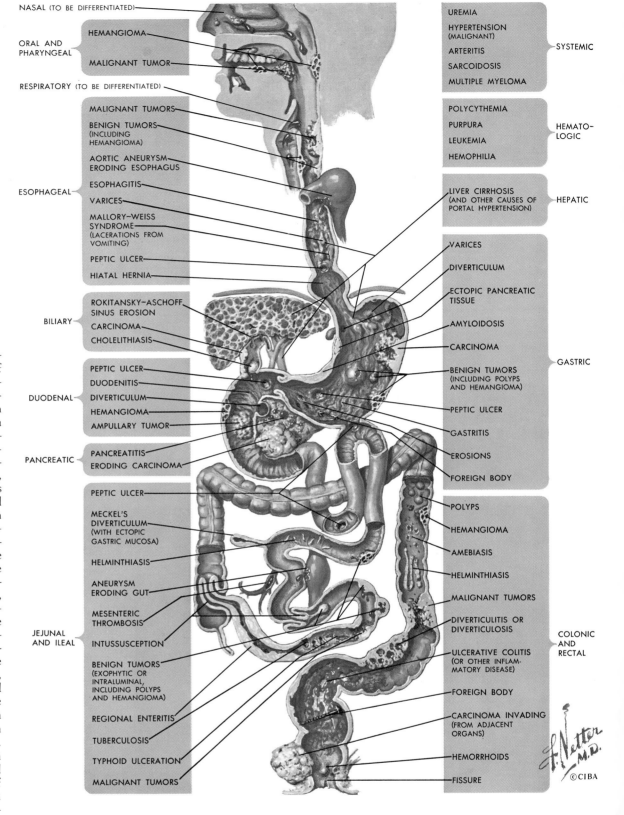

and melenemesis point to an extensive hemorrhage in the upper digestive tract, the cause of which is, in more than half of the cases, a *peptic ulcer;* the remaining cases result from *esophagitis, gastritis, carcinoma of the stomach, esophageal varices* and an endless variety of less frequent lesions anywhere between the pharynx and the ligament of Treitz. This, however, does not mean that all hemorrhages from ulcers, tumors, etc., must be accompanied by bloody vomiting. If the bleeding is not arterial or does not stem from the sudden opening of a large vein (*e.g.,* esophageal or gastric varices), blood does not usually accumulate in the stomach but passes into the small intestine. Infrequently, blood originating from the upper intestine, proximal to a point of obstruction, may regurgitate to the stomach and be ejected by vomiting.

Since saliva and sputum are often swallowed, *blood deriving* from the *oral* or *pharyngeal cavity* or from

hemorrhagic lesions in the *respiratory tract* may, depending on a variety of conditions, be vomited or appear in the feces. The same holds true for blood passing by gravity into the pharynx from the *nasal cavity*. It is usually not difficult to exclude these sources by appropriate examinations.

Adequate clinical skill and experience and the use of X-ray, esophagoscopy, gastroscopy, the string test (see CIBA COLLECTION, Vol. 3/1, page 99), intestinal intubation and sigmoidoscopy (see page 109), will localize and identify the cause of bleeding in all but a few cases. The precise point of the bleeding will, in many instances, be found only by performing an exploratory laparotomy, which must, however, be deferred if possible until blood volume has been restored.

In an occasional case bleeding from the gut will not be the result of a local disease but will be a manifestation of a systemic disorder, *e.g.,* a blood dyscrasia.

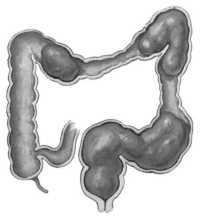

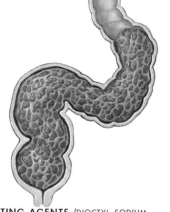

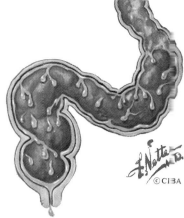

BULK AGENTS (AGAR, PSYLLIUM, METHYL-CELLULOSE) PROVIDE INCREASED RESIDUE, PROMOTE PERISTALSIS BY DISTENTION

WETTING AGENTS (DIOCTYL SODIUM SULFOSUCCINATE) SOFTEN STOOL BY COATING AND DISPERSION OF COMPONENT PARTICLES

MINERAL OIL LUBRICATES AND MIXES WITH STOOL TO SOFTEN IT

EFFECTS OF DRUGS ON INTESTINE

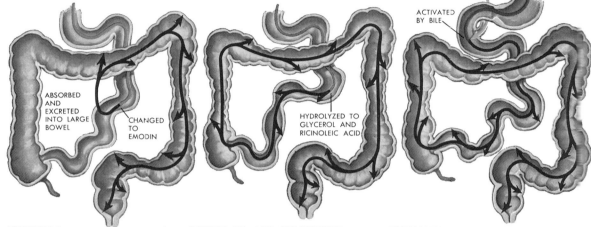

EMODINS (CASCARA, SENNA, ALOES) STIMULATE LARGE BOWEL PERISTALSIS AND SECRETION BY IRRITATION

CASTOR OIL AND DERIVATIVES STIMULATE ACTIVITY OF SMALL AND LARGE BOWEL BY IRRITATION

PHENOLPHTHALEIN STIMULATES PERISTALSIS AND SECRETION BY IRRITATION; SITE OF MAJOR ACTION UNDETERMINED, PROBABLY WIDESPREAD

The effects of drugs on the motor and secretory activities of the intestine are sometimes the primary therapeutic aim and sometimes an unwelcome by-product of therapy directed elsewhere. The *parasympathomimetic drugs* (*e.g., methacholine* or Urecholine®), including those agents that inhibit the hydrolysis of acetylcholine by blocking the action of cholinesterase (*e.g., physostigmine, neostigmine*), *stimulate* intestinal contractions. Pantothenyl alcohol stimulates propulsive motility, theoretically by facilitating the acetylation of choline; its action would, therefore, be classified as parasympathomimetic. *Atropine* and a legion of synthetic *anticholinergic drugs* block the transmission of parasympathetic stimuli to the effector organ and thus inhibit intestinal contractions. Drugs which either *stimulate* or *inhibit* the effects of *sympathetic nerves* are far less active on the gastro-intestinal tract than on other systems, so that, for the anticipated decrease in intestinal motility, sympathomimetic drugs (*e.g.,* ephedrine) would have to be used in doses which are poorly tolerated. *Ganglionic blocking agents,* interfering with the transmission of nerve impulses at both the sympathetic and parasympathetic ganglionic synapses, inhibit intestinal contractions.

Pituitrin,® the antidiuretic principle of the posterior pituitary, increases the motility of the bowel, more so in the large than in the small intestine.

Morphine and all related opiates, used for centuries as antidiarrheal drugs, generally decrease the propulsive motility and increase tonus, particularly of the

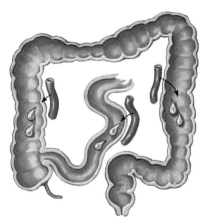

SALINES (MAGNESIUM SULFATE, CITRATE AND HYDROXIDE; SODIUM PHOSPHATE) DRAW AND HOLD FLUID IN LUMEN OSMOTICALLY, ALSO HAVE SOME IRRITANT ACTION

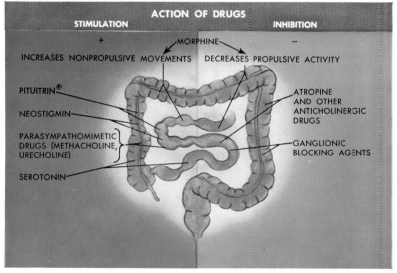

ACTION OF DRUGS

large intestine, sometimes to the point of "spasms", which may explain the abdominal discomfort arising from this kind of medication. Not all segments of the intestine may respond simultaneously and uniformly, so that, with one segment hypertonic, another quiescent and another manifesting continued propulsive activity, a condition of dyskinesia may result; the X-ray appearance of the bowel after morphine medication may resemble that of a string of sausages.

The endless number of drugs and preparations that promote defecation are called cathartics and were formerly classified, according to the intensity of their action, as laxatives, purgatives and drastics. Classification according to different mechanisms of action serves better as a basis for their selection in given clinical situations. The *bulk cathartics* include agents such as bran, agar, psyllium seeds and also the *saline purgatives* such as the sulfate, tartrate, phosphate and citrate salts of magnesium and sodium. The former provide an increased indigestible residue for stool formation; the latter increase the volume of the intestinal content, by the water they attract for their solution, to such an extent that the mechanical stimulus of distention furthers the propulsive activity. Among the *irritant cathartics* are cascara, senna and aloe, the active principle of which (*emodin,* an anthraquinone derivative) irritates the mucosa of the large intestine, thereby stimulating peristalsis. *Castor oil,* after hydrolysis, becomes an irritant to the small intestine, causing rapid propulsion and a watery stool from 4 to 6 hours after ingestion. *Phenolphthalein* is also an irritant, particularly of the large intestine. The emollient cathartics (*mineral oils* [liquid petrolatum] and wetting agents) counteract the hardening of the stool by mixing with the colonic content to render it better lubricated.

PHYSIOLOGY OF GASTRO-ENTERIC STOMAS

Gastrojejunostomy (simple anastomosis of the jejunum to the stomach) was the operation of choice in the surgical treatment of duodenal ulcer for 30 years, before the high incidence of recurrent ulceration made gastric resection the preferred procedure. With the introduction of vagotomy and the realization that a gastric drainage procedure was required to overcome the resulting gastric stasis, gastrojejunostomy was revived, and a large number of these operations are now being performed in connection with bilateral vagotomy. When, as occasionally happens, the vagotomy is incomplete, the result is essentially that of a simple gastrojejunostomy; it is therefore important to understand the physiology of this condition. When the jejunum is anastomosed to the stomach, the function of the neostoma is not significantly affected by the peristaltic direction of the intestine in relation to the stoma (*i.e.*, whether it is iso- or antiperistaltic), nor is it relevant whether the anterior or posterior wall is selected for the site of the anastomosis. The level of the stomach on which the anastomosis is placed may be of importance. The most dependent point of the stomach is not necessarily the best, because the stomach is not a passive bag emptying by gravity; furthermore, in pyloric obstruction — a frequent indication for gastrojejunostomy — the part appearing as the most dependent point of the distended or relaxed stomach is not the most dependent when the stomach regains its tonicity and contractile power. The new stoma should be of a caliber adequate to function as a stoma, and it would appear advantageous for it to be in a position to receive the gastric content in its most chymified condition, *i.e.*, in the pyloric portion. Theoretically, the stoma should not be in a position where distention of the stomach can stretch it and interfere with its function as a passage between the stomach and the intestine; thus, it should not be in the distensible fundic portion.

If a gastrojejunostomy is constructed in the presence of a patent pylorus, the gastric content may preferentially pass via the pylorus, in which case the stoma may become partially or completely nonfunctional. Furthermore, this arrangement may result in circulation of the gastric chyme via the afferent jejunal loop back into the stomach, resulting in indigestion, nausea and vomiting, which comprise the so-called "vicious cycle".

Regardless of how the gastrojejunostomy is constructed or placed, if a simultaneous vagotomy is not done or if it is incomplete, a high incidence of postoperative jejunal ulcer occurs for two reasons: (1) the jejunal mucosa is more susceptible to the ulcerating action of gastric juice than is the duodenal mucosa; (2) the net effect on the gastric secretory mechanisms brought about by a gastro-

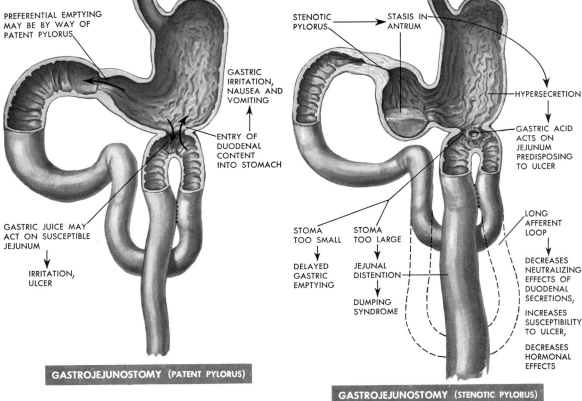

PREFERENTIAL EMPTYING MAY BE BY WAY OF PATENT PYLORUS

GASTRIC IRRITATION, NAUSEA AND VOMITING

ENTRY OF DUODENAL CONTENT INTO STOMACH

GASTRIC JUICE MAY ACT ON SUSCEPTIBLE JEJUNUM

IRRITATION, ULCER

GASTROJEJUNOSTOMY (PATENT PYLORUS)

STENOTIC PYLORUS

STASIS IN ANTRUM

HYPERSECRETION

GASTRIC ACID ACTS ON JEJUNUM PREDISPOSING TO ULCER

STOMA TOO SMALL → DELAYED GASTRIC EMPTYING

STOMA TOO LARGE → JEJUNAL DISTENTION → DUMPING SYNDROME

LONG AFFERENT LOOP → DECREASES NEUTRALIZING EFFECTS OF DUODENAL SECRETIONS, INCREASES SUSCEPTIBILITY TO ULCER, DECREASES HORMONAL EFFECTS

GASTROJEJUNOSTOMY (STENOTIC PYLORUS)

LOSS OF STORAGE CAPACITY

LOSS OF ABSORPTIVE CAPACITY

INCREASED BULK AND IRRITATING PROPERTY OF COLONIC CONTENT

LOSS OF PORTION OF COLON

LOSS OF ILEOCECAL SPHINCTER

UNREGULATED ENTRY OF ILEAL CONTENT INTO COLON

LOSS OF TERMINAL ILEUM

LOSS OF ABSORPTIVE CAPACITY

LOSS OF STORAGE CAPACITY

INCREASED FLUIDITY OF COLONIC CONTENT → DIARRHEA

ILEOTRANSVERSOSTOMY WITH RESECTION

MAY ACT AS SEQUESTERED LOOP → IMPAIRED VITAMIN B12 ABSORPTION

PRESERVATION OF STORAGE AND ABSORPTIVE FUNCTIONS

ILEOTRANSVERSOSTOMY IN CONTINUITY (BYPASS)

jejunostomy is an increase in gastric secretion. When a gastrojejunostomy is constructed in the presence of an obstructed pylorus, practically all the emptying of the stomach will be by way of the stoma, and the rate of gastric emptying will depend on the sensitivity of the jejunum to distention and to the physicochemical characteristics of the gastric content. Intermittent contraction of the jejunum in the region of the stoma will favor phasic emptying, and good tolerance of the jejunum for the gastric content will leave the emptying mechanism similar to that in the preoperative state. Some of the gastric content entering the jejunum may pass retrograde into the afferent loop and undergo peristaltic mixing there.

The site on the jejunum selected for the anastomosis is of significance in so far as the distance between the point of entry of bile and pancreatic juice to the point of emptying of the gastric content

into the intestine may influence the efficiency of intestinal digestion and the susceptibility to jejunal ulceration. It is therefore generally considered desirable to keep the afferent jejunal loop as short as possible. Emptying of the gastric content directly into the jejunum, besides predisposing to jejunal ulcer, as mentioned above, may also engender the syndrome of abdominal distress, sweating, weakness and syncope resulting from jejunal distention.

Ileocolostomy involves the resection or exclusion of some part of the ileum and colon. The functional changes following such an operation will depend upon the underlying condition for which the operation was performed, inasmuch as the type and extent of the disease will affect the length of ileum and colon resected or excluded. The loss of the ileocecal sphincter impairs the regulation of the emptying of the

(*Continued on page 105*)

PHYSIOLOGY OF GASTRO-ENTERIC STOMAS

(Continued from page 104)

intestinal content into the colon and thereby leads to: (1) a more rapid passage of intestinal content, (2) an irritation of the colonic mucosa by incompletely digested foodstuff and enzymes, (3) a diminished absorption and (4) a reflux of colon content into the small intestine. A diminished storage capacity of the colon, with acceleration of colonic passage time, diminished absorption of fluid and corresponding reduction in consistency of the fecal residues, results when the ascending colon is eliminated from the circuit. The loss of any significant segment of the distal colon intensifies the effects of the loss of the ileocecal sphincter in that it favors more rapid passage of the intestinal content into the colon, with again resultant diminution in the intestinal absorption and increased irritation of the colon.

When an ileocolostomy is performed for ileitis, the operation may consist of a side-to-side anastomosis in continuity or a resection with an end-to-end or end-to-side ileocolic anastomosis. The anastomosis in continuity preserves some function in the bypassed small intestine and colon, depending on the extent of the disease and the site of the anastomosis. This procedure has the disadvantage that diseased tissue remains in the body and that stasis in the bypassed loop may mean interference with vitamin B_{12} absorption. Resection of the diseased intestine, while it eliminates sequestration, sacrifices the distal ileum, the ileocecal sphincter and the right colon, and may lead to diarrhea, dehydration, electrolyte deficit, loss of weight, macro- or microcytic anemia, and peripheral edema even in the absence of hypoproteinemia.

Permanent *ileostomy* is done almost exclusively for ulcerative colitis (see pages 146 and 147) and for diffuse polyposis of the colon (see page 166). An ileostomy, if it functions satisfactorily, does not (contrary to numerous statements) develop any storage or increased absorptive capacity. If a dilatation develops adjacent to the stoma, it occurs only as a consequence of obstruction at the stoma. In the unobstructed ileal stoma no control of the discharge from the ileostomy ever develops, and a bag of adequate capacity must always be worn. Squirting of the contents from the stoma by vigorous peristaltic contractions may produce a "noisy" ileostomy. The ileal discharges are irritating to the peristomal skin, so that constant care is necessary to prevent excoriation. Satisfactory appliances and adhesive materials are available for the prevention of this complication. A high ileostomy, *i.e.*, one in which the stoma represents the terminus of a relatively short intestinal segment, poses problems of fluid and electrolyte balance sufficient, in some cases, to necessitate periodic intravenous administration of fluids and electrolytes.

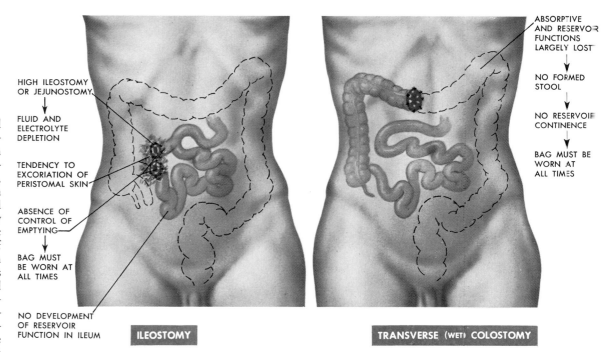

ILEOSTOMY

HIGH ILEOSTOMY OR JEJUNOSTOMY

FLUID AND ELECTROLYTE DEPLETION

TENDENCY TO EXCORIATION OF PERISTOMAL SKIN

ABSENCE OF CONTROL OF EMPTYING

BAG MUST BE WORN AT ALL TIMES

NO DEVELOPMENT OF RESERVOIR FUNCTION IN ILEUM

TRANSVERSE (WET) COLOSTOMY

ABSORPTIVE AND RESERVOIR FUNCTIONS LARGELY LOST

NO FORMED STOOL

NO RESERVOIR CONTINENCE

BAG MUST BE WORN AT ALL TIMES

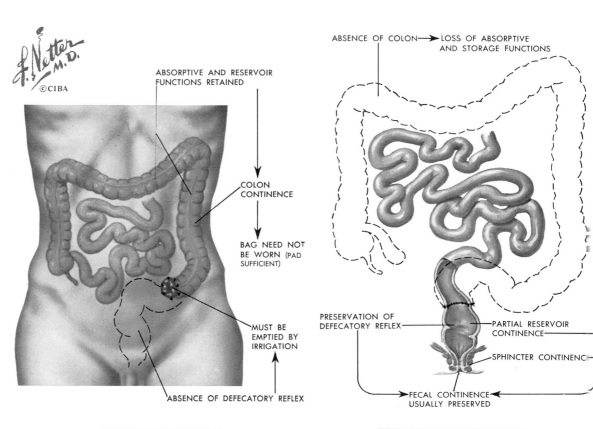

SIGMOID COLOSTOMY

ABSORPTIVE AND RESERVOIR FUNCTIONS RETAINED

COLON CONTINENCE

BAG NEED NOT BE WORN (PAD SUFFICIENT)

MUST BE EMPTIED BY IRRIGATION

ABSENCE OF DEFECATORY REFLEX

ILEORECTAL ANASTOMOSIS

ABSENCE OF COLON → LOSS OF ABSORPTIVE AND STORAGE FUNCTIONS

PRESERVATION OF DEFECATORY REFLEX

PARTIAL RESERVOIR CONTINENCE

SPHINCTER CONTINENCE

FECAL CONTINENCE USUALLY PRESERVED

Colostomy is usually performed for neoplasms of the sigmoid colon and for diverticulitis (see page 131). Since no defecatory reflex operates in the colon proximal to the rectum, the colostomy must be irrigated regularly to evacuate the fecal content mechanically. The colon motility is so sluggish that danger of a spontaneous discharge from the colostomy, except in instances of diarrhea, is small. Therefore, contrary to the situation prevailing with an ileostomy, a protective gauze and plastic or rubber sheet over the colostomy is usually sufficient to maintain satisfactory hygienic control. On the other hand, with a colostomy constructed in the transverse colon, where the fecal content has not yet been sufficiently inspissated to give it solid form and where "reservoir continence" is minimal, the situation is much the same as with an ileostomy and requires similar attention. It is fittingly termed a "wet colostomy".

Anastomosis of the ileum to the rectum — ileoproctostomy — is gaining rapid acceptance as the operation of choice in the surgery of ulcerative colitis. The aim of the procedure is to permit controlled defecation through the natural orifice by preserving the anal sphincters and an adequate rectal pouch. The fact that the intestinal chyme is discharged directly into the rectum will necessarily mean more frequent bowel movements. The irritating properties of the ileal content may initiate such vigorous contractions of the rectum as to exhaust the countercontractility of the external sphincter, making incontinence an ever-present concern, particularly during sleep when voltional control of the sphincter is diminished. Ileo-anal anastomosis brings the intestine down to the inner border of the anal sphincters. With this arrangement, continence is dependent on the efficient functioning of these muscles.

TESTS FOR SMALL-BOWEL FUNCTION

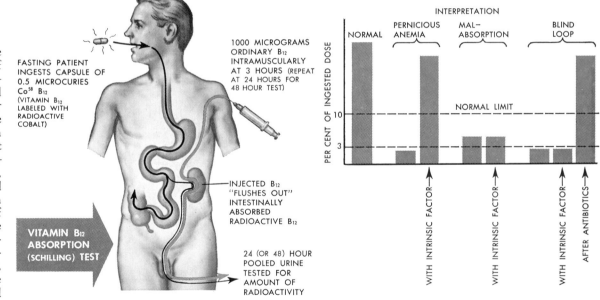

PATIENT INGESTS CAPSULE OF "RITO" (RADIO–IODINATED TRIOLEIN), 35 TO 50 MICROCURIES

TRIOLEIN DIGESTED BY PANCREATIC LIPASE

ABSORPTION

POOLED 72 HOUR STOOL TESTED FOR AMOUNT OF RADIOACTIVITY

RADIO–IODINATED TRIOLEIN (RITO) DIGESTION AND ABSORPTION TEST

PATIENT INGESTS CAPSULE OF RADIO–IODINATED OLEIC ACID, 35 TO 50 MICROCURIES

OLEIC ACID DOES NOT REQUIRE PANCREATIC DIGESTION PRIOR TO ABSORPTION

POOLED 72 HOUR STOOL TESTED FOR AMOUNT OF RADIOACTIVITY

RADIO–IODINATED OLEIC ACID ABSORPTION TEST

INTERPRETATION

PER CENT OF INGESTED DOSE

NORMAL — PANCREATIC INSUFFICIENCY — MALABSORPTION

NORMAL LIMIT — 5

TRI–OLEIN / OLEIC ACID

FASTING PATIENT INGESTS CAPSULE OF 0.5 MICROCURIES Co58 B12 (VITAMIN B12 LABELED WITH RADIOACTIVE COBALT)

1000 MICROGRAMS ORDINARY B12 INTRAMUSCULARLY AT 3 HOURS (REPEAT AT 24 HOURS FOR 48 HOUR TEST)

INJECTED B12 "FLUSHES OUT" INTESTINALLY ABSORBED RADIOACTIVE B12

VITAMIN B12 ABSORPTION (SCHILLING) TEST

24 (OR 48) HOUR POOLED URINE TESTED FOR AMOUNT OF RADIOACTIVITY

INTERPRETATION

PER CENT OF INGESTED DOSE

NORMAL / PERNICIOUS ANEMIA / MAL–ABSORPTION / BLIND LOOP

NORMAL LIMIT — 10

3

WITH INTRINSIC FACTOR / WITH INTRINSIC FACTOR / WITH INTRINSIC FACTOR / AFTER ANTIBIOTICS

Among the numerous tests which have been advocated for the evaluation of intestinal functions, only the well-established clinical diagnostic procedures will be included in this discussion. The *motor function* is studied by following the rate of passage of a radiopaque material taken on an empty stomach after an overnight fast. In situations where the visualization of mucosal detail is not essential, more physiologic conditions are achieved if the opaque medium is mixed with food, particularly for the evaluation of the effects of food intolerance. As the motility varies from time to time, depending on a diversity of conditions including the emotional state of the patient, repeated examinations will be more informative, in many cases, than would be a single one.

Reliable tests for intestinal secretion are not available, though indirect evidence of mucus hypersecretion can be obtained in cases of sprue, when sausage-shaped masses, as a result of barium precipitation by mucus, are visible in the X-ray films. In view of the dependence of absorption on adequate digestion of food, it is, at times, difficult to determine whether a patient suffers from a disturbance of digestion or of absorption. The appearance of excessive numbers of fat droplets, muscle fibers or starch particles in the feces, examined microscopically, indicates incomplete digestion. The most frequent causes of such digestive disorders are diseases of the pancreas, impeded influx of bile into the duodenum and

intestinal inflammations. Tests to diagnose these conditions have been described in CIBA COLLECTION, Vol. 3/III, pages 53, 57 and 58.

Techniques are now available to determine the degree of fat digestion without the cumbersome (though admittedly more accurate) fat analysis of the stool. Following the ingestion of a neutral fat labeled with I[131], the radioactivity of the blood, and particularly of the stool, provides a fairly reliable index of fat absorption. The details of the procedure vary to some extent in different laboratories. A representative method is as follows: The subject receives a capsule containing the equivalent of 35 to 50 microcuries in the form of radio-iodinated glyceryl trioleate (RITO, Trioleotope®), a quantity which, in view of the short half life of I[131] (8 days), is perfectly safe, even if all of the administered radioactivity is absorbed. Blood samples drawn at hourly intervals,

after administration of the test dose, show increasing radioactivity to a peak (1 per cent of the administered radioactivity per 1,000 ml. of blood is the lower limit of normal) between the fourth and sixth hours. The value of blood determinations, in contrast to the determination of fecal radioactivity, is controversial, because varying rates of the fat metabolism may influence the I[131] blood level.

The more reliable method consists of measuring the radioactivity of the total stool collected for a 72-hour period, the upper limit of normal being 5 per cent of the ingested dose. If the radioactivity of the stool is in excess of this figure, the differentiation between impaired digestion and impaired absorption is pursued by application of the *radio-iodinated oleic acid test*. The principle of this test is that oleic acid does not require the prior action of digestive enzymes for

(Continued on page 107)

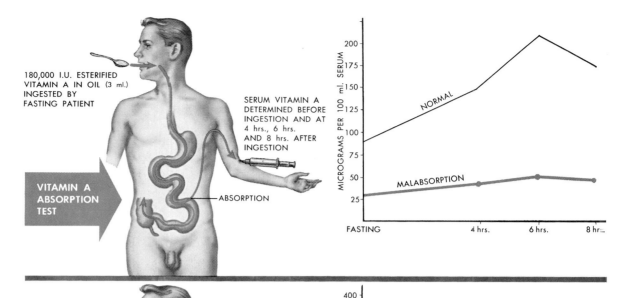

TESTS FOR SMALL-BOWEL FUNCTION

(Continued from page 106)

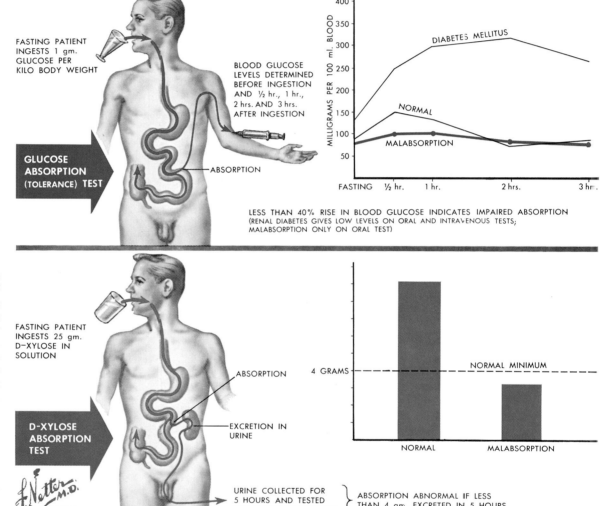

its absorption. The patient receives the equivalent of 25 to 50 microcuries of I^{131} in the form of radio-iodinated oleic acid, and the subsequent procedure is identical with that described above for radio-iodinated triolein. The tests with these two radioactive compounds have proved valuable in cases with steatorrhea, in which it is frequently difficult to differentiate between malabsorption and pancreatic deficiency.

Impairment of intestinal absorption rarely affects all substances that normally pass through the epithelium, or at least not all of them to the same extent. It is, therefore, rational to apply several tests as a guide to the qualitative and quantitative aspects of an absorption defect. The *Schilling test* (see Plate 22) measures the absorption of vitamin B12. It is based on the observation that the small amounts of intestinally absorbed B12 are "flushed" out with the urine when larger quantities, administered parenterally, are present in the organism. Thus it is possible to evaluate the B12 absorption by measuring the radioactivity in a 24-hour urine specimen after a patient has ingested a capsule containing 0.5 microcurie of radioactive cobalt (Co^{58} or Co^{60}) with which B12 (cyanocobalamine) has been labeled. Three hours after administration of the test dose, the patient receives a parenteral injection of 1 mg. of ordinary vitamin B12. In normal individuals, at least 10 per cent of the ingested radioactivity appears in the urine within 24 hours. In the absence of the intrinsic

factor, the radioactivity is minimal but will increase to normal levels when intrinsic factor (gastric mucosal extract) is administered simultaneously with the orally given B12. This differentiates pernicious anemia from the malabsorption syndrome in which radioactivity of the urine is not increased by the administration of the intrinsic factor.

To measure *vitamin A absorption,* which may be disturbed in states of impaired intestinal function, the vitamin A content in the blood can be determined colorimetrically or spectrophotometrically after ingestion of a test dose (180,000 I. U. of esterified vitamin A in oil). In cases of impaired absorption, vitamin A blood values tend to be lower than normal both in the fasting state and at 4, 6 and 8 hours after ingestion of the test dose.

The efficiency of *absorption of glucose* is estimated by determining the blood glucose level before and

after the ingestion of 1 gm. of glucose per kilogram of body weight. Less than 40 mg. per cent rise in the level of blood sugar indicates impaired absorption. Since a number of factors other than an absorptive defect may contribute to a "flat" glucose tolerance curve, the test may be validated by performing an intravenous glucose tolerance test.

According to recent observations, the *absorption of D-xylose* is a reliable indication of the status of intestinal absorption; in this respect, it has been said to parallel the results of fat absorption as determined by more complicated methods. If further intensive study supports these preliminary optimistic conclusions, a much simpler and cheaper method will be available. The patient is given a drink of a solution containing 25 gm. of D-xylose, and the urine is collected for the ensuing 5 hours. Absorption of D-xylose is normal if 4 gm. or more are excreted.

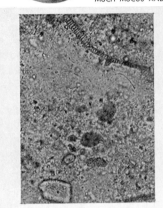

STOOL EXAMINATION

CLAY—COLORED STOOL (ACHOLIC)

TARRY STOOL (MELENA)

BLOOD—STAINED STOOL (LOCAL LESIONS OF LEFT COLON AND ANUS)

ULCERATIVE COLITIS STOOL (LOOSE, BLOODY, WITH MUCH MUCUS AND PUS)

RIBBON STOOL (SPASTIC COLITIS)

STEATORRHEA (MALABSORPTION)

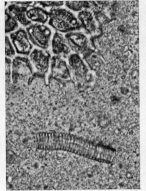

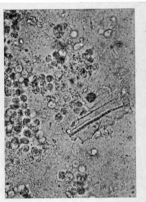

NORMAL STOOL: PARTIALLY DIGESTED MUSCLE FIBER (LOWER LEFT), SEVERAL VEGETABLE CELLS (CENTER), VEGETABLE FIBER (UPPER RIGHT) AMID AMORPHOUS DEBRIS, MOSTLY BACTERIA AND UNRECOGNIZABLE REMNANTS OF DIGESTION

NORMAL STOOL: SPIRAL VEGETABLE FIBER BELOW, PARTICLE OF LEAFY VEGETABLE ABOVE. NO INFLAMMATORY ELEMENTS PRESENT

ULCERATIVE COLITIS: NUMEROUS PUS CELLS, SINGLY AND IN CLUMPS. FRAGMENTED REMNANT OF VEGETABLE MATERIAL (RIGHT CENTER)

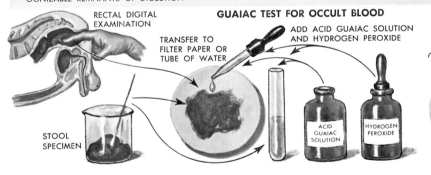

GUAIAC TEST FOR OCCULT BLOOD

RECTAL DIGITAL EXAMINATION — TRANSFER TO FILTER PAPER OR TUBE OF WATER — ADD ACID GUAIAC SOLUTION AND HYDROGEN PEROXIDE — POSITIVE RESULT (BLUE COLOR) — CONTROL (CONTAINING BLOOD)

STOOL SPECIMEN

ACID GUAIAC SOLUTION

HYDROGEN PEROXIDE

The value of stool examination has diminished as more direct methods for the diagnosis of gastro-intestinal disturbances have been developed, so that nowadays, in practice, the stool probably does not get the attention it merits. It must be admitted that the observation of appearance, consistency, color, etc., of the stool contributes only infrequently to the diagnostic information obtained by a carefully extracted past history and the application of appropriate tests. An *acholic stool* will certainly suggest biliary obstruction, but this is of little help in an obviously jaundiced patient. A *tarry stool* indicates gastro-intestinal bleeding (see page 102), usually from the upper levels, and a *stool colored red with blood* means bleeding in the lower intestinal tract. The shape of the stool is, as a rule, reliably reported by the patient, and the appropriate deductions may be made from this information without the physician having to observe the stool himself. The consistency of the feces is of interest when the patient complains of diarrhea and when suspicion of steatorrhea is entertained. In such instances, inspection of stool which has been collected in a glass jar may give valuable, if not indispensable, information in those instances where an oily deposit collects around the edges or at the bottom of the container. With these gross *steatorrheas,* the patient, if questioned, will report the same phenomenon in the toilet bowl in the form of a greasy ring around the edge of the water. Occasionally, a patient will mistake a long string of mucus for a parasite; this is one situation where the gross stool must be inspected to eliminate or verify the presence of a tapeworm (see below).

Chemical examination of the stool in a doctor's office consists of the *test for occult blood*. Many techniques and many reagents for carrying out this test have been proposed, and any one of them is acceptable. One of the simple procedures

which appears to be reliable is as follows:

The amount of stool which adheres to the end of an applicator stick is smeared on a piece of filter paper; onto it is dropped, in turn, a drop of glacial acetic acid, guaiac solution and hydrogen peroxide. The development of a distinctly blue color within a minute constitutes a positive reaction. The reaction is considered strongly positive if the blue color develops instantaneously. If bleeding lesions around the anus can be ruled out, a positive guaiac test means blood coming down from some place in the alimentary tract. Usually, the sequence of investigation is suggested by the symptoms which brought the patient to the physician in the first place. A negative guaiac or other test for occult blood does not, however, rule out a lesion.

A wet mount of the *stool for microscopic examination* is prepared by placing two separate drops of

saline on a large glass slide, mixing the stool into each of these drops until a cloudiness is obtained, adding a drop of one of the iodine stains to one of the stool suspensions and then covering each with a cover slip. The presence of undigested fibers of vegetable or muscle is not, in itself, diagnostic of anything, since these items are found to a variable extent in normal stool. In the presence of a diarrhea, the fact that the undigested material is increased does not explain the nature of the diarrhea. An *exudate of pus,* with or without red blood cells and macrophages, indicates an inflammatory process anywhere from the ileum to the rectum. Normally, the sigmoidoscope will point to the source of this exudate.

Both the unstained and the iodine-stained drops are scrutinized carefully for parasites; if any are detected, another smear of the stool must be made for fixation and appropriate staining (see page 184).

SIGMOIDOSCOPY

Sigmoidoscopy is the most important procedure for the diagnosis of diseases of the rectum and distal sigmoid colon; it should be included in the routine physical examination to detect asymptomatic neoplasms. The technique is simple. Prerequisites for the examiner are an adequate knowledge of the anatomy of the anorectosigmoid segment and a reasonably gentle hand, both of which can be acquired in a short training period. As far as the patient is concerned, the discomfort attending the procedure is not excessive and, in any event, is only transitory.

Sedation is indicated in excessively apprehensive patients. Parenteral administration of an opiate, or the local application of an anesthetic agent in a water-soluble base may be required when irritation of the anal region would render the instrumentation painful. Ordinarily, the procedure can be carried out on an examining table in the physician's office or in bed in the hospital or at home, with the patient in the knee-chest position or lying on his left side with the buttocks projecting well over the edge of the table or bed. The latter position is preferable in decompensated "cardiacs" or very ill and weakened patients.

Digital rectal examination preceding the introduction of a sigmoidoscope is obligatory to rule out any impediment to the free passage of the instrument. If a significant amount of stool is present, cleansing by means of a small, warm enema or postponement of the examination until larger fecal masses have been evacuated with the aid of a laxative may be necessary.

The tip of the warm, well-lubricated and properly obturated, 25-cm. standard sigmoidoscope (a 40-cm. instrument should be available in case one encounters a relatively convolution-free, redundant rectosigmoid) is *inserted* with steady pressure *into the anal ring* and slowly passed forward *through the sphincters* in the direction of the umbilicus; this part of the procedure may be facilitated by having the patient bear down as if defecating. Once the sphincters are passed, the tip of the *instrument is directed backward*. The obturator is removed and the sigmoidoscope is then advanced steadily, always with the lumen in view. Where the redundancy of the mucosa is such that the lumen cannot easily be identified among the opposed folds, a minimal puff of air from the insufflation bag will be helpful. The *sigmoidoscope* should be *advanced* as far as possible without torturing the patient; in the case of acute ulcerative colitis, this may mean only a few centimeters, but within that distance the diagnosis is readily apparent. In cases where the sigmoid angulates acutely just proximal to the rectosigmoid junction, it may not be possible to pass

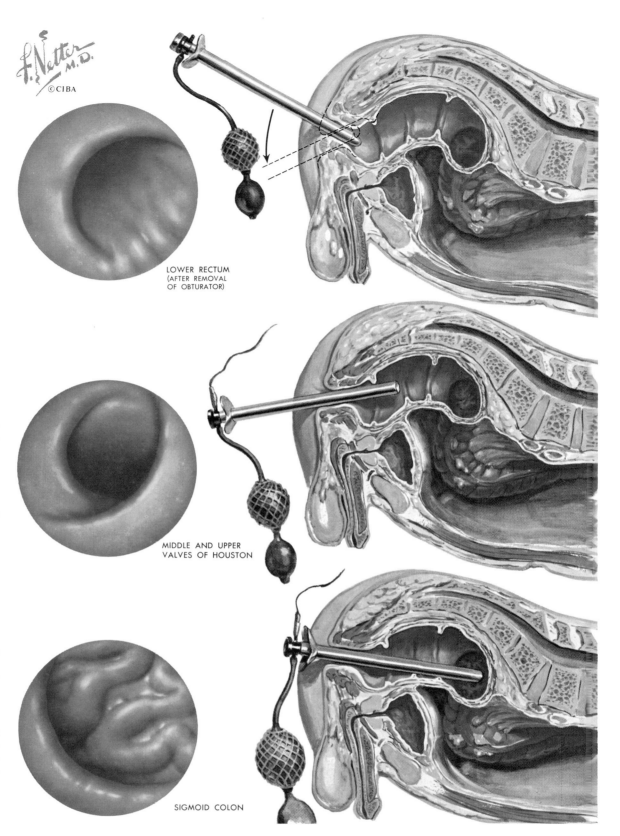

LOWER RECTUM
(AFTER REMOVAL
OF OBTURATOR)

MIDDLE AND UPPER
VALVES OF HOUSTON

SIGMOID COLON

more than 15 to 17 cm. In other cases, the angle to which the instrument must be maneuvered to bring the lumen into view may result in unbearable pressure on the coccyx. In the absence of conditions of this type, however, every reasonable effort should be made to introduce the sigmoidoscope to its full length in order to take fullest advantage of this approach to the diagnosis of neoplasms of the distal colon.

Except in painful diffuse inflammations of the rectosigmoid, the objective during the passage of the sigmoidoscope is to advance expeditiously as far as either the convolutions of the gut or the length of the instrument permits, leaving the careful scrutiny of the mucosa to be done as the instrument is withdrawn. This has the advantage of shortening the interval between the start of the procedure and the time when the patient can be told that the worst is over and that the tube is being taken out. It goes

without saying that the examiner should not ignore anything he may encounter on the way in and that if he encounters a constricting lesion, he should not insist on advancing beyond it.

The most important maneuver in the examination, particularly when it is performed as a part of the routine physical, is the careful inspection of all surfaces of the rectosigmoid mucosa during the steady withdrawal of the sigmoidoscope. This is accomplished by rotating the instrument through a circle, the diameter of which will depend on the part under scrutiny; e.g., it will be a smaller circle in the comparatively narrow sigmoid than in the rectal ampulla.

The technical manipulations are simple and are quickly mastered; the recognition and evaluation of pathology, excepting of course the grossly obvious lesions, depend on a thorough acquaintance with the range of normal variation.

PERITONEOSCOPY

Peritoneoscopy or laparoscopy is the direct inspection of the peritoneal cavity and its contents by means of an endoscopic instrument introduced through the abdominal wall. The procedure is used in gastro-enterologic and gynecologic disorders in which a positive diagnosis cannot be established by more simple methods; its value lies in the fact that it can frequently supply information which otherwise would be obtained only by exploratory laparotomy. The instrument with which the examination is carried out consists of a trocar (a sheath provided with a pointed obturator), the diameter of which varies in different available types from about 5 to 10 mm., and a telescope, armed on its tip with a lamp and made to fit airtight into the sheath. In most of the available models, the vision is in a forward-lateral direction, and the technique with which they are used is still essentially the same as devised by the inventors (Kelling, Jacobaeus). The examination is carried out in an operating room under all aseptic precautions, as if the patient were to be prepared for laparotomy. The first step in the procedure is insufflation of air into the peritoneal cavity through a pneumoperitoneum needle or cannula. The abdominal wall is thus separated from the viscera, and an air-filled space is formed which ensures good visualization and protection against injury of the abdominal organs. Ascitic fluid, if present, must be removed before the insufflation of air. All the layers of the abdominal wall are infiltrated with a local anesthetic at the point selected for the introduction of the instrument. A small skin incision is then made through which the trocar is inserted into the peritoneal cavity; the stylet is removed and replaced by the telescope through which the abdominal contents are visualized and examined. The usual site for introduction of the peritoneoscope is near the umbilicus, but other sites may also be chosen. The vicinity of operative scars (likelihood of adhesions), the upper right quadrant (because of the round ligament) and the midline of the musculi recti abdominis (the course of the epigastric vessels) should, however, be avoided. Through the telescope the parietal peritoneum of the wall, the anterior surface of the liver, parts of the stomach, the greater omentum, the intestines and the gallbladder can be seen. Turning the

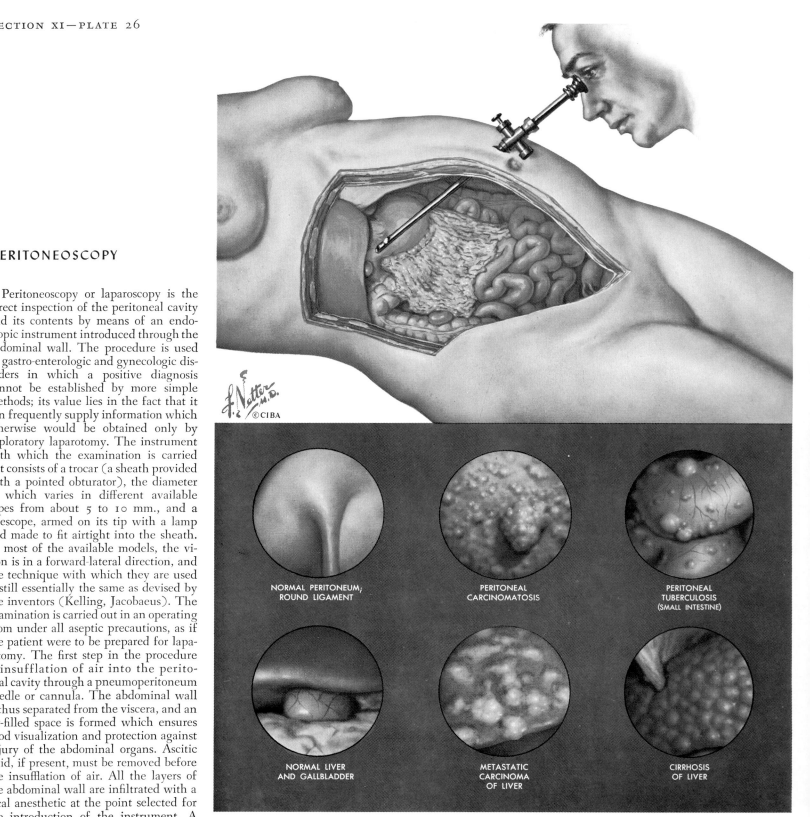

NORMAL PERITONEUM;
ROUND LIGAMENT

PERITONEAL
CARCINOMATOSIS

PERITONEAL
TUBERCULOSIS
(SMALL INTESTINE)

NORMAL LIVER
AND GALLBLADDER

METASTATIC
CARCINOMA
OF LIVER

CIRRHOSIS
OF LIVER

patient on his right side may help to expose the spleen, and by applying the Trendelenburg position the pelvic organs become visible. (The extraperitoneal organs buried deep in the cavity [pancreas, kidneys] as well as the lesions inside a viscus cannot, of course, be visualized.) Peritoneoscopy has proved its value in the diagnosis of peritoneal tuberculosis, abdominal malignancies and determination of their operability, in hepatobiliary diseases, identification of obscure abdominal masses, and in diseases involving the pelvic organs. The risks of peritoneoscopy are negligible; accidents such as air embolism, hemorrhage from a ruptured blood vessel, perforation of a hollow viscus, pneumothorax and pneumomediastinum can be avoided with a perfect technique and a proper selection of patients. Definite contraindications to the procedure are acute abdominal conditions, serious heart and lung diseases and dia-

phragmatic defects. It is also better to exclude from examination patients with extensive operative scars, as well as those who had a peritoneal disease in the past. During the peritoneoscopy biopsies can be performed under visual control, which obviously may be of great importance. Liver tissue is usually obtained with a needle (see CIBA COLLECTION, Vol. 3/III, page 46); other tissues are also recovered with special forceps. Specimens from tissues of a hollow viscus, however, cannot be taken because of the danger of perforation. With the aid of peritoneoscopy, a radiopaque substance can be injected into the gallbladder or into an intrahepatic bile duct. This procedure, called peritoneoscopic cholangiography, permits taking of pictures that facilitate the diagnosis of biliarytract diseases. Special photographic instruments with which color pictures can be taken are useful for documentation of peritoneoscopic findings.

Section XII

DISEASES OF THE LOWER DIGESTIVE TRACT

by

FRANK H. NETTER, M.D.

in collaboration with

C. EVERETT KOOP, M.D., Sc.D. (Med.)
Plates 1-14

H. E. LOCKHART-MUMMERY, M.D., M.Chir., F.R.C.S.
Plates 19-22, 30, 32 and 33

THE SÃO PAULO UNIVERSITY GROUP:

JOSÉ FERNANDES PONTES, M.D.
Plates 27, 31, 35-42

VIRGILIO CARVALHO PINTO, M.D., F.A.C.S.
Plates 15 and 23

DAHER E. CUTAIT, M.D., F.A.C.S.
Plates 52-55

MITJA POLAK, M.D.
Plates 16-18, 24-26, 28, 29, 34, 43-51, 61-71

JOSÉ THIAGO PONTES, M.D.
Plates 56-60

CONGENITAL INTESTINAL OBSTRUCTION I AND II

Intestinal Atresia, Malrotation of Colon, Volvulus of Midgut

Intestinal obstruction in newborn infants is caused by a variety of congenital anomalies and leads to the death of the infant within the first week of life if not treated surgically at the earliest possible moment, and that means, in some instances, within the first 24 hours after delivery. Under ordinary circumstances a newborn infant is an excellent operative risk and remains so during the first 48 hours, but its general physiologic reserve starts to diminish gradually and rapidly thereafter. Thus the earliest diagnosis and immediate efforts to correct the anatomic anomaly are of the utmost, and in many cases of lifesaving, importance. Only in some advanced cases, in which the correct diagnosis has not been made before onset of deterioration of the general status of the infant, a delay of a few hours to permit administration of fluids and plasma, while the baby is kept in an atmosphere of high oxygen concentration, may increase the chances of survival. When this delay is prolonged for more than a few hours, however, a point is reached at which the infant will benefit more from immediate surgery than from further supportive treatment.

The causes of such intestinal obstructions may be an atresia of the esophagus (see CIBA COLLECTION, Vol. 3/1, page 138), a diaphragmatic hernia (see page 123), an annular pancreas (see CIBA COLLECTION, Vol. 3/III, page 141), malrotation of the colon with volvulus of the midgut (see page 113), peritoneal bands mostly compressing the duodenum, internal or mesentericoparietal herniations, meconium ileus (see page 114), aganglionic megacolon (see page 118), imperforate anus (see pages 115 to 117) and *atresia* or *congenital stenosis* of the bowel.

Both atresia and stenosis probably result from an arrest in development during the second and third months of fetal life. As the intestine changes from a solid structure to a hollow tube (see pages 3 and 8), one or more septa may persist, leaving a diaphragm of tissue with only a minute opening and setting up a stenosis. If such persisting septa leave an intact diaphragm across the lumen, or when, during the solid stage, the intestine divides to form two or more blind segments entirely separate from each other or connected by threadlike fibrous bands, atresia ensues.

To wait for the diagnosis of intestinal obstruction until the classic triad of vomiting, absence of stool and abdominal distention has appeared means, in many instances, a loss of much valuable time for a lifesaving surgical intervention. Any one of these three signs should suggest obstruction, and careful exami-

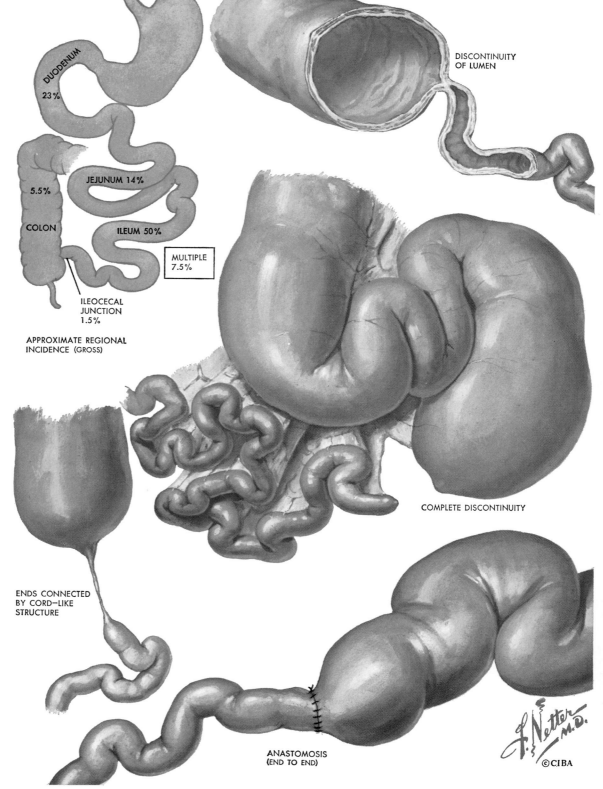

APPROXIMATE REGIONAL INCIDENCE (GROSS)

DUODENUM 23%

JEJUNUM 14%

5.5%

COLON

ILEUM 50%

MULTIPLE 7.5%

ILEOCECAL JUNCTION 1.5%

DISCONTINUITY OF LUMEN

COMPLETE DISCONTINUITY

ENDS CONNECTED BY CORD–LIKE STRUCTURE

ANASTOMOSIS (END TO END)

©CIBA

nation may lead to earlier diagnosis. X-ray study of the abdomen is indicated in the presence of persisting bile-stained vomitus, in the absence of meconium stools for more than 4 hours and when a stool is not produced by digital rectal examination. If an enema is indicated, it should be a diagnostic barium enema. It may be necessary to aspirate air from the stomach which might distort or obscure the pattern of gas distribution in the small bowel, or it may be advisable to introduce 20 ml. of gas into the stomach, if no gas is present, in cases of obstruction in the higher parts of the small intestine. Differentiation between the shadows of the small and large intestine is often difficult, because of an underdeveloped state of the circular folds of the jejunum as well as of the colonic haustrations. For this reason, the point of obstruction in an infant is commonly assumed to be lower than it actually is. Total absence of air in the abdomen is

indicative of esophageal atresia (see CIBA COLLECTION, Vol. 3/1, page 138, and of this book, pages 121 and 122) without tracheo-esophageal communication. Other obstructive lesions in the alimentary tract are, as a rule, marked by air distention above and complete absence of air below the point of obstruction, so, *e.g.*, in duodenal atresia the stomach and duodenum above the block are considerably dilated, with no air below.

Although every effort should be made to arrive at an accurate diagnosis and a determination of the location of an intestinal obstruction, one must, in many instances, be satisfied with the fact that any other diagnosis is unlikely and that the only reasonable course is to operate and to deal with the problem by the best possible means. Many methods are available for the management of intestinal atresia, but, (Continued on page 113)

Congenital Intestinal Obstruction I and II

Intestinal Atresia, Malrotation of Colon, Volvulus of Midgut

(Continued from page 112)

whichever is chosen, the mandatory principle remains, *viz.*, to preserve as great a part of the small intestine as possible. Unfortunately, in many instances the atretic portion of the intestine is so great that the lack of an adequate absorptive surface will sometimes bring about insurmountable difficulties in maintaining postoperatively the necessary nutrition.

The preferable surgical procedure is the *end-to-end anastomosis* between the two patent limbs of the bowel. Trying to resect no more than is absolutely unavoidable of the proximal, hypertrophied, dilated portion, the anastomosis is best carried out at the apex of the cone-shaped proximal segment, because the major thrust of propulsive peristalsis is, in this way, received by the anastomotic stoma, and proportionately little of the peristaltic wave is dissipated in the disproportionately large lateral parts of the proximal segment. Because of changes in the vascularity or of other mechanical difficulties, it is sometimes necessary to abandon the end-to-end anastomosis and perform an end-to-side anastomosis between the end of the proximal and the side of the distal segments. Side-to-side anastomosis will lead to the blind-loop syndrome, with mechanical and nutritional complications postoperatively. Fibrous stenotic areas must be resected. In dealing with only muscular narrowings, which could dilate with use, correction by plastic procedures, carried out on a portion of the circumference of the stenosis, may be attempted.

Volvulus, in general, is the term indicating the torsion and/or coiling of an organ about its attachment, which, in the specific case of the intestines, is the mesentery. It may occur at all ages when, for one reason or other, an intestinal segment becomes longer and the mesentery narrower. In the newborn, *volvulus of the midgut,* which leads to serious intestinal obstruction, is a complication of a *malrotation of the colon.* Normally, about the tenth week of fetal life, the ileocecal area rotates in counterclockwise direction, bringing the cecum into the lower right abdominal quadrant and permitting the mesentery of the ascending colon to be fixed posteriorly (see pages 7 and 8) and laterally to the parietal peritoneum. Arrest of this process results in a lack of attachment of the mesentery from the duodenojejunal junction to the middle of the transverse colon, so that this long mass of intestine remains suspended between the two points of fixation and may become twisted, to produce not only intestinal obstruction but also occlusion of the superior mesenteric vessels. The cecum may be held in this abnormal position in the upper right

1. SMALL INTESTINE PULLED DOWNWARD TO EXPOSE CLOCKWISE TWIST AND STRANGULATION AT APEX OF INCOMPLETELY ANCHORED MESENTERY. UNWINDING IS DONE IN COUNTERCLOCKWISE DIRECTION (ARROW)

2. VOLVULUS UNWOUND; PER TONEAL BAND COMPRESSING DUODENUM IS BEING DIVIDED

3. COMPLETE RELEASE OF OBSTRUCTION; DUODENUM DESCENDS TOWARD ROOT OF SUPERIOR MESENTERIC ARTERY; CECUM DROPS AWAY TO LEFT

quadrant by adventitious *peritoneal bands* and be fixed to the liver, parietal peritoneum or posterior abdominal wall in such a way as to compress the duodenum. Peritoneal bands, not associated with malrotation of the colon, may occasionally cause obstruction of the duodenum or, still more rarely, of other parts of the small bowel.

The clinical signs of these conditions are the same as those of any other cause of intestinal obstruction in the newborn. In the X-ray picture one may, in contrast to the completely gas-free section below the obstruction, observe a few air bubbles below this point, which passed along the intestinal tract before the volvulus occurred and were not completely absorbed. In operating these cases of volvulus of the midgut, the twisted portion of the bowel is unwound, and the Ladd procedure is carried out on the malrotated portion. Upon severing obstructing adventi-

tious bands or abnormal attachments, the colon will drop to the left side of the abdomen, leaving the small bowel on the right side.

Postoperative management of all these infants who have undergone emergency surgery because of intestinal obstruction is carried out independent of the specific cause and anomaly. It is outlined briefly on pages 122 and 124.

Internal (paraduodenal, duodenojejunal, etc.) hernia (see page 218) may also be responsible for intestinal obstruction in infants. A loop of bowel may become incarcerated, or perhaps even strangulated, by entering a defect in the mesentery or by passing between adventitious bands of peritoneum. The herniation can generally be diagnosed either by exclusion or on the operating table. The obvious procedure is to reduce any existing hernia and to divide any obstructing adventitious bands.

CONGENITAL INTESTINAL OBSTRUCTION III

Meconium Ileus

The condition known as meconium ileus may develop in infants born with fibrocystic disease of the pancreas (see CIBA COLLECTION, Vol. 3/III, page 142) or as a consequence of the absence of the pancreatic duct, which, however, is rare. Actually, this genetically determined disease is not restricted to the pancreas but is a generalized disorder involving the acinar structures of the intestinal, bronchial, salivary and sweat glands, as well as those of the pancreas. Infants with fibrocystic disease have a deficiency of the enzymes normally released into the intestinal tract by the pancreas (see CIBA COLLECTION, Vol. 3/III, page 55). This deficiency in utero causes the meconium to be tenacious and puttylike and to adhere to the intestinal mucosa, thus producing obstruction. The fact that less than 10 per cent of the infants with cystic fibrosis develop meconium ileus has so far remained unexplained.

If the intraluminal obstruction by abnormal meconium is complete, it presents a typical appearance. The bowel distal to the obstruction is generally empty and collapsed. More proximally, the *ileum* frequently *resembles a strand of beads,* as the bowel wall conforms to the contour of the *aggregations of meconium,* which is gray in color and of a dried, puttylike consistency. Just proximal to the occlusion, the *bowel is slightly larger* in caliber, and the meconium sticking to the wall is less firm but still so viscous as to prevent peristaltic propulsion. It is here still gray-green to green-black, and it contains so little fluid that it leaves no stain when held in the hand. Proximal to this region the *intestine is greatly distended, filled with gas, fluid and liquid meconium.* The great variation in size of the dilated loops presents, in the X-ray picture or on the screen, a characteristic sign. Some of the loops seem moderately enlarged, some are enormously ballooned, others appear normal and some are even smaller than normal. This is in marked contrast to intestinal obstruction from atresia, stenosis or aganglionic megacolon, where all the loops are likely to be extended with gas to the same extent. The inspissated meconium is seen on the X-ray film as a radiopaque mass, with a mottled appearance due to air bubbles which have been forced into it. How-

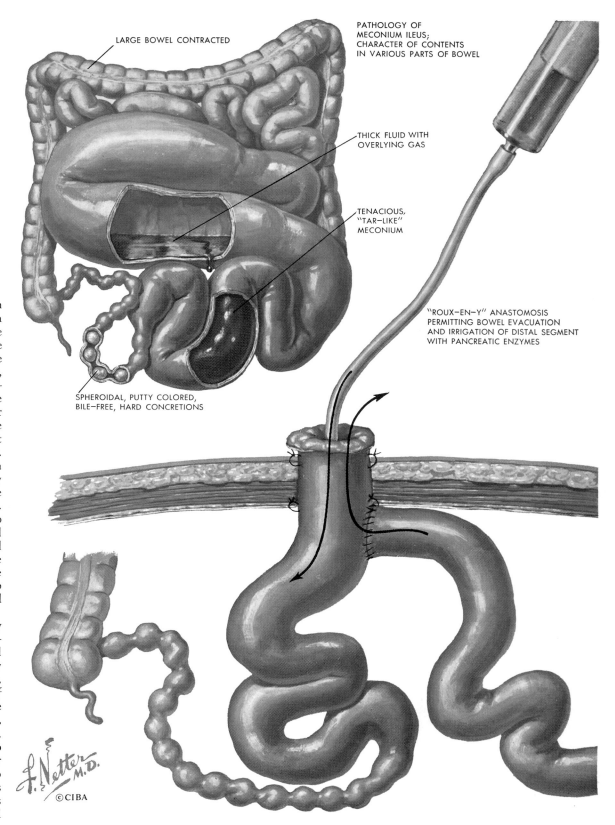

PATHOLOGY OF MECONIUM ILEUS; CHARACTER OF CONTENTS IN VARIOUS PARTS OF BOWEL

LARGE BOWEL CONTRACTED

THICK FLUID WITH OVERLYING GAS

TENACIOUS, "TAR–LIKE" MECONIUM

SPHEROIDAL, PUTTY COLORED, BILE–FREE, HARD CONCRETIONS

"ROUX–EN–Y" ANASTOMOSIS PERMITTING BOWEL EVACUATION AND IRRIGATION OF DISTAL SEGMENT WITH PANCREATIC ENZYMES

ever, it is important to remember that inspissated meconium may also be visualized in aganglionic megacolon (see page 118) and that both conditions, meconium ileus and aganglionic megacolon, may exist without any evidence of fecal shadows in X-ray examination. Flecks of calcium, either scattered throughout the abdomen or attached to the bowel wall, are diagnostic of meconium peritonitis caused by rupture of the intestine in utero.

The treatment of meconium ileus is surgical and, as with other causes of intestinal obstruction, must be performed at the earliest possible moment. As experience has demonstrated, the least traumatic procedure is the method of choice. For that reason the time-honored techniques, in which the small intestine is opened in an attempt to evacuate the puttylike meconium, have been, or should be, abandoned. Instead, the bowel should be divided at the point where the gas-filled portion meets the portion filled with thick, tenacious meconium, and a *"Roux-en-Y" type of anastomosis* should be carried out, which permits the deflating of the dilated proximal bowel as well as the introduction of pancreatic enzymes into the distal obstructed part. These enzymes soften the meconium and permit its expulsion by normal peristalsis. This method is successful in taking care of the acute obstruction, but the long-term results are, of course, disappointing, because, though the patients survive the meconium ileus phase of their disease, they succumb later to the pulmonary complications of this generalized disorder, which is appropriately classified as an "inborn error of metabolism" or deficiency disease, the meconium retention being only one of the manifestations of a general "mucoviscidosis" originating from the lack of some factor necessary to produce a normal mucus.

CONGENITAL INTESTINAL OBSTRUCTION IV

Imperforate Anus

Normally, by the eighth week of embryonic life, the cloacal membrane, which separates the rectum and the anal invagination, is absorbed, so that the anus and rectum become one continuous canal. When this membrane fails to rupture and be absorbed, an *imperforate anus* results (see page 8). This is one of the most common of congenital anomalies, incompatible with life in the newborn infant. Several varieties of this condition have been observed, and it is important to recognize which type prevails in a given case because of the different surgical approaches (see following pages) in the repair of this anomaly. In the first type, only a *thin membrane covers the anal opening.* Types 2 and 3 differ in so far as the *distance between the anal dimple and the blind pouch of the rectum* or *colon, respectively, is less or more than 1.5 cm.* In the fourth and rarest type, a normal anus and rectal canal end in a blind pouch a few centimeters proximal to the sphincter. This situation is really an *atresia of the rectum.*

Imperforate anus can be diagnosed by careful observation alone. The baby's buttocks should always be spread apart and the anal orifice inspected. If no meconium is seen, a thermometer, finger or soft rubber catheter should be inserted to ascertain the patency of the anus and to rule out the rare atresia of the rectal canal. The distance between the blind rectal pouch and the anal dimple can best be determined by roentgenographic studies. Usually, as the infant cries and swallows, sufficient air, essential for roentgenographic contrast, is taken into the gastro-intestinal tract and passed along by peristalsis toward the rectum, so that the level of the occlusion may be visualized within 24 hours after birth, though occasionally it may take as long as 36 hours. (Suction drainage, by means of a catheter placed in the stomach, should be instituted between 4 and 12 hours after birth as a precaution against excessive distention.) The roentgenograms for the diagnosis of imperforate anus are taken with the infant held by his heels and with an opaque object marking the location of the anal dimple (method of Wangensteen and Rice). Flexing the thighs on the abdomen (Rhodes's recommendation) may sometimes serve better to push gas into the distal bowel. A tight abdominal binder may also be helpful. Once the gas has reached the lowest end of the colon, the shadow increases in caliber on successive

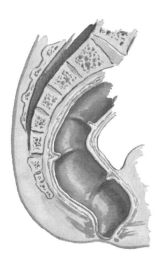

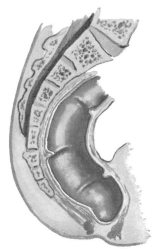

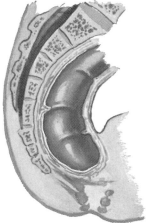

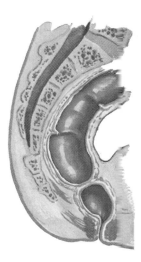

TYPE 1. THIN MEMBRANE OVER ANUS

TYPE 2. POUCH 1.5 cm. OR LESS FROM ANAL DIMPLE

TYPE 3. BLIND POUCH MORE THAN 1.5 cm. FROM ANAL DIMPLE

TYPE 4. ATRESIA OF RECTUM WITH NORMAL ANUS

TYPES OF FISTULA (ASSOCIATED WITH IMPERFORATE ANUS)

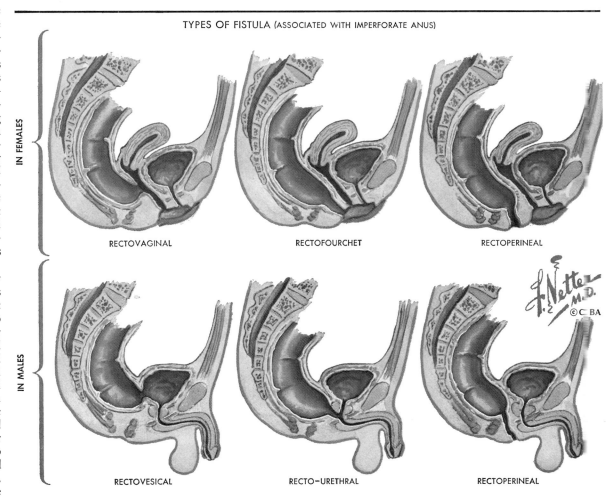

IN FEMALES

RECTOVAGINAL   RECTOFOURCHET   RECTOPERINEAL

IN MALES

RECTOVESICAL   RECTO-URETHRAL   RECTOPERINEAL

films, without farther descent toward the anus, and the decision to operate can be made as soon as the distance between the rectal or colonic pouch and the anal dimple has been established.

It is rather common that the malformation of the anal canal is accompanied by an incomplete separation of the rectum and urogenital sinus, so that, in fact, most infants with an imperforate anus have a fistula between the rectum and the perineum or the urinary tract in the male; or between the rectum and the vagina or perineum in the female. In the male the *fistula* may enter the bladder (*rectovesical*), the prostate or the urethra (*recto-urethral*), or may emerge in the skin of the scrotum or perineum (*rectoperineal*). In the female the fistula almost never enters the urinary tract but either opens into the vagina (*rectovaginal*) or emerges at the fourchet (*rectofourchet*) or perineum (*rectoperineal*). Usually, the

fistulas are easily demonstrated in the female but are more difficult to detect in the male. Furthermore in the female an imperforate anus with a fistula through which stool may pass does not necessarily present the emergency situation of acute intestinal obstruction that it does in the male. Certain diagnostic signs depend on both size and location of the fistula. Meconium may appear at the urethral meatus, or flecks of it may be found in the urine on microscopic examination. Air in the bladder, a rare demonstration by X-ray, indicates a communication between the intestinal and urinary tracts. It may also be possible to outline the entire fistula, or at least its point of entry, by radiopaque dye instilled into the bladder. Such studies, aiming to prove the presence of a fistula, necessitate, however, excessive handling of the infant and are, therefore, often more exhausting to the patient than is warranted by the information so obtained.

CONGENITAL INTESTINAL OBSTRUCTION V

Management of Imperforate Anus

The first type of imperforate anus (see preceding page), in which meconium can be seen behind the thin membrane covering the anal opening, seldom needs major surgical management. Perforation of the membrane with a blunt instrument is simple, safe and completely effective.

For the second type the *perineal approach* has, according to experience, proved adequate. The external sphincter is located, before the infant is anesthetized, by pricking with a pin the area around the dimple, stimulating contractions of the muscle. With the patient in the lithotomy position, any perineal fistula is dissected toward the rectum. A longitudinal incision in the perineum provides the best and safest exposure. Dissection in the operative area is kept close to the midline to avoid damaging the nerve and blood supply. The *fibers of the external sphincter muscle* appear as a rough horseshoe with the apex pointing posteriorly. The blind pouch of the rectum appears as a blue bulbous mass because it is filled with meconium. For the purpose of traction, the *most distal portion of the rectal pouch is grasped* (with hemostat or silk sutures). Dissection is continued, keeping as close as possible to the bowel and avoiding disruption of adjacent structures, until sufficient length of colon has been mobilized to permit the apex of the pouch to be brought to the skin edge without tension. The pouch is then opened and evacuated of meconium. *A row of simple sutures approximates the full thickness of the open bowel with the skin of the opened anal dimple.* The remaining anterior portion of the perineal incision is closed in layers.

When the separation between the colon and the anal dimple is greater than 1.5 cm., and if no contraindications to an immediate definitive operation (such as prematurity or a concomitant congenital anomaly) prevail, the recommended procedure is a combined *abdominoperineal approach.* Once the fact is established that such a procedure is necessary, the patient is placed on gastric suction drainage, and a plastic *catheter* is placed in a *right ankle vein* through a cutdown to facilitate administration of blood and fluids. The operative field is prepared to include the infant's left leg, making it possible to approach both the abdomen and the perineum.

The abdomen is opened by means of a *transverse incision* placed *between the umbilicus and the symphysis pubis.* The blind end of the colon is located and exteriorized. A fistula into the bladder or prostatic urethra, frequently present in infants requiring the abdominoperineal approach, is then repaired through the abdominal incision. If the colon contains

1. PERINEAL INCISION. FIBERS OF EXTERNAL SPHINCTER SEPARATED

2. BLIND END OF BOWEL ISOLATED AND PULLED DOWN; LINE OF AMPUTATION INDICATED BY BROKEN LINE

3. OPENED BOWEL END SUTURED TO PERINEUM, LEAVING SOME REDUNDANCY; PERINEUM SUTURED

COLOSTOMY

INCISION

OPENING COLOSTOMY ELECTROSURGICALLY

large amounts of gas and meconium, it also may be helpful to remove a portion of this material by suction through a small hole made in the blind loop of bowel.

Then a small longitudinal incision is made in the skin of the perineum directly over the anal dimple. This incision is first probed by means of a mosquito hemostat, then by a large hemostat, and finally by a Kelly clamp.

The latter is *passed* upward *through the perineal body and through the center of the sling formed by the levator ani muscles until it perforates the peritoneum in the true pelvis.* A finger is passed through the newly formed canal, and the blind loop of colon is pulled by a long, slender clamp through the canal to the aperture made in the anal dimple. *Several centimeters of colon* are left *hanging outside of the anus,* permitting the natural elasticity of the bowel to select the site of eventual fixation in the artificial

tunnel. The excess of colon is trimmed off later. This delayed procedure results in a better artificial anus than does immediate suturing.

When the site of the rectal pouch is uncertain, as happens occasionally, it is preferable to start the operation in the perineum, since it may be possible that the entire procedure can be adequately done from below. In this event, however, the dissection should not be carried cephalad for more than 1.5 cm. from the anal dimple.

A perineal fistula, when present, is dissected out. The colon is then brought down to the anal dimple in the middle of the external sphincter muscle.

Although the imperforate anus in females is not necessarily an emergency situation, it is preferable to operate the former also during the newborn period when a concomitant fistula in the perineum or the

(Continued on page 117)

CONGENITAL INTESTINAL OBSTRUCTION V

Management of Imperforate Anus

(Continued from page 116)

fourchet (see page 115) exists. These types of fistulas permit easier correction of the anomaly than does the rectovaginal type. A longitudinal incision is made in the perineum, and the fistulous tract is dissected far enough cephalad to bring it into position between the bundles of the external sphincter. The end of the bowel is trimmed to permit the full circumference of the colon to be sutured to the skin of the anal dimple. The perineum must be reinforced by approximating muscle and fascia in the midline, in much the same fashion as is done in colporrhaphy.

In infants with a true rectovaginal fistula, definitive surgery is usually postponed until the infant weighs 12 lb. or attains the age of 3 months. It is easier to handle the rectovaginal septum when the patient has grown somewhat. Wound complications are also less likely in this type of fistula than in those previously mentioned. It is frequently possible to make a transverse incision in the perineum and to mobilize the bowel by separating it from the posterior vaginal wall. The bowel is then moved posteriorly to its normal position in the middle of the anal dimple between the external sphincter muscles. A bridge of normal skin is left between the fourchet and the newly constructed anus. Obviously, the same precautions must be observed in closing the perineal body in the midline.

Experience has shown that the abdominoperineal approach is only necessary in female infants on the very rare occasions when the fistula actually enters the fornix of the vagina. Mention should be made of the fact that a female child with an imperforate anus and a perineal fistula just anterior to the anal dimple may be treated for months or even years for constipation or incontinence because the true condition has gone unrecognized. Defects in the perineal musculature make support of the anorectal canal difficult or impossible, and periodic incontinence in such a case may be expected.

Colostomy (see page 105) is a simple and often lifesaving operation which permits indefinite postponement of definitive surgery. Nevertheless, it is recommended that colostomy be avoided whenever possible, reserving this procedure for patients weighing less than 5 lb. or those with major concomitant problems, such as congenital heart disease or other anomalies of the bowel, contraindicating more extensive surgery than a colostomy. In those cases in which colostomy must be resorted to, it is much more practical to do the colostomy in the transverse colon rather than in the sigmoid portion. The pull-through procedure, described above, may be carried

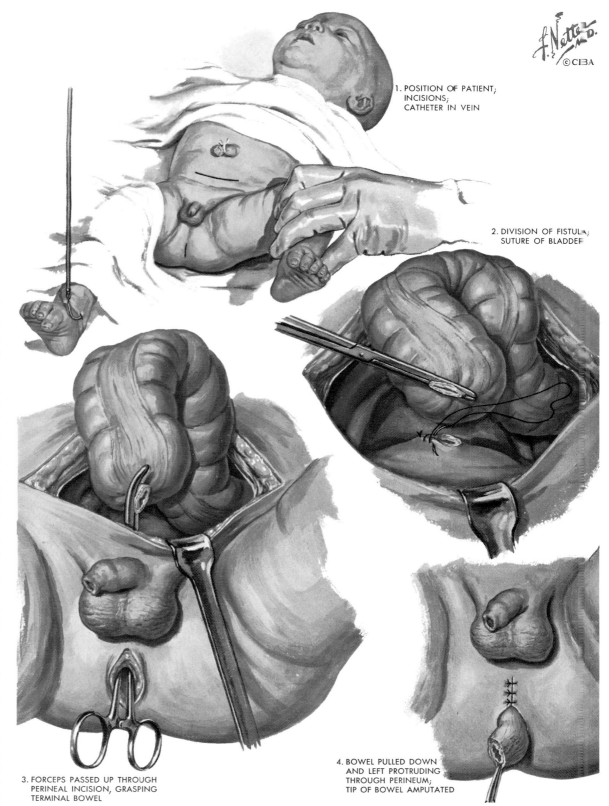

1. POSITION OF PATIENT; INCISIONS; CATHETER IN VEIN

2. DIVISION OF FISTULA; SUTURE OF BLADDER

3. FORCEPS PASSED UP THROUGH PERINEAL INCISION, GRASPING TERMINAL BOWEL

4. BOWEL PULLED DOWN AND LEFT PROTRUDING THROUGH PERINEUM; TIP OF BOWEL AMPUTATED

out at a later date, using the slack intact sigmoid colon to provide an adequate length of bowel. The colostomy may be closed at the same time or, preferably, by a later procedure. With better surgical technique and postoperative care, colostomy in infants does not carry the forbidding mortality of even a decade ago. If the surgeon has had little experience in the field, if safe and effective anesthesia is difficult to maintain or if adequate surgical assistance and postoperative care are not available, it would seem that the infant's future would best be served by the use of a transverse colostomy as a temporary measure. Later, the abdominoperineal procedure can be undertaken under optimal conditions.

Although male infants with imperforate anus do have complete intestinal obstruction, they do not present the dire situation existing when complete obstruction occurs higher in the intestinal tract. The

physician has a period of 36 to 48 hours after birth during which an operation may be performed without undue risk from the standpoint of neonatal physiology. However, when surgery is performed more than 72 hours after birth, the risk is considerably increased.

In practice, moderate delay in surgery is helpful if the physician is to assess the point of lowest descent of the colon with any degree of accuracy. On rare occasions, inspissated meconium in the distal end of the rectal pouch may be misleading. Since air cannot completely fill the pouch, the distance to the anal dimple appears greater than it actually is.

In patients where a fistula can be detected emerging in the scrotum or perineum, delay in operation is usually not necessary, because the fistula either indicates the location of the rectal pouch or permits demonstration of its location by instillation of a thin, water-soluble radiopaque dye.

Congenital Intestinal Obstruction VI

Megacolon (Hirschsprung's Disease)

Megacolon is a descriptive term which, unfortunately, has come to mean a number of clinical entities wherein the colon is dilated, hypertrophied or redundant. The diagnostic use of the term megacolon should be reserved for that specific clinical syndrome first described by Hirschsprung, the etiology of which remained obscure until the contributions of Swenson and Neuhauser and of Bodian. Since the etiology of the syndrome, as described by Hirschsprung, has been established as a terminal absence of ganglion cells in the myenteric plexus of the colon, the term *aganglionic megacolon* not only is descriptive but eliminates confusion with other anatomic and functional derangements of colonic function.

Aganglionic megacolon is a congenital lesion. Although diagnoses are being made with ever-increasing frequency in the neonatal period, an understanding of the pathologic physiology is best approached by a study of the full-blown clinical picture seen in later childhood.

Constipation is the symptom which drives the parent to seek medical advice for a child with aganglionic megacolon. Severe functional constipation brings far more children to medical attention than does aganglionic megacolon, and the differential diagnosis lies primarily between these two conditions. Although great variations in clinical signs and symptoms are expected, the typical situations are readily categorized. The child with chronic functional constipation is a healthy-looking youngster of normal physique for his age, whereas the child with aganglionic megacolon appears to be chronically ill, has a protuberant abdomen and bears the stigmata of malnutrition in growth and development. Parental concern and inability to cope with the constipation are frequently discernibly different in the two diagnoses. Where the child with aganglionic megacolon is the submissive recipient of the unsuccessful efforts of his mother, the child with functional constipation seems in control of the family's emotional problems, of which the constipated child is usually only one.

The history of bowel difficulty in the child with aganglionic megacolon goes back to birth, and frequently the history

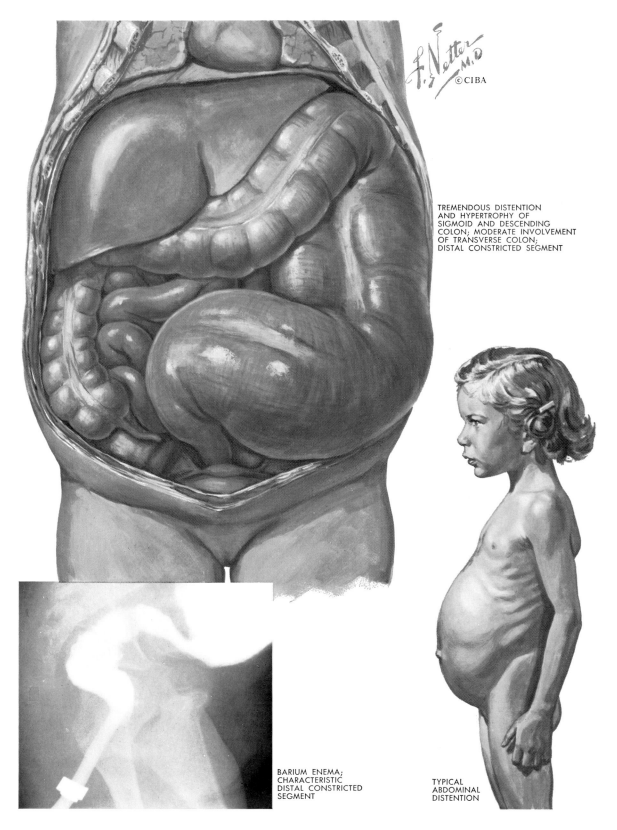

TREMENDOUS DISTENTION AND HYPERTROPHY OF SIGMOID AND DESCENDING COLON; MODERATE INVOLVEMENT OF TRANSVERSE COLON; DISTAL CONSTRICTED SEGMENT

BARIUM ENEMA; CHARACTERISTIC DISTAL CONSTRICTED SEGMENT

TYPICAL ABDOMINAL DISTENTION

includes a statement that the child has "never had a normal bowel movement". Enemas, laxatives, etc., have kept the bowel only relatively empty, and normal stools have not punctuated the history of obstipation. Occasionally, "diarrhea" has been noted, which is better described as liquid bowel content working its way around a fecal impaction and out. The youngster with chronic functional constipation usually has the onset of difficulty at the time of toilet training, has other emotional problems, may use constipation as a "weapon" against his family, gives a history of normal stooling intermittently and frequently has passed a stool the caliber of which is so large as to be unbelievable to the uninitiated. The passage of this stool of large caliber is never associated with aganglionic megacolon.

On physical examination the purely functionally constipated child has a relatively normal abdomen,

in which firm fecal masses may be felt in the sigmoid colon. On rectal examination the sphincter may be normal or loose, and feces are encountered at the sphincter or, if the bowel has recently been evacuated, the rectal ampulla is of huge dimensions. The child with aganglionic megacolon, on the other hand, has a *large abdomen,* and its musculature is somewhat lacking in tone. Tremendous fecal impaction of the bowel is palpable, and, at times, the diameter of the sigmoid is greater than the diameter of the child's thigh. Rectal examination reveals a tight sphincter; the rectal canal is empty and of normal caliber, and if feces can be felt at all, they are encountered high up at the point of junction between the rectosigmoid and the rectal ampulla.

On the basis of the afore-mentioned history, signs and symptoms, the diagnostician can separate most

(Continued on page 119)

CONGENITAL INTESTINAL OBSTRUCTION VI

Megacolon (Hirschsprung's Disease)

(Continued from page 118)

youngsters with aganglionic megacolon from the diagnosis of the chronically constipated child. The critical diagnostic study is the *barium enema*. Preparation for this must be time-consuming in the aganglionic megacolon, where bowel content is not readily removed by enemas. The technique of barium enema is specific if the diagnosis is to be made, and the routine barium enema, as undertaken by roentgenologists for study of the adult colon, may well miss the pathognomonic sign of aganglionic megacolon. The tip of the enema catheter must be inserted no higher than a point just within the rectal canal and at the proximal edge of the internal sphincter. Here the catheter is strapped in place, the mucocutaneous junction is indicated with a lead marker and the buttocks are taped together. Fluoroscopic guidance of the introduction of the barium must be made in the lateral as well as the oblique views, for, again, routine anterior-posterior examination may fail to visualize that segment of the bowel which is diagnostic.

In the chronically constipated individual, barium flows freely into a large ampulla, and the barium silhouette resembles the junction of a tulip bloom with its stem. Evacuation is complete. In aganglionic megacolon, however, the barium enters a colon of normal caliber and flows a short or long distance to a point where sudden transition to a tremendously enlarged colon occurs. This transition is abrupt and may be any place from 7 cm. above the sphincter to the rare situation where the entire colon is of small caliber and the aganglionic segment (for such is the narrow colon of normal caliber) extends to the small bowel. In the typical case the aganglionic segment is quite distal and does not extend proximal to the splenic flexure. On attempted evacuation in the patient with aganglionic megacolon, most of the barium remains behind, and the transition is prominent because peristalsis is normal to that point but absent distal to it.

In exploring the abdomen of the child with aganglionic megacolon, the surgeon is impressed with the *great dilatation of the sigmoid*, but for years other easily discernible signs were ignored: the presence of the distal bowel of normal caliber, the hypertrophy of the muscle bundles in the dilated segment and the relative

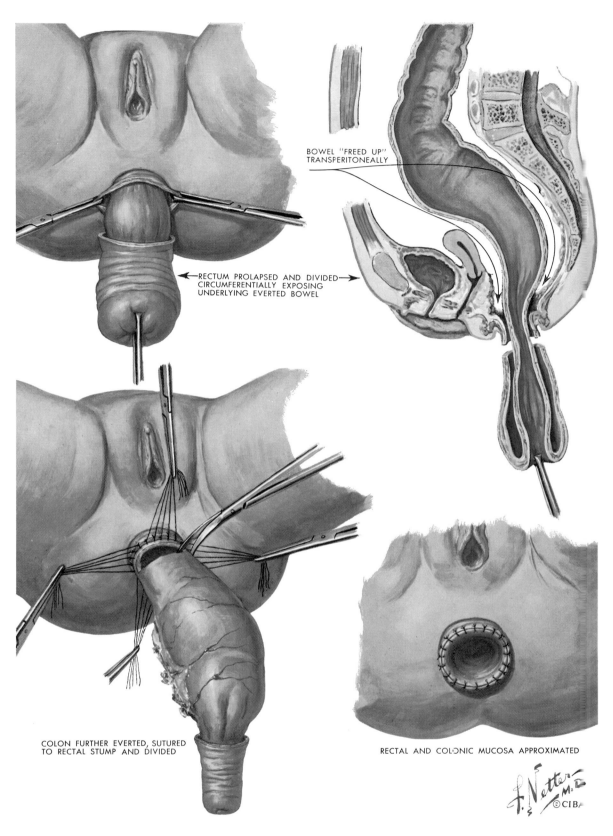

BOWEL "FREED UP" TRANSPERITONEALLY

← RECTUM PROLAPSED AND DIVIDED CIRCUMFERENTIALLY EXPOSING UNDERLYING EVERTED BOWEL →

COLON FURTHER EVERTED, SUTURED TO RECTAL STUMP AND DIVIDED

RECTAL AND COLONIC MUCOSA APPROXIMATED

localization of the extreme hypertrophy and dilatation in a typical situation where the aganglionic segment is distal to the sigmoid. Before the current correct concept of the etiology of aganglionic megacolon was developed, the surgeon directed his attention to this abnormal-appearing segment, *i.e.*, the dilated one, resected it and re-anastomosed the bowel without removing the distal segment which had initiated the whole process. In effect, the aganglionic segment, not being the site of a propulsive peristalsis, results in a work hypertrophy of the bowel just proximal to the transition, usually the sigmoid, which later gives way to dilatation with disruption of the hypertrophied circular and longitudinal muscle fibers. The hypertrophy is usually confined to that part of the left colon attached to a free mesentery, because the partial volvulus which follows impaction of the sigmoid with feces produces a variety of closed-loop

obstruction, with the aganglionic transition distally and the junction of fixed colon and loose sigmoid proximally. The abnormal-appearing loop of colon represents a physiologic response; the distal bowel which appears so normal is the etiologic culprit.

The only *operative procedure* which results in alleviating the child's clinical syndrome of aganglionic megacolon is an abdominoperineal pull-through procedure, with preservation of the sphincter. If the size of the colon is too great to permit a primary procedure because of the disproportionate calibers of the colon and rectum, colostomy should be performed, followed by a waiting period for the colon to shrink, through disuse, to a caliber suitable for anastomosis with the rectum. The colostomy may be either at the site of ganglion cell transition or proximal to it. The latter permits a safety valve at the time of definitive surgery,

(Continued on page 120)

CONGENITAL INTESTINAL OBSTRUCTION VI

Megacolon (Hirschsprung's Disease)

(Continued from page 119)

but its disadvantage is the need for an additional operation to close the colostomy.

The definitive procedure is much like that employed for resection of the rectum for carcinoma, except for the important difference in that the line of dissection for aganglionic megacolon stays as close to the bowel as possible to prevent disruption of the nerve and blood supply to the bladder and the ejaculatory mechanism in the male. Many children with aganglionic megacolon have an abnormal cystometrogram and are prone to urinary tract infection. For this reason the author avoids the use of a urethral catheter whenever possible. Dissection is carried into the pelvis to a point adjacent to the sphincter posteriorly and to the level of the vagina or prostate anteriorly. Following this, the bowel is intussuscepted, so that the aganglionic segment is completely delivered below the sphincter. Anastomosis is then carried out on the perineum, using a two-layer procedure with horizontal mattress sutures in the seromuscular layer and a catgut suture in the mucosa for hemostasis. When the final sutures are cut and the bowel retracts, the anastomosis should be just proximal to the sphincter. An anastomosis which lies more proximal to the mucocutaneous line than a distance twice the length of the sphincter may well result in nothing more than a temporary relief of symptoms, because of the length of aganglionic segment remaining.

In the newborn, aganglionic megacolon produces all signs and symptoms of an intestinal obstruction. The usual signs of vomiting, distention and failure to pass normal meconium are usually present. A flat film of the abdomen may show a ground-glass appearance of inspissated meconium. Differentiation must be made from meconium ileus (see page 114), where gas shadows in the bowel are of very irregular size, and the physiologic syndrome of the meconium plug. The surgeon's obligation is to relieve the intestinal obstruction, and, inasmuch as the infant cannot tolerate the definitive operation to remove the aganglionic segment, a colostomy is the procedure of choice. Here, as in the older child, the site of the *colostomy* may vary, with the same advantages and disadvantages. The surgeon need not fear that a right transverse colostomy will introduce difficult prob-

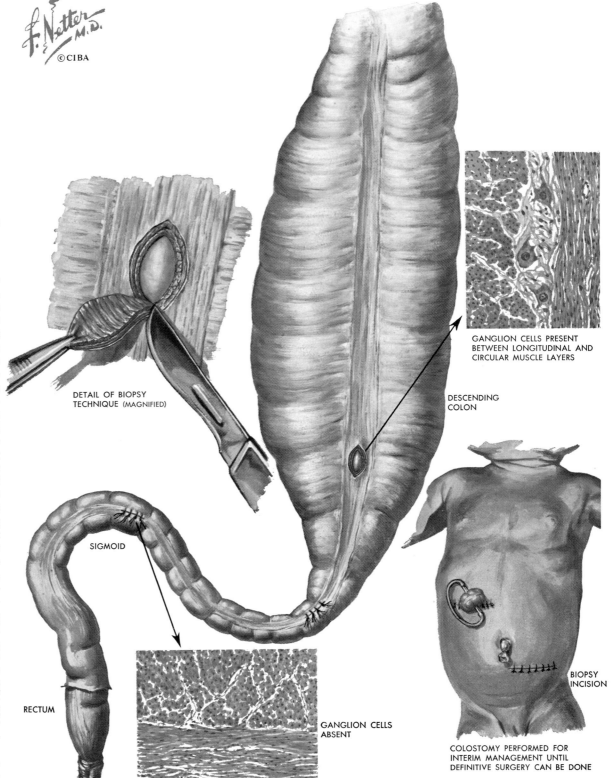

DETAIL OF BIOPSY TECHNIQUE (MAGNIFIED)

SIGMOID

RECTUM

GANGLION CELLS ABSENT

GANGLION CELLS PRESENT BETWEEN LONGITUDINAL AND CIRCULAR MUSCLE LAYERS

DESCENDING COLON

BIOPSY INCISION

COLOSTOMY PERFORMED FOR INTERIM MANAGEMENT UNTIL DEFINITIVE SURGERY CAN BE DONE

lems in therapy because of excessive fluid losses.

Barium enema at this age does not show the typical zone of abrupt transition between normal innervated bowel and the aganglionic segment. Instead, the bowel appears to have a somewhat serrated lining, and the aganglionic segment gradually emerges into the megacolonic portion by a symmetrical funnel-shaped enlargement.

At the time of the colostomy in the newborn, if the condition of the infant warrants it, the colon is examined and two or three *biopsies* of the wall are obtained through a transverse incision in the lower left quadrant of the abdomen. The information obtained through the microscopic examination of these biopsies aids the surgeon in determining the extent of the eventual resection of the aganglionic segment. At the time of the definitive operation, the zone of transition from the aganglionic to the ganglionic portion is not

evident, since the bowel distal to the colostomy has become uniform in caliber from disuse. This is also a helpful procedure in the older child, if a temporary colostomy is to be used awaiting collapse of the terminal colon from disuse. Without these initial biopsies, frozen-section diagnosis must be made, at the time of definitive surgery, to establish the level at which ganglion cells are present in the mesenteric plexus.

The technique of colostomy in the newborn should be carefully evaluated, and sutures must be taken at short intervals between the seromuscular layer of the bowel and the fascia through which the loop is withdrawn.

Unless the distention is great, the colostomy is not opened for approximately 24 hours postoperatively. Subsequently, when the infant weighs about 20 lb., the definitive operation is performed, as has been described above.

CONGENITAL INTESTINAL OBSTRUCTION VII

Management of Esophageal Atresia

Congenital atresia of the esophagus has been discussed in CIBA COLLECTION, Vol. 3/1, page 138, but its surgical management is described here in connection with other obstructions of the alimentary tract and their emergency treatment.

The presence of this life-endangering abnormality is suspected in infants with excessive amounts of mucus in the nasopharynx and with cyanosis, especially if this status recurs minutes or hours after the removal of the mucus and the administration of oxygen. The diagnosis becomes obvious at the first feeding, when the second swallow meets the first swallow, on its way back, in the nasopharynx, the infant choking, coughing and sneezing, and food being aspirated and forcibly ejected through the mouth and nose. To confirm the suspected diagnosis, one passes, through the nose into the esophagus, a No. 8 soft rubber catheter, which usually stops in the blind pouch. The possibility that it may coil in the pouch should be kept in mind. The physician should blow into the catheter and, at the same time, listen with a stethoscope over the infant's neck. Nothing will be heard if the end of the catheter is in the stomach, but a rush of air will be distinctly noticed if it is in an esophageal pouch. (This simple procedure should be routine for every newborn before it leaves the delivery room, in order to eliminate any delay in diagnosis and treatment.) Further confirmation of the diagnosis should be obtained by detecting roentgenographically the presence of the coiled catheter in the pouch. Instillation of radiopaque material is not only unnecessary but also dangerous. The presence of a fistula can be determined without radiopaque substances when air, which could only have entered by way of a fistula, is found in the gastro-intestinal tract.

Formerly, a retropleural approach with posterior resection of three rib segments was advocated to avoid respiratory embarrassment, secondary pleural infection and the inherent danger of empyema if leakage of the anastomosis should occur. Besides the fact that this approach provides a very small operative field, better techniques in anesthesia, the availability of antibiotics and the increased experience of surgeons now permit the use of a *transpleural approach through an intercostal space,* which furnishes a wider exposure of the field and also seems to carry a reduced mortality. With this technique, under endotracheal anesthesia and with the patient in the lateral recumbent position, an incision is made from the region of the costochondral junction to the region of the sacrospinalis muscle

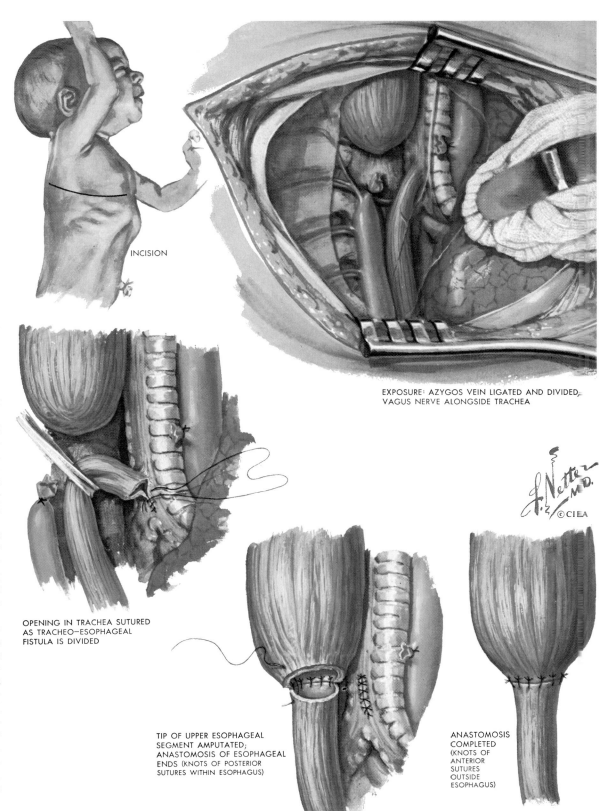

INCISION

EXPOSURE: AZYGOS VEIN LIGATED AND DIVIDED, VAGUS NERVE ALONGSIDE TRACHEA

OPENING IN TRACHEA SUTURED AS TRACHEO-ESOPHAGEAL FISTULA IS DIVIDED

TIP OF UPPER ESOPHAGEAL SEGMENT AMPUTATED; ANASTOMOSIS OF ESOPHAGEAL ENDS (KNOTS OF POSTERIOR SUTURES WITHIN ESOPHAGUS)

ANASTOMOSIS COMPLETED (KNOTS OF ANTERIOR SUTURES OUTSIDE ESOPHAGUS)

(erector spinae). Using a self-retaining retractor, the third or fourth costal interspace is entered without dividing any ribs. After opening the mediastinal pleura and *ligating and dividing the vena azygos,* the upper portion of the esophagus is mobilized as far cephalad as possible. To facilitate the identification of the upper pouch, a catheter should be inserted through the nose into the esophagus. The dissection of the lower esophagus and of the esophageal-tracheal fistula, which is usually present, must be performed with utmost gentleness, because this esophageal portion lacks both the blood supply and the muscular hypertrophy found in the upper segment. By exerting mild *traction on a strip of rubber drain placed around the lower esophagus,* the connection between esophagus and trachea is separated, and the defect in the trachea is closed by oversewing it with 5-0 silk, carefully avoiding constriction of the trachea as well as the

inclusion of esophageal tissue, which may later cause development of a diverticulum at the site of the former fistula. The tracheal closure should be tested under saline solution for air leaks.

Further steps depend upon the situation. If a reasonably well-developed lower esophagus is present, and if its distance from the upper pouches permit , an anastomosis of the upper and lower portions is undertaken, after trimming off any edges of the latter. Making every effort to minimize the trauma, the esophageal anastomosis is performed as a *one-layer closure, including the mucosa* with each of the twelve to fourteen stitches. If the anastomosis is not under great tension and seems tight, the mediastinal pleura is reapproximated, and the chest is closed without drainage. A small-diameter polyethylene tube with a smooth end is threaded down into the stomach in those

(Continued on page 122)

CONGENITAL INTESTINAL OBSTRUCTION VII

Management of Esophageal Atresia

(Continued from page 121)

cases in which the tension between the anastomosed parts seems great enough to make early feeding across it hazardous. This tube substitutes for the No. 8 catheter which, originally lying in the proximal segment, has been passed down after one third of the anastomosis has been secured, and which can be removed when the closure is completed.

In the absence of a lower esophagus or with too great a distance to permit an end-to-end anastomosis of the two pouches, a *cervical esophagostomy* and a feeding *gastrostomy* must be resorted to after the closure of any existing fistula. Subsequently, when the infant is 3 to 6 months old, either the right or the transverse colon is brought into the chest to connect the upper esophagus with the stomach. To attempt this *colonic replacement* of the esophagus as an emergency operation in the neonatal period is not recommended. In short, the essential points of the operation are: incision from the xiphoid process to the umbilicus; detachment of the right portion and hepatic flexure of the colon; division of the colic artery close to its origin, preserving as many arcades of mesenteric blood supply as possible; division of the ileum at or near the ileocecal valve; closure of the opening on the colonic side; mobilization of the esophagus toward the pharynx after detachment of the esophagostomy stoma from the skin by circumferential incision; exteriorization of the distal opening of the esophagus through a new transverse incision in the suprasternal notch; construction of a tunnel behind the sternum through the anterior mediastinum through which the cecum is passed and brought out through an incision in the suprasternal notch; amputation of the cecum, appendix and ileocecal valve if the remaining right colon is sufficient in length to permit tension-free anastomosis with the cervical esophagus, otherwise using the cecum to perform this two-layer end-to-end anastomosis; placement of a drain beneath the anastomosis and exteriorization through the incision; closure of the incision. The transverse colon is divided for anastomoses of its proximal end with the lesser curvature of the stomach and of its distal end with the terminal ileum. The gastrostomy is left in place until it has been ascertained that feedings can be taken well by mouth. Some surgeons prefer a two-stage procedure, completing all abdominal anastomoses during the first elective operation but reserving the esophago-colon anastomosis for a second operation; this, however, may sometimes

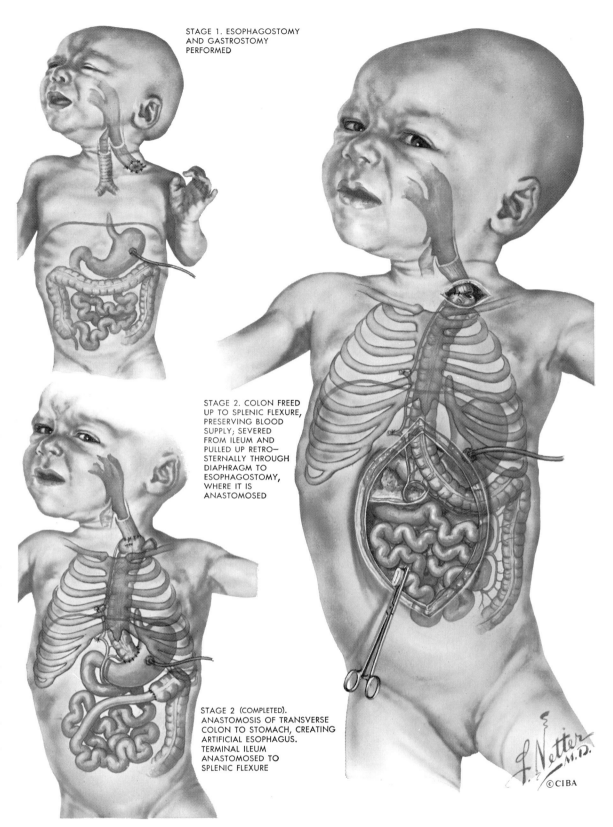

STAGE 1. ESOPHAGOSTOMY AND GASTROSTOMY PERFORMED

STAGE 2. COLON FREED UP TO SPLENIC FLEXURE, PRESERVING BLOOD SUPPLY; SEVERED FROM ILEUM AND PULLED UP RETRO-STERNALLY THROUGH DIAPHRAGM TO ESOPHAGOSTOMY, WHERE IT IS ANASTOMOSED

STAGE 2 (COMPLETED). ANASTOMOSIS OF TRANSVERSE COLON TO STOMACH, CREATING ARTIFICIAL ESOPHAGUS. TERMINAL ILEUM ANASTOMOSED TO SPLENIC FLEXURE

be more difficult because of an edema of the exteriorized cecum. Fistulas may develop at the esophago-colon anastomosis after the primary as well as after the secondary operation, but it seems that in the primary case they heal spontaneously, whereas in the latter case a third operation is necessary.

Postoperatively, particularly after the operation in the postnatal period, the infants are kept in an atmosphere of high humidity which is helpful in liquefying the copious, thick, tenacious mucus. The nasopharyngeal secretion is frequently aspirated by the attending nurse, and direct tracheal aspirations are carried out, when necessary, by the physician. Broad-spectrum antibiotics are given until the choice of a specific drug can be made, based on the kinds of organisms cultured from the mucus, obtained preoperatively in the blind pouch and later in the pharynx and upper esophagus, and on the organisms' sensitivity. Blood

or plasma is infused daily if necessary. Fluids are provided intravenously in minimum quantities and without salt, except for that amount needed to replace bases to avoid edema of the subcutaneous tissue. Isotonicity of parenteral fluid is achieved with glucose. Feedings are begun, either by mouth, through a tube in the esophagus or through the gastrostomy, on an average of 48 to 72 hours after operation, although some infants have been fed in less than 24 hours. Postoperative X-ray studies showing normal swallowing do not necessarily indicate that normal deglutition is established. The propulsive esophageal function in some infants remains disrupted for several weeks or months, as can readily be shown roentgenographically when a bolus of barium descends in the esophagus almost to the cardia, only to return promptly to the nasopharynx. Time alone will bring about normal functioning.

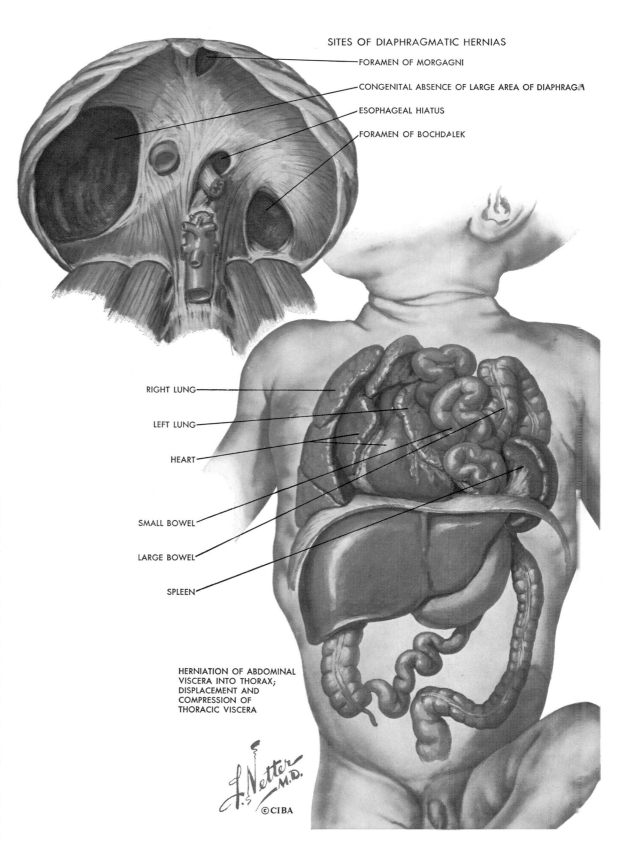

SITES OF DIAPHRAGMATIC HERNIAS

FORAMEN OF MORGAGNI

CONGENITAL ABSENCE OF LARGE AREA OF DIAPHRAGM

ESOPHAGEAL HIATUS

FORAMEN OF BOCHDALEK

RIGHT LUNG

LEFT LUNG

HEART

SMALL BOWEL

LARGE BOWEL

SPLEEN

HERNIATION OF ABDOMINAL
VISCERA INTO THORAX;
DISPLACEMENT AND
COMPRESSION OF
THORACIC VISCERA

DIAPHRAGMATIC HERNIA

Diaphragmatic hernia in the newborn is not an uncommon defect and seems to be reported more frequently than formerly, probably reflecting earlier diagnosis and more prompt treatment rather than increased incidence. If the diaphragmatic defect is not surgically repaired, most of these infants die within the first month of life as a result of respiratory embarrassment. It is generally agreed that, although such a hernia is not necessarily fatal, the mortality rate in untreated patients is so high as to justify placing this lesion in the category of congenital anomalies incompatible with life but amenable to corrective surgery if operated immediately. The hope that the infant may survive, grow and become a better surgical risk later should be abandoned, in view of the excessive and needless mortality. Even if the distress is not so great as to make an immediate operation imperative, or if the administration of oxygen is followed by periods of improvement, it is impossible to predict the future course, and it is dangerous to wait for the day when the infant's cardiorespiratory reserve may be upset by further crowding of the abdominal viscera into the pleural cavity and, consequently, further shifting of the mediastinum. Therefore, postponement of an operation in the expectation of more ideal conditions for surgery is inexcusable.

The most usual site of a congenital diaphragmatic hernia is the *foramen of Bochdalek* (fetal pleuroperitoneal hiatus) in the left posterolateral portion (see page 4). Less common are hernias at the esophageal hiatus, which have been discussed in Part 1 of this volume on the digestive system (pages 158 and 159), and at the *foramen of Morgagni* in the retrosternal portion of the diaphragm. Herniation through these latter abnormal openings usually does not produce severe respiratory distress. Still more rarely, the diaphragm may have completely failed to develop, or a large area on the right side may be absent, so that only a small rim of muscular tissue is present around the periphery; sometimes, even this rim may be lacking anterolaterally. Defects on the left leaf of the diaphragm are, statistically, twelve to fifteen times more common than defects of the right leaf, and the latter, in this author's experience, are always accompanied by some other major congenital anomaly.

Diaphragmatic hernia should be considered in any newborn in whom cyanosis persists after clearing the airways and making the usual efforts to establish respiration. The diagnosis can sometimes be made in the delivery room. The characteristic signs, *i.e.*, a relatively large chest, the left side of which lags behind the right in respiratory effects (if the hernia is on the left, as it is in most instances), and a small and frequently scaphoid abdomen, are recognized at birth. The heart is displaced to the right, often to an extreme degree. Breathing sounds are absent over the left chest and are heard only over the upper right thorax portion, where they are harsh in character. Gas fills the herniated bowel usually only later, so that the percussion sound over the chest is not necessarily tympanitic directly after birth. Auscultatory findings, suggestive of peristaltic movements in the chest, are at this point also unreliable. Some infants,

able to compensate for the presence of abdominal viscera in the chest, exhibit signs and symptoms only when the gas-filled intestines cause a greater mediastinal shift. Though the diagnosis can be made on physical findings alone, roentgenograms are taken almost universally to confirm the clinical impression, except when the severity of the infant's respiratory distress does not allow time for such a procedure. In those patients in whom the diagnosis is not clear on clinical grounds, the cardiorespiratory disturbances are less severe, so that the roentgenographic study is not an undue risk. The air in the bowel usually provides the necessary contrast, so that contrast media are superfluous and, indeed, even contraindicated. Anal instillation of a mixture of mineral oil and radiopaque oil to ascertain the nature of a small mass of abdominal viscera in the chest, which may

(Continued on page 124)

DIAPHRAGMATIC HERNIA

(*Continued from page 123*)

be colon alone, may, in some instances, be indicated.

Once the diagnosis of diaphragmatic hernia is made, immediate surgical intervention, in an effort to repair the defect, is the sole type of management. To avoid additional distention of the abdominal viscera, gastro-intestinal intubation of the infant before anesthesia is recommended. Succinylcholine administration and the insertion of an endotracheal tube are the only other preparatory measures. The abdominal approach is most commonly advocated, but this involves a number of difficulties. Working from the abdominal side, the surgeon is frequently hindered in the extraction of gas-filled loops of bowel through the defect, especially when removal is urgent. The repair of the defect from below may become difficult if the overhanging rib cage does not allow adequate exposure, and when the peritoneal cavity is to be closed but is not large enough to hold the replaced viscera. Experience with such infants has led to the recommendation of the *thoracic approach,* which is generally considered superior in adults with acquired or traumatic diaphragmatic hernias. The first advantage of the thoracic approach is achieved by a rapid intercostal incision, which gives immediate relief of cardiorespiratory embarrassment and permits instantaneous delivery of the displaced viscera. The mediastinum can return to the midline, the compressed lung can expand and the patient becomes a relatively normal cardiorespiratory risk under anesthesia, so that the remainder of the operation can be undertaken without the previous urgency. The replacement of the abdominal viscera through the diaphragmatic opening has been found not too difficult; certainly it is easier than closure of the peritoneum in instances of disproportion between the cavity and the mass of abdominal viscera. More adequate exposure of the defect and greater ease in repairing it are further advantages of the thoracic approach, which also permits postoperative aspiration of the pneumothorax without endangering the repaired diaphragm. Finally, postoperative ileus appears to occur less often when the bowel has no opportunity to come in contact with a large incision or with a raw surface, as in those cases in which the fascia must be left open and the cutaneous and subcutaneous layers alone are closed.

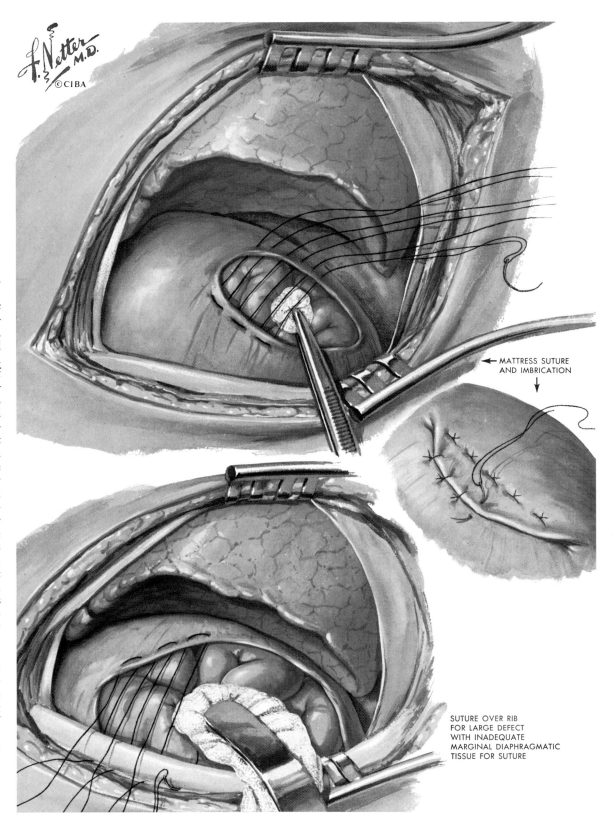

← MATTRESS SUTURE AND IMBRICATION

SUTURE OVER RIB FOR LARGE DEFECT WITH INADEQUATE MARGINAL DIAPHRAGMATIC TISSUE FOR SUTURE

The site of incision is the seventh right interspace. After opening the pleura and spreading the ribs apart with retractors, the abdominal viscera are evacuated from the chest, and the hole in the diaphragm is inspected. A hernial sac of pleuroperitoneum, if present, as is infrequently the case, should be preserved if possible but must be retracted to alleviate the pressure on the mediastinum. It may, however, be necessary to open the sac to replace the viscera, when adhesions between sac and its contents exist. Replacement of the herniated organs is a time-consuming procedure and must be done with the utmost care to avoid trauma. Once the viscera are replaced, closure of the diaphragmatic defect is not difficult if it is small. It is even frequently possible to imbricate the edges of the defect. Occasionally, the spleen may have to be removed in order to permit closure. In other instances it may be necessary to fracture one or two

ribs to make the lateral rim meet the medial rim of the defect, or to transplant other muscles to cover the diaphragmatic hole. After closure of the diaphragm, it will be noted that the underdeveloped lung will not fill the pleural space. The anesthetist should refrain from attempting to inflate the lung, in order to avoid pressure with consequent emphysematous changes. The lung will expand spontaneously within several days. The chest should be closed, with a tube in the pleural cavity to institute underwater suction if needed.

Gastric suction drainage, intravenous administration of fluids, plasma or whole-blood transfusion, when indicated, and measures to keep the nasopharynx and trachea clear of secretions are the essential features of postoperative care. Feedings may begin on the second or third postoperative day by gavage tube rather than by bottle in order to avoid gastric dilatation with swallowed air.

OMPHALOCELE

An *omphalocele,* or exomphalos, is a hernia of the bowel, and, occasionally, spleen and liver into the base of the umbilical cord. It originates, according to the most probable hypothesis, from a perpetuation of the physiologic, but normally transitory, protrusion of the embryonic celom between the sixth and tenth weeks of fetal life (see pages 3, 5 and 7).

The diagnosis of an omphalocele can usually be made by inspection, but an error may easily occur if the omphalocele is so small that it appears to be a normal part of the umbilical cord. The infant born with an omphalocele should be transferred directly to the nearest satisfactorily equipped operating room, because haste in getting to surgery prevents expansion of the bowel with swallowed air, averts drying out of the amniotic sac and minimizes contamination of the sac by air-borne bacteria. If the hernia is small enough to allow the viscera to be placed within the abdominal cavity, the usual *layered direct closure* of the abdominal wall will be found feasible, and the amniotic sac may be dissected away. If, however, the omphalocele is large, it may be impossible to place a large mass of abdominal viscera into an abdominal cavity developed only sufficiently to contain a much smaller quantity. With such disproportion between the sizes of the omphalocele and the abdominal cavity, a two-stage procedure is indicated. In the first, after incision at the junction of the amnion and the skin, *skin flaps* are raised *across the abdominal wall,* the dissection being carried far down *into the flanks* as well as cephalad and caudad. When the *skin flaps* can be *approximated in the midline over the amniotic membrane,* the procedure is completed by placing interrupted sutures in the skin. The amniotic sac must be preserved, if fascial closure of the abdominal wall is not possible, in order to prevent adhesions between the viscera and the skin.

Surprisingly, children without a fascial closure of the abdomen do not seem to have difficulties in defecation and micturition. The infant's trunk is supported with a broad (at least 15 cm.) elastic girdle until the time comes for a secondary closure of a skin-covered omphalocele. In general, the second step should be delayed for at least 2 years but should be performed when the viscera may be held in the abdominal cavity by manual pressure without signs of respiratory difficulties. It should be borne in mind that, without the pressure of the abdominal

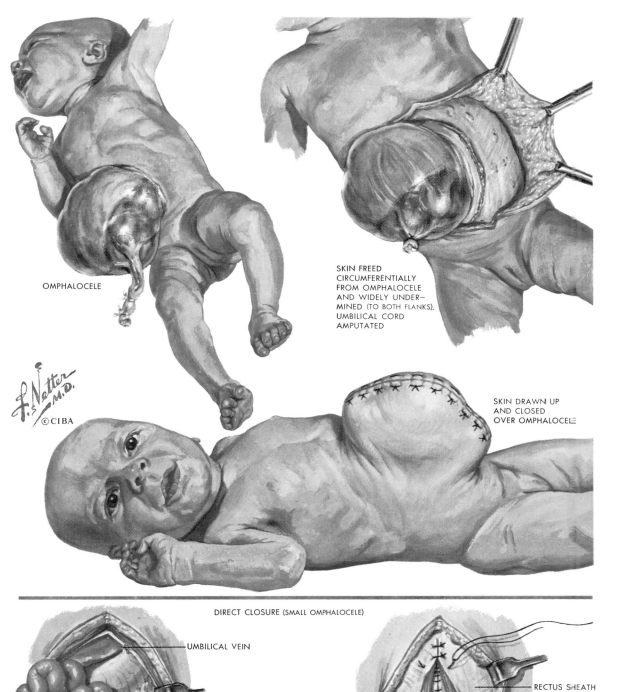

OMPHALOCELE

SKIN FREED CIRCUMFERENTIALLY FROM OMPHALOCELE AND WIDELY UNDER-MINED (TO BOTH FLANKS). UMBILICAL CORD AMPUTATED

SKIN DRAWN UP AND CLOSED OVER OMPHALOCELE

DIRECT CLOSURE (SMALL OMPHALOCELE)

UMBILICAL VEIN

LEFT UMBILICAL ARTERY

SAC AND ADJOINING RIM OF SKIN CUT AWAY; UMBILICAL ARTERIES AND VEIN LIGATED

RECTUS SHEATH

RECTUS ABDOMINIS MUSCLE

PERITONEUM

LAYERS OF ABDOMINAL WALL DISSECTED OUT AND SUTURED SERIALLY

musculature to force the liver upward and outward against the rib cage, the thorax lags behind in development for the child's chronological age.

At the second stage it should be possible to bring the medial edges of the rectus sheath together in the midline to form a linea alba. If this is not possible, the anterior sheath may be divided from the posterior sheath at the lateral border of each rectus muscle. The flaps of rectus fascia so formed are then folded medially and sutured together at the midline.

Management of an omphalocele may be complicated by various factors, *e.g.,* by rupture of the omphalocele sac either in utero or during delivery. The frequency of multiple congenital anomalies in these infants must also be borne in mind. Some variety of intestinal obstruction is commonly an associated finding, especially anomalies of rotation and fixation of the colon. Obviously, if intestinal obstruction is suspected from X-ray studies or from other signs such as vomiting, failure to pass a stool, or distention, the proper corrective intra-abdominal procedure must be undertaken before the closure is completed.

It is sometimes possible to obtain a fascial closure of the abdominal wall when it might have been more prudent to settle for a skin closure alone. When the abdominal viscera are overcrowded in a small peritoneal cavity, the diaphragm is elevated and the respiratory effort may be greatly increased. The patient may therefore succumb to the definitive operation, whereas he might have survived if only the first stage of a two-stage procedure had been undertaken.

The frequency of omphalocele has been estimated to be 1 in 3,200 births (McKeown *et al.*), and the surgical mortality 34 per cent (Gross), although a much lower mortality is the current experience in many hospitals.

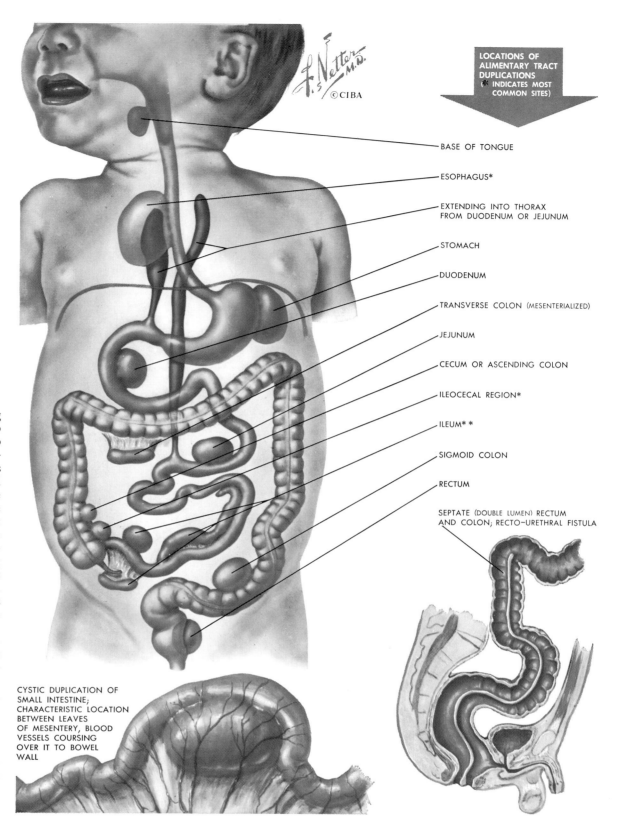

LOCATIONS OF ALIMENTARY TRACT DUPLICATIONS (* INDICATES MOST COMMON SITES)

BASE OF TONGUE

ESOPHAGUS*

EXTENDING INTO THORAX FROM DUODENUM OR JEJUNUM

STOMACH

DUODENUM

TRANSVERSE COLON (MESENTERIALIZED)

JEJUNUM

CECUM OR ASCENDING COLON

ILEOCECAL REGION*

ILEUM* *

SIGMOID COLON

RECTUM

SEPTATE (DOUBLE LUMEN) RECTUM AND COLON; RECTO–URETHRAL FISTULA

CYSTIC DUPLICATION OF SMALL INTESTINE; CHARACTERISTIC LOCATION BETWEEN LEAVES OF MESENTERY, BLOOD VESSELS COURSING OVER IT TO BOWEL WALL

DUPLICATIONS OF ALIMENTARY TRACT

Cystic structures, developing, during fetal life, in the mesentery adjacent to the intestine, are relatively rare and do not constitute an acutely life-endangering condition, as do other malformations (see pages 112 to 124). These spherical or elongated structures, which may be single or, more frequently, multiple, are equipped with all the layers of that part of the alimentary tract to which they are intimately attached, including the muscular coat, which, in contrast, is lacking in acquired diverticula. In view of this morphologic identity, particularly with regard to the mucosal layer, it seems that the designation "duplications of the alimentary tract" is the most suitable, though these malformations are also referred to as "mesenteric cysts", "giant diverticula", "enteric cysts" or other denominations.

Several theories have been propounded to explain the origin of the duplications, but none has been definitely proved. Duplications may be encountered in all parts of the digestive tube from the *tongue* to the *rectum* but are most frequently related to the *ileum,* and only very seldom to the *duodenum* and *jejunum.* They are always found on the mesenteric side of the bowel, being nourished or drained by the blood vessels which also supply the adjacent parts of the bowel. The walls of the two structures — intestine and its corresponding duplication — are not sharply separated but have muscular fibers in common; hence, it is difficult to remove the duplicated segment without damaging the blood supply or the wall of the contiguous intestine. The duplication, which can differ extremely in size and shape, furthermore, may at times communicate with the intestine at its proximal or distal end, or even at both ends. The *duplications* may, though rarely, extend into the *thoracic cavity,* where they may end blindly or may *communicate with the esophagus.*

Clinical manifestations of these duplications (partial bowel obstruction, dis-

tention, sense of fullness and discomfort) may set in within the first years of life. Frequently, it is possible to palpate a movable cystic mass in the region of the terminal ileum, which has not caused any disturbance. Anemia (blood loss into the intestinal tract) may occasionally be the only sign of a communicating duplication. X-ray examination may help in ascertaining the diagnosis, which is always rather difficult, except for the duplications extending into the thorax, which cause respiratory troubles and can be recognized by chest roentgenograms.

Once the diagnosis is established or even only seriously suspected, laparotomy is indicated, in order to remove the duplication, if present. The cystic form of duplication is resected, usually with the adjacent bowel, and the intestinal continuity is restored by a primary end-to-end anastomosis. Efforts to preserve the adjacent loop should not be made, because of the

inherent dangers resulting from the vascular situation and the wall structures which duplication and bowel have in common. With patients in poor condition, it is advisable to be satisfied with a simple exteriorization by the Mikulicz technique and to postpone the final repair to a later date. *Colon duplications,* the presence of which is relatively easily established with a barium enema, usually pose serious problems. Resection of large colonic segments should be avoided, and a more conservative technique, such as destruction of the septum separating the duplication from the normal colon, should be tried. The same holds true for *duplication of the rectum.* It is usually possible to perform a simple resection of the septum as long as it is restricted to the rectosigmoid region.

Duplications extending into the thorax are resected by means of a transpleural approach, after appropriate handling of their abdominal portions.

MECKEL'S DIVERTICULUM

Vitelline Duct Remnants

The vitelline or omphalomesenteric duct, connecting, in early embryonic stages, the yolk sac with the primitive tubular gut (see page 7), is normally obliterated at about the seventh week of fetal life. Failure of the vitelline duct to disappear in its entire extension results in a variety of remnants, the most common of which presents itself as a sacculation or pouch attached to the ileum and is best known as *Meckel's diverticulum*. This diverticulum, which, with an incidence of about 2 per cent, is the most frequent congenital anomaly of the gastro-intestinal tract, originates from the most proximal, *i.e.,* intestinal, end of the vitelline duct which, for reasons unknown, has remained patent and, in the course of fetal development, grows into an appendage of the ileum. Located from 30 to 90 cm. proximal to the ileocecal junction and always attached to the antimesenteric side of the ileal wall, the diverticulum varies in length (from 1 to about 10 cm.) and also in width (from 1 to 3, or even 4, cm. in diameter), though its shape usually resembles that of a finger of a glove. The artery supplying and the vein draining the diverticulum, both derivatives of the primitive omphalomesenteric (or vitelline) vessels, cross over the ileal wall and course subserously, or confined in an accompanying mesenteriolum, along the diverticulum to its tip.

In contrast to the acquired intestinal diverticula (see pages 129 and 130), the wall of Meckel's diverticulum is composed of all the layers—mucosal, muscular and serosal—characteristic of the gastro-intestinal tract and is thus considered a "true" or "complete diverticulum". The mucosal lining corresponds to that of the ileum, but it contains, in many instances, islands of heterotopic (jejunal, duodenal or gastric) mucosa and nodules of pancreatic tissue, which may give cause to serious complications (see below). The opening of the diverticulum is funnellike and, as a rule, wide enough not to give rise to occlusions, as do the "false diverticula" with a narrow neck (see page 131).

It is typical of the majority of individuals with Meckel's diverticulum that the rest of the former vitelline duct has become completely obliterated, so that no trace of its existence can be found, but in some cases a *nonpatent, fibrous cord* may have remained, which *attaches the blind end of the diverticulum with the umbilical site of the abdominal wall.* Occasionally, the diverticulum or the fibrous cord may be affixed to another intestinal loop or to another viscus. It may also happen that a rudiment of the

MECKEL'S DIVERTICULUM

MECKEL'S DIVERTICULUM WITH FIBROUS CORD EXTENDING TO UMBILICUS

FIBROUS CORD CONNECTING SMALL INTESTINE WITH UMBILICUS

UMBILICO–INTESTINAL FISTULA

UMBILICAL SINUS

FIBROUS CORD WITH INTERMEDIATE CYST

vitelline duct remains permanently in the form of a *solid fibrous cord without development of a diverticulum,* resulting in a fixation of an ileal loop to the umbilicus. The clinical significance of this fibrous cord, irrelevant of the presence or absence of Meckel's diverticulum, arises from the fact that it may become the starting point of a strangulation of bowel loops (see below).

The persistence of the entire vitelline duct as a permanent tube leads to an *umbilico-intestinal fistula,* which should be easily discovered soon after birth. The umbilical cord in such relatively rare cases is usually thicker at its base at birth than is normal, and, when its external structures have regressed and sloughed off, a reddish mass with a small opening in its center will be noted in the umbilicus. The fistula discharges intestinal contents, the amount and character of which depend upon the caliber of the duct

and the changes in the abdominal pressure. The discharge can vary from an occasional drainage of small amounts of mucus to continuous loss of chymous material. In such cases an umbilical polyp frequently forms at the external opening of the fistula. The most serious complication of an umbilico-intestinal fistula, however, is a prolapse of the ileum through a fistulous tube of large caliber. Increased abdominal pressure, incident to crying or coughing of the infant, may cause such a prolapse, which presents itself as a dark-red, protruding, sausagelike mass, being a portion of the bowel turned inside out, with the intestinal mucosa appearing at the external mouth of the fistula.

The vitelline duct may also remain open only at its outer portion. This results in an incomplete umbilical fistula, called *umbilical sinus.* The more proximal parts of the duct in such instances usually have

(Continued on page 128)

MECKEL'S DIVERTICULUM
Vitelline Duct Remnants

(Continued from page 127)

become transformed into a fibrous cord attached on one end to the sinus and on the other to the ileum. Finally, it may happen that the vitelline duct undergoes *fibrosis* on the *outer* as well as on the *inner ends,* while a central portion persists as a patent part, which develops into a *cyst* causing, in later life, a variety of symptoms.

Meckel's diverticulum, as well as other intra-abdominal structures as far as they concern remnants of the vitelline duct, may be present and remain quiescent and unobserved for a lifetime, but sometimes they may give rise to pathologic phenomena. *Acute inflammation of a diverticulum* may be produced by nonspecific infections, foreign bodies, parasites or trauma. The inflammatory changes may vary from mild catarrhal and transient alterations to the gangrenous type, with subsequent perforation and peritonitis. Both clinically and pathologically they are similar to those changes observed in the vermiform appendix (see page 148). The onset of symptoms with this diverticulitis is usually sudden. Severe pain of colicky character is localized around the umbilicus and accompanied by nausea, persistent vomiting, high temperature and — with impending gangrene — signs of toxinemia. The abdomen may be distended, with an area of tenderness around the umbilicus or in the right or left lower quadrant. The differentiation between a process in Meckel's diverticulum and appendicitis, acute cholecystitis, colonic diverticulitis, acute salpingitis or any other inflammatory condition of the abdominal viscera is rather difficult and, at times, possible only at a laparotomy.

It is obvious that Meckel's diverticula may also become involved in other processes that take place in the ileum or other parts of the small intestine, such as tuberculosis or typhoid.

As a result of heterotopic gastric mucosa in the lining of a diverticulum (see above), a *peptic ulcer* may develop, which also poses a serious diagnostic problem, whether it occurs as an isolated ulcer in the diverticulum or combined with peptic ulcers elsewhere. The ulcer forms usually in the ileal mucosa of the diverticulum in the neighborhood of the heterotopic mucosal island, or away from it in the neck of the diverticulum or even in the ileum proper. It resembles the marginal jejunal ulcer occurring after gastrojejunal anastomosis (see CIBA COLLECTION, Vol. 3/I, page 189). The symptoms are either vague or more or less similar to those of gastroduodenal ulcers, as are the complications, such as hemorrhage and perforation (see CIBA COL-

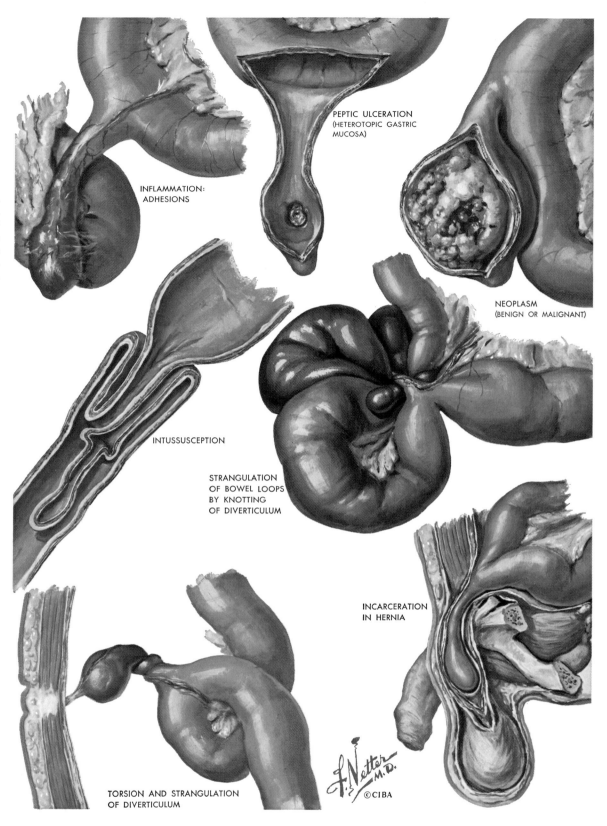

INFLAMMATION: ADHESIONS

PEPTIC ULCERATION (HETEROTOPIC GASTRIC MUCOSA)

NEOPLASM (BENIGN OR MALIGNANT)

INTUSSUSCEPTION

STRANGULATION OF BOWEL LOOPS BY KNOTTING OF DIVERTICULUM

INCARCERATION IN HERNIA

TORSION AND STRANGULATION OF DIVERTICULUM

F. Netter M.D. ©CIBA

LECTION, Vol. 3/I, pages 172 to 175).

The mouth of a Meckel's diverticulum may sometimes serve as the turning point of an *intussusception* (see page 134), the ileum playing the rôle of the intussusceptum, or an inverted diverticulum may serve as the leading point of ileal or ileocolic intussusception. A nodule of heterotopic tissue or a tumor situated near the fundus of the diverticulum may become the predisposing factor of an inversion, which, however, can be complete only when the diverticulum is in no way adherent to other structures. *Benign tumors* (myoma, lipoma, adenoma and neurogenic neoplasm), as well as malignant ones, develop occasionally in Meckel's diverticulum and may arise from the histologic elements that normally constitute this evagination or from the isles of heterotopic tissue. Different types of carcinoma, sarcoma and carcinoid tumors have been observed as in other parts of the

small intestine (see pages 163 to 165).

Strangulation of the diverticulum itself or *strangulation of a loop of the small intestine,* by a long diverticulum swinging around a loop and knotting, leads to intestinal obstruction. The mechanics of such an event have been explained by an extensive torsion of the diverticulum around its longitudinal axis. Strangulation of the diverticulum, which also may occur when it *enters the sac of an inguinal hernia* and becomes incarcerated, leads invariably to gangrene.

Correct clinical diagnosis of a Meckel's diverticulum and all its complications is seldom made preoperatively. X-ray demonstration of a diverticulum succeeds only in rare cases because of its wide neck and its complete muscular coat, both favoring a speedy emptying of the contrast medium. If the diverticulum is attached to the abdominal wall, it can be visualized by peritoneoscopy.

DIVERTICULA OF SMALL INTESTINE

A diverticulum is a blind outpouch of a hollow viscus, consisting of one or more layers of the part involved. In the jejunum and ileum, diverticula occur less frequently than in other segments of the alimentary canal, the stomach excepted (see CIBA COLLECTION, Vol. 3/1, page 161). Their incidence is estimated to be about 0.8 per thousand. In about 20 per cent of the cases, they are associated with diverticula in other parts of the digestive tract. The male sex is affected nearly twice as frequently as the female.

The small-intestinal *diverticula* may be single or multiple. The multiple diverticula can be so numerous as to involve nearly the entire small intestine. They are located almost always along the line of mesenteric attachment and are usually sessile. Their size varies from a few millimeters up to several centimeters in diameter.

The "complete" diverticula, formed by all the layers of the intestinal wall, are believed to be of congenital origin and are frequently associated with other malformations. The "incomplete" diverticula, consisting only of mucosa and serosa, represent, in fact, hernias of the mucous membrane protruding through the muscular coat of the intestinal wall. They are considered to be acquired deformities. The mechanism by which they come into existence has not been definitely established (see also page 130), though it has been recognized that the gap in the muscular coat caused by the entering of the blood vessels (see page 66) presents a weakened area through which the mucosa may be pushed by increased intraluminal pressure.

Diverticula of the small intestine are

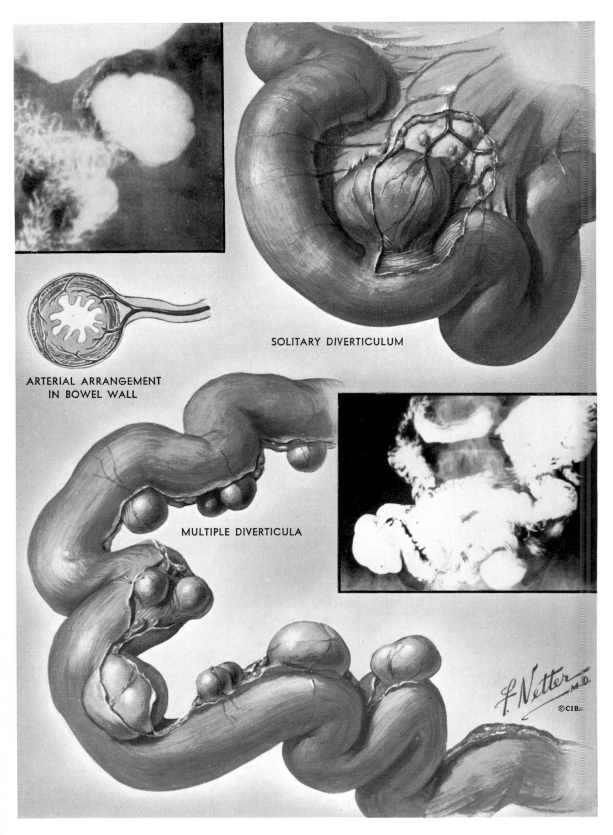

ARTERIAL ARRANGEMENT IN BOWEL WALL

SOLITARY DIVERTICULUM

MULTIPLE DIVERTICULA

frequently symptomless and are found incidentally in the course of an X-ray examination or at autopsy. In some cases the symptoms are limited to a vague abdominal pain and flatulence appearing a certain time after meals and attributed to retention of fecal matter in the diverticula. But the small-intestinal diverticula may also give rise to serious complications such as acute inflammation, intestinal obstruction, perforation and hemorrhage. Acute diverticulitis is usually the consequence of food rests, coproliths or parasites becoming trapped in the pouch and may present a symptomatology similar to that of an acute appendicitis. Intestinal obstruction may occur by strangulation, compression by an inflammatory tumor or, more rarely, intussusception. The perforation of a diverticulum is usually the consequence of an acute inflammation or traumatism produced by a foreign body which found its way into the pouch. The per-

foration may occur in the free abdominal cavity, the mesentery or another intestinal loop, resulting in a generalized peritonitis, a walled-off abscess or an intestinal fistula. A few cases are recorded in which aberrant pancreatic tissue and benign or malignant tumors were located in an intestinal diverticulum.

A massive diverticulosis of the small intestine may interfere seriously with the absorptive function of this organ and be responsible for the occurrence of steatorrhea, megaloblastic anemia and other symptoms that characterize the malabsorption syndrome (see pages 135 to 137).

Diverticula of the small intestine can be *diagnosed only* by means of X-ray studies. The X-ray demonstration is, however, rendered difficult when the wide neck of the diverticulum makes it empty readily or when the intestinal contents fill the diverticulum and prevent the entrance of the barium.

RELATIONSHIP OF DIVERTICULA
TO BLOOD VESSELS AND TAENIAE (SCHEMATIC)

DIVERTICULOSIS OF COLON I

Diverticulosis of the colon is an acquired condition which results from herniation of the mucosa through defects in the muscle coats. The defects are usually located at sites where the blood vessels pierce the muscular wall to gain the submucous plane. These vessels, the *"long circular"* arteries, enter at a very constant position just on the *mesenteric side of the two lateral taeniae coli,* so diverticula commonly occur in two parallel rows along the bowel. The *appendices epiploicae* are also situated in this part of the circumference; thus diverticula frequently enter the base of the appendices epiploicae.

The diverticula probably arise from pulsion as a result of increased intraluminal pressure from incoordinated peristalsis, but the etiology is not exactly known. Obesity and constipation may be aggravating factors but are not the primary causes.

Diverticula do not occur in the rectum but may be found throughout the *whole length of the colon.* They are, however, much more common on the left side and most frequently affect the sigmoid colon. Diverticulosis is rare under the age of 40, but its incidence increases with age, and it occurs in about 10 per cent of persons of middle age, being more common in males.

Diverticula of the colon are flask-shaped, with a narrow neck through the muscle wall and a wider body. As their wall lacks a muscular layer, the diverticula are unable to expel any fecal material which enters them and which, therefore, tends to harden within the sacs into firm *concretions*. The mucosa

of the diverticulum may become ulcerated by the hard fecalith, and organisms may enter the tissues and cause infection, which leads to the various forms of diverticulitis (see page 131).

The diagnosis of diverticulosis is made by radiologic examination after an opaque enema. The earliest radiologic change is a *fine serration of the wall* of the affected part of the colon, usually the sigmoid. This is called the "prediverticular state", it may be followed, in time, by the appearance of sacs and pouches arising from the bowel, which are at first retractile but, in fully developed diverticulosis, are permanently distended and extracolic.

Clinically, diverticulosis is a symptomless condition, often detected incidental to the administration of an opaque enema given for investigation of symptoms arising from some other lesion. No active treatment is usually required, but the patient should be

advised to take mineral oil regularly to ensure a soft stool, to abstain from much roughage in the diet and to avoid becoming fat.

Diverticulitis and its complications occur in only a small proportion of individuals with diverticulosis, and patients should not be alarmed unduly if diverticula are found on X-ray.

Sometimes, a solitary diverticulum is found in the cecum or the transverse colon, not associated with a generalized diverticulosis of the colon, and occurring in people of younger age. Should inflammation occur in such a solitary diverticulum, the patient may present clinically with abdominal pain which mimics appendicitis; the surgeon who operates usually finds a mass in the cecum, which is difficult to distinguish from carcinoma. However, if the correct diagnosis can be made at operation, excision of the diverticulum only, with repair of the bowel wall, suffices for cure.

DIVERTICULOSIS OF COLON II (DIVERTICULITIS)

Inflammation in and around the diverticula occurs in only a small percentage of patients with diverticulosis. The manner in which infection may arise has been discussed on the preceding page. Once infection occurs around one or more diverticula, the subsequent course varies according to the virulence of the organism and the resistance of the patient. Acute inflammation, in which all structures of the intestinal wall participate, may follow and terminate in perforation leading to general peritonitis, but, more commonly, a localized abscess forms, sealed off by the abdominal wall, the omentum and other viscera. A more usual course is that of a low-grade inflammatory process (peridiverticulitis), which leads to the formation of much *fibrofatty tissue around the affected part* of the bowel, resulting in *narrowing* of its *lumen,* shortening of the loop and its adherence to nearby structures. This thickening may extend over several inches of bowel, giving rise to a firm, tender mass along the line of the colon. Within this thickened tissue, infection persists, and recurrent activity of inflammation may lead to the further extension of small *abscesses,* which may open into the organs walling off the infection. In this way *fistulae* may form *on the anterior abdominal wall,* or *in the bladder, small bowel* or female pelvic organs.

The complications that may follow diverticulitis are, therefore, obstruction of the colon, more usually partial and chronic than complete; free perforation and general peritonitis; abscess formation; and the occurrence of internal or external fistulae. The most serious complication is the formation of a *vesicocolic fistula,* for this gives rise to persistent infection of the urinary tract; it rarely occurs in women, owing to the interposition of the uterus.

Clinically, acute diverticulitis presents with pyrexia and pain in the left lower quadrant of the abdomen, and examination will reveal a tender mass in that area, the lower edge of which may also be palpable per rectum. Patients with chronic diverticulitis usually complain of dull or recurrent pain in the same region, often associated with some alteration of bowel habit, a sense of distention and dyspepsia. Bleeding is unusual but is said to occur in about 10 per cent of the patients. Examination may reveal some tender enlargement of the sigmoid colon, and sigmoidoscopy may show rigidity

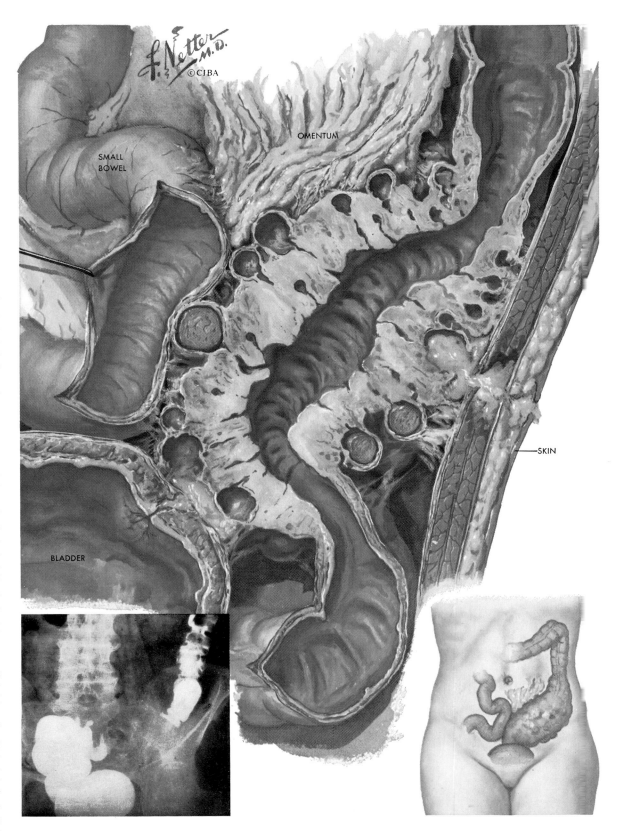

and edema of the bowel above the rectosigmoid junction. Should a vesicocolic fistula form, the classical symptom is pneumaturia, often associated with pain on micturition and with frequency of urination. An enterocolic fistula will give rise to severe diarrhea.

Radiologically, peridiverticulitis gives rise to an irregular "filling defect" after administration of a barium enema, and diverticula can usually be seen in the colon near the defect. Diagnosis between such a defect and that caused by a carcinoma may be difficult, but in the latter the defect is usually shorter and has more abrupt margins. Diverticulitis and carcinoma may rarely occur together in the colon, making diagnosis very difficult.

The milder forms of diverticulitis will respond to medical treatment, but surgery will be necessary if medical measures fail to control symptoms, if the disease progresses or recurs or if complications arise.

If surgery should be needed, its aims should be the resection of the diseased segment and anastomosis of normal colon to the remaining rectum. In cases with active inflammation, a staged operation with preliminary transverse colostomy is usually wiser, but in the easier cases a one-stage operation can usually be done with safety. In a patient who is unfit for major surgery, a proximal defunctioning colostomy will, in most cases, allow the infection to subside and will relieve symptoms, though it will probably need to be permanent.

Patients with a vesicocolic fistula should have a transverse colostomy established as a first stage. A few weeks later the diseased bowel is separated from the bladder and resected, the bladder is carefully closed and drained by an indwelling catheter and the intestinal continuity is restored. The colostomy may usually be closed 2 weeks later.

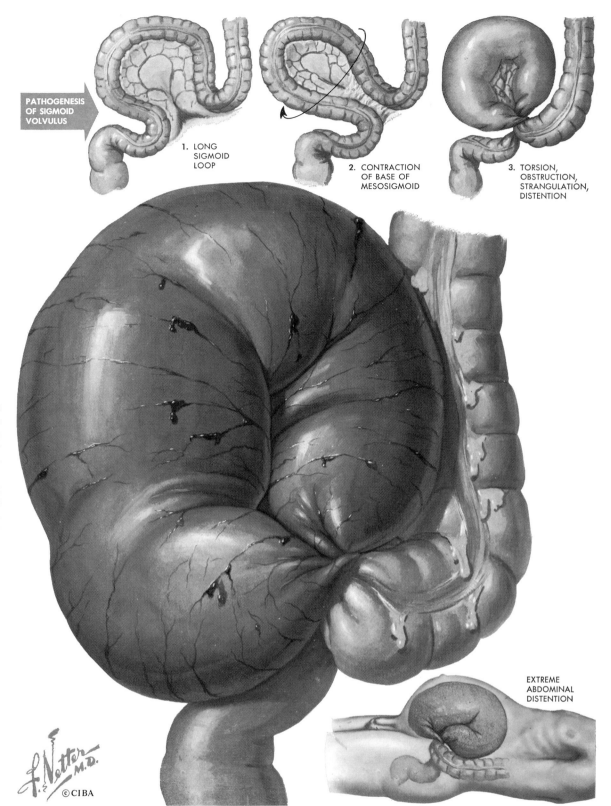

PATHOGENESIS OF SIGMOID VOLVULUS

1. LONG SIGMOID LOOP

2. CONTRACTION OF BASE OF MESOSIGMOID

3. TORSION, OBSTRUCTION, STRANGULATION, DISTENTION

EXTREME ABDOMINAL DISTENTION

VOLVULUS OF SIGMOID

Primary volvulus of the colon occurs only in the sigmoid colon and in the cecum, as the other parts of the large bowel are well fixed to the posterior abdominal wall. Volvulus is a comparatively rare form of intestinal obstruction in the Western world, usually occurring in middle-aged and elderly patients. It is more common in eastern Europe and Asia, and it is probable that the difference in incidence is due mainly to different dietary habits. A bulky vegetable diet is more common in less-developed and poorer parts of the world, and this diet results in a bigger fecal residue, which leads to a persistently loaded colon. In time, the loaded *sigmoid colon* may become chronically distended and *elongated,* and, as it elongates, its *two ends* tend to *approximate,* resulting in a narrower mesenteric attachment. Some fibrosis often occurs in the base of the mesosigmoid, accentuating the *narrow base.* These are the essential predisposing features of a volvulus, and, once they exist, the actual precipitating cause is often trivial, such as straining or coughing.

In its early stages a volvulus produces a "check-valve" effect, allowing flatus and some fluid feces to enter the loop but not allowing them to leave it. In this way, great and rapid distention is produced. If the twist becomes tighter, a complete "closed-loop" obstruction develops, and pressure on the vessels in the mesentery may lead to impairment of blood supply and *gangrene of the bowel.*

Clinically, the onset of the symptoms and signs of a sigmoid volvulus is usually sudden, with lower abdominal pain; constipation is absolute, but sometimes tenesmus with passage of a little mucus may occur. Vomiting is unusual. The general condition is commonly well maintained unless infarction and gangrene of the loop have started, in which case blood and fluid loss soon lead to shock. Distention occurs early, progresses rapidly and is always a dominant part of

the clinical picture; within a few hours it may be extreme, and no other features may be observed on abdominal examination.

The most valuable aid to diagnosis is a plain X-ray of the abdomen, both erect and supine. A single, enormous, gas-filled loop containing a little fluid is usually revealed, giving a characteristic picture (see following page).

Treatment should be tried first on nonoperative lines, in those patients who are not shocked, by attempting to pass a tube into the loop by means of a sigmoidoscope passed per rectum. If intubation is successful, decompression usually leads to spontaneous reduction of the volvulus, and operation is avoided; if unsuccessful, the attempt should be abandoned, and operation should be undertaken without delay. A long left paramedian incision is made, and the bowel can then be untwisted and fixed if it is

viable, or will need to be resected if it is gangrenous. Immediate anastomosis is hazardous, and the operation may be terminated either as a double-barreled colostomy for later closure (Paul-Mikulicz) or by oversewing the distal end and bringing the proximal end out as a colostomy; closure by anastomosis can be undertaken later. Deflation of the loop by aspiration through a needle puncture or by a tube passed per rectum greatly facilitates the operation.

In cases of a mild but recurrent type of volvulus, the patients complain of bouts of constipation, distention and abdominal pain, which are relieved spontaneously after some hours with the passage of much wind per rectum. In such instances, operation reveals a long sigmoid loop with a narrow base, as in the more severe forms of volvulus. The long loop should be resected, with immediate anastomosis to restore continuity.

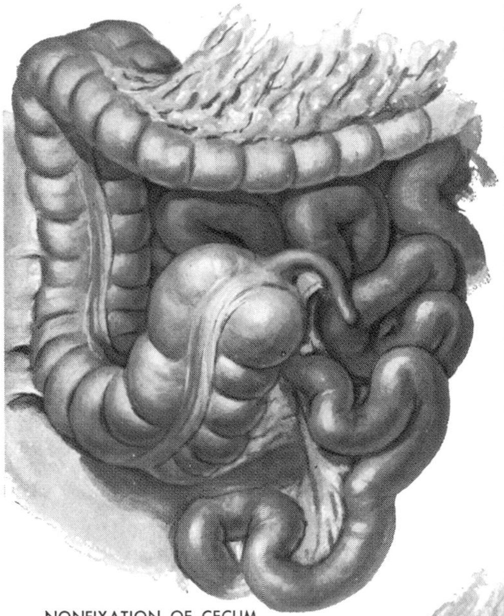

NONFIXATION OF CECUM

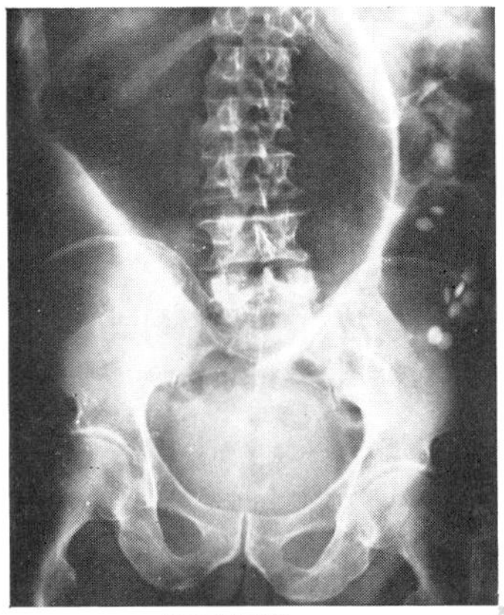

VOLVULUS
OF SIGMOID

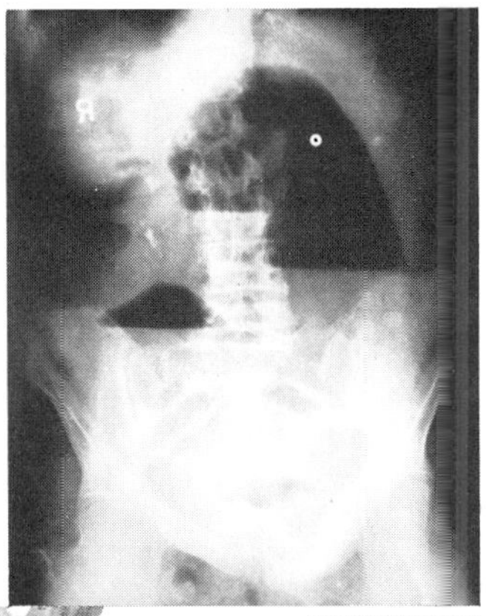

VOLVULUS OF
CECUM

VOLVULUS
OF CECUM

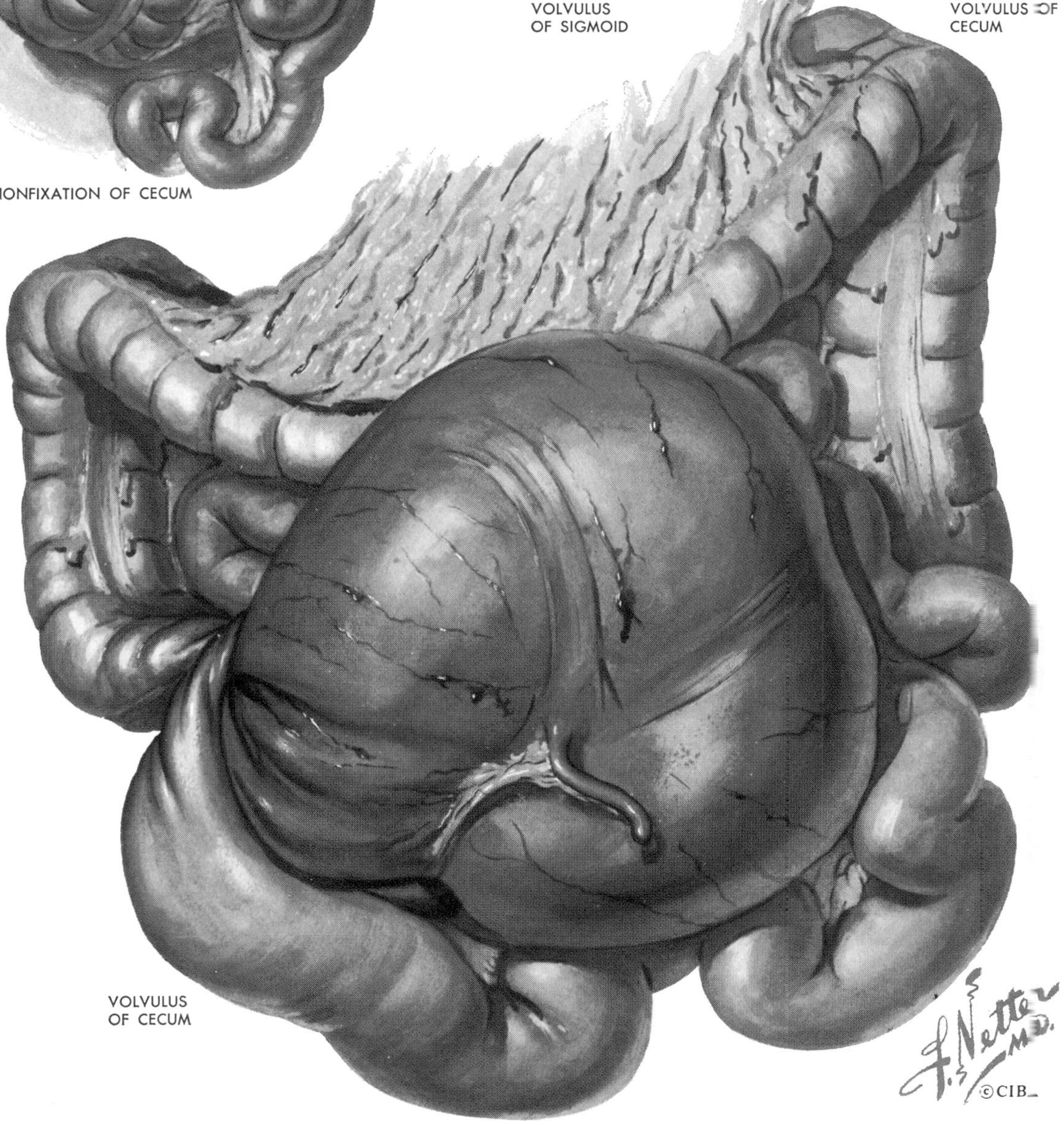

VOLVULUS OF CECUM

Volvulus of the cecum is an infrequent condition in the western part of the world, accounting for only about 1 per cent of the cases of intestinal obstruction. Like volvulus of the sigmoid colon (see page 132), it appears to be more common in those parts of the world in which vegetables and roughage form a greater part of the diet, and it is thought that persistent loading of the bowel with a big fecal residue may play a part in the etiology of this condition also.

The predisposing factor is *inadequate fixation of the cecum* and ascending colon to the posterior abdominal wall. Normally, in the third stage of intestinal rotation (see page 5), the cecum descends from the subhepatic region to lie in the right iliac fossa, and the ascending colon and most of the cecum become fixed to the posterior abdominal wall. If this last process is not fully completed, the cecum, a few inches of ascending colon and a few inches of terminal ileum may be attached by a mesentery with a relatively short base and may then be free to rotate around this axis. Should a twist occur, all these parts of the intestine are involved, and the condition should really be called "volvulus of the ileocecal segment".

As in volvulus of the sigmoid, the twist may not be tight at first and may untwist spontaneously. At this stage the "check-valve" effect will tend to lead to rapid distention of the cecum. If the twist becomes tighter, complete "closed-loop" obstruction is produced, and, finally, strangulation of the vessels will result in *gangrene of the bowel*, which is likely to occur more rapidly with a

volvulus of the cecum than with that of the sigmoid.

This condition usually occurs at a younger age than does volvulus of the sigmoid colon, most patients being between 20 and 40 years old. The onset is sudden, with severe central abdominal pain, and vomiting soon follows. The pain is constant, but intermittent "griping" pains also occur. Examination reveals some general abdominal distention as a result of an obstruction in the lower part of the small intestine, and in most cases the distended cecum may be distinguished as a palpable tympanitic swelling in the central part of the abdomen. On palpation a feeling of emptiness in the right iliac fossa may be encountered. The most valuable aid to diagnosis is the plain X-ray film, in which the *greatly distended central coil,* with perhaps a *fluid level* within it, is very conspicuous, if the X-ray study has been made in an erect position; distention of loops of ileum above

the point of obstruction may also be recognizable.

As soon as the diagnosis of cecal volvulus is made, a laparotomy is indicated. If possible, the bowel should be untwisted. Puncture and aspiration of the tensely distended cecum may be necessary before this can be attempted. If the bowel is viable after untwisting, and if the patient's condition permits, it is advisable to try to fix the cecum in its correct position with a few carefully placed sutures. If the bowel is not viable or viability is doubtful, immediate resection and anastomosis is the wiser course.

Cases of partial volvulus with spontaneous untwisting also occur, giving rise to recurrent attacks of lower abdominal pain. In such instances the diagnosis may be difficult, but the cause of the repeated attacks usually becomes apparent if laparotomy is undertaken; fixation of the cecum will then prevent further attacks.

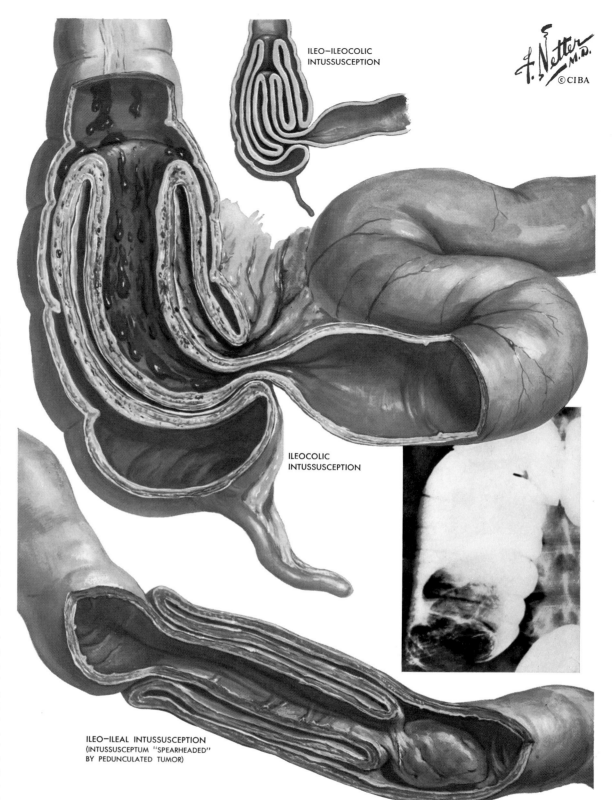

ILEO-ILEOCOLIC
INTUSSUSCEPTION

ILEOCOLIC
INTUSSUSCEPTION

ILEO-ILEAL INTUSSUSCEPTION
(INTUSSUSCEPTUM "SPEARHEADED"
BY PEDUNCULATED TUMOR)

INTUSSUSCEPTION

Intussusception is, by definition, the invagination of a portion of the intestine into the contiguous distal segment of the enteric tube. Much has been speculated about the etiology of this condition. The fact that intussusception occurs more frequently within the period of the fourth and tenth months of age suggested that the change from a pure milk diet to a more solid one plays a rôle by altering the intestinal peristalsis in such a way that the intussusception is initiated. Acute enteritis, allergic reactions and intestinal spasms — in short, any conditions with hypermotility — may result in an invagination. In older individuals it may be a *polyp,* an enlarged Peyer's patch or a diverticulum of Meckel which may mark the site at which the wall of the proximal segment turns and intrudes into its neighboring distal part. Whatever the etiologic factor may be, it remains undiscovered in more than 90 per cent of the cases.

Intussusceptions are classified according to the part of the digestive tube which telescopes into the "intussuscipiens", *i.e.,* the receiving part. Thus, one may encounter an *ileo-ileal,* jejuno-ileal, etc., invagination. The most frequent of them is the *ileocolic* (ileocecal) intussusception. A kind of double invagination or an intussusception within an intussusception (*e.g.,* an *ileo-ileocolic* intussusception) may also occur. How far the intussusceptum, *i.e.,* the part that becomes insheathed by the more distal portion, enters the intussuscipiens depends upon the length and motility of its mesentery, which, furthermore, is easily compressed and then causes the development of edema, peritoneal exudation, vascular strangulation and, finally, intestinal gangrene.

The clinical manifestations of the disease are almost always alarming and usually set in rather suddenly in generally normal, well-developed and well-nourished children. Colicky abdominal pains recur, as a rule, at intervals of 15 to 20 minutes and are accompanied by signs of acute shock, the child becoming extremely pallid. During the intervals the patient seems to recover, relaxes and behaves as if nothing had happened. In about 85 per cent of the cases, a movable mass may be palpated in the abdomen,

which can always be confirmed by rectal examination. In the more advanced stage of the disease, bloody stools are found, the sudden appearance of which may be considered pathognomonic. The diagnosis can be established by X-rays after administration of a barium enema, which, incidentally, may sometimes have also a therapeutic effect.

The safest method of treatment — thereby the method of choice — however, is laparotomy after adequate preparation of the patient, who is usually in shock. With two fingers introduced into the abdominal cavity, it will, in the majority, be possible to reduce a large portion of the invagination and to exteriorize the leading points of the intussusception through the incision. The reduction is completed by taxis with utmost gentleness to avoid intestinal disruption. About 95 per cent of the intussusception may be manually reduced in this fashion. The reduced por-

tion of the intestine and its adjacent parts must then be very carefully examined for their viability. Resection is indicated when the lesion is irreducible or when the intestinal loops have been irreparably damaged. Whether a primary end-to-end anastomosis should immediately succeed the resection and the decompression of the distended small intestine proximal to the intussusception or whether a temporary exteriorization of both the proximal and distal intestinal limbs is preferable depends on the condition of the patient as well as on the local conditions under which an emergency operation must be performed.

In general, the prognosis of this disease is favorable. The mortality after laparotomy and resection has decreased significantly in recent decades and will improve further with the ability to arrive at an early diagnosis and with increasing knowledge of supportive therapy.

PRIMARY MALABSORPTION

TROPICAL SPRUE

IDIOPATHIC STEATORRHEA (NONTROPICAL SPRUE)

CELIAC DISEASE

ATROPHY AND THINNING OF BOWEL WALL

FLATTENING, THICKENING AND CLUBBING OF INTESTINAL VILLI

SECONDARY MALABSORPTION

SYMPTOMATIC SPRUE

TUMORS (ESPECIALLY LYMPHOBLASTOMAS)

TUBERCULOSIS

REGIONAL ENTERITIS

INTESTINAL LIPODYSTROPHY (WHIPPLE'S DISEASE)

DIVERTICULOSIS

PNEUMATOSIS CYSTOIDES

SHORT CIRCUITS (SURGICAL OR PATHOLOGICAL)

EXTENSIVE INTESTINAL RESECTIONS

ENTEROGENOUS MALABSORPTION SYNDROME

(Sprue Syndrome)

The common denominator of a variety of clinicopathologic conditions is a defect in the absorptive functions of the small intestine. Two groups of such conditions can be distinguished. The first one comprises the so-called primary malabsorption conditions, the classification of which is difficult for the time being, because their etiology is obscure and also because the question as to whether or not they represent one and the same or several disease entities is still a matter of opinion. In any event, the diseases have so many features which are alike that they can be collectively discussed and classified, for practical purposes, under the headings: (1) *tropical sprue*, (2) *idiopathic steatorrhea* (nontropical sprue) and (3) *celiac disease*. From these must be separated the secondary malabsorption conditions in which the disturbances of absorption clearly result from anatomicopathologically well-defined organic diseases of the small intestine and/or mesentery, which, by damaging the epithelial cells or interfering with the motor activity of the gut or by blocking the pathways leading from the intestine, impair the absorption of food. The causes of such secondary malabsorption (symptomatic sprue) are numerous and include *tumors*, especially lymphoblastomas or lymphosarcoma (see page 163), *intestinal tuberculosis* (see page 159), *regional enteritis* (see page 143), *intestinal lipodystrophy* (see page 138), massive *diverticulosis* (see page 131), *pneumatosis cystoides* (a rare condition, characterized by gas-containing mucosal or submucosal cysts in the small and large intestine) and reduction of the absorptive surface eventuating from *extensive resections* or from surgical or *pathologic short circuits* (fistulas, anastomoses, blind loops). Needless to say, of course, impairment of the digestion resulting from lack of pancreatic enzyme or from hepatobiliary disease must also interfere with absorption, though only of fats, proteins and fat-soluble vitamins or fats and fat-soluble vitamins, respectively. Accordingly, the clinical syndrome of pancreatic and

hepatobiliary malabsorption includes only the symptoms related to deficient absorption of these substances and not, *e.g.*, of the water-soluble vitamins. Partial and total gastrectomy (first to a lesser and later to a greater extent) also interferes with absorption. This interference is due chiefly to the insufficient mixture of foods with digestive juices but also to loss of part of the intestinal absorption surface (blind loop). After total gastrectomy the lack of intrinsic factor disturbs also the absorption of vitamin B_{12}.

The disease termed *tropical sprue*, known for centuries but recognized as a separate clinical entity only since 1880 (Manson, van der Burg), is characterized chiefly by aphthous glossitis, *stomatitis*, by the passage of loose, pale and copious stools, by weakness and a *megaloblastic anemia*. This disease afflicts adults residing or having resided in certain tropical or subtropical regions, situated mainly in eastern and

southern Asia, where it is apt to occur in epidemic outbreaks, though sporadic appearance is the rule. It is important to realize that tropical sprue is a regional rather than a climatic disease; what makes it distinct from other primary malabsorption conditions is not the fact that it occurs in the tropics, but its regional and epidemic character, the usually sudden onset and rapid evolution to the full picture of the malabsorption syndrome, and the favorable response to the treatment with liver extract, folic acid and other supportive measures. Sporadic cases occur outside the endemic regions, namely in the West Indies and Central America, and, perhaps, even in nontropical countries. Idiopathic steatorrhea is the term applied nowadays to a form of primary malabsorption distinct from tropical sprue, though this name was originally (Thaysen) coined to cover all primary malabsorption

(Continued on page 136)

ENTEROGENOUS MALABSORPTION SYNDROME

(Sprue Syndrome)

(Continued from page 135)

conditions. Idiopathic steatorrhea, called also nontropical sprue (because it was observed first in nontropical countries), is a clinical entity (or entities) occurring sporadically in the temperate as well as in tropical climates, following a chronic course with remissions and exacerbations, and not responding to the treatment that is usually effective in tropical sprue. It is, however, of interest that a significant number of cases with idiopathic steatorrhea have a past history of intestinal disturbances extending back into childhood and may present, in fact, cases of celiac disease persisting into adult life (adult celiac disease). This possibility is further supported by reports indicating that about 40 per cent, or even more, of patients with idiopathic steatorrhea respond favorably to the strict withdrawal of gluten from the diet, as do the typical cases of celiac disease in children (Frazer, Green *et al.*). This latter disease, first described as "coeliac affection" (Gee), later better known as Gee's disease, Gee-Herter-Heubner syndrome, intestinal infantilism and other names, afflicts mostly children in the first 5 years of life and manifests itself by signs and symptoms not different from those characterizing tropical or nontropical sprue, except that the children exhibit no pronounced macrocytic anemia and respond in a less dramatic fashion to therapy with hematopoietic agents. A pronounced abdominal distention and, in line with the age of the patients, a stunting of growth, sometimes to the point of dwarfism, are also signs not seen in the adult forms of primary sprue. The certainly spectacular progress made in the management of celiac disease with the discovery of gluten (the protein of wheat, rye, barley and oats) or its alcohol-soluble fraction, named gliadin (Dicke *et al.*, Krainick and others), as the damaging (toxic or allergic) agent for these patients has not contributed to the fundamental etiologic problem of the malabsorption syndrome, but the observation that celiac disease occurs with increased frequency

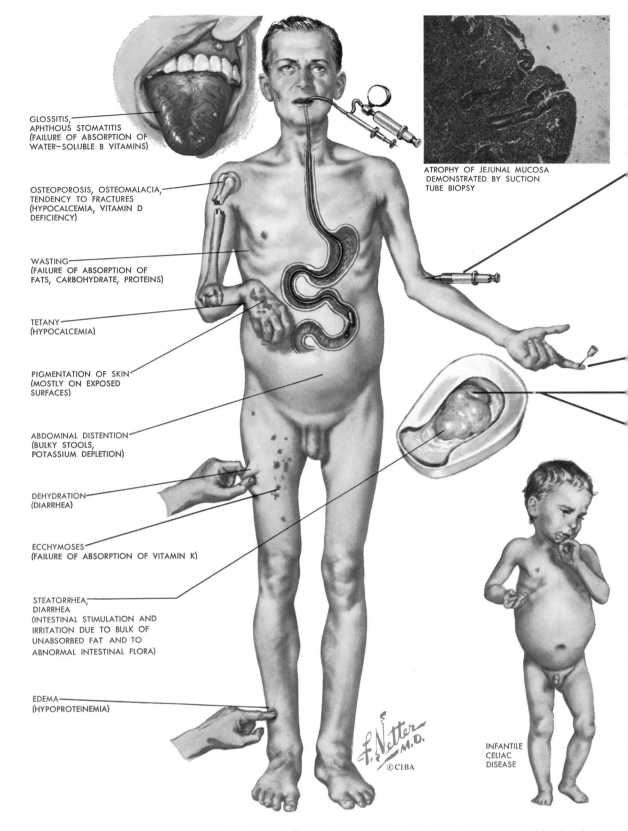

GLOSSITIS, APHTHOUS STOMATITIS (FAILURE OF ABSORPTION OF WATER–SOLUBLE B VITAMINS)

ATROPHY OF JEJUNAL MUCOSA DEMONSTRATED BY SUCTION TUBE BIOPSY

OSTEOPOROSIS, OSTEOMALACIA, TENDENCY TO FRACTURES (HYPOCALCEMIA, VITAMIN D DEFICIENCY)

WASTING (FAILURE OF ABSORPTION OF FATS, CARBOHYDRATE, PROTEINS)

TETANY (HYPOCALCEMIA)

PIGMENTATION OF SKIN (MOSTLY ON EXPOSED SURFACES)

ABDOMINAL DISTENTION (BULKY STOOLS, POTASSIUM DEPLETION)

DEHYDRATION (DIARRHEA)

ECCHYMOSES (FAILURE OF ABSORPTION OF VITAMIN K)

STEATORRHEA, DIARRHEA (INTESTINAL STIMULATION AND IRRITATION DUE TO BULK OF UNABSORBED FAT AND TO ABNORMAL INTESTINAL FLORA)

EDEMA (HYPOPROTEINEMIA)

INFANTILE CELIAC DISEASE

in siblings and other members of a family has pointed to the possibility that a genetic factor may be involved.

Anatomicopathologically, the primary malabsorption conditions present similar nonspecific changes, which may, however, also appear eventually in secondary malabsorption. The small intestine may be grossly normal or may be dilated, may show a thin wall and a more or less marked *atrophy* of the *mucosa*. The *villi* may be *flattened* and *thickened* and the epithelial cells may be reduced in size to low columnar cells with small, irregular nuclei and vacuolated cytoplasm.

The complex clinical picture of both the primary and secondary malabsorption conditions can be explained in all its details by the inadequate uptake by the intestinal epithelial cells of all foodstuffs (fat, proteins, carbohydrates, minerals, vitamins and even water) of biologic value, which pass through the bowel and are eliminated with the *pale, bulky and*

fatty stool. The caloric loss is responsible for the *wasting*. Diarrhea, flatulence and *abdominal distention* are related to the formation of irritating substances in the intestine, to potassium depletion and to an abnormal intestinal flora. Loss of water with the stool leads to *dehydration*. *Hypoproteinemia* and *edema* are explained by the deficient absorption of proteins. The fecal elimination of calcium due to the decreased permeability of the intestinal wall and the formation of insoluble calcium soaps in the intestine leads to a *calcium deficiency* which manifests itself in transient muscular cramps and, in more severe cases, in tetany, though the latter may fail to develop in the presence of hypoproteinemia, when the low calcium level is concerned more with the not-ionized than with the ionized calcium fraction. The calcium deficiency, together with the lack of vitamin D, causes

(Continued on page 137)

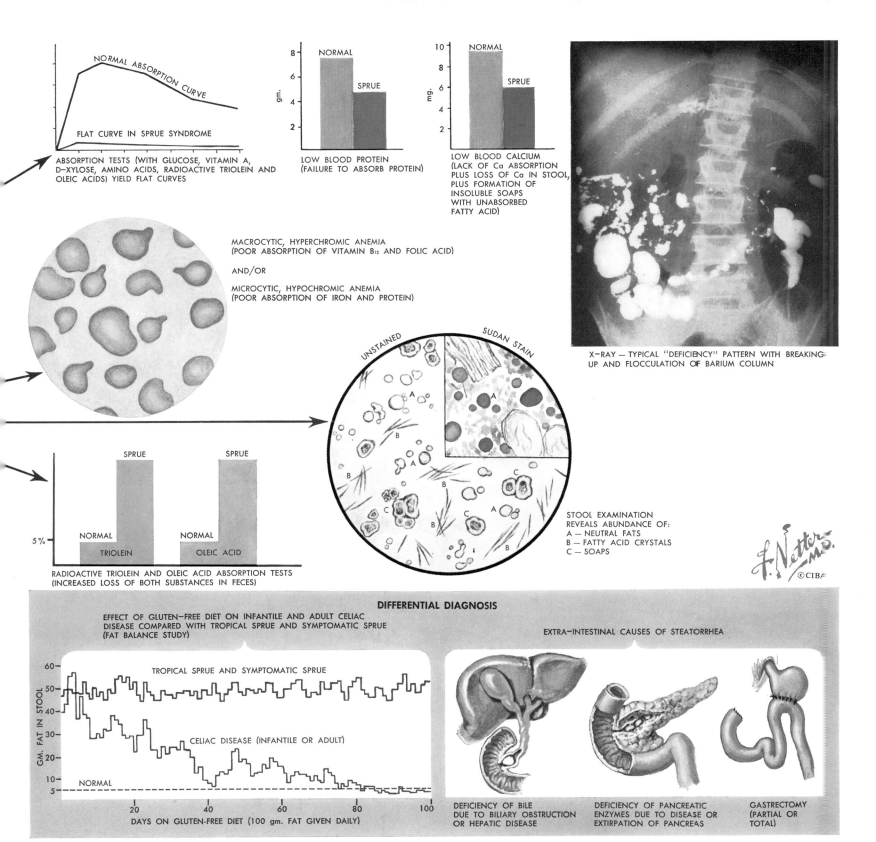

ABSORPTION TESTS (WITH GLUCOSE, VITAMIN A, D-XYLOSE, AMINO ACIDS, RADIOACTIVE TRIOLEIN AND OLEIC ACIDS) YIELD FLAT CURVES

NORMAL ABSORPTION CURVE

FLAT CURVE IN SPRUE SYNDROME

LOW BLOOD PROTEIN (FAILURE TO ABSORB PROTEIN)

NORMAL / SPRUE

LOW BLOOD CALCIUM (LACK OF Ca ABSORPTION PLUS LOSS OF Ca IN STOOL, PLUS FORMATION OF INSOLUBLE SOAPS WITH UNABSORBED FATTY ACID)

NORMAL / SPRUE

X-RAY — TYPICAL "DEFICIENCY" PATTERN WITH BREAKING UP AND FLOCCULATION OF BARIUM COLUMN

MACROCYTIC, HYPERCHROMIC ANEMIA (POOR ABSORPTION OF VITAMIN B_{12} AND FOLIC ACID)

AND/OR

MICROCYTIC, HYPOCHROMIC ANEMIA (POOR ABSORPTION OF IRON AND PROTEIN)

UNSTAINED / SUDAN STAIN

STOOL EXAMINATION REVEALS ABUNDANCE OF:
A — NEUTRAL FATS
B — FATTY ACID CRYSTALS
C — SOAPS

SPRUE / SPRUE

NORMAL / NORMAL
TRIOLEIN / OLEIC ACID

RADIOACTIVE TRIOLEIN AND OLEIC ACID ABSORPTION TESTS (INCREASED LOSS OF BOTH SUBSTANCES IN FECES)

DIFFERENTIAL DIAGNOSIS

EFFECT OF GLUTEN-FREE DIET ON INFANTILE AND ADULT CELIAC DISEASE COMPARED WITH TROPICAL SPRUE AND SYMPTOMATIC SPRUE (FAT BALANCE STUDY)

TROPICAL SPRUE AND SYMPTOMATIC SPRUE

CELIAC DISEASE (INFANTILE OR ADULT)

NORMAL

GM. FAT IN STOOL

DAYS ON GLUTEN-FREE DIET (100 gm. FAT GIVEN DAILY)

EXTRA-INTESTINAL CAUSES OF STEATORRHEA

DEFICIENCY OF BILE DUE TO BILIARY OBSTRUCTION OR HEPATIC DISEASE

DEFICIENCY OF PANCREATIC ENZYMES DUE TO DISEASE OR EXTIRPATION OF PANCREAS

GASTRECTOMY (PARTIAL OR TOTAL)

(Continued from page 136)

osseous changes (*osteoporosis, osteomalacia,* bone pains and fractures). Poor absorption of vitamin B_{12} and folic acid and/or of iron and protein causes a *macrocytic* and *hyperchromic* or *microcytic* and *hypochromic anemia,* respectively. Cheilosis, stomatitis, glossitis, the fiery red aspect of the buccal membranes and the multiple *aphthae* are typical expressions of the lack of the water-soluble B vitamins and so is, probably, the brownish-yellow pigmentation, mostly of the exposed skin areas, resembling sometimes the skin lesions of pellagra. Vitamin K deficiency may give rise to hemorrhagic phenomena (petechiae, ecchymoses and bleeding from orifices).

For the diagnosis of malabsorption conditions, it is necessary to verify the multiple absorption defects. As steatorrhea is the most constant mani-festation of these conditions, the most simple procedure is the microscopic demonstration of fat droplets, crystalline fatty acids and soaps in the feces (see page 108), which, however, because of the uneven distribution of fat in the feces is not always reliable. More conclusive, though somewhat cumbersome, is a fat balance study carried out during 4 or more days. On a diet containing 100 gm. of fat per day, an average daily fecal fat loss of more than 10 gm. is definitely abnormal. Most helpful, because it permits also the differential diagnosis between enterogenous malabsorption and pancreatic insufficiency, are the recently introduced test with radioactive triolein and oleic acid (see page 106) and the so-called tolerance tests (with vitamin A, B_{12}, D-xylose and glucose; see page 107), though the latter do not detect small absorption defects.

Disorders of intestinal absorption may be reflected also in abnormalities of the radiographic aspect of the small intestine, which were formerly thought to be associated with nutritional deficiency states and hence were called "deficiency pattern". The essential features are dilatation, alterations in the mucosal relief (especially jejunal), Kantor's "moulage sign" (obliteration of the markings of Kerckring's folds) and the breaking up (segmentation) of the barium column with flocculation of the barium suspension. The *atrophy of the jejunal mucosa* and the deformities of the villi may be demonstrated in a biopsy specimen obtained by a flexible biopsy tube. Such a procedure has also the advantage that it may eventually disclose the nature of the primary disease in secondary malabsorption conditions.

Intestinal Lipodystrophy

(Whipple's Disease)

Intestinal lipodystrophy is a rare fatal disease of unknown etiology, characterized anatomicopathologically by deposits of glycoprotein and lipid substances in the small-intestinal wall and mesenteric lymphatic tissue and clinically by a syndrome similar in many aspects to that of sprue (see pages 135 to 137). Exploratory surgery or autopsy performed in patients with this disease reveals a thickened small intestine, with *grayish, greasy serosa,* and *mucosa* that has *thickened folds* studded with yellowish-white flecks. The corresponding mesentery and retroperitoneal *lymph nodes* are enlarged, yellow or gray in color and of a soft, doughy consistency; on section they show many vacuolated spaces ("Swiss cheese" or *"honeycombed" appearance*), which are filled with a yellowish-white creamy material. *Histologically,* the small intestine shows a thickened lamina propria mucosae, containing a large number of mononuclear macrophages with foamy cytoplasm and eosinophilic granularity; with Schiff's periodic acid technique the granules stain a deep scarlet, identifying the phagocytosed material as a *glycoprotein.* In the *lymph nodes* the histopathologic picture is that of a *lipogranulomatosis.* The masses of fat are surrounded by multinucleated foreign-body giant cells and mononuclear foam macrophages. Sudan IV and periodic acid stain reveal that many of these cells contain lipids as well as a glycoprotein substance similar in all respects to that found in the macrophages which infiltrate the lamina propria. In the mesenteric lymphatic tissue no significant evidence of chylous obstruction can be observed. Extra-intestinal pathologic findings may include fibrous pleuritis, peri- and endocarditis, and polyarthritis.

Intestinal lipodystrophy affects, with a marked preponderance, men in the third, fourth and fifth decades of life. Clinically, the disease is characterized by intermittent chronic *diarrhea, steatorrhea,* ill-defined *abdominal pain, abdominal distention,* progressive *loss of weight, migratory* chronic *arthritis,* secondary anemia and hypotension, with systolic pressure being usually below 100. Rarer and less significant symptoms include *hyperpigmentation of the skin, purpura, generalized lymphadenopathy, edema, blood in stools,* chronic *cough,* fever, *chylous ascites, glossitis* and *tetany.* Physical examination may reveal an abdominal mass of doughy consistency. Most of the reported cases have succumbed to the disease, despite many attempted therapeu-

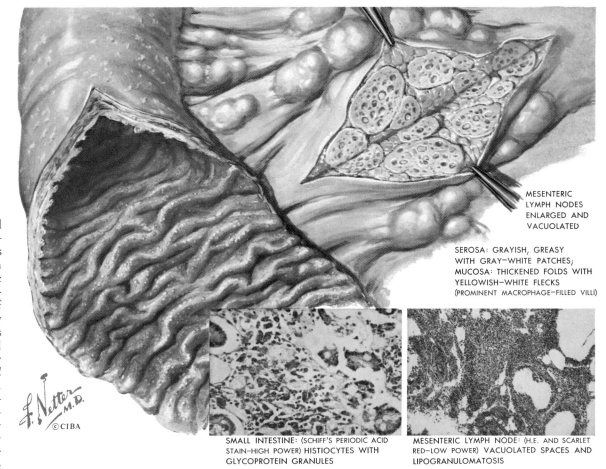

MESENTERIC LYMPH NODES ENLARGED AND VACUOLATED

SEROSA: GRAYISH, GREASY WITH GRAY–WHITE PATCHES; MUCOSA: THICKENED FOLDS WITH YELLOWISH–WHITE FLECKS (PROMINENT MACROPHAGE–FILLED VILLI)

SMALL INTESTINE: (SCHIFF'S PERIODIC ACID STAIN–HIGH POWER) HISTIOCYTES WITH GLYCOPROTEIN GRANULES

MESENTERIC LYMPH NODE: (H.E. AND SCARLET RED–LOW POWER) VACUOLATED SPACES AND LIPOGRANULOMATOSIS

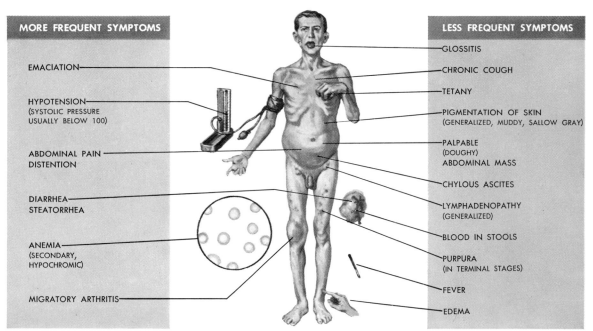

MORE FREQUENT SYMPTOMS

EMACIATION

HYPOTENSION (SYSTOLIC PRESSURE USUALLY BELOW 100)

ABDOMINAL PAIN DISTENTION

DIARRHEA STEATORRHEA

ANEMIA (SECONDARY, HYPOCHROMIC)

MIGRATORY ARTHRITIS

LESS FREQUENT SYMPTOMS

GLOSSITIS

CHRONIC COUGH

TETANY

PIGMENTATION OF SKIN (GENERALIZED, MUDDY, SALLOW GRAY)

PALPABLE (DOUGHY) ABDOMINAL MASS

CHYLOUS ASCITES

LYMPHADENOPATHY (GENERALIZED)

BLOOD IN STOOLS

PURPURA (IN TERMINAL STAGES)

FEVER

EDEMA

tic measures, within 5 years of the onset of symptoms.

Laboratory findings in intestinal lipodystrophy are similar to those encountered in sprue (see pages 135 to 137). Microscopic examination of the feces and fat-balance studies are useful in confirming the diagnosis of steatorrhea. The different absorption tests point frequently to an impaired absorption not only of fats but also of other food substances. With an analysis of gastric juice, achlorhydria may be detected. The serum protein and calcium values may be below the normal levels. Usually, a *secondary hypochromic* or normochromic *anemia* is present; so far no cases of intestinal lipodystrophy, with macrocytic anemia, have been reported. Roentgenologic study of the small intestine may show a so-called "deficiency pattern".

The diagnosis of intestinal lipodystrophy rests on demonstration of characteristic pathologic changes in the small intestine and mesenteric lymph nodes. Clin-

ically, a tentative diagnosis can be made when sprue-like manifestations, without macrocytic anemia, are accompanied by transient migratory polyarthritis. The suspicion that one is dealing with this disease is further strengthened should the physical examination reveal an abdominal mass of doughy consistency.

A number of other diseases, however, must be excluded by differential diagnosis. In the first place, it is necessary to distinguish tropical sprue, idiopathic steatorrhea, symptomatic sprue and pancreatic insufficiency. The diagnosis of some of these diseases, however, represents in itself a very difficult task and, not rarely, the ultimate differentiation can be made only with the aid of laparotomy. The diseases of pituitary and adrenal glands may present some resemblance to intestinal lipodystrophy; their recognition by means of clinical and laboratory examinations, however, is usually not difficult.

(*Illustration on pages 140 and 141*)

INTESTINAL DISTURBANCES DUE TO PSYCHIC FACTORS, ALLERGY AND ENDOGENOUS INFECTION

"Irritable colon syndrome", "spastic" or "unstable colon", "colonic neurosis", "common enteritis", "enterocolitis" or "colitis mucosa", "dysergia of the colon", "myxorrhea intestinalis" and "nonspecific enterocolopathy" are but a few of the many designations for a complex clinical syndrome, which cannot be sharply defined, but in which the most frequent characteristic is a generalized derangement of the muscular and secretory mechanisms of the alimentary tract. In many instances the colonic dysfunction — a pre-eminent feature of this syndrome — is accompanied by disturbances of the small intestine, of the stomach and of the biliary tract.

The syndrome is rather frequent and accounts for a large percentage of all consultations in which the gastro-enterologist is called. Etiologically, three distinct types can be recognized, of which the *psychogenic enterocolopathy* is by far the most common as compared with the other two — the allergic type and that attributable to endogenous infection. In view of the extensive cortical connections with the hypothalamic centers and the rôle of the latter as the source and terminus of the pathways concerned with visceral activities (see pages 76 and 77), it is easy to understand that psychogenic disturbances may produce hyper- or hypofunctions of the digestive tract. Emotional tensions, elicited by anger, resentment, guilt, anxiety, humiliation, conflicts and situations of being overwhelmed, bring about an increase in mucous and other secretions, increase in mucosal blood flow, increased muscular contractions, an increased mucous membrane fragility against various aggressive agents and intensification of the gastrocolic and other visceral reflexes (see page 95). Inversely, patients under symbolic or direct noxious stimulation, with feelings of depression, dissatisfaction, fear, dejection, futility or defeat will react by muscular relaxation, decreased mucosal blood flow, decrease of secretions, relaxation of the colon and depressed reflexes. The hyperdynamic state, when sustained or recurrent at short intervals, produces diarrhea, whereas the hypodynamic condition is usually characterized by constipation. The same or similar situations may, of course, result from local conditions, in so far as the hyperdynamic state may be brought about by active stimuli within the intestinal lumen (invasion by parasites, bacteria, increase of the bulk of the colonic contents) or may be produced or reinforced by parasympathetic drugs. The hypodynamic state, vice versa, may be elicited or augmented by sympathomimetic drugs, ganglion-blocking agents and parasympatholytic substances (see page 103).

The mucous membrane of the digestive tract in animals and in human beings can be sensitized to a variety of substances, and *allergic reactions* may set in when a specific antigen reaches the sensitized area of the mucosa either by the gastro-intestinal or hematogenous route or by both. The allergic response may express itself by hyperemia, edema, increased mucous secretion and muscular hyperactivity — in other words, in much the same way as, or at least in many aspects similar to, the psychogenic hyperdynamic state. The most common allergens are foodstuffs, followed by orally or hypodermically administered drugs, bacteria and, more rarely, by inhalants.

Endogenous infection, by which term an imbalance of the permanent intestinal flora is understood, results essentially from a cephalad migration of bacteria (Escherichia, Lactobacillus, Streptococcus and, perhaps, Clostridium) from their normal habitat to higher ones in the small intestine, where they adjust and grow luxuriantly. The cause of such abnormal behavior is unknown, though an alteration in the relative distribution of different strains of E. coli, the so-called "dysbacteriosis" (Nissle, Baumgärtel), may play a rôle. In the etiology of acute gastrointestinal disturbances, mainly in children, the significance of enteropathogenic E. coli has recently been demonstrated. It remains, however, to be ascertained that the bacteria are involved in the causation of chronic, recurrent enterocolopathies of children and adults. The old concept of "weak" and "strong" E. coli strains (Nissle) merits reconsideration, bearing in mind the modern knowledge of coliphages and colicin (Fredericq). That lysozyme and the gastric secretion may play a rôle is uncertain, although endogenous infection has been found very often in patients who have undergone partial gastrectomy (Pontes *et al.*). The result of the endogenous infection is that the normally almost bacteria-free jejunum becomes inhabited by a great number of microbes, and food substances become exposed, even in the proximal portion of the small intestine, to the complementary action of bacterial enzymes, producing increased amounts of gases, acids and volatile amines.

The *clinical picture* is almost the same in all three types of enterocolopathy, but numerous variations are encountered from patient to patient and in the same individual during the long course of the disease. Discomfort or pain in the lower abdomen, constipation and/or diarrhea are the major complaints. Borborygmus is another rather frequent symptom. The painful episodes may last for many days or for only a few minutes, to reappear at varying intervals, during which the patients may not suffer from intestinal symptoms. The mucus excreted with the feces varies in amount and may be the only material evacuated during an attack. (This, for the patient, very disturbing feature was taken in the past as characteristic of the secretory-type syndrome, which was responsible for the so-called "mucomembranous" or "mucous colitis".) The stool does not contain pus, and blood is present only when, as a result of or independent of the syndrome, hemorrhoids and fissures have developed or when the mucous membrane of the lower large intestine has been severely irritated by frequent evacuations accompanied by tenesmus, which, to some degree, are always present in severe episodes of bowel irritability. Though varying to a degree from day to day, the shape and consistency of the stool are abnormal in most cases of enterocolopathy. The same bowel movement may be partially composed of small, hard pellets and may contain, in another part, small, narrow pieces of soft consistency. Temporary relief from all symptoms may follow the expulsion of flatus, the act of defecation or the application of a small enema.

Pain may occur in different abdominal regions and may be misinterpreted. Tenderness in the left iliac fossa may suggest diverticulitis; in the epigastrium, ulcer; in the lower right quadrant, appendicitis. The differential diagnosis is frequently difficult, and unnecessary operations have been performed in patients with enterocolopathy. Pain in the upper abdominal region (more frequent in the upper left than in the upper right quadrant) may be accompanied by epigastric fullness, regurgitation, heartburn, eructation, aerophagia, nausea and vomiting and points to a gastroduodenal disease, all the more because in some cases it may have a time relationship with the ingestion of food. The exclusion of any organic disease of the gastro-intestinal tract is, of course, paramount before one arrives at the diagnosis of an enterocolopathy. All available diagnostic methods (X-ray, sigmoidoscopy, chemical and microscopic examinations, etc.) should be used, if necessary, repeatedly. Likewise should be excluded any organic disease outside the alimentary tract (genito-urinary affections, diseases of the nervous system, of the blood, endocrinopathies and nutritional disorders). The discovery of any organic disease, especially of the alimentary tract, does not exclude the syndrome of enterocolopathy, which may be present simultaneously, aggravating the signs and symptoms of the organic disease.

The diagnosis of the *psychogenic type* of syndrome is based largely on the finding of a close connection between emotional upsets and clinical manifestations. Generally, a state of anxiety antedates the onset of an attack, and relief follows a change of environment, isolation in a hospital or a vacation away from worries, home and business. Relief may also be achieved by supportive or analytic psychotherapy or simply after consulting a physician in whom the patient has confidence. Symptoms dependent on vasomotor instability (cold or sweating hands, numbness of the extremities, flushing of the skin, tachycardia or bradycardia, dizziness and headache) are typical of a psychogenic enterocolopathy. Cancerophobia, hypochondria, insomnia and easy fatigue likewise point to the primary psychogenic cause and irritability, which may also be reflected in complaints concerning the bladder, or by pruritus ani or vulvae, and dysmenorrhea. All symptoms may become more intense during menstruation.

The clinical picture of a gastro-intestinal allergy is extremely variable. It may be said that every sign and symptom encountered in other digestive diseases has been recorded in the allergic type of enterocolopathy. Certainly all the symptoms described for the psychogenic type may be present, a fact which makes the differential diagnosis between the two types very difficult; it may require prolonged periods of observation to arrive at a definite conclusion. The allergic origin of the gastro-intestinal symptoms gains in probability when other allergic disorders (*urticaria, angioneurotic edema,* anal and generalized pruritus, aphthae, cheilitis, sinusitis, *rhinitis,* asthma, hay fever and a histaminic type of *migraine*) are manifest simultaneously or at other times, when the gastro-intestinal complaints are less prevalent. The diagnosis is easily made when, within a few minutes or hours after ingestion of certain foods, a serious clinical picture develops, consisting of nausea, vomiting, diarrhea (sometimes sanguineous), violent pains, often urticaria, angioneurotic edema and circulatory collapse (the "grande anaphylaxie" of French authors). The establishment of a correlation between food and symptoms of an enterocolopathy syndrome is more difficult when the response to

(*Continued on page 40*)

INTESTINAL DISTURBANCES DUE TO PSYCHIC FACTORS, ALLERGY AND ENDOGENOUS INFECTION

(*Continued from page 139*)

an ingested allergen is delayed, appearing only many hours after its intake, and can be maintained only with time-consuming observations, demonstrating that relief of the symptoms derives from avoidance and that reappearance is prompted by ingestion of the suspected allergen. Blind or double-blind tests and also placebo techniques have sometimes been required for a final decision as to whether the complaints are of allergic or psychogenic origin. Except for the test eliminating diet components, other diagnostic procedures for the demonstration of antigen-antibody reactions are of little help. Skin tests by the scratch or puncture method are rarely positive. Slight or moderate responses are mostly meaningless with respect to food allergens (especially when the intracutaneous method is used), and only strongly positive reactions may point to an allergen whose elimination from the diet may bring about complete relief. The most frequent food allergens are milk, eggs, wheat, sea food, chocolate, strawberries, beans, bananas and oranges. Anamnestic data are of great importance. A *history of allergic diseases in the family* or a personal history of *allergy in infancy* and childhood with reference to milk rash, cyclic vomiting, asthma, unspecific diarrhea, etc., may point the way to the correct diagnosis.

The clinical picture of the *endogenous infection type* of nonspecific enterocolopathy resembles that of the two other conditions discussed above, so that the differential diagnosis is, in many instances, very difficult, all the more because the endogenous infection may be intimately related to the allergic type or may become related in the course of the disease. With an endogenous infection, intolerance to food substances with fermenting qualities, such as cakes, sweets, sugar, potatoes, acid fruits, etc., is observed rather commonly, and allergic reactions of the skin and of the mucous membranes may eventually appear, usually some time after the beginning of the gastro-intestinal symptoms. It seems, though it has by no means been proved, that the gastro-intestinal disturbances, *i.e.*, the change in the bacterial flora in the upper digestive tract (see above), promote sensitization to the organism by altering the permeability of the mucosa, which would permit the absorption of unaltered proteins. It is characteristic of patients with an endogenous infection that, in their personal history, no indication of allergy in infancy and childhood can be found, in spite of the appearance of allergic reactions. Likewise, psychologic instability or emotional situa-

COLLECTING APPARATUS IN PLACE

CONICAL PLUNGER RETRACTS WHEN SUCTION IS APPLIED, PERMITTING INTESTINAL CONTENTS TO ENTER

NORMAL: OCCASIONAL GRAM + BACTERIA

ENDOGENOUS INFECTION: GREAT NUMBER OF GRAM + AND GRAM — BACTERIA

LITMUS

pH METER

STOOL HIGHLY ACID (pH 4 to 6)

INFLAMMATORY PROCESS (INDICATED BY HEAVY CELLULAR EXUDATE) PLUS ENDOGENOUS INFECTION

tions, as described in relation to the psychogenic enterocolopathy, may be quite obvious in patients suffering for many years from an endogenous infection of the intestine. That, in such instances, disturbances of the mind are secondary to local reactions resulting from the bacterial overgrowth in the upper digestive tract may be concluded from the fact that the former vanish after treatment and disappearance of the enterocolic symptoms and also from the observation that irritation and distention of the small and large intestine may interfere with somatovisceral reflexes (see page 95) and may have a profound influence on other parts of the body. The diagnosis of endogenous infection rests upon the verification of a huge number of Gram-negative and Gram-positive bacteria in the jejunum. The jejunal contents may be collected by means of a capsule attached to a rubber tube. To avoid contamination of the capsule in

the duodenum and above, a conical plunger is firmly adapted to it, which retracts, when suction is applied to the tube, permitting the intestinal contents to enter the capsule. By controlling the location of the plunger and capsule in the jejunum on the X-ray screen, samples may be obtained from any place desired. The stool of patients with an endogenous infection frequently contains an increased amount of organic acids, which raises the acidity to pH values of 4 to 6. Some of the acids, being rather volatile, produce a specific "sour" odor of the feces.

True organic complications of nonspecific enterocolopathy are not known, but, during its enormously varying course, the syndrome may manifest signs and symptoms characteristic of almost every specific or organic intestinal disease. It is no wonder, thus, that in many cases the differential diagnosis poses formidable problems.

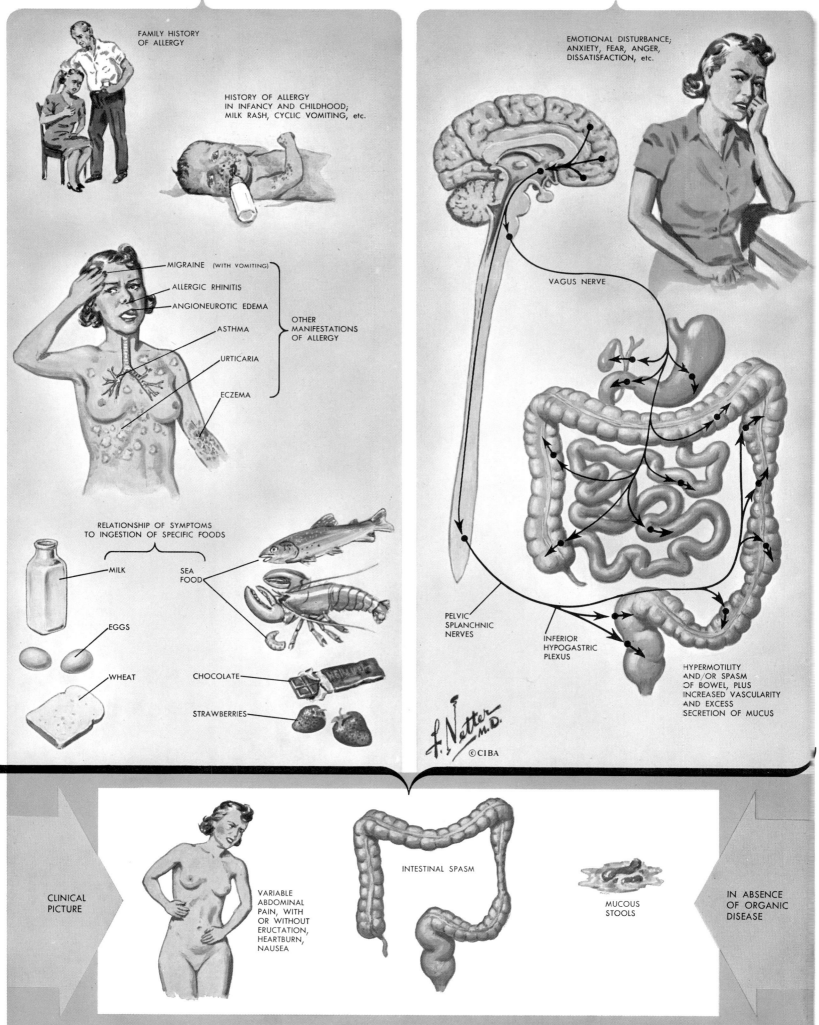

ALLERGIC

FAMILY HISTORY OF ALLERGY

HISTORY OF ALLERGY IN INFANCY AND CHILDHOOD; MILK RASH, CYCLIC VOMITING, etc.

MIGRAINE (WITH VOMITING)

ALLERGIC RHINITIS

ANGIONEUROTIC EDEMA

ASTHMA

URTICARIA

ECZEMA

OTHER MANIFESTATIONS OF ALLERGY

RELATIONSHIP OF SYMPTOMS TO INGESTION OF SPECIFIC FOODS

MILK

SEA FOOD

EGGS

WHEAT

CHOCOLATE

STRAWBERRIES

PSYCHOGENIC

EMOTIONAL DISTURBANCE; ANXIETY, FEAR, ANGER, DISSATISFACTION, etc.

VAGUS NERVE

PELVIC SPLANCHNIC NERVES

INFERIOR HYPOGASTRIC PLEXUS

HYPERMOTILITY AND/OR SPASM OF BOWEL, PLUS INCREASED VASCULARITY AND EXCESS SECRETION OF MUCUS

f. Netter M.D.
©CIBA

CLINICAL PICTURE

VARIABLE ABDOMINAL PAIN, WITH OR WITHOUT ERUCTATION, HEARTBURN, NAUSEA

INTESTINAL SPASM

MUCOUS STOOLS

IN ABSENCE OF ORGANIC DISEASE

REGIONAL ENTERITIS

(Crohn's Disease)

REGIONAL ENTERITIS
CONFINED TO TERMINAL ILEUM

REGIONAL VARIATIONS

TERMINAL ILEUM   INVOLVING CECUM   UPPER ILEUM OR JEJUNUM   "SKIP" LESIONS   AT ILEOCOLOSTOMY

Regional enteritis is a recurrent granulomatous disease of the intestinal tract, involving mainly the *terminal ileum;* isolated regional involvement of other *portions of the small bowel* or *colon* occurs also, though much less frequently. The etiology of this disease is obscure. It is not due to tuberculosis or other bacterial infections, and it is not a neoplastic phenomenon. The disease may occur in persons of any age, but it is predominantly one of young adults. Males are affected slightly more frequently than females. The frequency seems also to be higher in Hebrews than in other racial groups; it is rare among Negroes.

The initial pathologic changes probably occur in the intestinal submucosa. In the affected part of the intestine, the submucous coat becomes markedly thickened, owing to hyperplasia of the lymphoid tissue and obstructing lymphedema. The nodules of reacting lymphadenoid tissue, which may vary considerably in size, are scattered through the edematous submucosa; in some of them nothing more than nonspecific hyperplasia of reticulum cells and a sinus edema are detected; in others, however, the germinal centers are replaced by proliferating endothelial cells, in the midst of which Langhans' giant cells usually appear. Formation of such tubercles may also occur outside the lymphoid aggregations and follicles. The lymphatics of the submucosa are dilated and show areas of endothelial proliferation; their lumina may contain numerous lymphocytes and a number of histiocytes.

With the progress of the pathologic process, the affected segment of the intestine becomes thickened and rigid to such a degree that it resembles a hose pipe. The stenosis of the bowel may be so extreme that its lumen will admit only a medium-sized probe. The folds of the mucosa are disrupted by numerous ulcerations. Frequently covered with a shaggy, grayish-white exudate, the ulcers are usually located along the mesenteric border whence they extend in an irregular fashion; islands of intact mucosa between them may have a cobblestone appearance. The serosal surface varies in its color, according to the acuteness of the disease, from normal to bright red or even dusky blue, and may be covered with a fibrinous exudate. In time, numerous adhesions come into existence around the diseased intestinal portion. The mesentery of the involved portion is thickened and rubbery in consistency; it shows markedly enlarged lymph nodes. The gross lesion in the intestinal wall terminates usually rather abruptly, so that the demarcation of the involved from the uninvolved portion may be fairly sharp. In some instances the so-called *"skip" lesions* occur; *i.e.,* portions of diseased bowel are separated by areas of normal intestine of from a few inches to several feet.

The histopathologic picture in this stage of the disease is quite characteristic though not specific. In the vicinity of the lesions, the goblet cells of the intestinal epithelium have increased enormously, and a heavy cell infiltration, consisting mainly of plasma and neutrophil cells, has taken place in the regions adjacent to the ulcers, simultaneously with a variable degree of fibroblastic proliferation. In the submucosa, interstitial edema, lymphoid hyperplasia and dilated lymphatic vessels are seen, but the prominent feature is tuberculoid structures with giant cells, closely resembling those of tuberculosis or sarcoidosis. Caseation (as in tuberculosis), however, never occurs in regional ileitis. These tubercles may also be found in other intestinal coats in the mesentery and mesenteric lymph nodes.

Certain complications are typical of this disease. An ulcerous lesion may penetrate through the intesti-

(Continued on page 143)

REGIONAL ENTERITIS

(Crohn's Disease)

(Continued from page 142)

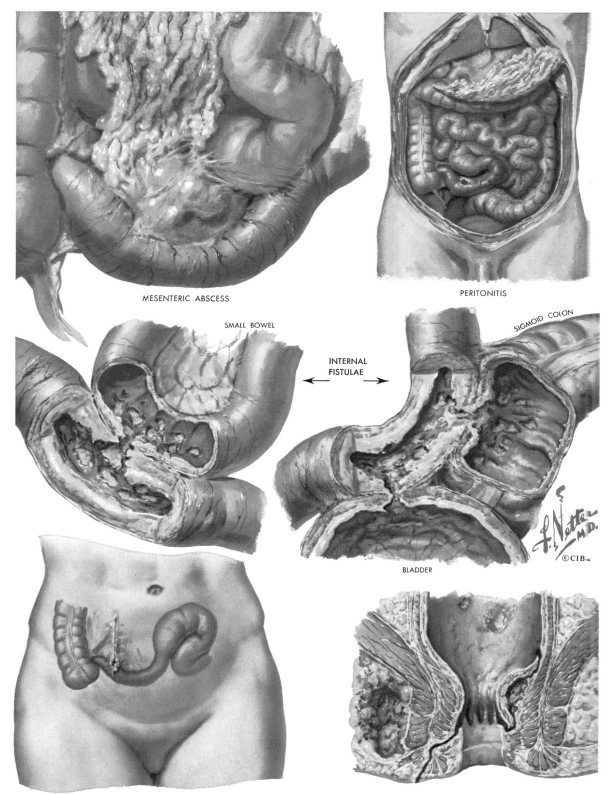

MESENTERIC ABSCESS

PERITONITIS

SMALL BOWEL

INTERNAL FISTULAE

SIGMOID COLON

BLADDER

EXTERNAL FISTULA (VIA APPENDECTOMY INCISION)

PERI—ANAL FISTULAE AND/OR ABSCESSES

nal wall and, if the peritoneal space is obliterated, may produce a blind fistula. The process, however, may extend to a neighboring hollow viscus, giving rise to *internal fistulae,* the most common of which connect *ileum to ileum,* ileum to cecum and *ileum to sigmoid. Fistulae* to *urinary bladder* and vagina are less common. *External fistulae to the anterior abdominal wall* appear most frequently at a scar of a previous laparotomy. In the absence of firm peritoneal adhesions around the affected part of the bowel, the penetration of an ulcer through the intestinal wall may result in an abscess which may extend in various directions and eventually rupture into an adjoining viscus. An ulcer or an abscess may also perforate, though rarely, into the free abdominal cavity and give rise to *peritonitis.* Regional enteritis sometimes involves the appendix and obstructs its outlet; an acute inflammation may result and cause gangrene and rupture of the appendix. The appearance of lesions in the anus, rectum and sigmoid colon, in the course of regional enteritis, is surprising, because they cannot be explained by direct connections with the main lesions. But such pathologic changes at the lower end of the colon, including mucosal edema, hyperemia, ulcers, abscesses and fistulae in peri-anal and perirectal regions are by no means rare exceptions and appear with a certain frequency. *Fistula-in-ano* may precede for years the onset of the characteristic symptoms of regional enteritis.

The clinical picture of regional enteritis is related to the character and extent of the anatomic-pathologic lesions. The disease has usually a long and chronic course, marked by recurrent attacks often separated by longer or shorter periods of well-being. The remissions of the disease are probably due to the reversible nature of the early lesions. Repeated exacerbations, however, lead to irreversible changes and complications. The multitude of symptoms include abdominal pain, diarrhea, constipation, intestinal bleeding and fever. The abdominal pain is colicky and is attributable to functional obstruction early in the course of the disease and, later, to organic obstruction. Once the pathologic process involves the serosa, and especially when abscesses and fistulae have formed, the pain becomes increasingly severe. Diarrhea varies from mild to intense but may, at the onset, alternate with normal bowel function or constipation. The movements are usually semiliquid or soft and may contain mucus and blood; if bleeding is profuse, the stools are colored red or black. High fever is usually associated with severe or extensive inflammation and complications such as fistulae and abscesses. Physical examination may reveal a usually moderately firm mass in the lower right quadrant of the abdomen, without well-defined margins. In some patients signs of intestinal obstruction, with visible peristalsis and distention of intestinal loops, may be present. Anemia of varying severity, but generally microcytic and hypochromic, is frequently encountered. In patients with extensive involvement of the small intestine and mesenteric lymphatic tissue, the absorptive function may be seriously impaired, giving rise to malabsorption syndrome (see page 135). Arthritis, usually of the rheumatoid type, and erythema nodosum may occasionally accompany regional enteritis; their severity seems to parallel the activity of the intestinal disease.

The X-ray examination of the intestine may reveal mucosal changes, filling defects, narrowing of the intestinal lumen (Kantor's "string sign"), dilatation of intestinal loops proximal to the lesion and, eventually, fistulous tracts. In the differential diagnosis of regional enteritis must be considered intestinal tuberculosis, sarcoidosis, lymphopathia venereum, tumors and systemic reticulo-endothelial and collagen diseases.

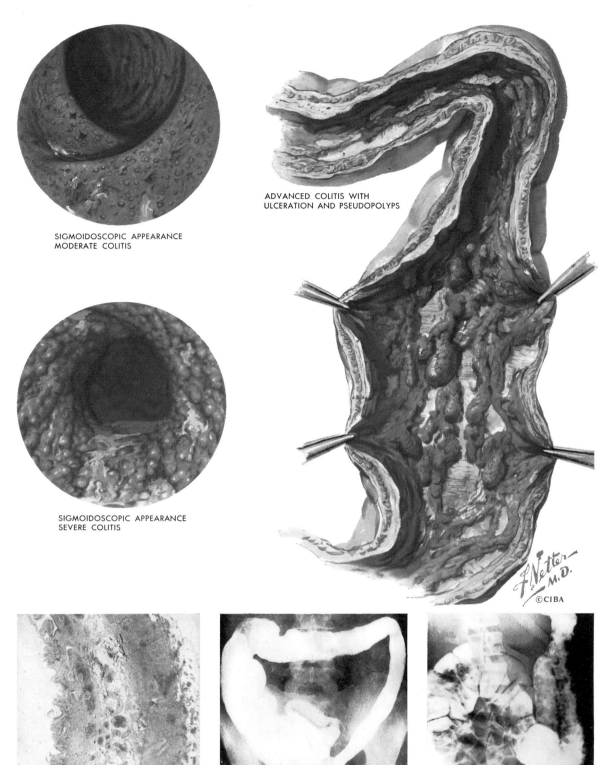

SIGMOIDOSCOPIC APPEARANCE
MODERATE COLITIS

ADVANCED COLITIS WITH
ULCERATION AND PSEUDOPOLYPS

SIGMOIDOSCOPIC APPEARANCE
SEVERE COLITIS

MICROPATHOLOGY

CONTRACTED BOWEL

PSEUDOPOLYPOSIS

Nonspecific Ulcerative Colitis I

Pathology and Diagnosis

Ulcerative colitis is a disease of unknown etiology characterized by diffuse inflammation of the large bowel. The disease is variable in its extent, severity and clinical course, and our knowledge of many aspects of it is still incomplete.

In nearly all cases of ulcerative colitis, the rectum and the rectosigmoid region are involved; in most cases the disease appears to start in this part of the bowel and to extend proximally. In the majority of severe cases, the disease process has spread over the entire colon, but in some cases only the descending and more distal colon takes part, while the right colon remains unaffected. In about 10 per cent of the cases, the disease not only involves the whole colon but spreads in continuity to affect several inches of the terminal ileum; in such instances the ileocecal valve always becomes dilated and incompetent.

The earliest microscopic changes in ulcerative colitis are confined to the mucosal layer, which becomes considerably infiltrated with round cells and increasingly vascular. This leads to a *rough and granular appearance of the mucosa,* which bleeds easily on touch. This characteristic appearance of ulcerative colitis in its milder stages may be seen on *sigmoidoscopic examination.* In *more advanced stages* the round-cell *infiltration* extends, and *abscesses* form in dilated crypts, which discharge on the mucosal surface, with the formation of small ulcers. The changes in the bowel wall are still mainly superficial, but all layers show an augmented blood supply and some round-cell infiltration, and the bowel is somewhat contracted. In the most severe active cases the crypt abscesses burst through the wall of the crypt and spread in the submucosa, undermining areas of mucosa which are deprived of blood supply and which subsequently shed. In this way extensive serpiginous ulcers are formed, often deep enough to expose the muscle coat; the remaining mucosa is edematous and partly undermined, leading to the appearance of pseudopolyps. In acute cases the bowel may be edematous and friable, and is sometimes dilated. In more chronic or recurring disease, the intestine tends to be both shortened in length and reduced in diameter, which is the result not of fibrosis but of hypertrophy and tonic contraction of the muscle coats.

The course of ulcerative colitis is commonly one of remissions and relapses. During remissions, considerable repair and healing occur in the colon. The vascularity and edema subside, a thin epithelial cover grows over the granulation tissue of the denuded areas and the rough and granular appearance of the mucosa may revert to normal. A contracted and shortened bowel may relax, and haustrations may reappear.

The *earliest sigmoidoscopic changes* are loss of the normal vascular pattern and the presence of a pink and finely granular mucosa. In *more severe cases,* the mucosa is darker red, more roughly granular and bleeds easily. A variable amount of mucus, blood and pus may be seen in the lumen of the bowel, which may be somewhat contracted. It is less usual to see ulcers and pseudopolyps, but severe cases may show these changes, even in the rectum.

Barium enema and *X-ray studies* will give information about the state of the colon above the reach of the sigmoidoscope. The changes to look for are the loss of mucosal pattern, ulceration and pseudopolyps, loss of haustration and contraction of the bowel. In this way the severity and extent of the disease may be established and, thereby, decisions for treatment and an assessment of the prognosis may be obtained.

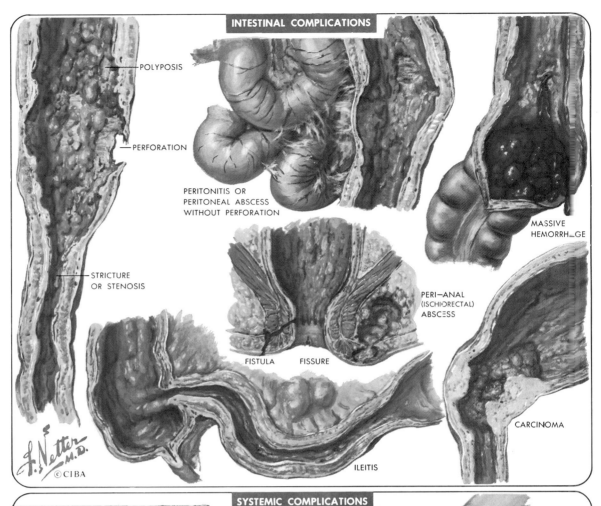

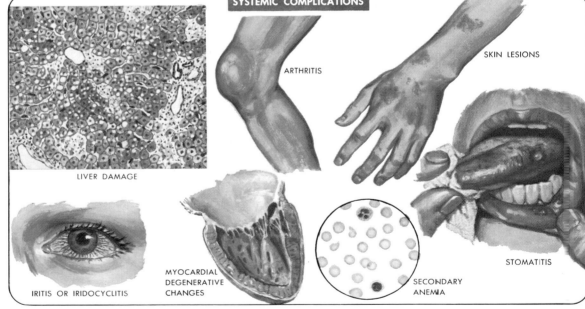

NONSPECIFIC ULCERATIVE COLITIS II

Etiologic Factors, Complications

Lacking proof of a primary etiologic rôle of bacteria in ulcerative colitis, it has been claimed that pathogenic microorganisms may act secondarily as invaders in a colon previously damaged by an unknown agent or an unknown process (psychogenic or allergic), or that bacteria may produce primarily a hypersensitive state in the colon, with the lesions resulting from an antibody-antigen reaction. Another theory that has been entertained to explain this enigmatic condition is that ulcerative colitis may be a systemic collagen disease with a peculiar localization in the large intestine. In support of this theory, it was pointed out that the many complications that have been observed with this disease include *arthritis*, erythema nodosum, *iritis* or *iridocyclitis* and that, furthermore, treatment with adrenal corticoids or the adrenocorticotropic hormone (ACTH) may bring to a swift stop an acute attack of ulcerative colitis. The frequent association of the disease with neurosis has led many observers to the belief that it is, at least partially, a psychosomatic disorder. Indeed, in the majority of patients, it is not difficult to establish the presence of characteristic neurotic traits. The patients are usually emotionally immature; they evidence reduced ability to tolerate frustration or to assume responsibility, or they manifest a dependent attitude toward other people (mother and substitute figure) and an inability to face situations demanding aggressive and decisive action. Though often ambitious and intelligent, the patients are unsuccessful but demonstrate a certain obsessiveness or compulsion, and they may be haunted by perfectionism, fastidiousness, overpunctuality, obstinacy or conformity. These neurotic features are usually present before the first attack of the disease, frequently even in childhood. Patients who do not improve from other therapeutic measures have, not infrequently, benefited from psychotherapy. This, however, does not explain why the colon is specifi-

cally affected and how psychic stress acts to produce structural tissue damage in the colon.

Ulcerative colitis usually begins with diarrhea and colicky, diffuse or mainly hypogastric pain, which progressively becomes severe. The bowel movements (accompanied by tenesmus) are fluid, containing little fecal material but large amounts of mucus, pus and blood. Fever may be present in varying degrees. In the most acute or fulminating type, the patient gradually becomes toxemic and emaciated and may die within a short time. Less severe cases drift into the chronic form, with remissions and exacerbations alternating. In a continuous type the patient may never experience actual relief of symptoms. Remissions in the relapsing type may last for several years, and attacks may recur only at intervals of 1, 2 or more years.

Laboratory findings depend on the severity of the disease. The blood picture may show hypochromic

anemia, leukocytosis, shift to the left with predominance of nonfilamented forms, rapid sedimentation rate of erythrocytes, hypo-albuminemia and hypo-prothrombinemia.

Complications arising from the bowel changes in ulcerative colitis include intestinal *perforation, peritonitis, peritoneal abscess, massive hemorrhage, ileitis, stricture* or *stenosis, ischiorectal abscess, fistulae* and *fissures,* and occurrence of *carcinoma.* Remote complications include *liver damage, arthritis, skin lesions, stomatitis, iritis* and *iridocyclitis, myocardial degenerative changes* and *secondary anemia.*

In the differential diagnosis of ulcerative colitis must be considered specific infections of the colon such as bacillary dysentery, amebic colitis, tuberculous enterocolitis, lymphopathia venereum, colonic diverticula, regional enteritis and enterocolitis and new growths, mainly familial polyposis.

NONSPECIFIC ULCERATIVE COLITIS III

Principles of Operative Treatment

Treatment of nonspecific ulcerative colitis is primarily medical, but surgical intervention may become necessary when the patient does not respond to medical management, or does so poorly, or when he has been rendered a chronic invalid by the severity of the disease or by continuous relapses which have occurred in spite of medical care. A severe acute episode may give the indication for an emergency operation to save the life of the patient, when all previous efforts to treat medically have failed. The most frequent indications for operative treatment are intractable diarrhea, massive hemorrhage, chronic inanition, perforation of the distended colon, stricture or fistula formation, abscesses, increasing signs of pseudopolyposis and malignant changes (carcinoma), which develop in long-standing cases, though relatively rarely in a case of ulcerative colitis of less than 10 years' duration. The chances for the development of a carcinoma of the large bowel increase with time and are statistically more common in the younger patients in whom the disease started relatively early and who developed a marked pseudopolypoidosis. Of the systemic complications in this disorder, a progressive or persistent arthritis (see page 145) may also present an indication for surgery.

Once the decision for surgery has been reached, it is usually advisable to remove the entire large bowel and to establish an ileostomy. In most cases it is to be recommended that this procedure be carried out in two stages; ileostomy and subtotal colectomy being done as a first stage, followed by excision of the remaining rectocolic segment a few months later. Total proctocolectomy can be done with safety in one stage in a very small portion of patients, whose general condition is so good that a single operation promises a better risk than two.

The operation of ileostomy and subtotal colectomy is best done through a long left *paramedian incision*. After exploration and assessment, the terminal ileum is mobilized and divided between clamps in healthy bowel, as near to the cecum as possible; the blood supply to this future ileostomy being carefully preserved. The colon is then mobilized from its lateral attachments, and from the stomach by division between ligatures of the gastrocolic (greater) omentum. Mobilization of the splenic flexure may be difficult unless the whole colon has been much shortened by disease, and care and good retraction and lighting are necessary if damage to the spleen or the

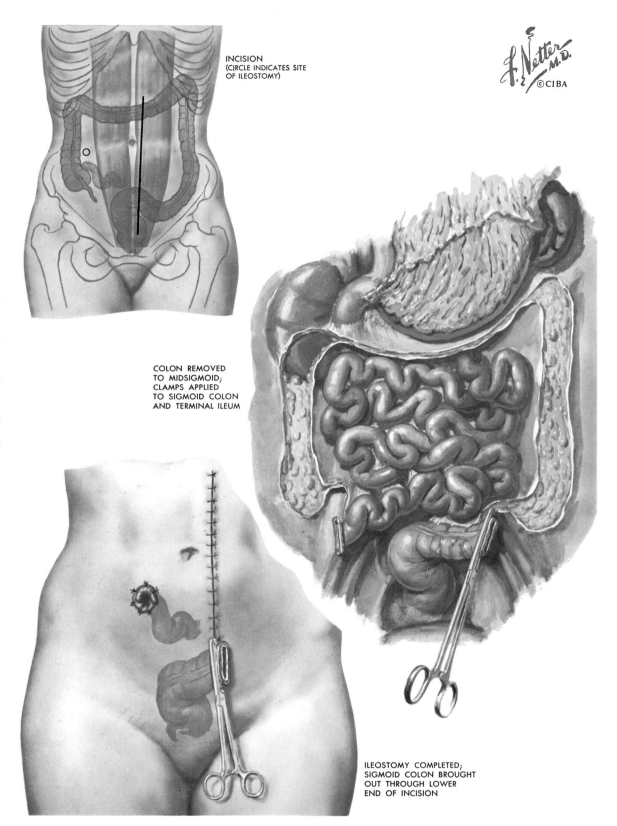

INCISION (CIRCLE INDICATES SITE OF ILEOSTOMY)

COLON REMOVED TO MIDSIGMOID; CLAMPS APPLIED TO SIGMOID COLON AND TERMINAL ILEUM

ILEOSTOMY COMPLETED; SIGMOID COLON BROUGHT OUT THROUGH LOWER END OF INCISION

colon is to be avoided. Once mobilized, the *colon* may be *removed,* starting at the proximal end; by transilluminating the mesocolon with a strong light, the vessels are clearly seen and may be picked up easily with hemostats before division. The bowel is removed to the level of the lower sigmoid colon, preserving enough distally to allow the cut distal end to reach to 2 in. above the surface of the abdominal wall without tension and with good blood supply. At this level it is again divided between clamps and the specimen is removed.

The terminal ileum should be brought out as an ileostomy, through a separate "trephine" incision, in an area of smooth and healthy skin at least 2 in. away from the umbilicus or any bony prominence. As a belt will probably be worn with the appliance, the ileostomy site should be on or only just below the belt line. At the point selected, a circle of skin ¾ in.

in diameter is removed, and the layers of the abdominal wall are then dissected and stretched until a *circular hole* has been made through all layers. The *terminal ileum* is brought through this until about 1½ in. protrude beyond the skin surface. The mesentery of the ileum should be sutured to the parietal peritoneum within the abdomen, and the space between the emerging ileostomy and the lateral abdominal wall should be closed by sutures if possible.

After closure of the abdomen and sealing of the main wound, the clamp on the ileostomy is removed, and the bowel is everted and sewed to the skin edges with interrupted catgut stitches, so that the final protrusion is only about ¾ in. The clamp on the distal colon is left on for several days until sound fixation of the bowel to the abdominal wall has taken place.

Patients usually improve rapidly in general health

(Continued on page 147)

NONSPECIFIC ULCERATIVE COLITIS III

Principles of Operative Treatment

(Continued from page 146)

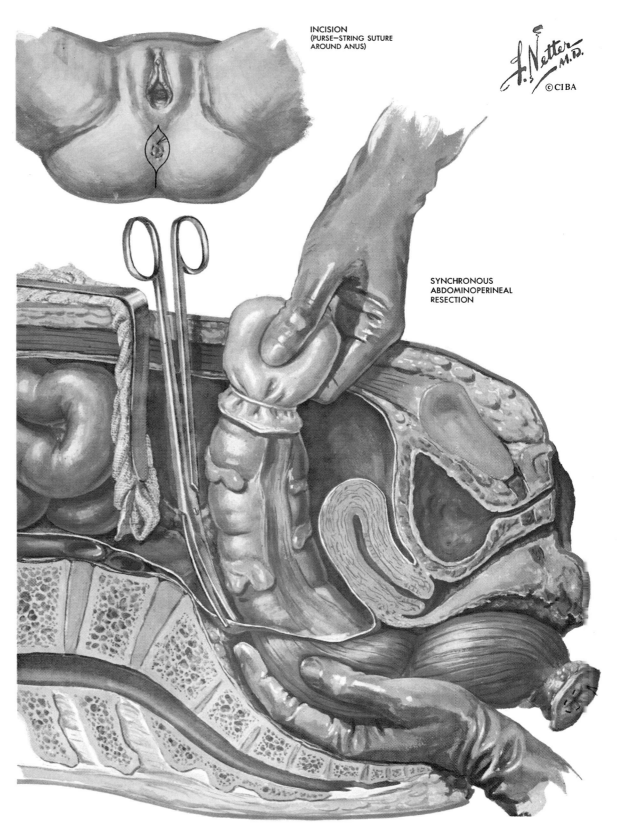

INCISION (PURSE—STRING SUTURE AROUND ANUS)

SYNCHRONOUS ABDOMINOPERINEAL RESECTION

after subtotal colectomy and the establishment of an ileostomy (see pages 104 and 105), but it is advisable to remove the remaining large bowel at some later time, because the persistence of the disease in the most distal part of the colon and rectum prevents a return to full health and remains a possible source of trouble and complications. It is usual to wait a few months before undertaking this second stage, allowing the patient to regain strength.

Excision of the remaining sigmoid colon and rectum can be most conveniently done by the synchronous combined method (Lloyd-Davies, 1939), *i.e.*, with the patient in lithotomy-Trendelenburg position, using special supports to hold the legs in abduction with little flexion. Using this method, an abdominal operator and a perineal operator can work simultaneously, and the operation can be completed quickly and with good control of bleeding.

The abdominal operator reopens the lower half of the previous left paramedian incision and extends it down to near the pubis. In doing this the bowel is freed from the abdominal wall, and a sterile swab is tied firmly over the upper end to prevent soiling. After gentle exploration and assessment, the small bowel is packed out of the pelvis, with the table tilted from 10 to 15 degrees, head down. The peritoneum around the rectum is incised, and the superior hemorrhoidal (rectal) vessels are defined, doubly ligated and divided as they cross the pelvic brim (see page 67). Dissection then proceeds downward, freeing the rectum posteriorly from the sacral curvature first, then anteriorly from the cervix and vagina, or from seminal vesicles and prostate, respectively, and, lastly, dividing its lateral attachments. It is important, when excising the rectum for benign conditions, to keep the plane of dissection quite close to the bowel and to avoid taking too much perirectal tissue; in this way, damage to pelvic autonomic nerves can be avoided, and urinary and sexual functions are not affected.

The perineal operator, having sewed up the anus with an encircling stitch, makes an oval incision around the anus and extends it an inch or so in the midline, both forward and backward. Dissection then proceeds through the fat of the ischiorectal fossa, the levator ani muscles are divided and the presacral fascia to the rectum is incised. A little further dissection posteriorly will lead to the same plane to which the abdominal operator has progressed. Similarly, dissection anteriorly,

through the perineal body or recto-urethralis muscle, will lead to the plane between vagina and rectum or between prostate and rectum, respectively, and will also meet the field the abdominal operator has dissected. The lower parts of the lateral attachments are then divided, again keeping close to the bowel, so that the entire specimen is completely free. Bleeding points are controlled easily by both surgeons working in cooperation. The abdominal surgeon closes the pelvic peritoneal floor and then the abdominal wall. The perineal surgeon closes the skin and subcutaneous tissues but leaves the central part of the wound open, with a large soft drain in the space anterior to the sacral curvature.

In certain toxic patients with severe acute ulcerative colitis, considered too ill to withstand colectomy, ileostomy alone may be done as a first stage. A left paramedian incision is made, the terminal ileum is

divided and the distal end is closed. The proximal end is brought out through a separate "trephine" incision and sewed to the skin, as already described. An ileostomy must always be most meticulously fashioned, otherwise complications are frequent, and in these sick patients any complication may be fatal.

In a few patients the rectum may be preserved, and the ileum anastomosed (see page 105) to it after removal of the colon, the anastomosis being made about level with the sacral promontory. Selection of patients for this procedure is not easy, and the operation is sometimes unsuccessful, mostly because the retained rectum is involved in the pathologic process, and the absorption of toxic material continues. Such an ileosigmoid or ileorectal anastomosis may be attempted in young people and in those in whom the rectum has been proved to be not at all or not badly affected by the disease.

DISEASES OF THE APPENDIX

Inflammation, Mucocele, Tumors

Inflammatory changes of the vermiform appendix—the most frequent cause of laparotomy—can be classified into different stages, according to the intensity of the pathologic process and its progress in involving the various tissue layers. Infection and obstruction of the lumen are, in all instances, the most important exciting factors. In *acute catarrhal appendicitis, i.e.,* the first stage, the inflammation is, at least initially, confined to the mucous membrane, which displays edema and hyperemia and, microscopically, proliferation of the glandular epithelial cells and small-cell infiltration. If the inflammatory process does not subside in this stage, the submucosa and other coats become involved, and that occurs, in many cases, rather rapidly, so that in the next stage, *i.e.,* in acute suppurative appendicitis, the whole organ appears enlarged and thickened and assumes a bright- or dark-red color. The mucosa is extremely congested, eroded and ulcerated, and the lumen is filled with mucopurulent material. A fibrinous or fibrinopurulent exudate covers the serosal surface, and the meso-appendix shows all signs of an acute peritoneal infection. Abscesses form in the appendiceal wall and may lead to a *gangrenous appendicitis.* The necrosis and putrefaction of the entire appendiceal tissues are probably the result of thrombosis of, or pressure on, the vessels by the inflammatory swelling or by concretions. In this acute suppurative stage perforation may occur at the site of an *abscess* or of the gangrene or as the consequence of a gradual erosion of all the layers. Once infected material has spilled into the abdominal cavity, the development of a localized walled-off or a generalized peritonitis is inevitable. The former occurs most commonly in the form of a peri-appendiceal abscess. A retroperitoneal abscess may develop if the appendix happens to be located retrocecally (see page 53). Infected material may also reach the cul-de-sacs, giving rise to pelvic abscess, and a subdiaphragmatic abscess may be produced as a result of a generalized peritonitis. Further complications include thrombophlebitis in the region of the cecum, which may lead to pyelophlebitis and, by discharge of septic emboli, to the production of multiple abscesses in the liver and lungs.

Acute appendicitis in other instances, however, may also have a more favorable course and evolve without the above-described complications. The inflammatory process may subside, and healing

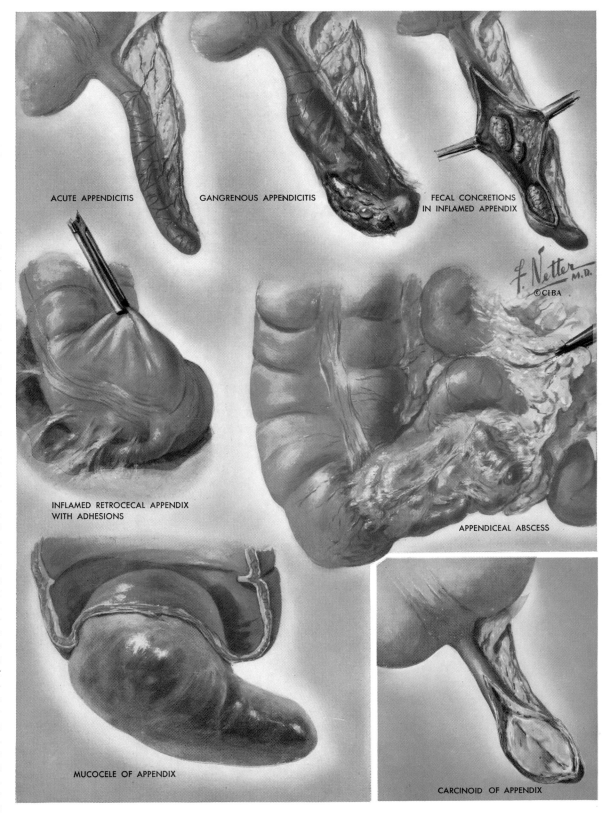

ACUTE APPENDICITIS   GANGRENOUS APPENDICITIS   FECAL CONCRETIONS IN INFLAMED APPENDIX

INFLAMED RETROCECAL APPENDIX WITH ADHESIONS

APPENDICEAL ABSCESS

MUCOCELE OF APPENDIX

CARCINOID OF APPENDIX

may ensue. The mucosa and also other coats may become fibrosed, and the lumen of the appendix may be partially or totally obliterated. If, in partial obliteration, the mucosal epithelium of the distal portion remains viable and continues to secrete, a cyst containing sterile mucoid material, known as a *mucocele,* may form. This type of mucocele must be distinguished from the malignant type which represents a true cystic tumor, usually a cystadenocarcinoma. Either type of mucocele may rupture and spill the mucoid material into the abdominal cavity, but it is probably only the malignant one that produces the grave condition of pseudomyxoma peritonei (see page 195).

A typical attack of acute appendicitis is characterized clinically by increasing abdominal pain, which, at the onset, may be diffuse, epigastric or midabdominal but which, after a short time, tends to localize in the right lower quadrant. The pain is accompanied by nausea, vomiting, fever and, eventually, constipation or diarrhea. Physical examination reveals tenderness on palpation in the right lower quadrant. When the appendix is retrocecal or in the pelvis or high in the abdomen, the area of maximum tenderness may be confined to the right flank, middle lower abdomen or right upper quadrant. The most important laboratory finding is a marked increase in the total leukocyte count and an increase of immature neutrophils in the differential count (shift to the left).

Other primary malignant tumors, besides the previously mentioned malignant mucocele, may arise in the appendix. They include *carcinoids,* adenocarcinomas and lymphosarcomas. Carcinoids are the commonest appendiceal tumors; they have marked local invasive properties, but their tendency to metastasize is slight. Metastatic deposits may give rise to a peculiar clinical syndrome (see page 165).

TYPHOID FEVER

Paratyphoid Fever, Enteric Fever

The designation "typhus" (from the Greek, meaning smoke, fume, stupor) has been applied for many centuries, since the time of Hippocrates, to a great number of diseases, which, during their course, have in common partial or complete loss of consciousness. With the conceptual changes that took place in clinical medicine 200 to 300 years ago, the term became restricted to two disease entities still known as "typhus abdominalis" and "typhus exanthematicus", which were not separated as different pathologic conditions until the nineteenth century and were finally established etiologically as salmonella infection in 1880 and as Rickettsia infection no earlier than the second decade of the twentieth century.

Typhus abdominalis, or *typhoid fever,* as it is generally called in the Anglo-Saxon countries, is caused by a specific microorganism, classified as Salmonella typhosa (or typhi, also Eberth's bacillus), which belongs to the rather large group of Gram-negative, nonsporing, peritrichously flagellated bacilli known as the salmonella group (D. S. Salmon, American pathologist). Some species of this group, particularly the Sal. paratyphi A, B and C and Sal. typhimurium, may bring to pass pathologic and clinical conditions very similar to typhoid fever, though in many instances they produce only an acute gastro-enteritis (food poisoning, see pages 152 and 153). Many other organisms of the salmonella group, such as Sal. choleraesuis, Sal. dublin, Sal. blegdam, Sal. enteritidis var. Chaco, etc., give rise, as a rule, to food poisoning but may, occasionally, depending on the pathogenicity of a specific type of germ or a variety of host factors, create a systemic illness, with manifestations much like those characteristic of typhoid fever. This similarity to the clinical symptomatology of infections from Sal. typhosa and other salmonellae gave rise to the suggestion that all these diseases be grouped under the common name of "enteric fever".

Epidemiologically, the important facts to keep in mind are that typhoid and paratyphoid fever are specifically human diseases and that the primary source of infection is always the excreta of an infected human being, though the passage of the infectious material (*stool and urine*) from one individual to the mouth of another may be direct or indirect. The indirect transmission occurs mainly through polluted *drinking water* and, less frequently, through dairy products or other food articles, in the preparation of which food handlers who are carriers of the pathogenic organism become involved. These carriers, without clinical signs or symptoms, are, in any event, a far greater danger in the transmission of

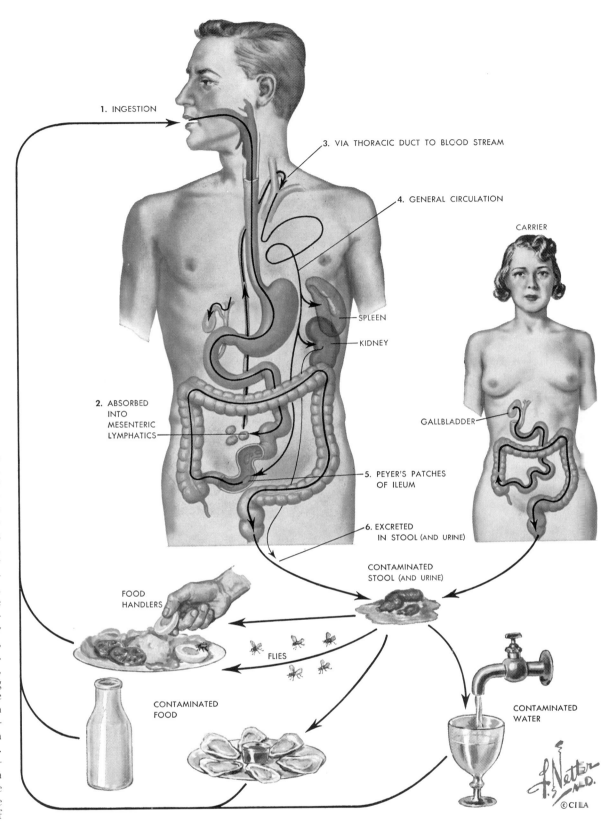

1. INGESTION
3. VIA THORACIC DUCT TO BLOOD STREAM
4. GENERAL CIRCULATION
CARRIER
SPLEEN
KIDNEY
2. ABSORBED INTO MESENTERIC LYMPHATICS
GALLBLADDER
5. PEYER'S PATCHES OF ILEUM
6. EXCRETED IN STOOL (AND URINE)
CONTAMINATED STOOL (AND URINE)
FOOD HANDLERS
FLIES
CONTAMINATED FOOD
CONTAMINATED WATER

the disease than are the patients with the active disease. They are the principal agents in the direct conveyance of bacilli to food, but *flies*, carrying bacilli on their feet and proboscises, or even for several days within their intestinal canals, may also act as transferring intermediates. These and other possibilities, *e.g., the eating of shellfish* collected in areas of sewage disposal, should not detract from the prevalence of enteric fevers as water-borne diseases, a characteristic they share with cholera and which explains, in both cases, the usually explosive onset of epidemics in a military, as well as a civilian, population.

The port of entry for the bacilli is the gastro-intestinal tract, from whence they invade the intestinal lymphatics, though some authors maintain that the tonsils and the pharyngeal lymphoid tissue may sometimes also be the site of entry. From the lymphatic tissue the bacilli enter the blood stream. This primary bacter-

emia is of only short duration, because the reticulo-endothelial cells, mainly those of the spleen, liver and mesenteric lymph nodes, remove the bacilli by means of their phagocytic activity. But the bacilli multiply within the lymphatic tissue, and a second bacteremia occurs, usually coinciding with the beginning of clinical manifestations and the appearance of antibodies. The events up to this phase correspond to the incubation period, which lasts, in the case of typhoid fever, 10 to 12 days, with variations from 5 to 25 days. With the second bacteremia the upper part of the small intestine becomes invaded, probably via the gallbladder and bile ducts, and bacteria begin to settle in other tissues, such as skin, bone marrow, etc.

The characteristic lesions of typhoid fever are seen in the intestinal lymphatic tissue, especially in the terminal portion of the ileum. They begin with a

(Continued on page 150)

TYPHOID FEVER
Paratyphoid Fever, Enteric Fever

(*Continued from page 149*)

hyperplasia of *Peyer's patches* and hyper-emia, edematous swelling of the follicles, which increase in size because of a pro-liferation of endothelial and reticular cells. The mucosa, at first adjacent to the follicles and then also farther away, par-takes in the process and the muscularis mucosae becomes dissociated. These changes may, in milder cases, revert within 10 days by absorption of the inflammatory tissue components and cell regeneration. More commonly, however, the process continues, and necroses appear in the superficial parts of the hyperplastic lymphoid tissue, which then slough, resulting in *ulcers* of varying extent and depth. The shape of the ulcers is usually oval, with the longest diameter parallel to the long axis of the intestinal lumen. The edges are soft, swollen and irregular, but not undermined. The floor is usually smooth and is formed by the muscular coat. Near the ileocecal valve, where perforation occurs more com-monly, the ulcers become deeper than elsewhere in the ileum. The large intes-tine is involved in only one third of the cases, and seldom extensively. The lesions tend to decrease in severity the more dis-tant they are from the ileocecal valve. Starting with the fourth week of the dis-ease, the ulcers heal by granulation tissue filling the floor and mucosal epithelium growing inward from the edges, resulting in a slightly depressed, pigmented, but smooth cicatricial tissue, without causing strictures or intestinal obstruction. The process in the mesenteric lymph nodes is identical with that in the intestinal lym-phoid tissue. The *spleen* participates in the disease from its very beginning by becoming congested and palpable by the end of the first week. Its pulp is very soft and interspersed with multiple, small, necrotic foci and regions of hyperplastic reticular cells of the malpighian bodies. The liver also is enlarged and infiltrated by lymphocytes, plasma cells and mono-nuclear cells. The characteristic change is a focal necrosis (see CIBA COLLEC-TION, Vol. 3/III, pages 64 and 65). In both spleen and liver, typhoid bacilli can be found scattered through the organs.

Owing to the success with prophy-lactic vaccination of military personnel in World War I, and thereafter also of the civilian population in times and at places of epidemics, and owing also to vastly improved sanitation methods, the frequency of typhoid fever has decreased remarkably. The availability of effective antibiotics has, furthermore, altered the medical situation to an extent that the classical clinical picture and the typical course of this disease are encountered far more seldom than in former times. How-ever, for didactic purposes, it is still use-ful to remain cognizant of the traditional four periods or stages of the disease (each

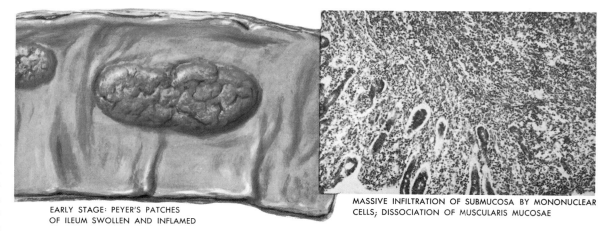

EARLY STAGE: PEYER'S PATCHES
OF ILEUM SWOLLEN AND INFLAMED

MASSIVE INFILTRATION OF SUBMUCOSA BY MONONUCLEAR
CELLS; DISSOCIATION OF MUSCULARIS MUCOSAE

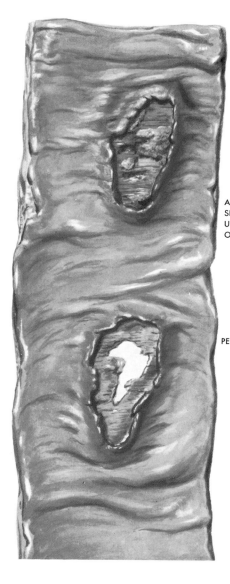

ADVANCED:
SLOUGH CAST OFF;
ULCER BASE
ON MUSCULARIS

PERFORATION

MODERATELY ADVANCED: SLOUGHING OF PEYER'S PATCH

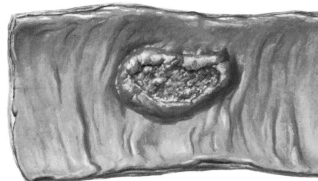

SPLEEN: SWOLLEN,
INTENSELY CONGESTED

of approximately 1 week's duration) as it runs its course uninfluenced by a specific therapy. After the incubation period (see above), the disease sets in insidiously, with malaise, sensation of chills, weak-ness, languor, anorexia, persistent and severe head-ache, and abdominal pain. Constipation is more common than diarrhea. *Epistaxis* is a frequent though rarely serious symptom. The *temperature* rises stead-ily, step by step, to reach, around the fourth or fifth day, 104° F. (40° C.). The pulse may be dicrotic and is slow in proportion to the fever, rarely exceeding the rate of 105 in adults. During the first week, typhoid bacilli usually grow in culturing blood specimens. Between the seventh and tenth days, with the spleen becoming palpable, "*rose spots*" (roseolae), 2 to 4 mm. in diameter, with a small, palpable central peak, erupt over the face and trunk. The second week, in untreated patients, is characterized by the increasing

severity of all symptoms and signs. Anorexia becomes more intense; constipation may persist or give way to numerous diarrheic, "pea soup" stools. The abdomen is distended and very tender. The mental state deteri-orates in stages, from a defective memory to complete confusion, torpor and, finally, stupor. The patient's face is pale except for a malar *flush*, the expression is dull, the pupils are dilated, the lips are dry and the tongue is furred. The temperature reaches its maxi-mum, remaining at a plateau, with little daily change. Serious complications, such as hemorrhages and per-foration of the ulcers, may be expected by the end of the second week and during the third. First signs of improvement tend to appear, under favorable circum-stances, toward the second half of the third and the beginning of the fourth weeks. The temperature diminishes gradually, the mental and abdominal signs

(*Continued on page 151*)

TYPHOID FEVER

Paratyphoid Fever, Enteric Fever

(Continued from page 150)

subside, the appetite returns and the tongue assumes a more normal appearance. The status of those 8 to 12 per cent of typhoid fever patients who died from the disease in the pre-antibiotic era usually worsened in the third week, all the signs persisting and increasing in severity. The causes of death were extreme weakness, heart failure, pneumonia and, of course, complications such as intestinal hemorrhage and perforation. Other complications, including thrombosis (femoral), cholecystitis, bone lesions (abscesses, periostitis), vulvitis, orchitis, mastitis, meningitis, peripheral neuritis, etc., were frequent phenomena. Relapses occurred a week or two after the temperature had returned to normal, or even before that period in about 8 to 10 per cent of the cases, either in a milder or, sometimes, in a more severe form than that of the original disease. These experiences have all changed since the development of a highly effective specific drug (chloramphenicol), which controls the bacteremia within a few hours and brings about dramatic improvement when the regimen is continued for 7 to 10 days.

The diagnosis of typhoid fever depends essentially on the observation of the early, suggestive clinical signs, as mentioned, supported by laboratory findings, such as neutropenia and eosinopenia, and, naturally, by the demonstration of Sal. typhosa in the blood, feces and urine. This bacillus grows readily in all usual media at a temperature of 37° C. It is destroyed in 15 minutes at 60° C. and more rapidly at 100° C. It can survive freezing and drying, and remains alive in sterile water. Its inability to ferment lactose and to produce gas in any carbohydrate-containing medium, as well as its other special properties in relation to carbohydrate transformation, have been widely used to identify Sal. typhosa and to separate it from other members of the salmonella group and Enterobacteriaceae. Blood culture is the method of choice during the first week, after which time the chance of finding Sal. typhosa in the blood diminishes progressively. Cultures with fecal material and urine become positive usually in the second week of the disease and may remain positive even after the disappearance of the clinical signs. The formerly widely used bacteriologic differentiation methods have lost ground somewhat in practical significance, because they are time-consuming and require well-equipped laboratories and highly experienced technicians.

Examination of the blood for specific agglutinins (*Widal test*), which gives positive results within the seventh to tenth days, has proved to be more helpful. Typhoid and paratyphoid bacteria

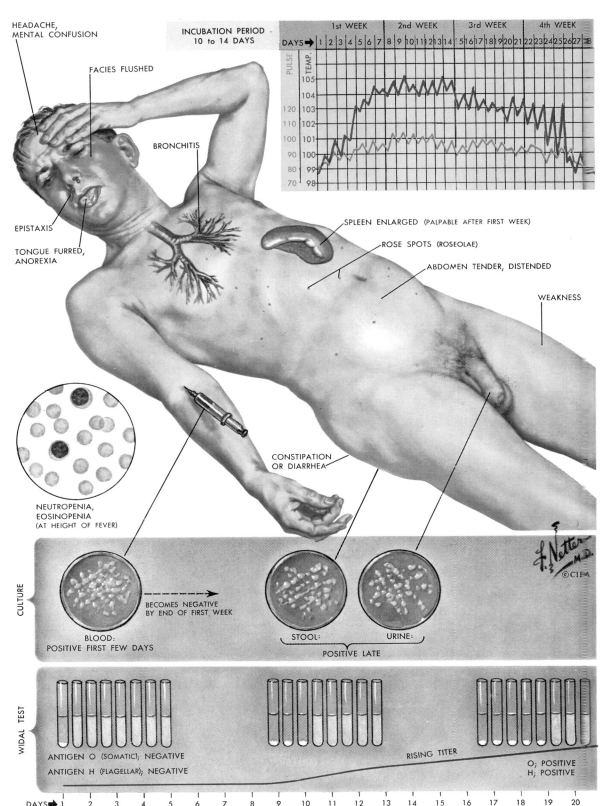

possess *three antigens*, designated *O, H and Vi* (located on the surface of the bacterial body, in the flagella or in the extreme periphery of the body, respectively, and preparable by specific serologic techniques). The corresponding antibodies (agglutinins) are found in the serum of patients and carriers. Their *titers rise in the second week*, reaching, between the sixteenth and twenty-second days, the highest level, falling slowly afterward but remaining detectable for months after convalescence. Normal agglutination varies greatly from one geographic region to another, but the sera of healthy individuals previously not vaccinated usually agglutinate H antigen of Sal. typhosa in dilutions up to 1:20 and O antigen up to 1:100. Both agglutination titers rise progressively during the disease; as to whether the O titer rises earlier than the H titer, or vice versa, discrepant answers are given by various authors, prob-

ably because the available antigen preparations and the agglutination techniques need standardization. Typhoid fever vaccination produces a greater increase of H than of O agglutinins. Therefore, tests in which O agglutinins are found in high titers, with H agglutinins absent or in low titer, strongly suggest the disease even in a vaccinated person. The opposite, *i.e.*, high H agglutinin titer and O absent or low, indicates previous typhoid vaccination but not an acute infection. Nevertheless, a very high titer for H, *e.g.*, 1:1280, may be significant even in vaccinated people, because it is unusual for H agglutinins to persist in titers higher than 1:640 for longer than 6 months after immunization. The determination of Vi agglutinins is useful in the detection of carriers; the persistence of Vi agglutinins for more than 6 months after an attack of enteric fever is strongly indicative of the continued presence of infection.

FOOD POISONING

The term "food poisoning" denotes a clinical situation which arises after the ingestion of certain contaminated foodstuffs. The concept of its etiology, however, has changed somewhat with the passing of time. Up to the beginning of this century, food poisoning was believed to be caused by the consumption of proteinic decomposition products, called ptomaines, which are basic amines. As a result of epidemiologic studies and animal experiments, this concept has changed. Presently, food poisoning designates a condition characterized chiefly by an acute gastro-enteritis developing within a few hours after ingestion of food or drinks which contain one of the following three types of pathogenic material:

1. Food or drinks contaminated with living micro-organisms, which, while multiplying in the intestine, release toxins (*infection type*).

2. Food containing no living organisms but toxins formed outside the body (*toxic food poisoning*).

3. Food or drinks adulterated with poisonous chemicals (*e.g.*, salts of arsenic, antimony, lead, zinc, etc.) or substances consisting of plants or animals which are in themselves toxiferous, such as certain mushrooms, poisonous fish or mussels living on an alkaloid-containing plankton.

In the *infection type* of food poisoning, mainly the small intestine is affected. The incubation period varies from 7 to 30 hours, but in the majority of the cases symptoms appear within 10 to 24 hours after ingestion of the causal organism, the most important of which belong to the *salmonella* group of bacteria, which includes Salmonella typhi, the organism responsible for "enteric fever" (see pages 149 to 151), and Salmonella paratyphi A, B and C. The salmonella organisms most frequently isolated from patients suffering from food poisoning are Sal. typhimurium, Sal. newport, Sal. montevideo and Sal. tennessee. It is characteristic of almost all species of salmonella that they grow rapidly in a great variety of human food. They are usually motile, equipped with peritrichous flagella. Although not forming spores, they are surprisingly resistant to a variety of disinfectants and to freezing. They can survive for long periods outside animal bodies. Susceptible animals are *birds, pigs, cattle, rats, mice, cats* and *dogs,* and these infected carrier animals or the products derived from some of them, such as eggs, meat and milk, present a major source of salmonella infections in man and animals. *Human* chronic or temporary *carriers* are of much less importance. *Flies, cockroaches* or other insects may be instrumental in the transmission of the infection, and human handling, as necessary in the production of food articles such as ice cream, cakes, pies, custard and other trifles, may play a significant rôle.

The main symptoms of salmonella

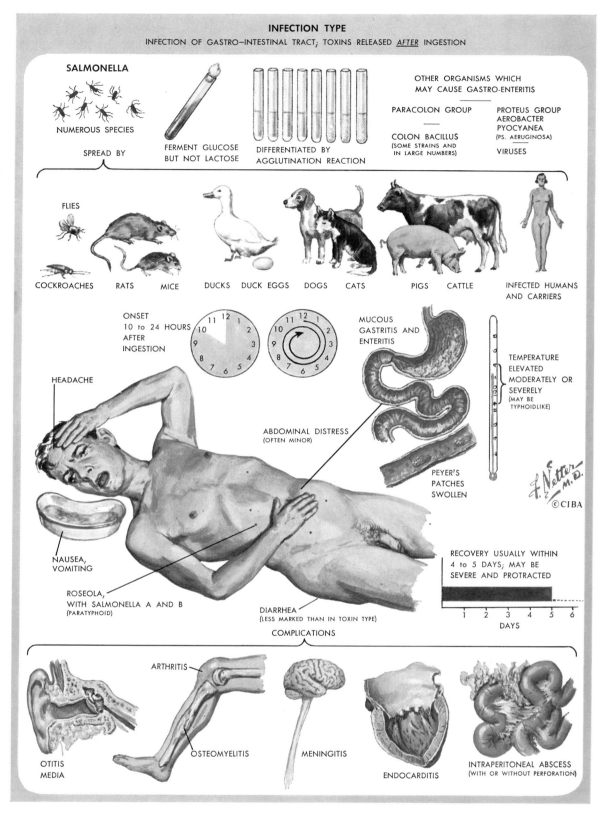

infections are *headache, nausea, vomiting, diarrhea* and *pyrexia*. The stools are usually fluid, and contain mucus, fairly well-conserved pus cells and eventually blood, the amount of which, however, is small in comparison with that in typical dysenteric stools (see page 154). The severity of the symptoms varies from case to case, even among victims of one and the same epidemic. For some patients the clinical picture may be indistinguishable from that of a true enteric fever. Few or no signs of an intestinal disease, except those of a generalized septicemia, may be present in some sporadic cases in which, not seldom, a special strain, Sal. choleraesuis, can be isolated from the blood. Typically, patients with salmonella food poisoning recover in about 5 days, though sometimes an extremely toxic condition may evolve terminating with death (1 to 2 per cent). When the disease has abated clinically, the patients continue to excrete the organisms for about 6 weeks. In general, the diagnosis of salmonella food poisoning can be made on clinical grounds and is established with isolation of the pathogens from vomit, blood or food rests. The importance of isolating the causal organisms in suspected food in sporadic cases and in the early ones of an epidemic is obvious.

The salmonella bacilli produce a thermostabile endotoxin, chemically believed to be a polysaccharide-lipid-protein complex, which irritates the mucosa of the stomach and the small and large intestine, found at autopsy to be covered with a slimy exudate, small hemorrhages and superficial ulcers. *Peyer's patches* are usually *swollen,* and the liver may show fatty degeneration. Only exceptionally do the salmonellas invade the mesenteric glands and spleen in adults, though the latter may be enlarged and soft in patients

(Continued on page 153)

FOOD POISONING

(Continued from page 152)

with septicemia. In infants the local lymphatic glands are more commonly affected, and complications such as *osteomyelitis, otitis media, purulent arthritis,* subacute *bacterial endocarditis, meningitis* and *intraperitoneal abscess* may occur.

For the *toxin type of food poisoning,* the most important enterotoxin-producing organisms belong to some of the coagulase-positive, gram-positive *staphylococcus* strains, which grow readily in many, particularly in carbohydrate-containing, foodstuffs. The organisms themselves are destroyed easily at comparatively low temperatures, but their enterotoxins resist boiling for 30 minutes and more.

The characteristic clinical feature of the staphylotoxin poisoning is the abrupt and immediately severe *onset* of *abdominal pain, vomiting, diarrhea, weakness,* sometimes *collapse, pallor,* cold skin and *sweating,* usually no later than 2 to 5 hours (rarely, 7 hours) *after ingestion* of the contaminated food. The body temperature rarely rises above normal but is often subnormal. The patients recover rapidly, as a rule within 24 hours. Based on this sequence of clinical events, the diagnosis can and should be made, because a bacteriologic confirmation presents considerable difficulty, except when the causal food article is available and still contains an adequate number of viable staphylococci for culture and phage typing to establish the presence of an enterotoxin-producing strain. Kittens, being the only animals sensitive to these essentially human parasites, have been advocated for an inoculation test, but such tests have been found unreliable.

A toxin-producing variety of *streptococci* has been isolated from suspected food in many outbreaks of food poisoning. The clinical appearance is much the same as in those cases with the staphylococcus toxin, except for the incubation period which may take a few hours more (3 to 12 hours).

The two other organisms responsible for the toxin type of food poisoning belong to the spore-forming, anaerobic, Gram-positive group of bacilli, classified as clostridia. One of them, *Cl. welchii* (Cl. perfringens, according to more recent nomenclature), is considered one of the most common species causing gas gangrene. The type involved in food poisoning is widely distributed in soil but has been found also as a parasite, causing no ill effects, in the intestines of about 2 to 5 per cent of normal, healthy people. Massive infection is required to set up symptoms in man. Meat dishes, cooked and allowed to stand overnight, particularly when kept moist by gravies, are the most frequent sources of contamination; meat, being a poor heat conductor, favors the survival of the relatively heat-resistant spores and, when cooked in large portions, prevents the penetration of air oxygen, thus providing the anaer-

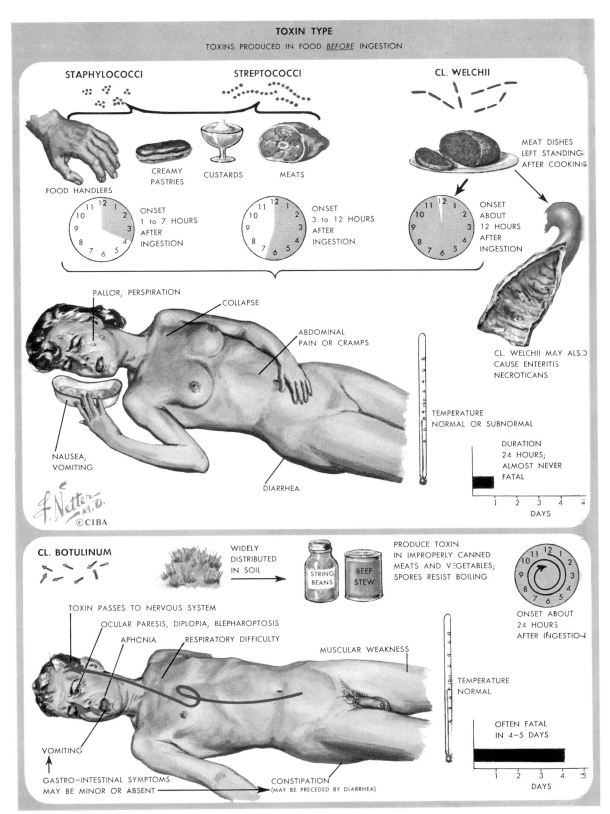

TOXIN TYPE

TOXINS PRODUCED IN FOOD *BEFORE* INGESTION

STAPHYLOCOCCI — STREPTOCOCCI — CL. WELCHII

FOOD HANDLERS — CREAMY PASTRIES — CUSTARDS — MEATS

MEAT DISHES LEFT STANDING AFTER COOKING

ONSET 1 to 7 HOURS AFTER INGESTION

ONSET 3 to 12 HOURS AFTER INGESTION

ONSET ABOUT 12 HOURS AFTER INGESTION

CL. WELCHII MAY ALSO CAUSE ENTERITIS NECROTICANS

PALLOR, PERSPIRATION — COLLAPSE — ABDOMINAL PAIN OR CRAMPS

NAUSEA, VOMITING — DIARRHEA

TEMPERATURE NORMAL OR SUBNORMAL

DURATION 24 HOURS; ALMOST NEVER FATAL

DAYS

CL. BOTULINUM — WIDELY DISTRIBUTED IN SOIL — STRING BEANS — BEEF STEW — PRODUCE TOXIN IN IMPROPERLY CANNED MEATS AND VEGETABLES; SPORES RESIST BOILING

ONSET ABOUT 24 HOURS AFTER INGESTION

TOXIN PASSES TO NERVOUS SYSTEM — OCULAR PARESIS, DIPLOPIA, BLEPHAROPTOSIS — APHONIA — RESPIRATORY DIFFICULTY — MUSCULAR WEAKNESS

TEMPERATURE NORMAL

VOMITING — GASTRO-INTESTINAL SYMPTOMS MAY BE MINOR OR ABSENT — CONSTIPATION (MAY BE PRECEDED BY DIARRHEA)

OFTEN FATAL IN 4-5 DAYS

DAYS

obic conditions required for the growth of this microorganism. The incubation period in this type of food poisoning is about 12 hours, after which time clinical manifestations, much the same as from other types of food poisoning only comparatively much milder, set in and last one or two days, provided that the number of surviving clostridia or spores are not so large as to cause an enteritis necroticans. The heat-resistant form of the pathogen can be cultivated from stools of about 90 per cent of the patients.

The other clostridium, *Cl. botulinum,* produces the most potent exotoxin known. The toxin, "Botulin", has been isolated in crystalline form. One milligram of it contains 20 million mouse lethal doses, so that the lethal dose for man is probably less than 1 microgram. Cl. botulinum is a natural soil inhabitant and, from this source, enters canned foods improperly prepared, with the result that the heat-

resistant spores survive. The organism itself does not infect the human body, but the toxin is absorbed from the digestive tract to act, about 24 hours after ingestion, on peripheral nerve endings. *Vomiting, ataxia, constipation, ocular paralysis, aphonia,* difficult deglutition and other neuromuscular signs are the leading manifestations. The patients remain conscious until near the time of death, which, in approximately 65 per cent of the cases, occurs within a week.

Five strains of Cl. botulinum have been isolated, each one producing a different toxin, but only three, namely, A, B and, rarely, E, are etiologically responsible for botulism. Early or prophylactic (for persons probably exposed) use of an antitoxin effective against all three (or two) toxins has been recommended. Both types of food poisoning, the infection and the toxin type, are "reportable diseases" in the United States.

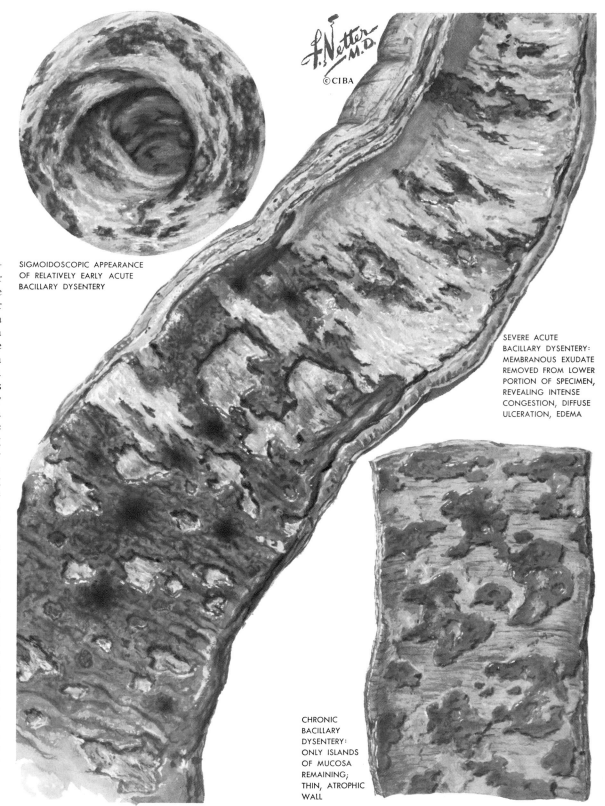

SIGMOIDOSCOPIC APPEARANCE
OF RELATIVELY EARLY ACUTE
BACILLARY DYSENTERY

SEVERE ACUTE
BACILLARY DYSENTERY:
MEMBRANOUS EXUDATE
REMOVED FROM LOWER
PORTION OF SPECIMEN,
REVEALING INTENSE
CONGESTION, DIFFUSE
ULCERATION, EDEMA

CHRONIC
BACILLARY
DYSENTERY:
ONLY ISLANDS
OF MUCOSA
REMAINING;
THIN, ATROPHIC
WALL

BACILLARY DYSENTERY

Nonmotile, nonsporing, Gram-negative bacilli of the genus Shigella (together with Salmonellae; see page 149) are the most frequent cause of an acute or chronic relapsing enterocolitis. Shigella dysenteriae (Shiga-Kruse), excreting a potent exotoxin, produces a very acute and severe dysentery. Other Shigella strains (Sh. flexneri, Sh. sonnei), which on autolysis release endotoxins, are less pathogenic. Shigellae are transmitted by "food, fingers, feces and flies" from man to man (Jawetz *et al.*). The chief source is carriers, *i.e.*, convalescents passing viable bacilli with the feces, or incompletely cured persons who excrete bacilli, possibly for years. Though occurring throughout the year, the disease is more common in summer and more frequent in the tropics and subtropics, especially in countries with poor sanitary conditions.

The pathologic lesions in Shigella infection are restricted essentially to the large intestine, especially to the rectum and sigmoid colon. In severe, prolonged cases the last portions of the small intestine may eventually become affected. The early stages are characterized by a variable degree of mucosal edema and hyperemia, hypersecretion of mucus by the goblet cells and hyperplasia of the intestinal lymphatic tissue and mesenterial lymph nodes. A *diphtheric type* of *inflammatory reaction*, with fibrinopurulent exudate covering areas denuded of epithelium, follows. The ulcers, which may involve the submucosa and the muscular coats, are separated by variously sized spots of seemingly intact mucosa, which are infiltrated, however, by mononuclear and polynuclear leukocytes. From these islands of mucosa which have escaped destruction, the process of repair of the mucous membrane takes place. Extensive, not undermined, serpiginous ulcerations, rarely penetrating beneath the muscular layers in spite of a usually thin, atrophic wall, are typical of what is known as chronic bacillary dysentery. Peritonitis resulting from perforation of a dysenteric ulcer is very rare.

The incubation period is short, rarely more than 48 hours. The disease, as a rule, starts with colicky abdominal pain followed within minutes by a diarrhea, which varies in degree from a few to as many as 40 (or more) movements per day. The stools are watery, contain blood-stained mucus or may consist of gross blood. Tenesmus, accompanied by diffuse cramp-like abdominal pain, is present. The body temperature rises early and may fluctuate from 38° to 40° C. (100° to 104° F.). The patient's general condition can be severely affected as a result of dehydration and fever (rapid pulse, hypotension, coated tongue, mental torpor). A fulminating, toxic, choleralike picture may develop, which may be fatal within 2 or 3 days (mainly in children and old people) from the time of onset. Since the event of sulfonamides and antibiotics, the disease can, however, be relatively easily controlled, and death from bacillary dysentery has become rare. In the mild form the symptoms may be restricted to an attack of diarrhea with a few loose stools, with or without a small amount of flecked bloody mucus, and fever. A chronic form of bacillary dysentery, better called chronic shigellosis, is characterized by an irregular functioning of the intestine, with constipation alternating with diarrhea, and by a tender abdomen, meteorism and diffuse colicky pains. Complications that may occur rarely in bacillary dysentery include arthritis, peripheral neuritis, iritis and iridocyclitis. Though bacillary dysentery may be suspected on the ground of clinical symptoms and the *sigmoidoscopic appearance* of the mucosa, the final diagnosis is reached by the cultural identification of the specific organism in the feces. Radiology is not contributory to the diagnosis of the disease. The blood count may show a secondary anemia and, in acute cases, a leukocytosis with shift to the left. The differential diagnosis must take into consideration every intestinal disease capable of producing the clinical syndrome of dysentery and diarrhea. One must also keep in mind that bacillary dysentery may occur conjointly with other dysenteric or chronic diarrheic disorders such as ulcerative colitis, carcinoma, polyposis and diverticulitis of the colon.

AMEBIASIS

Amebiasis is a man-to-man-transmitted, infectious disease produced by Entamoeba histolytica (Schaudinn, 1903), a protozoan of the class Rhizopoda and of the genus Entamoeba, to which genus other nonpathogenic human parasites also belong (see page 185). Although more frequently observed in warm climates, amebiasis is ubiquitous and by no means limited to the tropics. The global incidence has been estimated at about 13 per cent of the total population. In the United States of America, the infestation rate is about 10 per cent (Craig) but varies locally, as indicated by figures as low as 3.9 per cent (McHardy). Surveys in Brazil (Amaral, Pontes and Pires, 1947) disclosed an infestation rate of 17.4 per cent. The incidence is certainly related to sanitation.

The *life cycle of E. histolytica* is characterized by several stages. The motile and vegetative form, or *trophozoite*, multiplies by fission in the intestinal lumen and within the tissues of the host and perishes when eliminated in the feces. It varies in size from 15 to 60 microns and is made up of two distinguishable portions of cytoplasm — the clear, glasslike ectoplasm and the finely granulated endoplasm, in which the nucleus is located and which contains ingested substances such as erythrocytes. The trophozoite moves by means of pseudopodia, formed by the ectoplasm, as may be observed microscopically in fresh and still-warm stool specimens. In cool stool the motility is absent or very sluggish. In the second stage of the cycle, the mature trophozoite encysts and develops into the *precystic form,* which still may be equipped with pseudopodia. Out of this form the amebic cyst arises. The encystation occurs only in the intestinal lumen and never in other host tissues. Once cysts have come into existence in the host, they probably never undergo excystation in the same individual but are excreted with the stool. The cysts are the infective material which transfers the disease from one individual to another. Ingestion of trophozoites is not infectious, because they are not resistant to the digestive power of the gastric juice. In contrast, the cysts are very resistant and survive in nature under the most unfavorable conditions. They are the infective form of E. histolytica and are ingested with *food* and *drinks* contaminated either by the handling of the food, milk, etc., by infected persons, or by the droppings of *flies* and other insects which had access to human excrements or by

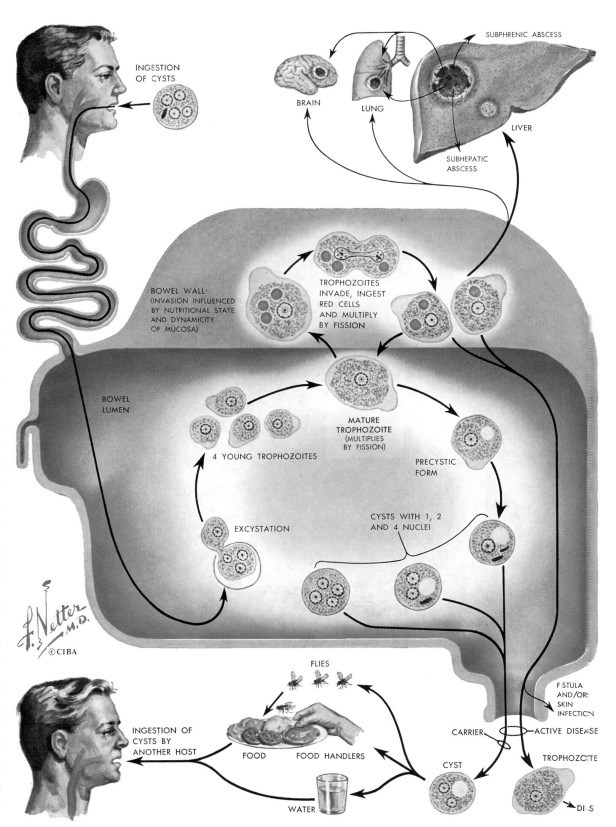

vegetables fertilized by feculent manure. "Carriers" or "cyst passers", who have no or only slight symptoms, are the most important source of infection. The *cysts* contain 1 to 4 (rarely, 6 to 8) nuclei, passing through a tear in the cyst's membrane (*excystation*) after the ingested cysts have reached the lower small bowel. From each nucleus and accompanying cytoplasm, young and subsequently mature trophozoites develop, which are able to invade the colonic mucosa and to multiply either in the lumen or, usually, within the gut's wall.

The pathogenicity of E. histolytica depends on many factors, the degree of tissue invasion being the result of a complex balance between parasites and the environment offered by the host. Excystation, e.g., requires a favorable intestinal medium, as does the growth into a mature trophozoite, otherwise the swallowed cysts (still infective) or the trophozoites may

be voided with the feces. Some strains seem to have a greater invasive capacity than do others. Strains with smaller cysts are believed to be less virulent than are those with larger ones. Food elements, irritating agents in the chyme and the bacterial flora seem also to influence the aggressive ability of the trophozoites.

The *lesions produced by E. histolytica* are located in the large intestine, mainly cecum, sigmoid and rectum. The small bowel is rarely affected, and then only in the terminal ileum. By way of the blood stream, rarely through the lymphatics, amebae may be carried to the *liver, lung* and *brain,* where they incite abscesses (for the hepatic involvement, see CIBA COLLECTION, Vol. 3/III, page 102). Invasion of the skin occurs almost always by contiguity, from drainage of liver abscess, from rectal or anal lesions and, rarely, by way of the circulation. The incidence of extra-

(Continued on page 156)

AMEBIASIS

(Continued from page 155)

intestinal amebiasis has dropped considerably, probably because of the availability of effective amebicides and antibiotics. The earliest lesions in the mucosa consist of pinhead-sized, hyperemic and edematous areas or small yellow papulae, which evolute to ulcers containing often actively motile trophozoites in a viscid necrotic tissue. Inflammatory reactions around the ulcers are usually the result of secondary bacterial invasion. The *amebic ulcers,* smaller but deeper than the more diffuse ones caused by Shigellae (see page 154), spread in the submucosa, producing *undermined edges* and even *tunnels,* which connect adjacent lesions. They may reach the muscular and sometimes the peritoneal coat.

The majority of people infected by E. histolytica have no symptoms even though, as reported by several observers, they may suffer from deep and extensive ulcerations. In others amebic dysentery begins insidiously with vague abdominal sensations. The classical clinical picture of the acute form, nowadays seen less frequently than formerly, is characterized by mucous, bloody bowel discharges, tenesmus, abdominal pain, fever, sometimes vomiting. More common are chronic, nonspecific gastro-intestinal disturbances such as constipation alternating with bouts of diarrhea, abdominal tenderness, generalized or confined either to the lower or to the upper quadrants, combined with epigastric fullness after meals, nausea, malaise, aerophagia and eructations.

An amebic infection should be considered in every person presenting himself with diarrhea of long standing. The diagnosis is established by demonstrating the trophozoites (see page 185) in a freshly passed, still-warm fecal specimen. *Rectosigmoidoscopy* permits recognition of the pathognomonic, scattered, pinpoint ulcers or, in the early stages, of petechiae or yellowish elevations with hyperemic margins marking the site of future ulcers. Very rarely, large, undermined, oval-shaped ulcers are encountered. In the chronic stage the mucosa may appear normal or may have a granular surface with scattered red areas which bleed easily. Radiologic examination can only seldom contribute positively to the diagnosis. The complement fixation test, though helpful in confirming extra-intestinal lesions, is of questionable assistance in intestinal amebiasis, all the more because a stable, reliable antigen preparation is difficult to obtain.

The differential diagnosis may pose

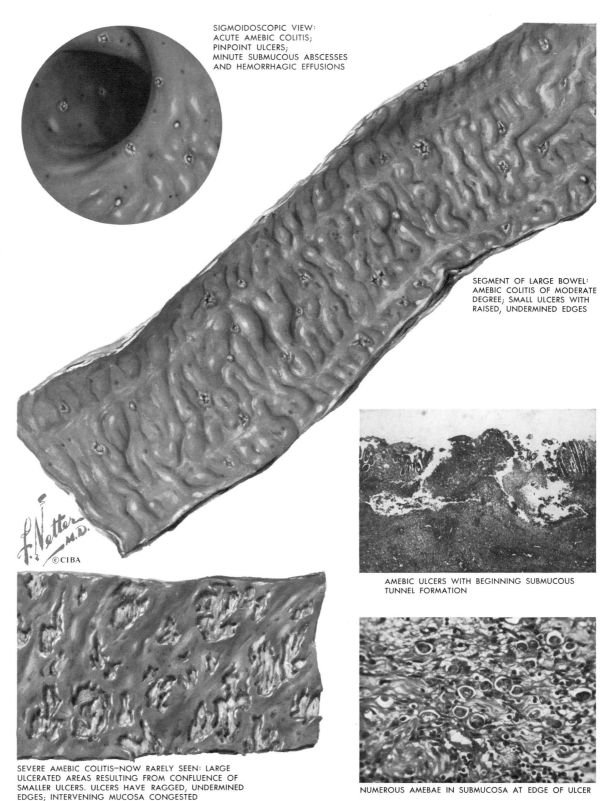

SIGMOIDOSCOPIC VIEW: ACUTE AMEBIC COLITIS; PINPOINT ULCERS; MINUTE SUBMUCOUS ABSCESSES AND HEMORRHAGIC EFFUSIONS

SEGMENT OF LARGE BOWEL: AMEBIC COLITIS OF MODERATE DEGREE; SMALL ULCERS WITH RAISED, UNDERMINED EDGES

AMEBIC ULCERS WITH BEGINNING SUBMUCOUS TUNNEL FORMATION

SEVERE AMEBIC COLITIS—NOW RARELY SEEN: LARGE ULCERATED AREAS RESULTING FROM CONFLUENCE OF SMALLER ULCERS. ULCERS HAVE RAGGED, UNDERMINED EDGES; INTERVENING MUCOSA CONGESTED

NUMEROUS AMEBAE IN SUBMUCOSA AT EDGE OF ULCER

problems because of the many diseases accompanied by diarrhea, which must be taken into consideration. Bacillary dysentery (see page 154) can be excluded by microscopic examination of the feces and bacteriologic techniques. Whereas in amebic dysentery the intestinal exudate is composed of mucus, erythrocytes and very little cellular debris, in bacillary dysentery it is rich in neutrophils and phagocytic endothelial macrophage cells. Care must be taken in differentiating amebiasis from Balantidium coli infection, ulcerative colitis, polyposis, diverticulitis and, particularly, tuberculosis of the intestine, when the small bowel lesions of this condition are missing. In chronic amebic dysentery, amebic granuloma (or "ameboma"), resulting from an exuberant granulating fibroblastic response to repeated local amebic invasion, may easily be confused with malignant intestinal tumors or inflammatory granuloma of other origin. The clinical differentiation between a chronic amebic typhlitis and chronic appendicitis is almost impossible except by the success of anti-amebic therapy. The differentiating considerations are complicated by the fact that most, if not all, conditions named above and many others may coexist in patients with both a symptomatic or asymptomatic amebic infection and that the problems are by no means settled by finding trophozoites in the feces. If, as repeatedly described, manifestations such as nervousness, asthenia, easy fatigue, anorexia, weight loss, migraine, character changes and insomnia — all of them rarely ever produced by an amebic infection alone — are present or even govern the clinical picture in a patient with proved amebiasis, it is most likely that the amebic infection is a condition concomitant to a nonspecific enterocolopathy (see pages 139 to 141).

INTESTINAL TUBERCULOSIS

Tuberculous infections of the intestine occur most frequently in individuals suffering from pulmonary tuberculosis with cavitation. Pathologic studies carried out a few decades ago disclosed that from 50 to 90 per cent of autopsied cases of pulmonary tuberculosis had also intestinal involvement. Intestinal tuberculosis was especially frequent in patients who had had advanced active pulmonary tuberculosis for several years. The incidence of tuberculous lesions in the bowel has markedly declined since the introduction of specific antituberculous therapy.

Bowel infection secondary to phthisis is, in most instances, attributable to the *swallowing of sputum* carrying the tubercle bacilli to the intestine, where they first cause the production of inflammatory exudate in the depths of the tubular mucosal glands. Passing through the epithelial lining, the bacilli are carried by way of the submucosal lymphatics to the lymphoid tissue in which the typical granulomatous lesion will develop. The second but less frequent pathway, by which a secondary intestinal tuberculosis can arise, is the hematogenous route; lymphogenous spread and infection by direct contiguity from adjacent infected organs seem to be very rare occurrences.

The infectious organism in secondary intestinal tuberculosis is nearly always the human type of tubercle bacillus (Mycobacterium tuberculosis hominis). Primary intestinal tuberculosis, nowadays seldom encountered in countries with modern public health control, is, in the majority of instances, the result of an infection by the bovine variety (Myco. tuberculosis bovis) ingested through infected food, essentially dairy products. Primary intestinal tuberculosis has declined in frequency as a consequence of numerous public health measures, chiefly concerned with the elimination of infected milk and milk products, by the eradication of tuberculous cows and the pasteurization of milk. The fact that primary intestinal tuberculosis is more often encountered in children than in adults is probably explained by an acquired resistance on the part of the latter or other factors of the very complex host-parasite relationship.

The tuberculous lesions developing in the alimentary tract are most commonly located in the terminal ileum, cecum and ascending colon. Other sites in the gastrointestinal tract may be involved, but much less frequently. Predilection of *tuberculosis* for the *ileocecal region* may possibly be related to certain anatomic and physiologic characteristics of this portion of the alimentary canal. Lym-

PATHWAYS OF INFECTION

PRIMARY BY INGESTION OF INFECTED FOOD

SECONDARY FROM PULMONARY TUBERCULOSIS BY SWALLOWING OF SPUTUM CONTAINING TUBERCLE BACILLI

SECONDARY FROM LUNGS BY HEMATOGENOUS ROUTE

HISTOPATHOLOGY; TUBERCULOUS ULCER

EXTENSION TO REGIONAL LYMPH NODES

GENERALIZED INVOLVEMENT OF PERITONEUM BY CASEATION AND RUPTURE OF LYMPH NODES

EXTENSION TO OTHER PARTS OF BOWEL VIA LUMEN OR LYMPHATICS

DIRECT EXTENSION TO SEROSAL SURFACE BY PENETRATION

INFECTION OF GASTRO–INTESTINAL TRACT USUALLY ORIGINATES IN ILEOCECAL REGION

EXTENSION TO OTHER PARTS OF BOWEL VIA LUMEN AND/OR LYMPHATICS

ROUTES OF SPREAD

phoid tissue, for which the tubercle bacilli have a special affinity, is particularly abundant in the terminal ileum and cecum (see page 75). The progress of the intestinal contents is slower in the ileocecal region (see page 85) than in other portions of the bowel, thus facilitating the invasion of this area by the longer exposure of tubercle bacilli. The high degree of digestion of intestinal contents in the lower ileum permits also a freer contact of the bacilli with the intestinal lining. In the solitary lymph follicles and Peyer's patches characteristic tuberculous lesions develop. The overlying mucosa usually undergoes necrosis and is cast off, the underlying caseous tissue is discharged, and an ulcer is formed. The infection tends to spread in the bowel wall by way of the lymphatics, the course of which (see page 49) can explain the tendency of the ulcerative lesions to be of elliptical shape, extending laterally and partially

encircling the bowel. From the site of initial lesions, the infection may spread by contiguity and by way of the lymphatics in either direction, up or down the intestinal tract, and may involve, to a varying extent, the small intestine and colon.

From the lesions in the intestine, the tubercle bacilli may be carried to mesenteric lymph nodes which drain the affected segment of the bowel and may produce there a specific lymphadenitis. Tuberculous infection may extend from the intestine and mesenteric lymph nodes to the peritoneum. Tuberculous ulcers, especially those located in the small intestine, may penetrate as deep as the visceral peritoneum and may give rise to formation of tubercles on the serosal surface of the bowel. Generalized involvement of the peritoneum is usually produced by rupture of a caseated lymph node.

(Continued on page 58)

INTESTINAL TUBERCULOSIS

(Continued from page 157)

Tuberculosis of the bowel, from the pathologic point of view, may be divided into two distinct forms — the ulcerative and the hypertrophic. The development of one or the other form seems to depend on factors involving, among others, resistance of the host, type and virulence of the tubercle bacilli and duration of the disease. The *ulcerative form* is by far the more common. The initial lesions, most frequently seen at the lower end of the ileum and in the cecum, usually affect Peyer's patches and solitary lymph follicles, which appear enlarged, somewhat gray and translucent. These initial tubercles become yellow and soft on caseation; the overlying mucosa undergoes necrosis, sloughs off and leaves small lenticular ulcers, which tend to extend laterally, following the course of the lymphatics. The ulcers, however, may extend also into the long axis of the intestine, especially when confined to Peyer's patches. The *margins* of the ulcers are usually *irregular*, ragged and slightly *undermined*. The floor of the ulcers may be covered with necrotic material or may show small gray tubercles. Intestinal mucosa adjacent to ulcers becomes thickened, and its proliferation may lead to formation of small pseudopolyps. The ulcers penetrate the intestinal wall in varying degrees. The subserosal tissue often contains tubercles which can be seen from outside. The peritoneal coat is thickened and may show minute gray tubercles and patches of fibrinoplastic exudate.

Histologically, the base of the ulcer often shows a nonspecific inflammatory reaction due to secondary invasion of the intestinal bacteria. Deeper in the intestinal wall, however, and particularly beneath the serosa, typical tubercles with lymphocytes, epithelioid cells, giant cells and caseous necrosis are found. By means of special staining methods, acid-fast bacilli may be demonstrated in a good percentage of the cases.

The mesentery is invaded both directly and along the lymph vessels; formation of a thick, tuberculated tissue results. The mesenteric lymph nodes become enlarged, though some of them undergo nonspecific inflammatory changes. In other lymph nodes the typical tuberculous lesions develop to the point that they become completely caseous. Reparative processes may ensue and may give rise to fibrosis and calcification.

Tuberculous intestinal ulcers may heal by filling of the defect with cicatricial tissue, which, as a rule and particularly

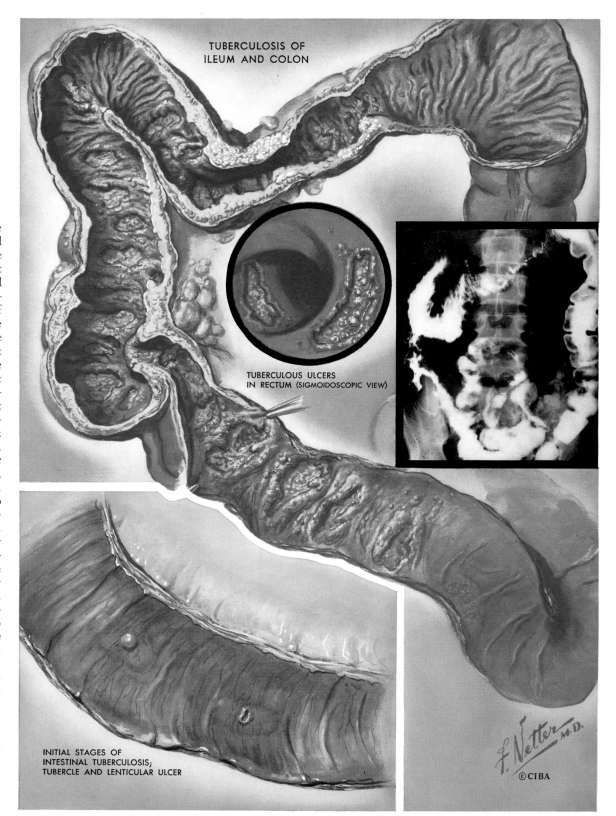

TUBERCULOSIS OF ILEUM AND COLON

TUBERCULOUS ULCERS IN RECTUM (SIGMOIDOSCOPIC VIEW)

INITIAL STAGES OF INTESTINAL TUBERCULOSIS; TUBERCLE AND LENTICULAR ULCER

when the tissue destruction has been extensive, produces a marked contraction effect, so that, on account of the encircling position of the original ulcer, a bowel stenosis results. Since the ulcers are frequently multiple, it happens that the intestine becomes stenosed at several points with the interspaced intestinal segments showing dilatation.

The *hypertrophic form* of intestinal tuberculosis is rare. It is believed to be, in the majority of cases, a primary infection of the bovine type. Hypertrophic tuberculous lesions are most commonly located in the ileocecal region. They are characterized by the predominance of the productive over the destructive processes. The affected segment of the bowel is greatly thickened, forming a tumorous mass, with extensive formation of tuberculous granulation tissue in the submucosa. The mucosa is folded and nodular and projects into the lumen of the intestine. It may eventually become ulcerated, though this is not a conspicuous feature. The regional lymph nodes are enlarged.

The histopathologic picture of the hypertrophic lesions shows the pathognomonic giant cells in the granulomatous inflammatory tissue. Typical tubercles and caseation occur less commonly than in the ulcerative form. The presence of acid-fast organisms in the granulation tissue may be demonstrated in a certain number of cases by special staining methods or, better, by animal inoculations.

Primary hypertrophic intestinal tuberculosis must be distinguished from the nonspecific granulomatous diseases of the intestine, particularly regional enteritis (see pages 142 and 143). Since in these diseases the gross and histologic appearances may be very similar, the differentiation can often be made only by careful bacteriologic studies.

(Continued on page 159)

INTESTINAL TUBERCULOSIS

(Continued from page 158)

Complications of intestinal tuberculosis include intestinal obstruction, perforation of the bowel and impairment of the absorptive function. Intestinal obstruction may be brought about by different mechanisms. Extension of the infection to the serosal surface of the bowel leads to a localized fibrinoplastic peritonitis and, subsequently, to *adhesions*, which may cause kinking of the bowel loops. Another cause of intestinal obstruction, partial or complete, is the stenosis of the bowel produced by retraction of the scar tissue in the healed ulcers (see above). In the hypertrophic form of the enteric tuberculosis, the intestinal obstruction may occur through the occlusion of the bowel lumen by the tumorous mass.

Perforation of a tuberculous ulcer leads to either a localized or a generalized peritonitis. The localized, "walled-off" peritonitis is a more common event owing to the dense peritoneal adhesions, formation of which usually precedes the perforation. The "walled-off" perforation occurs most frequently in the right iliac fossa, where it may lead to a fecal abscess. A tuberculous ulcer may also perforate, though rarely, into another bowel loop and produce an intestinal short circuit.

Extensive tuberculous involvement of the small intestine and/or mesenteric lymphatics may seriously impair the absorption of food materials and be responsible for the occurrence of the *malabsorption syndrome* (see also page 135).

Intestinal tuberculosis has no definite or specific symptomatology. In patients suffering from pulmonary tuberculosis, the appearance of abdominal symptoms may indicate the involvement of the digestive tract; but it must be remembered that not all gastro-intestinal symptoms occurring in patients with phthisis are due to intestinal tuberculous lesions. In pulmonary tuberculosis, symptoms of the kind often seen in intestinal tuberculosis may also be the result of toxin production in the lung lesions, neurogenic disturbances or other concomitant organic diseases. It also happens that the intestinal process may have progressed to the stage of considerable ulcerations in patients whose complaints never suggested any abdominal manifestations.

At the onset the tuberculous infection of the bowel may manifest itself with vague abdominal discomfort, nausea and regurgitation. The temperature may rise without any relation to the course of the lung lesion. A short attack of mild diarrhea may be followed by constipation. With the progress of the disease, and

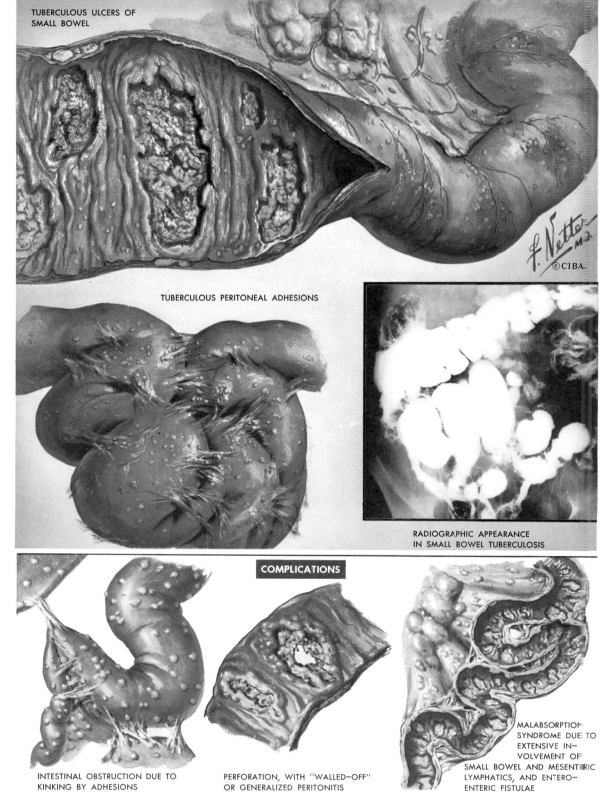

TUBERCULOUS ULCERS OF SMALL BOWEL

TUBERCULOUS PERITONEAL ADHESIONS

RADIOGRAPHIC APPEARANCE IN SMALL BOWEL TUBERCULOSIS

COMPLICATIONS

INTESTINAL OBSTRUCTION DUE TO KINKING BY ADHESIONS

PERFORATION, WITH "WALLED-OFF" OR GENERALIZED PERITONITIS

MALABSORPTION SYNDROME DUE TO EXTENSIVE INVOLVEMENT OF SMALL BOWEL AND MESENTERIC LYMPHATICS, AND ENTERO-ENTERIC FISTULAE

especially with its spread in the colon, the diarrhea may become frequent or even continuous. The stools are usually liquid or semiliquid, foul, and may contain mucus, pus and, seldom, blood. Massive bleeding from the intestine is very rare. Generalized abdominal pain or pain localized in certain areas, most frequently in the lower half of the abdomen and peri-umbilical region, is a complaint which, in patients with a pulmonary infection, should arouse suspicion of an intestinal involvement. When due to spasm or exaggerated peristalsis in the area of the disease, the pain is colicky; it may appear after eating and be somewhat relieved by defecation. A more localized, constant abdominal pain may point to peritoneal irritation or to acute swelling of the mesenteric lymph glands. The symptoms and signs, in instances of bowel obstruction or perforation, are not specific and are the same as in other conditions of this kind.

In patients with ulcerative intestinal tuberculosis, the physical examination of the abdomen may be negative, or it may reveal an area of tenderness over the site of the intestinal lesion. In the hypertrophic form a circumscribed mass may be palpated, usually in the right lower quadrant.

X-ray studies may be of great help in the diagnosis of intestinal tuberculosis. In the ulcerative form the radiograms may show persistent tendency of the cecum and/or the ascending colon to empty itself promptly of the barium, indicating a great irritability of these bowel segments (Stierlin sign). In the hypertrophic form a filling defect may be found in the cecum. Other intestinal roentgen findings include irregularities of contour, narrowing alternating with dilatation, and matting together of intestinal loops.

Rectosigmoidoscopic examination may occasionally reveal tuberculous ulcers in the rectum or sigmoid.

BENIGN TUMORS OF SMALL INTESTINE

and Peutz-Jeghers Syndrome

Benign tumors of the small intestine are not a common occurrence. In a series of 22,810 autopsies, an incidence of 0.16 per cent was found (Buckstein). The neoplasm may be located anywhere in the small bowel, but the ileum is affected more frequently than is the jejunum. In both sexes the incidence is about the same. For some types of benign adenomas, neurofibromas and hemangiomas, it is established that their occurrence is familial.

Benign tumors of the small bowel may arise from any of its histologic elements. They may be single or multiple. According to their location, they may be classified into intraluminal, extraluminal and intramural types. In size they may vary from that of a grain of wheat to that of a fetal head, or even exceeding it. In their form they may be globular, polypoid, plaquelike or annular. The more common benign neoplasms are adenomas, lipomas, myomas, hemangiomas and neurogenic tumors. They account for more than two thirds of all small-intestinal benign new growths. Rarer tumors include true fibromas, lymphangiomas, myxomas and osteomas. Many of the so-called fibromas reported in the literature have been actually mixed tumors such as fibromyomas, fibromyxomas, fibro-adenomas, etc.

Adenomas, the most common of benign tumors of the small intestine, are usually sessile or pedunculated intraluminal tumors. They may be single or multiple. Their size varies in most instances between a few millimeters and about 3 cm.; greater size is rarely reached. Histologically, the adenomas are made up of intestinal epithelium which shows some irregularity in its arrangement. The cells lining the surface are mucus-secreting and form glands similar to those seen in normal mucosa. Edematous, vascularized connective tissue and usually some mononuclear cells are seen beneath the epithelium. In the polypoid adenomas, a stalklike connective tissue central structure arises from the submucosa and, sometimes, extends into the growth, separating it into lobules.

Lipomas (see Plate 47) can be divided into submucous and subserous types, the former being more common than the latter. In rarer instances they may be both submucous and subserous. The submucous lipomas tend to grow inwardly, whereas the subserous lipomas expand in the outward direction and sometimes reach great dimensions. Whether the submucous lipomas are sessile or pedunculated, the mucosa covering the growth may be normal in appearance or thinned and atrophic, and the submucosal connective tissue may develop into a thin or a comparatively thick capsule, from

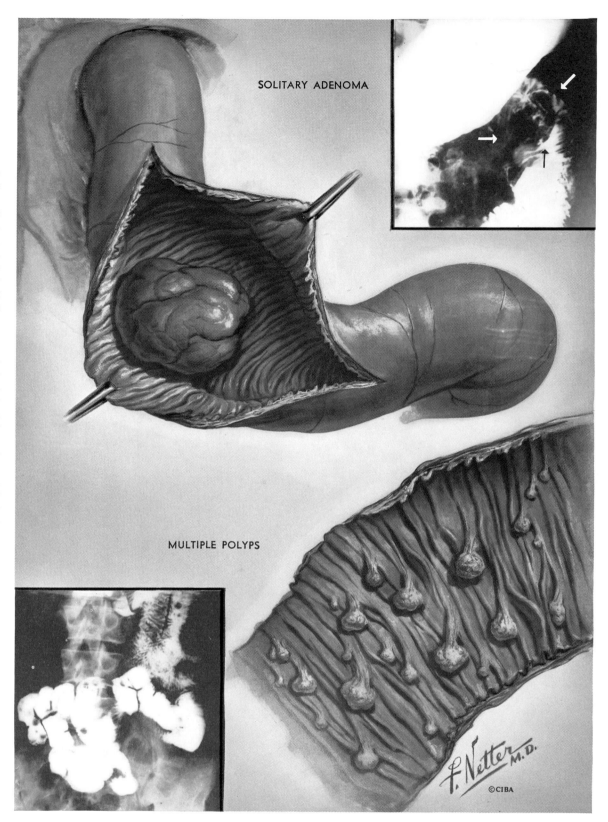

SOLITARY ADENOMA

MULTIPLE POLYPS

which septa may enter the fatty tissue and divide it into lobules. In the smaller sessile tumors, the mucosal and muscular layers are usually displaced about equally in the opposite directions. If the lipoma is attached by a broad base, its form may vary from that of a disk to that of a pear. If it is attached by a fibrous pedicle, the tumor may be oval, or it may be flattened and elongated. The surface may be rounded and smooth or irregular and lobulated.

Leiomyomas of the small intestine are usually single tumors; multiple growths occur but rarely. Starting in the muscle coats, they grow toward or away from the lumen of the bowel, or in both directions. Tumors of small size may remain intramural. Leiomyomas of the small intestine are firm, well-defined, usually rounded, sometimes lobulated, sessile or pedunculated masses of varying size; those growing outwardly may attain very great dimensions. The cut

surface presents a grayish-pink, whorled appearance. Regressive and inflammatory changes, attributable chiefly to the relative avascularity of the tumor, supervene rather commonly and are the cause of fibrosis, necrosis, cavitation, calcification and abscess formation within the tumor. The mucosa overlying the tumorous mass not rarely becomes ulcerated. The histology of the small-intestinal leiomyomas is similar to that of smooth muscle tumors located in other parts of the body. The smooth muscle cells, with their myofibrils and an accompanying framework of connective tissue, are arranged in bundles which tend to interlace.

The small-intestinal benign tumors arising from the nerve elements are reported in the medical literature under a great variety of terms, such as neurinoma, *neurofibroma, neurilemmoma,* schwannoma,

(Continued on page 161)

BENIGN TUMORS OF SMALL INTESTINE
and Peutz-Jeghers Syndrome

(Continued from page 160)

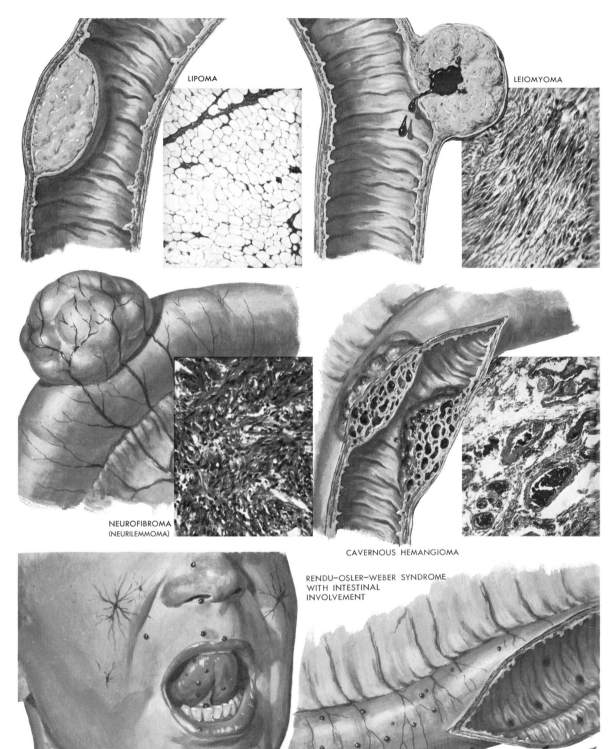

LIPOMA

LEIOMYOMA

NEUROFIBROMA (NEURILEMMOMA)

CAVERNOUS HEMANGIOMA

RENDU–OSLER–WEBER SYNDROME WITH INTESTINAL INVOLVEMENT

schwannoglioma, lemmoblastoma, peripheric glioma, etc. The neurogenic tumors may be located anywhere in the small intestine; they may be single or multiple; extraluminal, intraluminal or intramural. The outward-growing tumors may be found on the serosal surface as ovoid or globular, smooth nodules. The inward-growing tumors may be sessile or pedunculated; the overlying mucosa may thin out and ulcerate. The cut surface shows a grayish-yellow or pinkish-gray color, in which cavities containing clotted blood may be encountered. The histologic examination reveals fasciculated spindle cells with palisading of nuclei, and thin-walled vascular spaces and areas of old and recent hemorrhages. Since the neurogenic tumors may closely resemble other connective tissue tumors, special staining methods are required for their identification. The neurogenic tumors encountered in the small intestine may be part of a generalized neurofibromatosis (von Recklinghausen's disease) (see, e.g., CIBA COLLECTION, Vol. 3/1, pages 133 and 178).

Benign vascular tumors of the small intestine comprise true tumors of blood vessels or angiomas, and congenital vascular malformations or hamartomas. It is extremely difficult to differentiate between these two types of tumors. The small-intestinal angiomas may be solitary or multiple, and they may be classified into capillary, compact and cavernous types, and are composed of a meshwork of capillaries, dilated or nondilated, and separated by few or abundant fibrous strands. The compact hemangiomas are composed of solid alveolar masses of endothelial cells and less obvious blood spaces. The *cavernous hemangiomas* consist of large blood-filled communicating spaces lined by endothelium, and have little stroma. The larger tumors may have a racemose or varicose structure, consisting of ramified blood vessels. In some instances only small telangiectasia may exist; in others large hemangiomas may extend considerably along the bowel.

The hemangiomatous lesions localized in the small intestine may be part of a general vascular dysplasia (hemangiomatosis). The best known of such conditions is the *Rendu-Osler-Weber syndrome* (multiple hereditary telangiectasis, with recurring hemorrhages). This disease is characterized by the appearance of angiomatous lesions on the skin, mucous membranes and viscera, and a history of familial occurrence. In its typical form it runs the following course: In childhood or in early adult life, only recurrent epistaxis may pose a diagnostic problem. In early or middle adult life, angiomatous lesions appear on the skin, particularly of the face, ears and fingers, and on the mucous membrane of the nose, tongue and lips. The trunk and limbs may also be affected. The vascular lesions tend to increase in number and bleed readily, and may cause severe anemia; visceral lesions may become manifest, especially in the stomach, small intestine and rectum. The liver, peritoneum and trachea are also known to be affected. It is possible that the visceral lesions may be present without external manifestations of the disease and may be the cause of an unexplained melena, hematemesis, hemoptysis or hematuria. The vascular lesions present themselves in two main types: the *spider telangiectasis,* consisting of a punctiform central area from which radiate small vessels; it is bluish or red, and it fades partially on pressure. This type of lesion can be found, particularly, on the nose, cheeks, ears, eyelids and fingers, and on the mucosal surfaces of the lips, tongue and nose. The *nodular angiomas* are solid-looking tumors, 1 to 3 mm. in diameter; they do not disappear on pressure and are situated, particularly, on the tongue, lips, face and fingers. Regression of individual vascular lesions may occur, especially after bleeding. The Rendu-Osler-Weber syndrome seems to be a Mendelian-dominant hereditary disease, affecting both sexes equally.

The hemangiomatosis may be associated with other congenital anomalies. As an example of such an association, mention may be made of the so-called hemangiectatic hypertrophy of limbs (Klippel-Trenaunay-Weber syndrome) in which hemangiomatosis and hypertrophy of one or more limbs coexist.

In general, many of these benign lesions may never cause symptoms during life or may cause only such vague symptoms that a diagnosis cannot be established. If serious clinical manifestations develop,

(Continued on page 162)

BENIGN TUMORS
OF SMALL INTESTINE
and Peutz-Jeghers Syndrome

(Continued from page 161)

they are, as a rule, the result of complications, namely, intestinal obstruction, necrotic changes in the tumor, with resultant hemorrhage, infection or rupture, and malignant degeneration. The occurrence of complications depends largely on the type of growth and its size. The intraluminal tumors are liable to cause symptoms earlier than do extraluminal tumors, which sometimes attain enormous dimensions before giving the first indication of their existence. The slow-growing intraluminal sessile tumors may bring about a partial, gradually progressive obstruction. The polypoid tumors lead usually to obstruction by *intussusception*. The extraluminal tumors cause the obstruction by compression of the intestine, kinking or volvulus. The small-intestinal obstruction manifests itself by abdominal colic, vomiting, constipation (sometimes alternating with bouts of diarrhea), abdominal distention and blood loss in stools (occult or visible blood, or melena). The severity of symptoms depends on the degree of obstruction. The *bleeding* of intraluminal tumors derives from ulceration of the overlying mucosa or rupture of a blood vessel draining the tumor. In the fast-growing tumors, particularly in the extraluminal leiomyomas and neurofibromas, the bleeding may result from a central hemorrhagic necrosis, with cavitation and formation of a fistula connecting the cavity with the intestinal lumen. Extraluminal tumors may rupture into the peritoneal cavity or may become necrotic following torsion of a pedicle, and thus may lead to intra-abdominal hemorrhages. In rare instances fistula formation may occur through intramural or extraluminal tumors connecting the intestinal lumen with the abdominal cavity and resulting in peritonitis.

Malignant degeneration of benign tumors of the small intestine seems not to be a frequent occurrence. In contrast to the adenomatous polyps of the colon, which are widely regarded as precancerous, the small-intestinal polyps undergo malignant changes only rarely and usually do not give rise to secondary deposits in lymph nodes, liver or other organs.

A clinical entity which was identified about 40 years ago but the importance of which has been fully recognized only in recent years is the *Peutz-Jeghers syndrome*, characterized by association of *gastro-intestinal adenomatous polyposis*, a distinctive type of *mucocutaneous pigmentation* and inheritance through a Mendelian-dominant gene. The factor has a high degree of penetration and is carried by both sexes, which appear to be affected about equally. The polyposis may involve any part of the gastro-intestinal tract, but the small intestine is

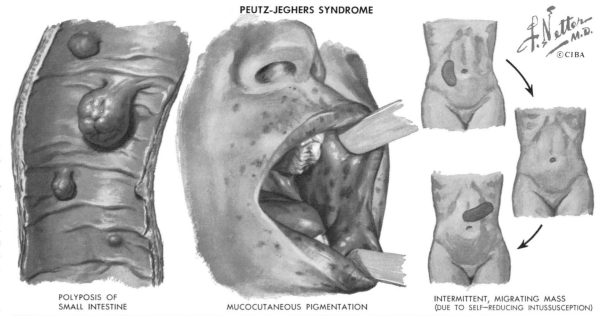

PEUTZ-JEGHERS SYNDROME

POLYPOSIS OF SMALL INTESTINE

MUCOCUTANEOUS PIGMENTATION

INTERMITTENT, MIGRATING MASS
(DUE TO SELF—REDUCING INTUSSUSCEPTION)

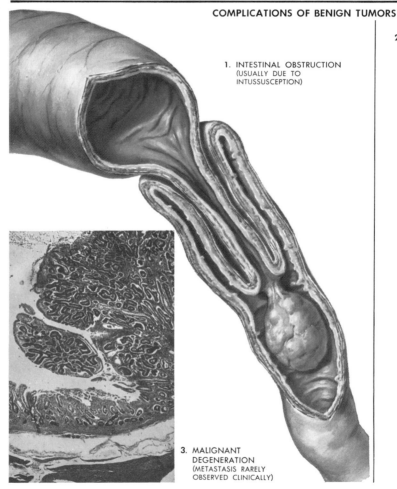

COMPLICATIONS OF BENIGN TUMORS

1. INTESTINAL OBSTRUCTION
(USUALLY DUE TO INTUSSUSCEPTION)

3. MALIGNANT DEGENERATION
(METASTASIS RARELY OBSERVED CLINICALLY)

2. HEMORRHAGE
(MOST OFTEN IN LEIOMYOMA)

FIRST STAGE: INTERSTITIAL HEMORRHAGES

SECOND STAGE: CONFLUENCE OF NECROTIC, HEMORRHAGIC AREAS

THIRD STAGE: EVACUATION INTO INTESTINE; BLEEDING PERSISTS OWING TO FIRM, "NONCOLLAPSING" CAVITY WALLS

Modified after O. N. Smith

always affected. The cutaneous pigmentation consists of sharply demarcated dark-brown or black macules grouped around the mouth, eyes and nostrils. The fingers and palms, the toes, the forearms and the umbilical region may also be involved. The mucosal pigmentation is a constant finding and consists of macules located on the lips and buccal mucosa, occasionally also on the gums, the palate, the fauces and the nasal mucosa. The pigmented spots, containing melanin deposits, are level with the skin or mucosa; they are nonvascular and nonhairy. Various other disorders and congenital deformities (bladder polyps, bronchial adenomas, congenital heart disease, nasal polyps, diverticulosis, skeletal and cutaneous malformations, retarded development, and ovarian cysts and tumors) may occasionally be associated with this syndrome.

The symptoms of the Peutz-Jeghers syndrome

include some remarkable abdominal manifestations which are the result of transient, self-reducing and recurrent enteric *intussusceptions*. The patients experience attacks of colicky abdominal pain accompanied by borborygmi; at first these attacks tend to be mild and of short duration and may recur for years at intervals of months or weeks only, but gradually they grow more prolonged and severe, and the remissions become shorter. During the attack the physical examination of the abdomen may reveal an area of tenderness or a mass which disappears as soon as the crisis is over. At the next attack such an ephemeral mass may appear again at another location. In case of multiple intussusceptions, more than one mass may be palpated. Surgical repair of the intussusception (see page 134), if it is not reduced spontaneously within a few hours, is necessary. Elective polypectomy may in some cases be the treatment of choice.

MALIGNANT TUMORS OF SMALL INTESTINE I AND II

Malignant tumors of the small intestine are rare, their frequency in a huge number of autopsies recorded over many decades remaining below 0.1 per cent (Shallow *et al.*). Of all neoplasms (carcinoma, malignant lymphoma, sarcoma and carcinoid) in the entire gastro-intestinal tract, only about 5 per cent are located in the small bowel. The reason for this unique situation with regard to that part of the intestine is no less obscure than is the pathogenesis of the tumors there and in other parts of the body.

Carcinomas of the small bowel occur more frequently in males than in females (approximately 2:1) and are most common in patients between the ages of 40 and 60 years. They present two main gross forms, that of a tumor infiltrating the bowel wall, usually in an encircling manner, and that of a polypoid mass proliferating into the lumen. According to their histologic characteristics, they are classified into glandular, medullary, scirrhous and colloid types. The glandular type (adenocarcinoma) arises from the epithelial cells of the mucous membrane and grows into the intestinal wall in sheets and strands, displacing the normal elements and forming cell nests with glandular structure. The cells are commonly of the tall columnar variety but may be cuboidal or even stratified. They have a moderate amount of cytoplasm and a large, oval, hyperchromatic nucleus; mitotic figures are frequent. Adenocarcinoma does not, however, always exhibit a pure glandular structure; the cells may be irregular in form, closely packed together, and may be arranged in nests and sheets that bear only a rough resemblance to true acinar formations. The medullary type of carcinoma arises also from the epithelium of the mucous membrane, but the cells do not show the tendency to reproduce glandular structures; they are closely packed and formed in solid sheets and strands. Their cytoplasm is scant; the nucleus is large and contains numerous hyperchromatic particles. In the scirrhous type, as with carcinoma of the stomach (see CIBA COLLECTION, Vol. 3/1, page 183) or of the colon (see page 168), the fibrous elements predominate over the epithelial components, imparting to the growth a very hard consistency. Colloid carcinoma, again in analogy to the gastric colloid carcinoma (see CIBA COLLECTION, Vol. 3/1, page 182), is an adenocarcinoma that has undergone mucoid degeneration. Such tumors consist of lobulated gelatinous material, their cut section showing numerous cystlike structures filled with semisolid mucoid masses.

Malignant lymphomas, arising from the lymphatic tissue, are usually a manifestation of a generalized systemic disease but may sometimes remain restricted to certain organs. Thus, lymphomas found limited to the small intestine may denote only a primary focus of

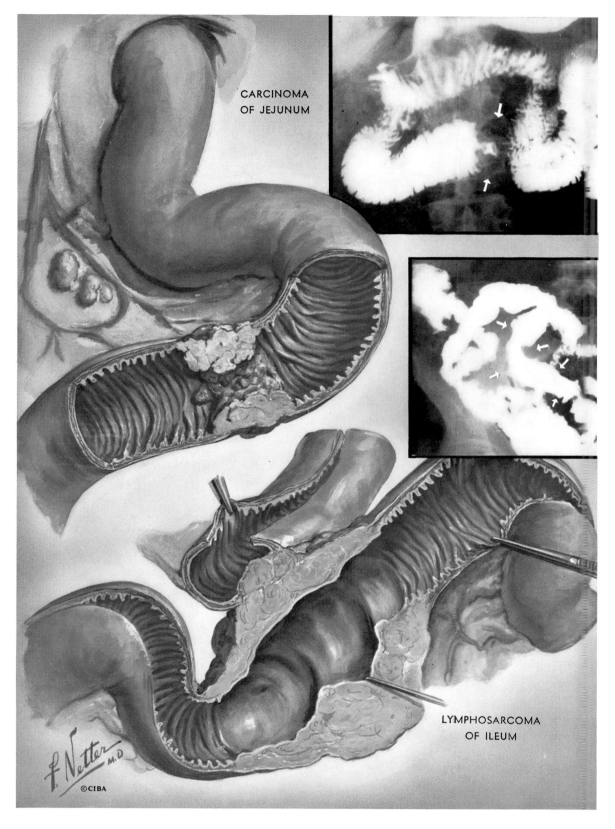

CARCINOMA OF JEJUNUM

LYMPHOSARCOMA OF ILEUM

a predestined general systemic disorder; occasionally, however, they may remain localized and are, theoretically, susceptible to cure by extirpation. The gross appearance of the intestinal malignant lymphomas, occurring at any age, though most frequently in the third and fourth decades and about twice as often in men as in women, is extremely variable. The most common form assumed by the tumor is that of an infiltrating, constricting growth encircling the lumen; its surface may or may not be ulcerated. Extension of the growth may also proceed in the longitudinal direction of the bowel; in the middle portion of such an extensive infiltrative growth, the intestine may become dilated and present an aneurysmal appearance. Not rarely, the tumor grows into the intestinal lumen as a fungating, polypoid mass. The texture of a malignant lymphoma is firm, the cut surface is bluish-white and central necrosis with excava-

tion may be present. Histologically, the malignant lymphomas are characterized by multiplication of one or more elements normally present in the lymphatic organs. Numerous attempts to subdivide and classify this group of tumors have been made; they have resulted, however, in an extraordinary confusion of terminology and controversial theses. The classification most frequently used, though with different modifications, is based, in essence, on the predominant cell type found in the growth (Gall and Mallory). It subdivides the malignant lymphomas into: (1) reticulum-cell sarcomas (stem-cell lymphoma and clasmatocytic lymphoma), (2) lymphosarcomas (lymphoblastic lymphoma and lymphocytic lymphoma), (3) Hodgkin's lymphomas (Hodgkin's lymphoma and Hodgkin's sarcoma) and (4) follicular lymphomas.

The small intestine is, in rare instances, the seat of

(Continued on page 174)

MALIGNANT TUMORS OF SMALL INTESTINE I AND II

(Continued from page 163)

leiomyosarcoma and fibrosarcoma. Leiomyosarcomas, arising from the muscular coat, tend to grow outward, to undergo central necrosis and to form cysts, which become connected with the intestinal lumen and cause bleeding. The behavior of leiomyosarcoma is, thus, very similar to that of leiomyoma (see page 161); the histopathologic pictures may also be similar, sometimes making extremely difficult the differential diagnosis between the benign and malignant varieties. Fibrosarcomas arise from the connective tissue of the intestinal wall. They also tend to grow outward, sometimes attaining very great dimensions. The gross form is usually rounded and lobulated; their consistency is hard or, in case central necrosis has occurred, soft and spongy; the cut section is white and translucent. Microscopic examination reveals the tumor to be composed of whorls and strands of spindle-shaped cells of fibrous connective tissue. Myxosarcoma of the small intestine is believed to be a degenerate form of fibrosarcoma.

Malignant tumors of the small intestine have no specific symptomatology. They simulate so closely other intra-abdominal lesions that a correct diagnosis can hardly be made on the basis of symptoms and physical signs alone. Symptoms of small-intestinal malignancy are largely the result of local mechanical conditions and, to a lesser degree, of constitutional effects of the tumor on the patient. The most important mechanical condition produced by the tumor is the *obstruction* (partial or total) of the intestinal lumen and interference with the normal progression of the intestinal contents. The mechanism by which the obstruction is brought about varies with the gross morphology of the tumor. An infiltrating *annular growth* produces a gradually progressive constriction of the intestine, which may become so great that only a tiny distorted tubule of the former lumen will remain. An inward-growing, sessile or pedunculated, *polypoid tumor* may be responsible for the occurrence of a sudden obstruction by *intussusception*. *Infiltrative growth,* extending in the longitudinal direction, may cause obstruction by disturbing peristaltic function. *Exophytic tumors* may produce obstruction by compressing the intestine from the outside or by causing kinking of a bowel loop. The symptoms of obstruction vary. In cases of sudden total obstruction (usually intussusception), the patients feel a sudden, sharp, agonizing abdominal pain. If the obstruction is localized in the proximal parts of the intestine, the pain will be followed soon by nausea and repeated vomiting, which may eventually become stercoraceous; diarrhea may appear accompanied by tenesmus and discharge of bloody mucus. If the obstruction is localized in the distal parts of the small intestine, the pain may be accom-

MORPHOLOGIC TYPES OF GROWTH

ANNULAR
(GRADUAL, PROGRESSIVE OBSTRUCTION)

POLYPOID
(SUDDEN OBSTRUCTION DUE TO INTUSSUSCEPTION)

INFILTRATING
(OBSTRUCTION DUE TO DISTURBANCE OF PERISTALSIS)

EXOPHYTIC
(OBSTRUCTION DUE TO KINKING OR PRESSURE)

LOCAL CONSEQUENCES

ANNULAR OBSTRUCTION

INTUSSUSCEPTION

HEMORRHAGE
(FROM ULCERATION OR CENTRAL NECROSIS)

PERFORATION

FISTULA

MALABSORPTION

EXTENSIVE OR MULTIPLE

panied mainly by abdominal distention and ceasing of bowel movements. If the obstruction is not reduced spontaneously, the patient may go into a state of shock within a few hours after the onset of symptoms. In cases of slowly progressive obstruction, a dull or sharp, cramplike pain may, for a certain time, be the only complaint before other symptoms of obstruction gradually set in. Malignant tumors may manifest themselves by *bleeding,* owing to either erosion of the tumor's surface or a central hemorrhagic necrosis, with cavitation and formation of a *fistula* connecting the cavity with the intestinal lumen. Necrosis of the tumor tissue may lead to intestinal *perforation* and peritonitis. Perforation may occur also into another intestinal loop, producing a fistula which, by short-circuiting the intestine, may cause a disturbance in the absorption of food materials. Extensive involvement of the small intestine by a malignant growth

may also seriously impair the absorptive function and give rise to a malabsorption syndrome (see page 135). Constitutional symptoms of small-intestinal malignancy include anorexia, malaise, loss of weight, emaciation, anemia and, eventually, fever. Physical examination of the abdomen may reveal a localized tenderness or a mass, if the tumor has reached a sufficient size; in cases of intestinal obstruction, visible peristalsis and distention of intestinal loops may be observed. X-ray studies may be of help in diagnosis by showing the existence of a small-intestinal lesion, but, unfortunately, a growth that does not produce a marked obstruction remains frequently undetected by this examination.

Metastases of the malignant tumors of the small intestine occur by direct extension to neighboring structures, via lymphatics to regional and distant lymph nodes and by hematogenous route to distant organs.

Malignant Tumors of Small Intestine III

Carcinoid Tumors, Malignant Carcinoid Syndrome

From the argentaffine cells (of Kultschitzky) in the crypts of the intestinal mucosa (see pages 49, 50 and 55), known also as enterochromaffin or chromaffin cells, bright yellow, nonencapsulated but circumscribed tumors may arise. These so-called "carcinoid tumors" resemble carcinomas in their histologic structure and invasiveness. The *primary carcinoid tumors* occur in the gastro-intestinal tract from the cardia to the anus and, occasionally, in the gallbladder, gonadal teratoma and, presumably, in the pancreas. Preferentially located in the appendix (see page 148) and jejuno-ileum, they usually appear as small (0.5 to 2 cm.), occasionally multiple, subepithelial nodules, which, when expanding, may invade all the intestinal coats, grow outward, encircle the gut or proliferate into its lumen. The carcinoids grow very slowly and metastasize late, commonly into the regional lymph nodes and, less commonly, into more distant organs, especially the *liver*. *Histologically,* these neoplasms are composed of columns, sheets and clumps of epithelial cells, sometimes forming acinar structures. Three types of cells — (1) round, or polygonal, cells, (2) "palisade" cells and (3) cells lining the small acini — can be differentiated (Masson), essentially by means of the distribution of the chromaffin granules they contain.

The physiologic significance of the argentaffine cells and the pathologic significance of the carcinoid tumors rest upon their property to contain or, very probably, produce *5-hydroxytryptamine* (enteramine, serotonin), a metabolite of tryptophan. Though its functional rôle in the healthy organism has not been established as yet, this compound is classified nowadays as "tissue hormone" (Hedinger and Labhart), and its presence has been demonstrated in the intestinal chromaffin cells as well as in the hypothalamus, spleen and blood platelets. It is degraded enzymatically in the liver, kidney, brain, lungs and intestinal mucosa to *5-hydroxyindole acetic acid,* which appears as a urinary excretion product. In pharmacologic doses, *i.e.,* in the presence of amounts certainly higher than those found under normal circumstances, serotonin has marked effects on the smooth musculature of vessels and viscera (vasoconstriction or vasodilatation, bronchoconstriction, antidiuresis, peristalsis increase) and also on the central nervous system. Some of these effects

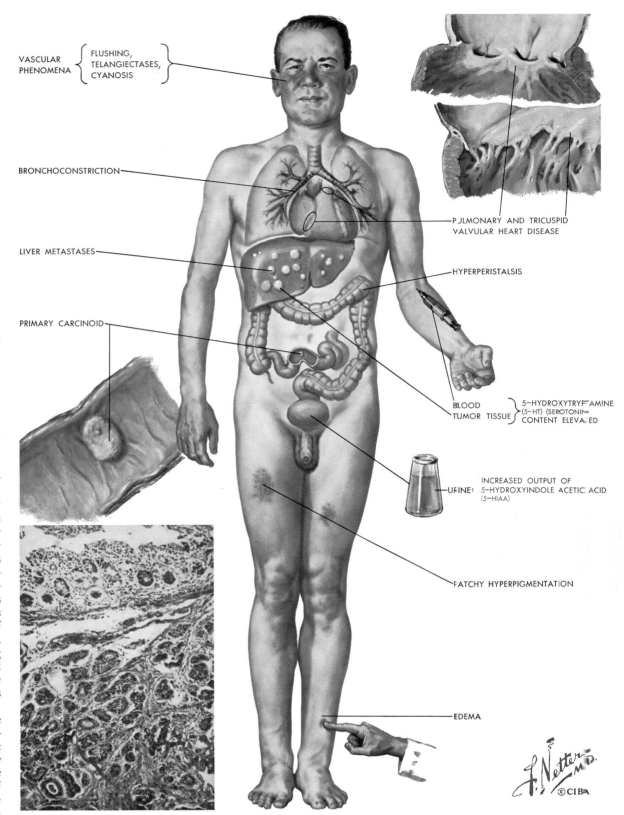

VASCULAR PHENOMENA { FLUSHING, TELANGIECTASES, CYANOSIS }

BRONCHOCONSTRICTION

LIVER METASTASES

PRIMARY CARCINOID

PULMONARY AND TRICUSPID VALVULAR HEART DISEASE

HYPERPERISTALSIS

BLOOD TUMOR TISSUE } 5-HYDROXYTRYPTAMINE (5-HT) (SEROTONIN) CONTENT ELEVATED

URINE: INCREASED OUTPUT OF 5-HYDROXYINDOLE ACETIC ACID (5-HIAA)

PATCHY HYPERPIGMENTATION

EDEMA

can be clearly related to the symptoms of the *malignant carcinoid syndrome,* as it is observed in the presence of metastases of carcinoid tumors.

This syndrome, also known as the Thorson-Biörck syndrome, is characterized by paroxysmal flushing of the face and neck and, variably, of other skin areas, patchy cyanotic discoloration and telangiectases, colicky abdominal pain, diarrhea and, eventually, asthmalike *respiratory distress.* Not all symptoms need be directly dependent on 5-hydroxytryptamine overproduction. *Patchy* (pellagralike) *hyperpigmentation of the skin, edema,* ascites and pleural effusion may be the results of nutritional disturbances, hypo-albuminemia, portal hypertension and other factors. Late in the course *endocardial lesions* may develop, especially involving the *pulmonary* and *tricuspid valves.* They consist of fibrous thickening of the endothelial lining and shortening and fusion of the chordae tendinae,

leading subsequently to cardiac failure.

The malignant carcinoid syndrome, when fully manifest, can be readily recognized and can be established by determination of 5-hydroxyindole acetic acid in the urine. Values above 15 mg. per day are suggestive; values of 30 mg. and over are diagnostic.* The diagnosis of a primary carcinoid tumor presents, in the absence of endocrine manifestations, the same or even greater difficulties than do other intestinal neoplasms, because they produce no or only local effects. The primary growth cannot be visualized by X-ray. Hepatomegaly points to the presence of liver metastases, and peritoneoscopy, with liver biopsy, will establish the diagnosis.

*The patient should be on a banana-free diet, because bananas contain a considerable amount of serotonin (Connell *et al.,* Waalkes *et al.*).

FAMILIAL POLYPOSIS OF LARGE INTESTINE

The same types of benign tumors occur in the colon and rectum as are encountered in the upper gastro-intestinal tract (see pages 160, 161 and CIBA COLLECTION, Vol. 3/1, pages 177 to 179). Summing up the single, multiple, sessile and pedunculated polypoid tumors, the adenomatous polyp is the most common. The practical significance of these neoplasms is attained by their great tendency to undergo malignant changes (see page 167).

A distinct disease entity, that must be separated from the more frequent polyp formation in the large intestine, is the diffuse *familial intestinal polyposis,* also known as multiple familial adenomatosis, adenomatosis coli, hereditary multiple polyposis or multiple papillomas. It is characterized by an *excessive proliferation of the glandular epithelium all over the mucous membrane of the colon and rectum,* which leads to the formation of *sessile,* flat or *pedunculated polyps,* depending upon the stage of the individual growth. The red or purplish-red, soft polyps, with a smooth or lobulated surface, vary in size from a few millimeters to several centimeters, and in number from a few in a small, confined area to several hundred covering the length of the entire large bowel. The rectum is involved in 95 per cent of the cases. The continuity of the polyp's stalk with the submucous fibrous tissue and the continuity of the epithelial covering with the intestinal surface epithelium can be demonstrated microscopically. A stalk of a polyp may consist of a single strand of well-vascularized connective tissue or may be divided into many fingerlike branchings. Numerous goblet cells are usually seen in the epithelial lining.

The most important feature, clinically and pathologically, is the frequency with which the adenomas, though they all appear at first nonmalignant, undergo *malignant degeneration.* Cancer is most likely to develop about 15 years after the onset of symptoms (Dukes). In some patients more than one primary focus of carcinoma may be present. Histopathologically, the degenerated adenomatous polyps show an atypical cell arrangement, a localized occurrence of anaplastic cells ("carcinoma in situ") or frank invasive cancer.

The hereditary character of familial polyposis has been clearly established. As a rule, it is inherited as a simple, nonsexlinked, dominant Mendelian trait, which manifests itself not at the time of birth but only after several years, in most cases not until late in the second decade of life.

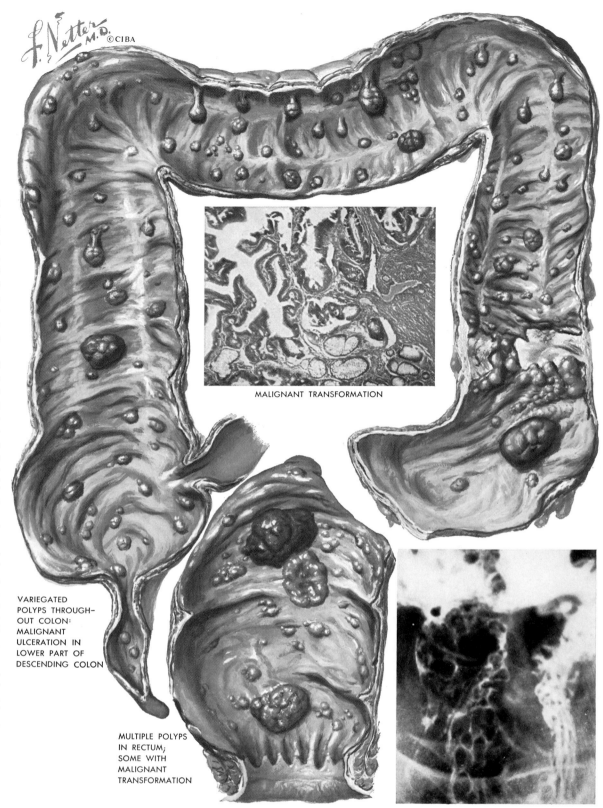

MALIGNANT TRANSFORMATION

VARIEGATED POLYPS THROUGHOUT COLON: MALIGNANT ULCERATION IN LOWER PART OF DESCENDING COLON

MULTIPLE POLYPS IN RECTUM; SOME WITH MALIGNANT TRANSFORMATION

Familial polyposis presents no single symptom or symptom complex that could be considered pathognomonic. The mild, early signs, such as a trifling melena and loose stools, may remain unnoticed until several years have passed. With the progress of the disease and, particularly, when malignant degeneration has started, the mentioned symptoms become more pronounced, and the patient may complain of a more or less constant colicky pain. The stools become liquid, fetid, truly hemorrhagic, mixed with mucus and, eventually, pus. At times, the bleeding may be severe, so that the patient becomes anemic and loses weight and appetite. He suffers, furthermore, from nausea, indigestion, easy fatigue, tenesmus and frequent desire to evacuate. The abdomen, on physical examination, offers no definite findings, except when a palpable mass points to an already well-developed malignant growth. Clubbing fingers,

with manifestations as mentioned, should support a suspected diagnosis of polyposis, as, of course, does the family history indicating that individuals in the same or previous generations had the disease. Though rectal digital examination can decide the issue, rectosigmoidoscopy will establish the diagnosis in practically all cases. X-ray examination with a barium enema and double contrast studies will show the extension of the disease.

Radical surgery is the only efficient treatment for familial polyposis. A few cases with good response to high voltage X-ray therapy have been reported (Bassler). Multiple epidermoid cysts, fibromata and osteomata occasionally accompany familial polyposis of the colon. Their presence should prompt a proctoscopic examination and double contrast X-ray study of the rectosigmoid in order to ascertain or exclude polyps.

RELATIVE REGIONAL INCIDENCE OF CARCINOMA OF LARGE BOWEL

MALIGNANT TUMORS OF LARGE INTESTINE

ADENOCARCINOMA

CARCINOMA OF CECUM

About one third of the malignant lesions of the gastro-intestinal tract are localized in the large bowel. They are encountered in any part of this intestinal segment, but the relative regional distribution is different. About 50 per cent of the malignant tumors of the large intestine are found in the rectum and 25 per cent in the sigmoid colon; the remaining 25 per cent are distributed about equally through the cecum, ascending colon, hepatic flexure, transverse colon, splenic flexure and descending colon.

The disease is more common in the male, the sex ratio being about 3:2. The neoplasms develop at any age but are most frequent between the ages of 50 and 70. However, it is important to realize that in about 10 per cent of the cases the patients affected are under the age of 30, and most of these have not yet entered the second decade of life.

Adenocarcinomas are the most frequent malignant new growths of the large bowel. The lesion is single, as a rule, but may sometimes be multiple. One or more benign adenomas are found, not rarely, in their neighborhood or elsewhere in the colon, suggesting that the malignant lesion arose from a primary benign polyp. The possibility of cancer degeneration of benign adenomas is demonstrated by the following facts: (1) Percentual incidence of benign adenomas in the different segments of the large bowel is the same as that of adenocarcinomas. (2) Follow-up of the untreated benign adenomas reveals malignant degeneration in a large number of cases. (3) Histopathologic studies of the adenomas reveal atypical cell arrangements, carci-

noma "in situ" or invasive carcinoma in a fair percentage of cases. (4) In the familial polyposis of the large intestine (see page 166), the degeneration of one or more adenomas is frequently observed.

Chronic inflammatory conditions, such as lymphogranulomatous rectitis and ulcerative colitis, are also considered to be lesions that may eventually give rise to malignancy. In lymphogranulomatous rectitis more than 10 per cent of the untreated cases show squamous cell carcinoma infiltration of the rectal wall. In ulcerative colitis, adenocarcinoma is observed in more than 5 per cent of the cases that had the disease for 10 years or longer; some authors reported this occurrence in even more than 30 per cent of their cases. The concept of the origin of these malignancies is still controversial. Though some authors believe that the malignant growth arises in the pseudopolyps, the appearance of the malignant features seems rather

dependent upon the pre-existence of an inflammatory lesion. This assumption is borne out by three main considerations: (1) In a large number of cancer cases with a history of ulcerative colitis, pseudopolyps are not observed. (2) No adenomatous glandular arrangement is seen histopathologically in pseudopolyps in contrast to the true adenoma. (3) The neoplasm in the great majority of instances, is of the infiltrative type, the proliferative, bulky type being only rarely observed.

Adenocarcinomas of the large bowel occur usually as nodular proliferating or as *scirrhous infiltrating tumors*. Both varieties may, occasionally, undergo mucoid degeneration (colloid adenocarcinoma). The nodular adenocarcinoma represents a bulky fungating mass, projecting into the lumen and becoming ulcerated rather speedily. In the well-differentiated tumor

(*Continued on page* 68)

CONSTRICTING
ADENOCARCINOMA
OF TRANSVERSE COLON

SESSILE POLYPOID
ADENOCARCINOMA
OF RECTOSIGMOID
REGION

INFILTRATING
ADENOCARCINOMA
OF SIGMOID COLON

Malignant Tumors of Large Intestine

(*Continued from page 167*)

one finds histopathologically well-formed glands lined by large, columnar cells with darker-than-normal cytoplasm and vesicular, hyperchromatic nuclei showing mitoses here and there. In poorly differentiated tumors the glandlike structures are much less in evidence; the cells vary in size and display mitoses relatively frequently. The scirrhous type of carcinoma infiltrates the bowel wall rather than projecting into the lumen. It tends to encircle the gut and give rise to stenosis. In this type of tumor, the fibrous elements predominate over the epithelial, producing an extremely hard, contracted mass. The carcinomas that have undergone mucoid degeneration display a gelatinous appearance, because of their rich content in mucinous material. A rare variety of tumor is the papillary adenocarcinoma, which presents, on its surface, villous processes and resembles the papilloma. Infection superimposed on a tumor may cause a suppurative process which may eventually spread and lead to formation of fistulous tracts, perforation and peritonitis.

Malignant tumors of the large intestine present no pathognomonic symptoms. The difficulty of an accurate diagnosis is, in many cases, enhanced by the fact that the large bowel is frequently the site of other pathologic processes which resemble carcinoma in their main clinical manifestations. Moreover, the clinical features of carcinoma are often found to vary widely in different cases, the symptomatology depending largely on the location and size of the tumor and the presence of complications such

as ulceration, infection and obstruction. Abdominal pain, diarrhea or constipation, or both, ease of fatigue, weight loss and blood in the stools are the most common symptoms. With a tumor on the right side the patients may, in addition to the mentioned symptoms, report localized pain, nausea, inappetence and occasional vomiting. Sometimes, the patient himself accidentally palpates a mass in the right iliac fossa. Weakness, loss of weight and severe anemia are, in many instances, the leading signs. Increasing constipation is conspicuous in patients with a tumor on the left side, although in such cases diarrhea too, usually mild, either persistent or alternating with constipation, is characteristic of the early stages, in which a tumor should be suspected when blood and mucus are found in the stool. Since the lumen of the colon on the left side is somewhat smaller than on the right, the intestinal content is more consistent and formed

and the tumors belong more frequently to the scirrhous type, signs of intestinal obstruction (see page 191) become manifest with a left-sided cancer far more frequently and earlier than with a tumor on the right. Obstruction, of course, when present, dominates the clinical picture and dictates the management of the case.

When the tumor is located in the rectum, the prominent signs are discharge of blood mixed with mucus, tenesmus and frequent desire to defecate. Bleeding and persistent anal pain are the most important symptoms of malignant lesions of the anal canal.

For the diagnosis of malignant growth of the large bowel, the most important methods are digital examination, proctosigmoidoscopy and X-ray studies with barium enema. Almost every case of rectal cancer can be easily detected by a careful, methodical palpation

(*Continued on page 169*)

ADENOCARCINOMA
COMPLETELY ENCIRCLING
LOWER RECTUM
(SIGMOIDOSCOPIC VIEW)

ULCERATED
CRATERIFORM
ADENOCARCINOMA
OF UPPER RECTUM

MELANOMA

EPITHELIOMA
OF ANAL CANAL

MALIGNANT TUMORS OF LARGE INTESTINE

(*Continued from page 168*)

of the entire rectal wall, from low down to as far up as possible. With a digital examination one feels the tumor as a bulky, indurated mass of irregular surface or as an ulcerated area, with a hard, raised, irregular border. Blood of a bright- or dark-red color on the examiner's finger, sometimes mixed with mucus, and with a peculiar sickly, offensive smell, reinforces the suspicion of the presence of a carcinoma.

The rectum and terminal sigmoid should be visualized directly by the procto- or sigmoidoscope (see page 109) in every suspicious case preceding radiologic examination. Such examination will reveal the characteristics of the growth, its size, its mobility and the degree of obstruction of the bowel, if any is present. When the tumor is situated above the reach of the sigmoidoscope tube, one can suspect the presence of the growth by finding blood in the upper part of the rectum or in the sigmoid. Biopsy should be taken in every case to determine the histopathologic type and grade of the lesion. Sometimes, the histopathologic study of what seems to be a malignant tumor may reveal an amebic or other granulomatous inflammatory lesion.

Roentgen examination should be done by means of barium enema and double contrast studies. Oral administration of barium is of little use for morphologic studies of the large bowel, because of the irregular distribution of the contrast medium throughout the intestinal lumen; furthermore, barium given by the oral route is a menace in the presence of constrictive lesions. After a barium enema the X-ray picture will reveal an annular narrowing, with regular contours at the level of scirrhous carcinoma or an irregular mucosal pattern, with a filling defect in the presence of a proliferative, polypoid variety of growth.

Epitheliomas of the anal canal are tumors that originated in the cutaneous coat and are nearly always of the squamous cell variety; only seldom is a basal cell type encountered. They appear as a piled-up nodule or as an ulcerated lesion with a soft or firm base and irregular, undermined edges. The growth may be very small, resembling a fissure, or it may show a greater extension and, eventually, involve the entire circumference of the anus.

Malignant melanoma is a rare and highly malignant growth of the anorectal region. It usually arises from the anal verge or canal, but in some cases it seems to originate from the rectum itself. It is considered a variety of sarcoma, containing special tumor cells, the melanoblasts, which show variable amounts of iron-free pigment, the melanin. Malignant melanoma is a dark, sessile or pedunculated tumor, resembling a thrombosed hemorrhoid. It grows rapidly and metastasizes widely. It presents no specific symptoms. Blood in the stools, frequent desire to defecate, tenesmus and pain are the usual complaints.

Other malignant tumors that may occur in the large bowel, though very rarely, include carcinoid, leiomyosarcoma, fibrosarcoma, angiosarcoma and lymphoblastomas.

Metastases of cancer of the large bowel occur in three ways: (1) by direct extension to contiguous structures, (2) via the lymphatics to regional and distant lymph nodes and (3) through hematogenous dissemination to distant organs. The most common sites of metastases are the regional lymph nodes, the liver and the lungs.

169

PROCTOLOGIC CONDITIONS I

Hemorrhoids

Hemorrhoids are varicose dilatations of the radicles of the hemorrhoidal (rectal) veins (see page 73), in either the superior or the inferior plexuses, or both, accompanied in varying degrees by hypertrophy and round cell infiltration of the perivascular connective tissue. Hemorrhoids are present in about 35 per cent of the population. They usually occur between the ages of 25 and 55, and only seldom under the age of 15. Both sexes are affected equally.

To explain the formation of hemorrhoids, a great variety of factors have been considered. A hereditary predisposition seems to play a rôle in some individuals. Man's erect posture, the absence of valves in the portal venous system, the arrangement of the collecting veins in the rectal submucosal space (see pages 58 and 59), the veins being liable to compression in passing through the anorectal musculature and other biologic and anatomic conditions are contributory elements. More direct causes are all the various events that produce transient or constant increased pressure or stasis within the rectal venous plexuses, such as straining at stools because of constipation or diarrhea, tumors or strictures of the rectum, pregnancy, tumors and retroversion of the uterus, hypertrophy and tumors of the prostate, and portal hypertension.

In line with the anatomic situation (see pages 60 and 73), the external and internal hemorrhoids must be differentiated. Varicosities of the inferior hemorrhoidal plexus present the *external hemorrhoids,* situated below the pectinate line and covered by the modified skin of the anus. Thrombotic external hemorrhoids are an acute variety of external hemorrhoids, resulting from the formation of a thrombus within a vein or, more frequently, from the rupture of a vein with extravasation of blood into the cellular tissue, constituting, strictly speaking, a hematoma. The *thrombotic variety* occurs usually as the result of strain. The patient complains of a sudden painful lump at the anus, and inspection reveals a rounded, bluish, tender swelling. Thrombosed external hemorrhoids finally result in the so-called *"skin tabs",* consisting of one or more folds of the anal skin and composed of connective tissue and a few blood vessels. Skin tabs may form also by imperfect healing of the skin after hemorrhoidectomy or as a consequence of an inflammatory process in the anal region.

Internal hemorrhoids are the varicose

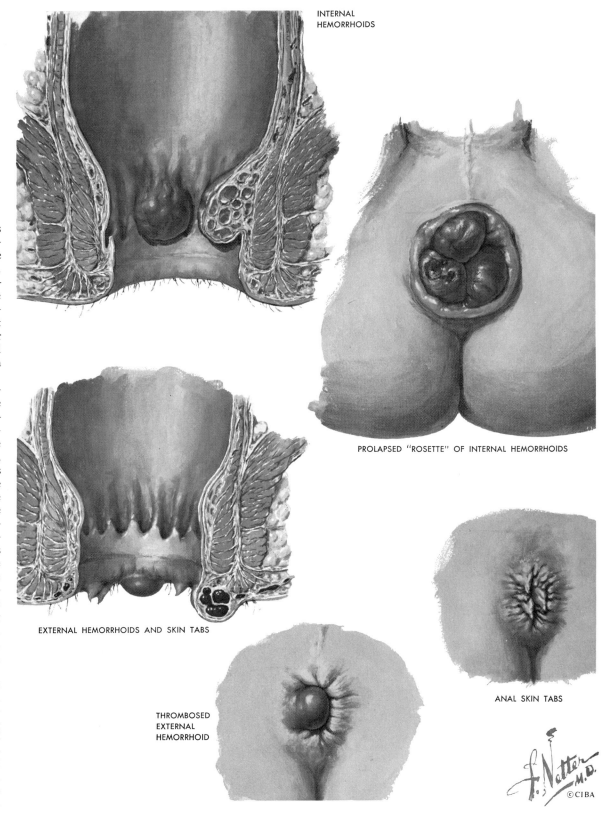

INTERNAL HEMORRHOIDS

PROLAPSED "ROSETTE" OF INTERNAL HEMORRHOIDS

EXTERNAL HEMORRHOIDS AND SKIN TABS

THROMBOSED EXTERNAL HEMORRHOID

ANAL SKIN TABS

enlargement of the veins of the superior hemorrhoidal plexus. In their early stage (first degree), they do not protrude through the anal canal and can be detected only by proctoscopy, where they appear as globular, reddish swellings. The superior rectal veins being fairly constantly distributed, internal hemorrhoids are usually located in the right and left posterior and right anterior quadrants. Histologically, the walls of the dilated veins are atrophic and surrounded by a perivascular inflammatory infiltrate. In a later stage internal hemorrhoids may protrude through the anal canal. Initially, the protrusion may occur only at defecation, receding afterward spontaneously (second degree); in time, the protrusion becomes more pronounced, occurring on any extra exertion and receding only by manual reduction (third degree). Finally, the *hemorrhoids* may become permanently *prolapsed,* in which instance the mucosal surface of

the hemorrhoids is constantly subjected to trauma and may become ulcerated. Increased mucoid discharge may also cause irritation of the peri-anal skin, producing burning and itching.

The earliest symptom of internal hemorrhoids is usually intermittent bleeding, occurring during or following defecation. Pain is not a characteristic symptom, being present only in cases with complications (thrombosis, strangulation) or other concomitant conditions (fissure, abscess).

The so-called "strangulated hemorrhoids" constitute the most common and also the most painful complication of internal hemorrhoids. This complication occurs when the prolapsed hemorrhoids cannot be reduced because of sphincteric contractions and because of the blockage of the thrombosed internal varices by the simultaneously or subsequently thrombosed inferior hemorrhoidal veins.

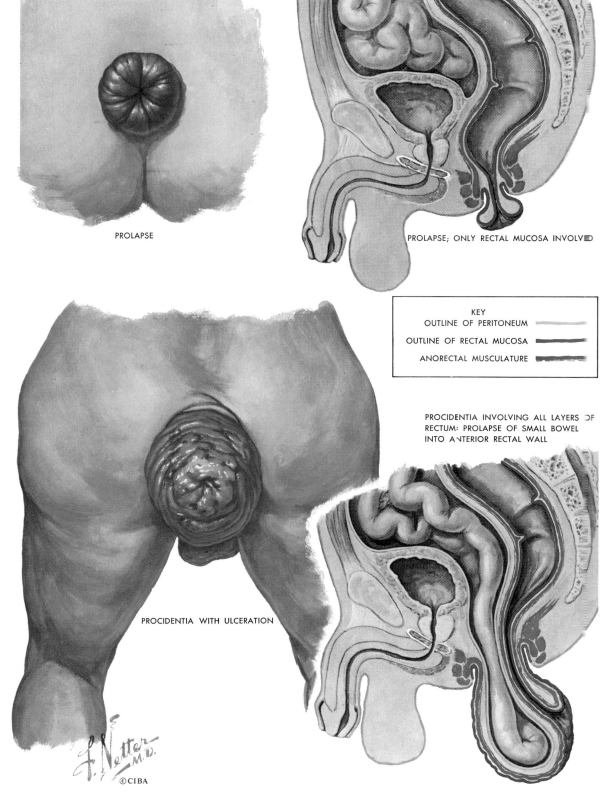

PROLAPSE

PROLAPSE; ONLY RECTAL MUCOSA INVOLVED

KEY
OUTLINE OF PERITONEUM
OUTLINE OF RECTAL MUCOSA
ANORECTAL MUSCULATURE

PROCIDENTIA INVOLVING ALL LAYERS OF
RECTUM: PROLAPSE OF SMALL BOWEL
INTO ANTERIOR RECTAL WALL

PROCIDENTIA WITH ULCERATION

Proctologic Conditions II

Prolapse and Procidentia

Prolapse of the rectum, as ordinarily understood, is a condition in which one or more layers of the rectum or/and the anal canal are protruded through the anal orifice. A prolapse can be partial or complete. In partial prolapse (usually called simply *prolapse*), only the mucosa is involved; it extends usually not more than ½ to 1 in. In total prolapse (called *procidentia*), all the layers of the rectum are involved; it presents a larger, bulbous mass, which may eventually contain a hernial sac of peritoneum with a segment of bowel in its interior.

In procidentia, in addition to the descent of the rectal tissues, an eversion of the lining of the anal canal takes place, so that the covering of the displaced tissues becomes continuous at approximately a right angle with the peri-anal skin. When only the rectal tissues descend, while the anal structures remain in their normal position, a sulcus will surround the protruded rectum.

Some authors speak of sigmoidorectal intussusception (concealed or protruded) as a procidentia, but this is a different entity. The confusion arises when the intussusception protrudes through the anal orifice. However, digital examination will easily differentiate this condition from rectal procidentia. In the former the finger will pass into the rectal ampulla. In the latter the finger will meet a blind end in the anal canal, or the displaced tissue is continuous with the peri-anal skin.

The etiology of prolapse and procidentia is unknown. A defect in one or more of the supporting structures of the anorectum seems to be the chief predisposing factor; it is not likely that an increased abdominal pressure, in the absence of alterations in the supporting structures of the anorectum, will result in prolapse or procidentia.

Prolapse occurs most frequently in childhood and in old age. In children the majority of cases are between 1 and 4 years of age, and a shallow sacral curve and reduction of the supporting fat, as may occur in wasting diseases, are the

chief predisposing causes. In old or debilitated subjects, the prolapse is usually due to the loss of sphincter tonus. It is obvious that some lesions within the bowel that drag down the mucous membrane, such as polyps, hemorrhoids and tumors, and anatomic or neurologic disturbances of the sphincters may favor the occurrence of prolapse.

Procidentia may occur at any age, but it is uncommon in children. It is now commonly accepted that the disorder is, in reality, a sliding hernia of the pouch of Douglas through a weakened or damaged pelvic fascia and levator muscles, the occurrence of which is possibly favored by an abnormally mobile rectum. Recently, attention has been called to the importance of some neurologic and rectal sensory factors related to the defecation mechanism (Todd). Faulty sensorial rectal appreciation, either as a result of poor interpretation of the normal stimulus (see page 87)

or as a result of a rectal-wall abnormality with an associated hypo-excitability, leads to a lack of coordination between the appreciation of the full-rectum stimulus and straining.

The most common complaint in patients with prolapse or procidentia is the protrusion of a mass from the anus, during defecation or walking, that will become more and more difficult to reduce. Other symptoms are a sensation of fullness, incontinence, diarrhea and bleeding.

The examination is best carried out with the patient in a standing or squatting position; he should be asked to strain so that the full extent of the protrusion can be observed. In prolapse the inspection reveals a relatively small mass with *radially* arranged folds. In procidentia the protruded mass is bulky, showing a congested, eventually *ulcerated* mucosa with folds arranged in a *concentric* pattern.

PROCTOSCOPIC VIEW OF
VARIOUS STAGES
IN HYPERTROPHY
OF ANAL PAPILLAE:
HOOK RETRACTING
ANAL VALVE TO
EXPOSE CRYPTITIS

FIBROUS
POLYP
(MARKEDLY
ENLARGED,
FIBROTIC
PAPILLA)

PROCTOLOGIC CONDITIONS III

Papillitis, Cryptitis, Adenomatous Polyps, Villous Tumor, Fissure and Pruritus Ani

Inflammatory processes of the papillae, which usually start in one of the crypts, give rise to extreme pain (and tenesmus) out of all proportion to the size and severity of the lesion. In *acute papillitis* the structure is *swollen, edematous* and *congested,* becoming later, in the chronic stage of the papillitis, *fibrosed* and *hypertrophied.* Gradually, the hypertrophic papilla may develop a stalk and may change into a so-called *fibrous polyp,* which may produce the sensation of a foreign body in the anal canal, a dissatisfied feeling after defecation, itching and objective signs of irritation.

The crypts of Morgagni (see pages 58 and 59), in which fecal material can collect and which are continuously exposed to traumatism, become easily involved in infectious inflammatory processes. The *cryptitis* may remain restricted to circumscribed reactions in and around the crypts or may spread to the surrounding tissues, inducing the formation of abscesses and fistulae (see next page). The symptoms of cryptitis — sometimes resembling those of a fissure ("phantom fissure") — are anal formication, itching and radiating pain, which are aggravated by defecation and ambulation. Anoscopy, under anesthesia, permits recognition of the affected crypt, a purulent discharge or granulation tissue, and enlargement of the related papilla.

Benign tumors of epithelial origin occur in the rectum in two varieties, the simple adenomatous polyp and the villous tumor (also termed papilloma, papillary tumor, papillary adenoma, papillary polyp, villous polyp and villoma). The usually lobulated *adenomatous polyps* may be sessile or pedunculated; they may vary in size from a few millimeters up to about 2 cm. in diameter, only rarely becoming larger. The less common *villous tumor* is mostly attached to the mucosa by means of numerous papillary stalks and is soft and velvety to the touch. Both of these benign epithelial tumors tend to undergo malignant degeneration and may manifest themselves by bleeding, mucous discharge, diarrhea, tenesmus and protrusion through the anal canal.

An *anal fissure* is a crack or splitlike

ADENOMATOUS
PEDUNCULATED,
LOBULATED POLYP
AND SESSILE POLYP

VILLOUS TUMOR

VILLOUS TUMOR

ADENOMATOUS POLYP

ANAL FISSURE WITH SENTINEL PILE

PERI-ANAL IRRITATION DUE TO PRURITUS ANI

ulcer of the anal canal lining below the pectinate line, extending often as far as the anal verge. It starts rather suddenly, and the lesion is usually associated with severe pain. If untreated, it tends to run a course of exacerbations and remissions. Fissures occur at all ages, particularly in middle life, and somewhat more frequently in women. When single, it is most commonly located at the posterior commissure. Multiple fissures, also more frequent in women, involve usually the anterior and posterior commissures and only rarely the lateral margins. Mechanical traumatic factors (overdistention of the anal canal at defecation) and anal infection are the most frequent pathogenic causes. The typical anal fissure is racket-shaped and has sharply defined edges; at the lower, wider, rounded end, the skin forms frequently an edematous tab (*sentinel pile*); the upper end, quite close to the anal valves, is often guarded by one or two hypertrophied

papillae. Pain related to defecation is the main symptom; occurring during passage of the stools or shortly thereafter, it may be extremely severe and may persist for some time. The diagnosis can be made by simple inspection of the anus.

Pruritus ani is a symptom which may accompany every known anorectal disease, as well as other organic or systemic affections. Not seldom, however, no evident primary cause is found. Peri-anal itching without any apparent cause — by some authors believed to be a neurodermatitis, by others simply designated as "cryptogenetic" — is usually more intense at night in bed and during warm weather. The peri-anal skin is hyperemic and will show superficial abrasions from scratching. In more chronic cases a whitish discoloration of the skin, accentuation of the folds, rhagades, lichenification, hyperkeratosis and patchy parakeratosis are characteristic.

PROCTOLOGIC CONDITIONS IV

Anorectal Abscess and Fistula

A localized infection with collection of pus in the anorectal area is designated as *"anorectal abscess"*. It results from the invasion of, usually, the normal rectal flora (Bacillus coli, B. proteus, B. subtilis, staphylococci and streptococci) into the perirectal or peri-anal tissues. The pathologic process seems to start, as a rule, with an inflammation of one or more crypts (cryptitis, see page 172). From the crypt (portal of entry) the infection may spread to the anal ducts and anal glands (see page 59) and from there submucously, subcutaneously or transsphincterally to the surrounding tissue. This sequence of events closes with a spontaneous rupture of the abscess, either into the anorectal canal or through the peri-anal skin, if the abscess has not been drained surgically. Once the abscess has perforated, the cavity, as well as its outlet, shrinks, leaving a tubelike structure, an *"anorectal fistula"*, which invariably is the result of an abscess.

The levator ani plane, demarcating the various perineopelvic spaces (see pages 31 to 33), is also used to classify the anorectal abscesses according to their localization. To the *supralevator abscesses* belong the *retrorectal, pelvirectal* and *submucous abscesses,* located in and affecting tissues that have a visceral rather than a somatic sensory nerve supply, causing a sensation of discomfort and pressure, rather than pain, in the anorectal region. They can be felt by digital examination or observed through the proctoscope as swellings encroaching the rectal lumen. In contrast to the infralevator abscesses, they may produce signs of toxemia and extreme prostration. The retrorectal and, more so, the pelvirectal abscesses, in most instances, originate from infectious processes in other pelvic organs and are thus not anorectal lesions in the strict sense, though they usually rupture into the rectum or anal canal, or sometimes through the levator ani.

The infralevator abscesses are divided, according to their site, into *subcutaneous, intermuscular, ischiorectal* and *cutaneous abscesses,* though the last mentioned is such a superficial lesion that it amounts to no more than a *furuncle.* The infralevator abscesses are clinically easily recognized. Pain is, in all instances, the prevailing symptom.

The course of a fistula, which will

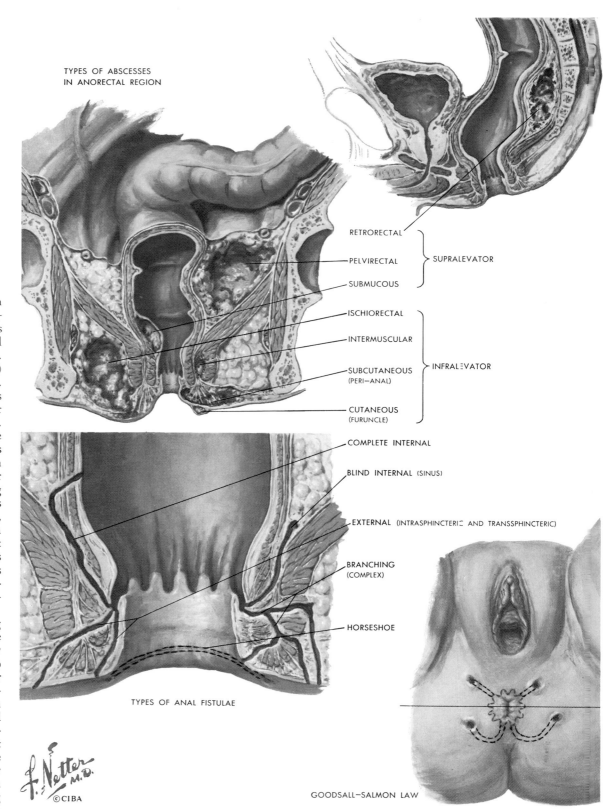

TYPES OF ABSCESSES IN ANORECTAL REGION

RETRORECTAL
PELVIRECTAL — SUPRALEVATOR
SUBMUCOUS

ISCHIORECTAL
INTERMUSCULAR
SUBCUTANEOUS (PERI–ANAL) — INFRALEVATOR
CUTANEOUS (FURUNCLE)

COMPLETE INTERNAL
BLIND INTERNAL (SINUS)
EXTERNAL (INTRASPHINCTERIC AND TRANSSPHINCTERIC)
BRANCHING (COMPLEX)
HORSESHOE

TYPES OF ANAL FISTULAE

GOODSALL—SALMON LAW

eventually remain as the end phase of the abscess formation, evacuation and healing, will essentially depend on the original localization and point of drainage of the abscess. A *fistula* is called *"complete"* when both openings, the primary (cryptic) and the secondary, can be detected and are accessible. Such a complete variety usually connects the rectal lumen with the anal or peri-anal skin. If only one opening, either the primary or, as is more often the case, the secondary, can be determined, one deals with a *"blind"* fistula, also designated as a *"sinus"*, which may discharge either into the lumen of the bowel or through the peri-anal skin; accordingly, it is named an internal or external sinus, respectively. The former comes into existence when the abscess has drained spontaneously through the crypt from which the infectious process started. The external sinuses are, in principle, always complete fistulae, in spite of the fact that the primary

(cryptic) opening cannot be demonstrated. Applying *Goodsall-Salmon's law*, one may obtain a rough idea of the course of the fistulous tract and the probable location of its primary opening. Drawing an imaginary transverse line across the center of the anus, one may expect a curved tract and the primary opening posterior to the midline when the secondary opening is situated posteriorly to this line, whereas a straight tract and an anteriorly located primary opening may be expected when the secondary opening is anterior to this proposed line.

A branched fistulous tract with several openings, so-called *"complex"* fistula, may be encountered. A *"transsphincteric"* fistula passes through the musculature, and an *"intrasphincteric"* fistula runs submucously or subcutaneously, leaving the sphincter intact. A curved tract partially encircling the anus is known as a *"horseshoe"* fistula.

PROCTOLOGIC CONDITIONS V

Lymphogranuloma Venereum and Syphilis

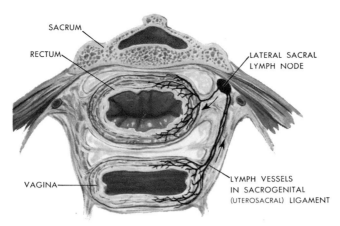

PATHWAY OF SPREAD OF LYMPHOGRANULOMA (LYMPHOPATHIA) VENEREUM FROM UPPER VAGINA AND/OR CERVIX UTERI TO RECTUM VIA LYMPH VESSELS

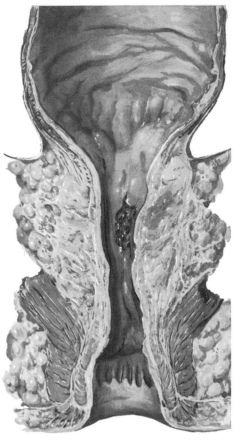

LONG TUBULAR STRICTURE OF RECTUM

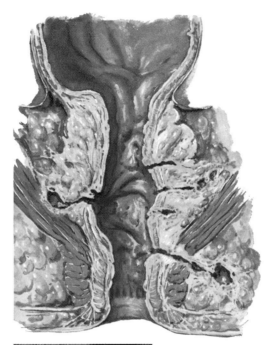

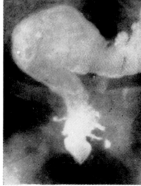

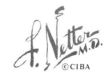

STRICTURE OF RECTUM WITH MULTIPLE BLIND SINUSES

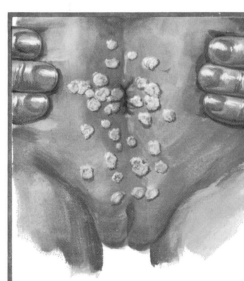

CONDYLOMATA LATA (2° SYPHILIS)

Lymphogranuloma venereum (venereal lymphogranuloma, lymphogranuloma inguinale [not to be confused with granuloma inguinale], climatic or tropical bubo, lymphogranulomatosis inguinalis, Durand-Nicolas-Favre disease, lymphopathia venereum, etc.) is an infectious disease caused by a filtrable virus, producing lesions in the genital tract, inguinal region and/or anorectocolonic tube (see CIBA COLLECTION, Vol. 2, page 133). In the male it is characterized by suppurative inguinal adenitis (see CIBA COLLECTION, Vol. 2, page 39), occasionally by rectal stricture and uncommonly by elephantiasis of the penis and scrotum. In the female it is characterized by rectal stricture, abscess, fistulae, anovulval esthiomene (elephantiasis), less frequently by suppurative inguinal adenitis. The primary lesion, usually unnoted by the infected person, appears on the glans penis or prepuce in the male and on the fourchette, posterior vaginal wall or posterior lip of the cervix in the female.

Inguinal adenitis (bubo) marks the second stage in men, because the lymphatic drainage of the external genitalia, the common site of the initial lesion, is by way of the inguinal nodes. In women, the second stage manifestations are more apt to be *rectal stricture* and abscesses and fistulae, because the site of the primary lesion is commonly vaginal or cervical, and invasion of the perirectum and rectal wall is much easier. The predilection for rectal stricture in women is not the result of any difference in the genitoanorectal lymphatics in the two sexes, for, in this respect, no difference exists (see CIBA COLLECTION, Vol. 2, pages 17 and 102). Rectal strictures in the male are less frequently encountered and are probably the consequence of primary infection of the rectum in sexually perverted individuals.

The essential pathologic changes in the rectum are those of an ulcerative *inflammatory process with an extensive production of contracting connective tissue* in the mucosa and deeper tunics of the bowel. When the entire intestinal wall and the perirectal tissues become involved, the affected segment is transformed into a *firm, fixed, narrowed canal*. Multiple *blind sinuses* and not-infrequent perirectal abscesses may form, which can perforate into the vagina, bladder or perianal skin. Occasionally, other segments of the large intestine (particularly left-sided colon) may also be involved by the disease. In the acute prestricture stage, the signs and symptoms are those of an intensive purulent proctitis. Digital examination may disclose only a rough anorectal lining and slight fixation. Endoscopy shows almost complete destruction of the mucous membrane with abundant bloody, purulent discharge. The ulcerated surface bleeds easily. In the fully developed stricture stage, the signs and symptoms are typical, and a digital exploration will reveal a definite narrowing in nearly every instance. Proctoscopic study in this phase is possible only with a stricturoscope.

The definite diagnosis of lymphogranuloma venereum is established by the intradermal Frei's test, complement fixation test and biopsy. X-ray studies are helpful in determining the extension of the process.

Syphilitic affection of the anorectum occurs in the form of early or late lesions. In adults, chancre (primary lesion) is usually located at the posterior commissure, very rarely at a higher level within the anal canal or rectum, and has a peculiar indurated base. The diagnosis can be readily established by dark-field examination of the secretion, which will reveal the presence of Treponema pallidum. The manifestations of secondary syphilis occur usually in the form of peri-anal *condylomata lata* (flat warts), which have a flat surface rather than the pedicle and cauliflower lobulations of the condylomata acuminata. Treponema pallidum may be demonstrated in the former. Serologic tests are generally positive at this stage of the disease.

In late syphilis, ulcerated gummas may occur in the anus and rectum; this condition, however, has become extremely rare in recent years. In infants, multiple superficial fissures may indicate congenital syphilis.

Parasitic Diseases I

Trichuriasis

Trichuriasis is parasitism produced by the worm Trichuris trichiura (Trichocephalus trichiurus, Trichocephalus dispar, human whipworm). This worm is cosmopolitan in distribution but is more common in warm, moist regions. Man seems to be the only host, although whipworms obtained from pigs and monkeys are morphologically similar. The *male worm* measures 30 to 45 mm. in length and the *female* 35 to 50 mm. In both sexes the pinkish body of the parasite shows two portions: the cephalic, which is longer and attenuated (whiplike), containing the esophagus, and the caudal, which is shorter and thicker, containing the intestine and sex organs. The posterior end of the male is coiled, while that of the female is comma-shaped.

The *adult parasites, male and female,* live *in the cecum* and in the appendix; only rarely do they infest other parts of the colon and, very rarely, the small intestine. After fertilization the female lays *eggs,* which are expelled in the feces. The number of eggs produced by a female has been estimated at from one to several thousand per day. The eggs are barrel-shaped and measure approximately 50 microns in length and 23 microns in breadth. They have a double shell, which is perforated at the poles; the polar orifices are closed by prominent, colorless, refractive albuminous plugs (see page 184). At oviposition, the fertilized ova show unsegmented granular contents. Embryonic development takes place outside the host, in the soil. Under favorable conditions of temperature and moisture, the ova reach the motile embryo stage in about 3 to 4 weeks; under unfavorable conditions, especially at low temperature, the embryonation takes from several months to 1 year. The ova are not very resistant to dessication, cold or heat, and are killed in a short time at 54° C. and −12° C.; they also do not survive direct sun's rays. Human beings become infested on *swallowing fully embryonated eggs* obtained directly or indirectly from the soil. Food (especially uncooked vegetables), water and hands may become contaminated directly by infested soil or indirectly by domestic animals, flies and other insects. The ingested embryonated egg reaches the intestine and becomes softened; the *embryo escapes* by forcing

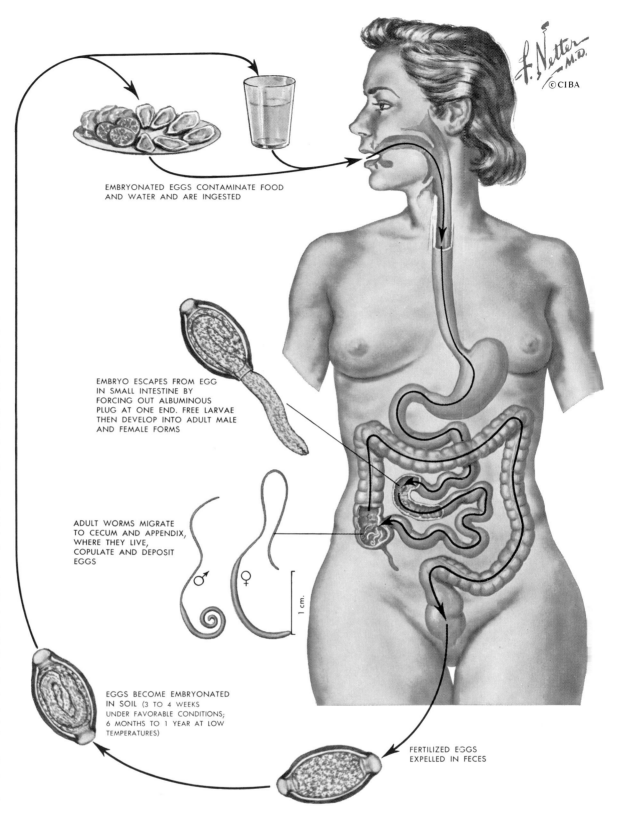

EMBRYONATED EGGS CONTAMINATE FOOD AND WATER AND ARE INGESTED

EMBRYO ESCAPES FROM EGG IN SMALL INTESTINE BY FORCING OUT ALBUMINOUS PLUG AT ONE END. FREE LARVAE THEN DEVELOP INTO ADULT MALE AND FEMALE FORMS

ADULT WORMS MIGRATE TO CECUM AND APPENDIX, WHERE THEY LIVE, COPULATE AND DEPOSIT EGGS

EGGS BECOME EMBRYONATED IN SOIL (3 TO 4 WEEKS UNDER FAVORABLE CONDITIONS; 6 MONTHS TO 1 YEAR AT LOW TEMPERATURES)

FERTILIZED EGGS EXPELLED IN FECES

one of the two albuminous plugs at the poles. The free larval worms develop into mature adult worms; after copulation the female lays eggs, and a new cycle begins. The adult worm is attached to the intestinal wall with the thin anterior portion embedded in the mucosa. In most cases the infestation is not very intense, the number of parasites being usually not greater than ten. Occasionally, however, a thousand or more worms may be harbored in the intestine.

The pathologic effects of a whipworm infection are usually mild, if at all existent; they are chiefly due to traumatism of the intestinal mucosa and to toxic substances produced by the parasites, if they are present in large numbers. Although the anterior portion of the worm is buried in the intestinal mucosa, using its secretions' lytic effects upon the neighboring cells, the damage is slight. At the site of the worm's penetration into the mucosa, however, a secondary

invasion by intestinal bacteria may occur and may give rise to inflammatory reactions. It is believed that in this way the whipworms may induce an acute appendicitis. Toxic substances released by the parasite may occasionally produce allergic reactions. Some parasitologists believe also that Trichuris trichiura may suck blood and, in cases of intense infestation, be responsible for manifestations of anemia.

The clinical signs of trichuriasis vary with the intensity of infestation, extent of intestinal penetration and secondary bacterial infection. In most instances no noticeable or only vague digestive disturbances occur. Pronounced symptoms are associated with massive infestation or bacterial invasion; they include diarrhea, dysenteric syndrome, constipation, abdominal pains, abdominal distention, weakness, emaciation and anemia. The diagnosis is made by recovery of the characteristic eggs in the patient's stools.

PARASITIC DISEASES II

Ascariasis

Ascaris lumbricoides (the large intestinal roundworm) is the causal agent of one of the most common and cosmopolitan helminthic diseases. The white or pinkish *adult worms* are elongated nematodes, tapering anteriorly and posteriorly to conical ends. Their smooth cuticle is finely striated, and two faint whitish streaks run along either side of the entire body length. The adult male (15 to 25 cm. by 2 to 4 mm.) is smaller than the female and is characterized by a ventrad curvature of its posterior extremity. The adult female measures 20 to 35 cm. in length and 4 to 6 mm. in breadth. Specimens of both sexes, however, sometimes may reach a considerably larger size. The adult worms live, as a rule, in the lumen of the small bowel, obtaining their nourishment from the semidigested food of the host. A mature female worm produces about 200,000 eggs a day. The *fertilized ova,* measuring from 45 to 70 microns in length and 35 to 50 microns in breadth, contain a mass of coarse lecithin granules. They have an outer coarsely mammillated, albuminous covering and a thick, hyaline shell, composed of several layers. The *unfertilized ova* are longer and narrower, usually have a thinner shell and an irregular albuminous coating and contain refractive granules of various sizes. In both fertilized and unfertilized eggs the albuminous covering is easily broken or may be absent. The ova are expelled with the feces and must undergo a process of maturation before becoming infective. Under favorable conditions (moist, shady soil and a temperature of about 25° C.) infective larvae develop in the fertilized eggs in about 2 to 3 weeks. If the conditions are unfavorable, the ova may remain dormant for several years and embryonate with the return of a favorable environment.

Human infestation occurs by swallowing mature ova, which are conveyed to the mouth by contaminated fingers, water, green vegetables or other food, and possibly by inhalation. In the small intestine the larvae are liberated, penetrate the intestinal wall and pass into the portal circulation; via the liver and heart they reach the lungs, penetrate the capillaries and enter the alveoli. From there they are carried up the bronchi and trachea to the glottis, are swallowed and pass down to the small intestine, where they develop into adult male or female worms.

In the lungs the larvae give rise to petechial hemorrhages. Clinically, symp-

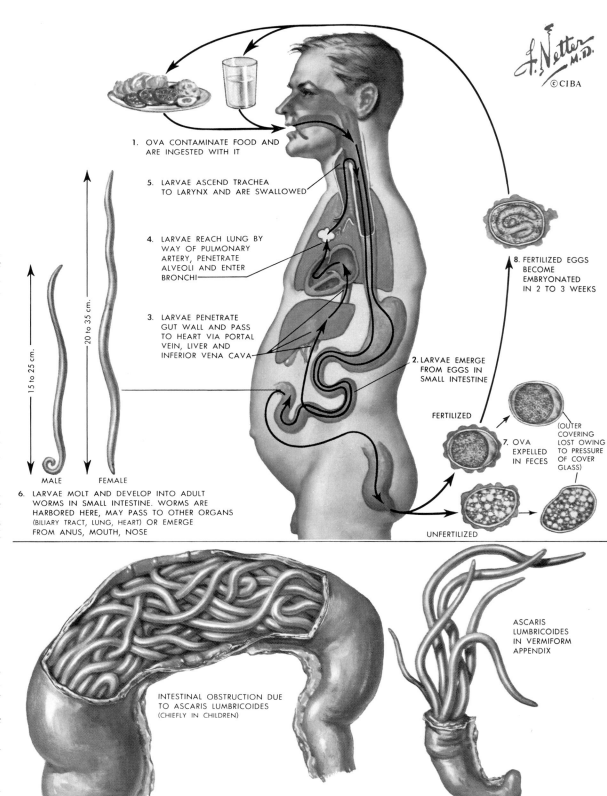

1. OVA CONTAMINATE FOOD AND ARE INGESTED WITH IT

5. LARVAE ASCEND TRACHEA TO LARYNX AND ARE SWALLOWED

4. LARVAE REACH LUNG BY WAY OF PULMONARY ARTERY, PENETRATE ALVEOLI AND ENTER BRONCHI

3. LARVAE PENETRATE GUT WALL AND PASS TO HEART VIA PORTAL VEIN, LIVER AND INFERIOR VENA CAVA

2. LARVAE EMERGE FROM EGGS IN SMALL INTESTINE

8. FERTILIZED EGGS BECOME EMBRYONATED IN 2 TO 3 WEEKS

FERTILIZED

7. OVA EXPELLED IN FECES

(OUTER COVERING LOST OWING TO PRESSURE OF COVER GLASS)

UNFERTILIZED

15 to 25 cm.

20 to 35 cm.

MALE FEMALE

6. LARVAE MOLT AND DEVELOP INTO ADULT WORMS IN SMALL INTESTINE. WORMS ARE HARBORED HERE, MAY PASS TO OTHER ORGANS (BILIARY TRACT, LUNG, HEART) OR EMERGE FROM ANUS, MOUTH, NOSE

INTESTINAL OBSTRUCTION DUE TO ASCARIS LUMBRICOIDES (CHIEFLY IN CHILDREN)

ASCARIS LUMBRICOIDES IN VERMIFORM APPENDIX

toms of a pulmonary affection may become manifest, and a marked eosinophilia will appear in the blood. An extensive alveolar exudation of red blood cells, neutrophils, eosinophils and fibrin may evolve, resulting in a lobular pneumonia; eventually, an entire lobe may become consolidated (ascaris pneumonitis). Sensitive individuals react to the larvae with an allergic edema and eosinophilic infiltration of the lungs (Löffler's syndrome). Larvae, entering the circulation, may be deposited in various organs (kidney, brain, eyeballs, etc.), where they die, leaving behind some inflammatory tissue alterations.

Infestation with a few adult worms in the intestinal lumen is usually asymptomatic. Heavier infestations may cause local disturbances, such as a mechanical hindrance or generalized toxic and allergic effects, owing to absorption of the worms' metabolic products. In most cases the symptoms consist of abdominal dis-

comfort, pain, loss of appetite, nausea, diarrhea or constipation. Occasionally, masses of ascarides may obstruct the intestinal lumen, especially in children. Having migratory tendencies, the adult worms may wander up or down the intestinal tract and be passed per anus or emerge from mouth or nose or, sometimes, may penetrate into the appendix, bile ducts, gallbladder, pancreatic duct, peritoneal cavity (especially after gastro-intestinal surgery), pharynx or middle ear, giving rise to serious complications. Invasions of the lungs, genito-urinary tract and even of the heart are on record.

The diagnosis is usually made by recovery of the characteristic eggs in the feces (see page 184) but must rest tentatively on clinical manifestations if male worms are present. Following an opaque meal the X-ray examination may reveal the worms as characteristic filling defects.

Parasitic Diseases III

Enterobiasis

Enterobius vermicularis, known also as Oxyuris vermicularis, human pinworm or seatworm, belongs to the phylum of nematodes and common parasites of man in all parts of the world. The small, spindle-shaped, round adult worms inhabit the cecum, appendix and adjacent portions of the large and small intestine, with their heads attached to the intestinal mucosa. The *male worm* measures 2 to 5 mm. in length and 0.1 to 0.2 mm. at its greatest diameter, and has a sharply curved posterior end. The *female worm*, 9 to 11 mm. in length and 0.3 to 0.5 mm. at its greatest diameter, has a pointed tail. The female produces eggs in its ovary and releases them into a reservoir, the "uterus", where fecundation takes place. When the reservoir is filled, the worm detaches itself from the bowel wall, migrates down the colon to the rectum, and from there through the anal canal to peri-anal and perineal regions. Some of the parasites are expelled from the host's rectum passively with the feces. Migration beyond the anal sphincter occurs at night; the female worm, while crawling on the skin, deposits eggs in the peri-anal and genitocrural folds. The average number of eggs deposited by a single female has been found to be about 11,000. At the time of laying, the eggs are already embryonated, containing tadpolelike embryos, which, within a few hours, develop into the infective vermiform stage. The embryonated eggs measure 50 to 60 by 20 to 30 microns and are flattened on one side. They have a translucent shell that consists of an outer, albuminous covering and an inner, embryonic, lipoidal membrane. The eggs require no intermediate host for their subsequent development; they become infective within a few hours after being laid and may remain viable for weeks or months. From the peri-anal region the ova are transferred to clothes and bed linen; the hands of the patient, particularly the fingernails, may become contaminated through scratching the peri-anal regions or handling clothing. The ova may be transferred to the same or another host either by hand to mouth or indirectly through food and drink. The eggs from bed linens and clothes may also be blown into the air and get indirectly into the mouth or be inhaled and swallowed. Female parasites that are expelled in the feces empty their "uteri" outside the host; part of the discharged ova become infective and may be ingested with contaminated foods or water. When

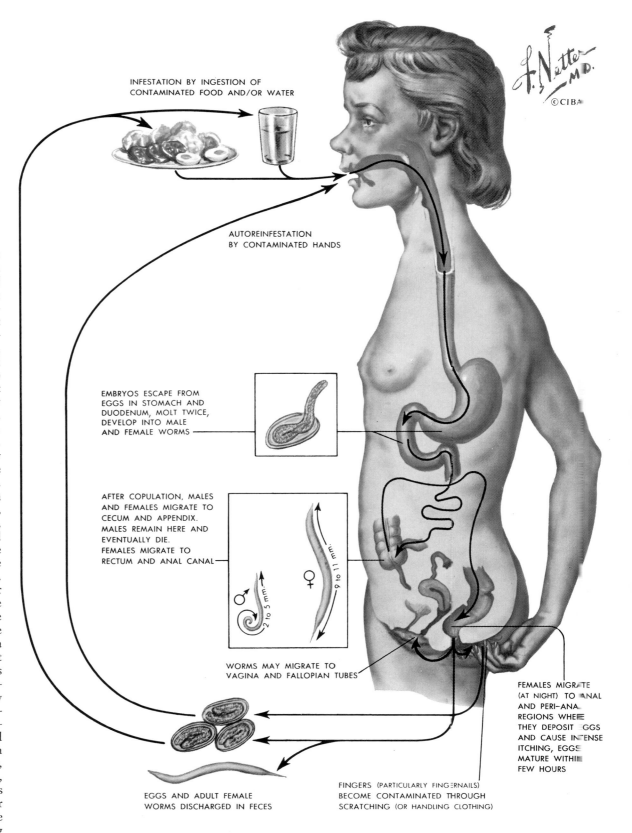

INFESTATION BY INGESTION OF CONTAMINATED FOOD AND/OR WATER

AUTOREINFESTATION BY CONTAMINATED HANDS

EMBRYOS ESCAPE FROM EGGS IN STOMACH AND DUODENUM, MOLT TWICE, DEVELOP INTO MALE AND FEMALE WORMS

AFTER COPULATION, MALES AND FEMALES MIGRATE TO CECUM AND APPENDIX. MALES REMAIN HERE AND EVENTUALLY DIE. FEMALES MIGRATE TO RECTUM AND ANAL CANAL

WORMS MAY MIGRATE TO VAGINA AND FALLOPIAN TUBES

FEMALES MIGRATE (AT NIGHT) TO ANAL AND PERI-ANAL REGIONS WHERE THEY DEPOSIT EGGS AND CAUSE INTENSE ITCHING, EGGS MATURE WITHIN FEW HOURS

EGGS AND ADULT FEMALE WORMS DISCHARGED IN FECES

FINGERS (PARTICULARLY FINGERNAILS) BECOME CONTAMINATED THROUGH SCRATCHING (OR HANDLING CLOTHING)

eggs, containing infective larvae, reach the stomach and duodenum, the digestive secretions soften the eggs' walls and the larvae are set free. These larvae pass down the small bowel, molt twice and develop into mature male and female worms. After copulation the female becomes "gravid", and a new cycle begins. The duration of the cycle from the ingestion of the ovum to the development of a mature worm is variously given as from 2 to 7 weeks.

Enterobius vermicularis is a relatively innocuous parasite that only seldom produces serious lesions. A mild catarrhal inflammation of the intestinal mucosa may result from the attachment of the worms and mechanical irritation. In sensitive individuals their by-products, when absorbed, may produce allergic reactions. A heavy infestation and secondary bacterial invasion may, occasionally, lead to inflammation of the deeper layers of the intestine and, eventually, be

responsible for the occurrence of an acute appendicitis. In female patients the parasites may enter the vagina, producing vulvitis and vaginitis with violent pruritus and leukorrhea. A few cases are on record where the female parasites *migrated to the Fallopian tubes* and became encysted there, or wandered out into the peritoneal cavity and became encysted on the peritoneum. Infection of the bladder is extremely rare. The most common and most disturbing symptom of enterobiasis is pruritus ani, which can vary in degree from mild to extreme. Scratching of the irritated region may lead to excoriation, eczema and pyogenic infection. The infested individuals, particularly children, may lose appetite, suffer from insomnia and become restless, irritable and emotionally unstable. The diagnosis of enterobiasis is made by discovery of the worms or the characteristic eggs in peri-anal scrapings or swabs, or in feces (see page 184).

PARASITIC DISEASES IV

Strongyloidiasis

Strongyloides stercoralis (Anguillula stercoralis or Anguillula intestinalis, threadworm), the causative agent of human strongyloidiasis, is a cosmopolitan nematode parasite but is encountered mostly in the tropics and subtropics. The adult parasitic female, a delicate, filiform worm measuring about 2.2 mm. in length and 30 to 75 microns in diameter, lives within the mucosa of the small intestine, laying several dozens of embryonated eggs a day, from which *rhabditiform larvae* hatch. These are expelled in the feces. Under favorable conditions (as in warm climates) the rhabditiform larvae may develop in the soil into free-living, sexually mature and sexually active *rhabditiform males and females* (measuring about 0.7 and 1 mm. in length, respectively). The fertilized, free-living female discharges eggs, from which a *second generation of rhabditiform larvae* hatch, which then may develop into infestive *filariform larvae* (indirect, or long, sexual life cycle). However, favorable conditions persisting, the second rhabditiform larvae may develop again into free-living adults, from which another generation of rhabditiform larvae evolve. When conditions in the external environment are not favorable, the rhabditiform larvae, expelled with the feces and deposited on soil, metamorphose within a short time directly into *infestive filariform larvae* (direct, or asexual, life cycle). When in contact with human skin, the infestive filariform larvae penetrate the cutaneous blood vessels and are carried into the *capillaries of the lungs,* where they break through the alveoli, *ascend the respiratory tree* to the pharynx, are swallowed and reach the intestine. During this migration the filariform larvae change into the adolescent stage and may copulate (heterogonic development). *In the duodenum and jejunum,* occasionally also in the ileum, appendix and colon, the mature parasitic females *burrow into the mucosa* and start *oviposition.* The males, not being tissue parasites, after a brief stay in the intestine, are voided in the feces. The females that were not inseminated during the migration seem to be able to produce their progeny parthenogenetically (hologonic development). The heterogonic development and the existence of a parasitic male (Kreis, Faust) are, in the view of many parasitologists, still considered an unsettled matter. At times, the life cycle of S. stercoralis may occur in an abbreviated direct form, known as auto-infection or hyperinfection, in which the rhabditi-

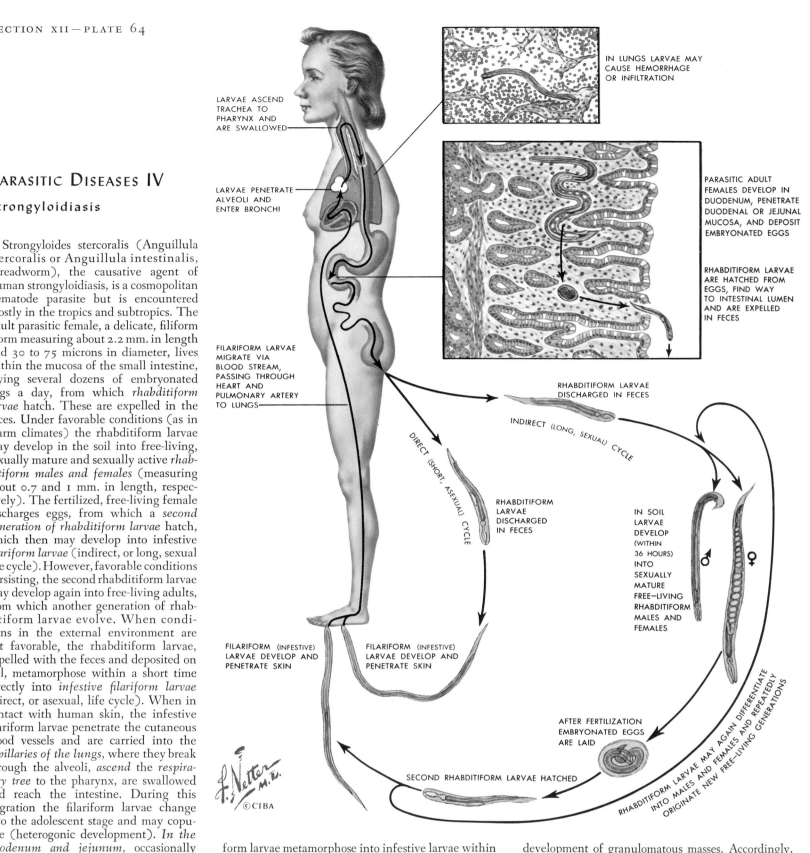

IN LUNGS LARVAE MAY CAUSE HEMORRHAGE OR INFILTRATION

LARVAE ASCEND TRACHEA TO PHARYNX AND ARE SWALLOWED

LARVAE PENETRATE ALVEOLI AND ENTER BRONCHI

PARASITIC ADULT FEMALES DEVELOP IN DUODENUM, PENETRATE DUODENAL OR JEJUNAL MUCOSA, AND DEPOSIT EMBRYONATED EGGS

RHABDITIFORM LARVAE ARE HATCHED FROM EGGS, FIND WAY TO INTESTINAL LUMEN AND ARE EXPELLED IN FECES

FILARIFORM LARVAE MIGRATE VIA BLOOD STREAM, PASSING THROUGH HEART AND PULMONARY ARTERY TO LUNGS

RHABDITIFORM LARVAE DISCHARGED IN FECES

INDIRECT (LONG, SEXUAL) CYCLE

DIRECT (SHORT, ASEXUAL) CYCLE

RHABDITIFORM LARVAE DISCHARGED IN FECES

IN SOIL LARVAE DEVELOP (WITHIN 36 HOURS) INTO SEXUALLY MATURE FREE-LIVING RHABDITIFORM MALES AND FEMALES

FILARIFORM (INFESTIVE) LARVAE DEVELOP AND PENETRATE SKIN

FILARIFORM (INFESTIVE) LARVAE DEVELOP AND PENETRATE SKIN

AFTER FERTILIZATION EMBRYONATED EGGS ARE LAID

RHABDITIFORM LARVAE MAY AGAIN DIFFERENTIATE INTO MALES AND FEMALES AND REPEATEDLY ORIGINATE NEW FREE-LIVING GENERATIONS

SECOND RHABDITIFORM LARVAE HATCHED

form larvae metamorphose into infestive larvae within the intestinal canal or on the peri-anal skin, and reinfestation of the individual takes place without these organisms leaving the host's body.

Penetration of the larvae into the skin is usually asymptomatic, but in hypersensitive individuals it may cause a pruriginous eruption. The migration of the larvae through the lungs may give rise to inflammatory reaction in the air sacs and in the bronchial epithelium. Occasionally, bronchial congestion may prevent the escape of larvae from the lungs, so that some of them may develop at this site into adult worms, causing more pulmonary damage and, eventually, invading the pleural and pericardial cavities. Depending upon the degree of infestation, the reaction of the intestinal mucosa varies from a light inflammatory cellular infiltration to patchy necrosis, with sloughing, followed by fibroblastic repair or the

development of granulomatous masses. Accordingly, the clinical manifestations vary also from an asymptomatic course to pronounced dysenteric disturbances, with alternate diarrhea and constipation prevailing in moderate infestations. The general condition of the patient is usually not greatly affected; the blood picture reveals no or only a slight anemia and eosinophilia. Chronic, recurrent and severe infestations, however, may lead to progressive emaciation and, eventually, may culminate in death (Kyle *et al.*). Erratic migration of larvae, especially in conjunction with auto-infection, may occur, and they may be found in the myocardium, liver, gallbladder, brain, urogenital organs and other foci, producing tissue damage and corresponding symptoms. The diagnosis of strongyloidiasis rests upon recognition of the characteristic rhabditiform larvae in the feces or duodenal content (see page 184).

PARASITIC DISEASES V

Necatoriasis and Ancylostomiasis

Necator americanus (Uncinaria americana, American hookworm) and *Ancylostoma duodenale* (Uncinaria duodenalis, "Old World" hookworm) are nematodes that produce the human hookworm disease (necatoriasis and ancylostomiasis, respectively). These helminths are widely diffused throughout the tropical and subtropical zones; in temperate climates they are found only in places (mines, tunnels) where suitable conditions of warmth and moisture exist. N. americanus is the species which predominates in the Western Hemisphere, in Central and South Africa, southern Asia, in the East Indies, Polynesia, Micronesia and Australia, whereas A. duodenale is the predominant species in coastal North Africa, the Mediterranean, southern Europe, northern India, northern China and Japan. N. americanus is a cylindrical, fusiform worm, grayish-yellow or reddish in color, the *adult male* measuring 7 to 9 mm. in length by 0.3 mm. in breadth and the *female,* 9 to 11 mm. in length by 0.4 mm. in breadth. The posterior end of the male is extended into a bell-shaped bursa, whereas that of the female is cone-shaped. The position assumed by N. americanus is very characteristic: the body describes an arc, with the ventral surface on the inner side, while the anterior extremity curves sharply backward over the body. The chief morphologic characteristics by which N. americanus and A. duodenale can be differentiated concern the *mouth parts* and *copulatory bursae.* The buccal capsule of N. americanus is provided on the upper (ventral) side with two semilunar cutting plates, whereas that of A. duodenale shows at this place two pairs of teeth. Copulatory bursae of the two species present morphologic differences in regard to muscular digitations (the function of which is to hold the female during copulation) and copulatory spicules.

The life cycles of N. americanus and A. duodenale are essentially the same. The adult worms live in the small intestine, where they attach themselves to the mucosa by their buccal capsules and feed on the blood and lymph of their host. The *fertilized* female lays *eggs,* the average daily output of which has been estimated at about 10,000 for N. americanus and twice as many for A. duodenale. The eggs, ovoid in shape, measuring 60 to 70 microns in length and having a thin shell, are usually passed in the feces in the 2- to 8-cell stage of segmentation.

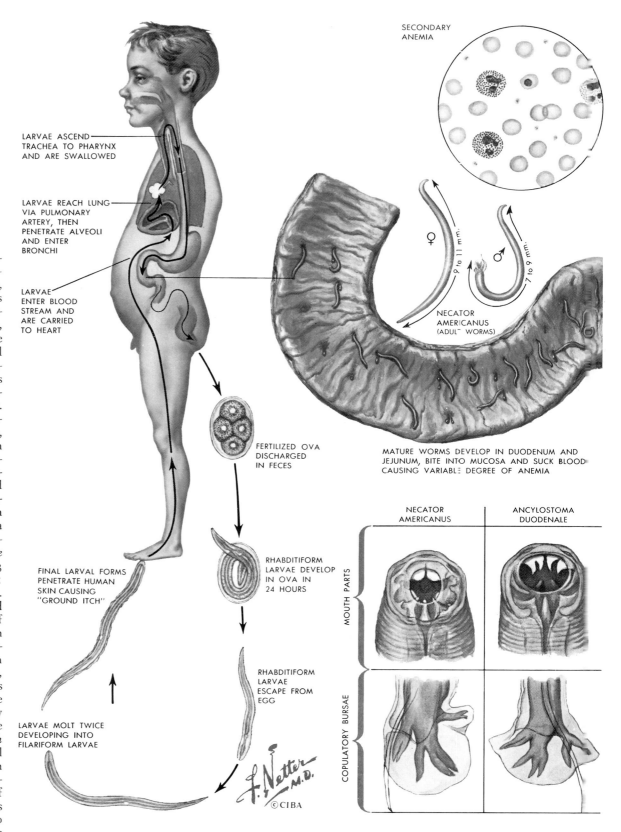

SECONDARY ANEMIA

LARVAE ASCEND TRACHEA TO PHARYNX AND ARE SWALLOWED

LARVAE REACH LUNG VIA PULMONARY ARTERY, THEN PENETRATE ALVEOLI AND ENTER BRONCHI

LARVAE ENTER BLOOD STREAM AND ARE CARRIED TO HEART

FINAL LARVAL FORMS PENETRATE HUMAN SKIN CAUSING "GROUND ITCH"

LARVAE MOLT TWICE DEVELOPING INTO FILARIFORM LARVAE

FERTILIZED OVA DISCHARGED IN FECES

RHABDITIFORM LARVAE DEVELOP IN OVA IN 24 HOURS

RHABDITIFORM LARVAE ESCAPE FROM EGG

♀ 9 to 11 mm.   ♂ 7 to 9 mm.

NECATOR AMERICANUS (ADULT WORMS)

MATURE WORMS DEVELOP IN DUODENUM AND JEJUNUM, BITE INTO MUCOSA AND SUCK BLOOD CAUSING VARIABLE DEGREE OF ANEMIA

	NECATOR AMERICANUS	ANCYLOSTOMA DUODENALE
MOUTH PARTS		
COPULATORY BURSAE		

Under favorable conditions of aerated soil, moderate moisture and an optimal temperature, *rhabditiform larvae* hatch from the eggs within 24 hours. For about 3 to 5 days they grow while feeding on fecal material, molt twice and develop into infective *filariform larvae.* When human *skin* comes in contact with infested soil, the filariform larvae penetrate it, enter the lymphatics or venules and are carried in the blood through the heart to the lungs, where they pass from the capillaries into the alveoli, ascend the respiratory tree, pass to the pharynx, are swallowed and reach the duodenum and jejunum, where they grow up into male and female worms.

The clinical manifestations caused by N. americanus and A. duodenale are also similar. Penetration of the larvae into the skin may occasionally give rise to a local pruriginous dermatitis (*"ground itch"*), with edema, erythema and papular or vesicular erup-

tion. The blood-lung migration of the larvae causes minute hemorrhages and cellular infiltration in the alveolar tissues, which, however, remain of subclinical grade unless large numbers of larvae are migrating simultaneously. In the intestinal phase, the adult worms may eventually provoke hyperperistalsis with cramps and diarrhea. By sucking blood and by producing *small erosions in the mucosa,* the parasites may be responsible for development of secondary (hypochromic and *microcytic*) anemia. A severe anemia is, however, likely to occur only in cases of heavy infestation and when the food intake is deficient in iron and protein. At times, a single massive infestation may induce acute symptoms that include headache, nausea, prostration, pulmonary and circulatory disturbances, severe abdominal pain and dysentery. The diagnosis of hookworm disease is made by recovery of characteristic eggs in the feces (see page 184).

PARASITIC DISEASES VI

Taeniasis Saginata

Taeniasis saginata is a parasitosis produced by Taenia saginata (beef tapeworm), a cestode of the phylum Platyhelminthes. The definitive host of this cosmopolitan parasite is man, who harbors the adult worm, while the intermediate host is the bovine, which harbors the larval form called *Cysticercus bovis*. The adult worm measures from 4 to 10 m. in length, but it may be even longer. It inhabits the small intestine, attached to the mucosa by means of the *scolex*. Usually, only one parasite is harbored by the host, but on rare occasions two or even more may be present. The small, elongate and quadrangular scolex, measuring 1 to 2 mm. in diameter and having four hemispherical suckers, is connected by a short and narrow neck to a great number of *proglottids*. In the short and wide (called "immature") proglottids that lie behind the neck, the genital organs are not yet developed. Gradually, the proglottids increase in breadth and width until they reach a maximum diameter of about 12 mm.; at this stage they are mature, containing functioning male and female organs. In mature proglottids, ovules are produced and fertilized hermaphroditically. Still more distally the proglottids become elongated and slightly narrowed; they contain a uterus that has a large number of branched lateral arms and is crowded with eggs. Gravid proglottids become detached successively from the parent worm, pass through the colon into the sigmoid and rectum and are either expelled passively in the feces or emerge by means of their own motility through the anus. Outside the intestine, but eventually also inside, the gravid proglottids rupture and set free the *eggs*. They are of spherical shape, measure 30 to 40 microns in diameter and have a thick, radially striated shell that contains the embryo (oncosphere) which has three pairs of delicate, lancet-shaped hooklets. The eggs are originally enclosed in a thin, easily detachable hyaline membrane. When gravid proglottids or eggs, dropped on pasture or grazing land, are ingested by cattle, the hexacanth embryos hatch in their intestines, bore into the venules and lymphatics and are

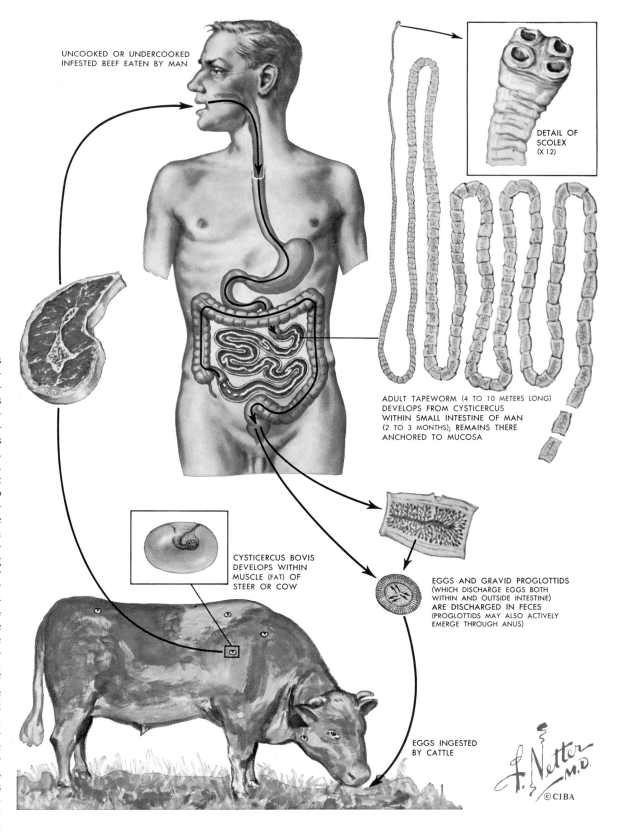

UNCOOKED OR UNDERCOOKED INFESTED BEEF EATEN BY MAN

DETAIL OF SCOLEX (X 12)

ADULT TAPEWORM (4 TO 10 METERS LONG) DEVELOPS FROM CYSTICERCUS WITHIN SMALL INTESTINE OF MAN (2 TO 3 MONTHS); REMAINS THERE ANCHORED TO MUCOSA

CYSTICERCUS BOVIS DEVELOPS WITHIN MUSCLE (FAT) OF STEER OR COW

EGGS AND GRAVID PROGLOTTIDS (WHICH DISCHARGE EGGS BOTH WITHIN AND OUTSIDE INTESTINE) ARE DISCHARGED IN FECES (PROGLOTTIDS MAY ALSO ACTIVELY EMERGE THROUGH ANUS)

EGGS INGESTED BY CATTLE

carried to the skeletal muscles, heart, tongue, diaphragm, adipose tissues and other regions, where they develop in 2 to 2½ months into the cysticercus stage. *Cysticercus bovis* (bladder worm) measures about 5 to 10 mm. and has a miniature head like that of the adult worm, invaginated into the fluid-filled vesicle. The larvae remain viable in cattle for about a year, after which they become calcified. When uncooked or undercooked infested beef is eaten by man, the membranes of cysticerci are digested. The embryos evaginate their heads, attach themselves to the mucosa of the small intestine and grow into adult worms in about 2 to 3 months.

The infestation with T. saginata is frequently symptomless, the patients complaining only about the inconvenience resulting from gravid proglottids crawling out of the anus. Some patients, however, experience vague abdominal discomfort, exaggerated appetite or, the contrary, loss of appetite, nausea, indigestion, diarrhea or constipation, pruritus ani and nervous disturbances, including headache, dizziness, irritability and change of character. Proglottids lodged in the lumen of the appendix may sometimes produce symptoms of appendicitis. Occasionally, the diarrhea becomes severe and prolonged, and may even endanger the life of the patient. A rare but serious complication may evolve when a mass of tangled proglottids causes intestinal obstruction. The diagnosis of taeniasis saginata is made by recognition of gravid proglottids in the feces. Examined under low-power magnification, they can be differentiated from those of T. solium (see page 181) by the number of main lateral arms of the uterus (15 to 20 on each side). Less frequently, the diagnosis is made by recovery of eggs in the feces; they are, however, morphologically indistinguishable from those of T. solium.

Parasitic Diseases VII

Taeniasis Solium
(Cysticercosis Cellulosae)

Taenia solium (pork tapeworm) is a cestode parasite occurring in countries where raw or inadequately processed pork is consumed. The adult worm, living in the small intestine of man, usually attains a length of 2 to 3 m., rarely more. The globular *scolex,* measuring about 1 mm. in diameter, is provided with four cup-shaped suckers and a rostellum carrying a double row of 22 to 32 large and small hooklets, arranged alternately. As in T. saginata (see page 180), a long chain of immature, mature and terminal *gravid proglottids* follow the scolex. Man infested with T. solium *expels* gravid segments, singly or in short chains, in the *feces;* unlike those of T. saginata, they are flabby and inactive. The *ova,* consisting of a hexacanth embryo surrounded by a spherical, radially striated shell, 30 to 40 microns in diameter, are liberated by the rupture of the proglottids before or after leaving the host. When the eggs are *ingested by hogs,* the hexacanth embryos hatch in the intestine, bore into blood or lymph vessels and are carried to different parts of the body. They *settle* most commonly in the skeletal *muscles,* tongue and heart, where they develop in about 2 to 3 months into cysticerci (bladder worms). *Cysticercus cellulosae,* as this larval form is called, measures about 5 by 10 mm. and consists of an ellipsoidal, fluid-filled vesicle and an invaginated scolex bearing four suckers and an apical crown of hooklets. When uncooked or undercooked pork containing viable cysticerci is eaten by human beings, the cysticerci are digested, and the heads evaginate from the vesicle, attach themselves to the mucosa of the small intestine and grow, in about 2 to 3 months, into adult worms. The adult T. solium in the small intestine produces the same clinical manifestations as T. saginata (see page 180). Because of the shorter length of the chain of proglottids, however, it is less likely that intestinal obstruction will occur. The diagnosis of taeniasis solium is made by the discovery of gravid proglottids in the feces; they can be readily differentiated from those of T. saginata, because the uterus they contain has only 5 to 10 main lateral arms on each side of the longitudinal stem.

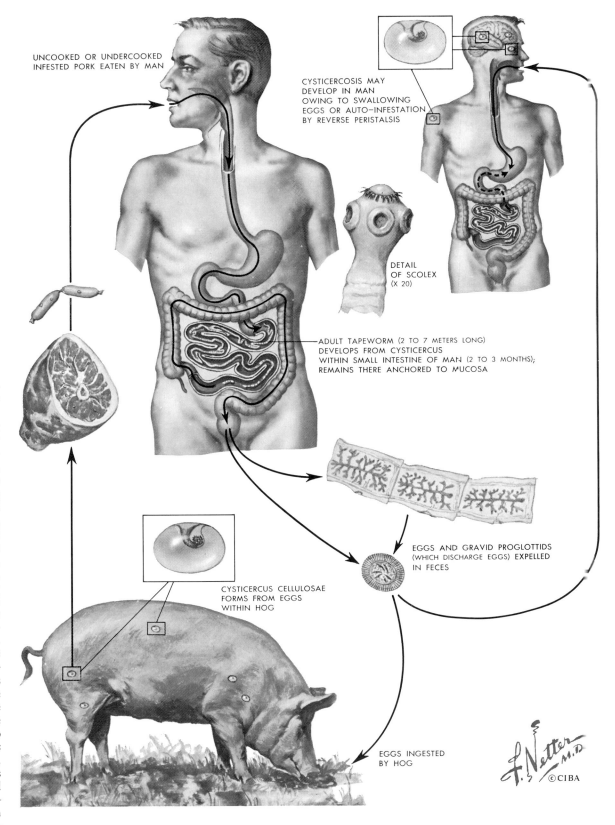

UNCOOKED OR UNDERCOOKED INFESTED PORK EATEN BY MAN

CYSTICERCOSIS MAY DEVELOP IN MAN OWING TO SWALLOWING EGGS OR AUTO-INFESTATION BY REVERSE PERISTALSIS

DETAIL OF SCOLEX (X 20)

ADULT TAPEWORM (2 TO 7 METERS LONG) DEVELOPS FROM CYSTICERCUS WITHIN SMALL INTESTINE OF MAN (2 TO 3 MONTHS); REMAINS THERE ANCHORED TO MUCOSA

EGGS AND GRAVID PROGLOTTIDS (WHICH DISCHARGE EGGS) EXPELLED IN FECES

CYSTICERCUS CELLULOSAE FORMS FROM EGGS WITHIN HOG

EGGS INGESTED BY HOG

The eggs, morphologically indistinguishable from those of T. saginata, may also be found in the feces.

T. solium may give rise to another much more dangerous morbid condition, known as cysticercosis cellulosae, resulting from the development in man of larval forms of this parasite. Human cysticercosis, like that of the hog, results from ingestion of mature eggs. This may occur by swallowing eggs passed by another infested person, by the transmission of eggs from anus to mouth by the individual who is harboring T. solium, or by internal auto-infestation when the ova or gravid proglottids reach the stomach by reverse peristalsis. Cysticerci may develop in any tissue or organ of the body but do so most commonly in the subcutaneous tissues (where they can be palpated as smooth, firm nodules the size of a pea or larger), and in the brain, eyes and muscles. Around the larvae a cellular reaction takes place that leads to the forma-

tion of a fibrous capsule; later, the center of the lesion, including the larvae, may caseate or calcify. The symptomatology of cysticercosis varies according to the location and number of parasites. Most serious consequences result from involvement of the brain, particularly after the death of larvae. The symptoms, which may simulate those of brain tumor, meningitis, general paralysis and other nervous diseases, include severe headache, epileptiform seizures, motor and sensory disturbances, visual disturbances, deafness, aphasia and psychic changes. Though clinical signs may be indicative of cysticercosis, the definitive diagnosis is made by the excision and microscopic examination of a larva. Roentgenograms may be helpful in locating the lesions after calcification of the larvae has occurred. Intradermal and precipitin tests are group specific and, therefore, useful only in the absence of other cestode infestation.

PARASITIC DISEASES VIII

Hymenolepiasis Nana

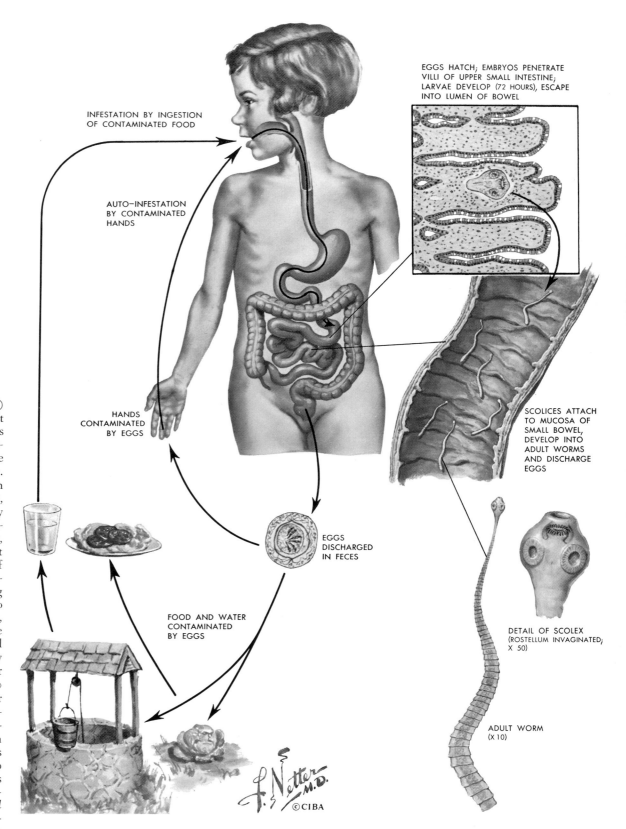

INFESTATION BY INGESTION OF CONTAMINATED FOOD

AUTO-INFESTATION BY CONTAMINATED HANDS

EGGS HATCH; EMBRYOS PENETRATE VILLI OF UPPER SMALL INTESTINE; LARVAE DEVELOP (72 HOURS), ESCAPE INTO LUMEN OF BOWEL

HANDS CONTAMINATED BY EGGS

SCOLICES ATTACH TO MUCOSA OF SMALL BOWEL, DEVELOP INTO ADULT WORMS AND DISCHARGE EGGS

EGGS DISCHARGED IN FECES

FOOD AND WATER CONTAMINATED BY EGGS

DETAIL OF SCOLEX (ROSTELLUM INVAGINATED; X 50)

ADULT WORM (X 10)

Hymenolepis nana (dwarf tapeworm) is the commonest tapeworm in man. It is cosmopolitan in its distribution but is encountered in warm climates more frequently than in cold ones. In man, the *adult worm,* measuring from 5 to 45 mm. in length and from 0.5 to 1 mm. in breadth, inhabits the small intestine, where it is attached to the mucosa by means of the scolex. The minute globular *scolex,* about 0.3 mm. in diameter, bears four cup-shaped suckers and a short rostellum, armed with a single ring of 20 to 30 hooklets, capable of invagination into the apex of the organ. A long and slender neck connects the scolex to a chain of about 200 or more immature, mature and gravid proglottids, which are more broad than long. The most distal gravid proglottids disintegrate gradually and set free the eggs. The spherical or subspherical, hyaline *eggs,* measuring 30 to 50 microns in diameter, have an outer and an inner envelope; the inner envelope (embryophore) has two polar thickenings, from each of which arise from four to eight thin, wavy, polar filaments that lie in the space between the two membranes. The embryophore encloses the embryo that has three pairs of lancet-shaped hooklets. These eggs are *passed in the feces* and are immediately infective for the same or another person; no intermediate host is required for the completion of the life cycle. Infestation of man occurs either by *ingestion of food or water* contaminated by eggs or by anus-to-mouth auto-infestation through contaminated hands. In the small intestine the embryo is liberated and *penetrates a villus,* where, in about 3 to 4 days, it develops into a cysticercoid larva. This larva then migrates into the intestinal lumen and becomes attached by its scolex to the mucosa farther down in the small intestine, where, in the course of 2 weeks or more, it grows into an adult worm. The infestation with H. nana may be intense; the presence of several hundred worms is not unusual; infestations with several thousand specimens are on

record. It has been suggested that heavy infestations may be due to internal auto-infestation; in such cases the ova would hatch within the intestine soon after being liberated, and larvae would penetrate the villi and develop into adult worms without reaching the outside.

The majority of persons infested with H. nana have no clinical manifestations. These occur usually only in the presence of a large number of parasites. Irritation of the intestinal mucosa may result in diarrhea and cramps. The absorption of the metabolic wastes of the worms, particularly in children, may give rise to headache, dizziness, insomnia and, rarely, to epileptiform seizures. A slight to intense eosinophilia may be present. The diagnosis of hymenolepiasis nana is made by the recovery of the characteristic eggs from the feces.

Certain rodents, especially rats and mice, are hosts

of a tapeworm that is morphologically identical with H. nana. It is believed that this tapeworm, called H. fraterna, and H. nana represent two biologically different strains of the same parasite, one of which is better adapted to life in the intestines of rodents, the other to life in the intestines of man. Cross infestation, however, seems to be possible. Cysticercoid larvae of H. nana and H. fraterna have been found also in certain species of fleas and beetles; this seems to indicate that the dwarf tapeworm may eventually have also an indirect life cycle, certain insects being the intermediate hosts. Hymenolepis diminuta, a common tapeworm of rats and mice (having various arthropods as intermediate hosts), may, occasionally, infest man also. The eggs of this parasite, passed in the feces, have a certain resemblance to those of H. nana; they can, however, be identified by their greater size and the absence of polar filaments (see page 184).

PARASITIC DISEASES IX

Diphyllobothriasis

Diphyllobothriasis is parasitism produced by the adult form of the cestode Diphyllobothrium latum (Bothriocephalus latus, fish or broad tapeworm). This parasite is found chiefly in the northern temperate regions where fresh-water fish constitute a major portion of the diet of the population. In Europe the most important foci are situated in the Baltic countries, in the region of the Alpine lakes of Switzerland, France, Italy and Germany, and in the delta of the Danube. In Asia this tapeworm is found throughout extensive areas in Siberia, northern Manchuria, Japan and in the vicinity of Lake Tiberias in Palestine. In North America several foci are known, particularly in the Great Lakes region. In South America a focus was discovered recently in Chile. D. latum inhabits the intestines of man, dogs, cats, bears, foxes, minks and other fish-eating mammals. The *adult worm* ranges in length from 2 to 10 m., but it may be even longer. The elongated, almond-shaped *scolex,* by means of which it is attached to the mucosa of the small intestine, measures from 2 to 3 mm. in length by 1 mm. in breadth and is provided with a dorsal and a ventral sucking groove (bothrium). An attenuated neck, several times the length of the scolex, is followed by a chain of more than 3,000 *proglottids.* The distal part of the strobila is formed by mature proglottids that contain minute spherical testes, a bilobate ovary, and a coiled rosettelike uterus provided with an opening (*laying orifice* or birth pore) in the midventral line just behind the *genital pore.* Through the laying orifice fertilized eggs are evacuated periodically; it is estimated that a single worm may discharge as many as one million eggs daily. The gravid proglottids normally do not separate from the parent worm; they are sloughed off only after completing their reproductive function. The ovoid *eggs,* their mean size being 70 by 45 microns, have a single shell with an inconspicuous operculum at one end; when expelled in the feces, they contain immature embryos. Reaching water, the eggs hatch at a favorable temperature in about 2 weeks. The embryo (called *coracidium*), surrounded by a ciliated embryophore, escapes through the opercular opening and swims

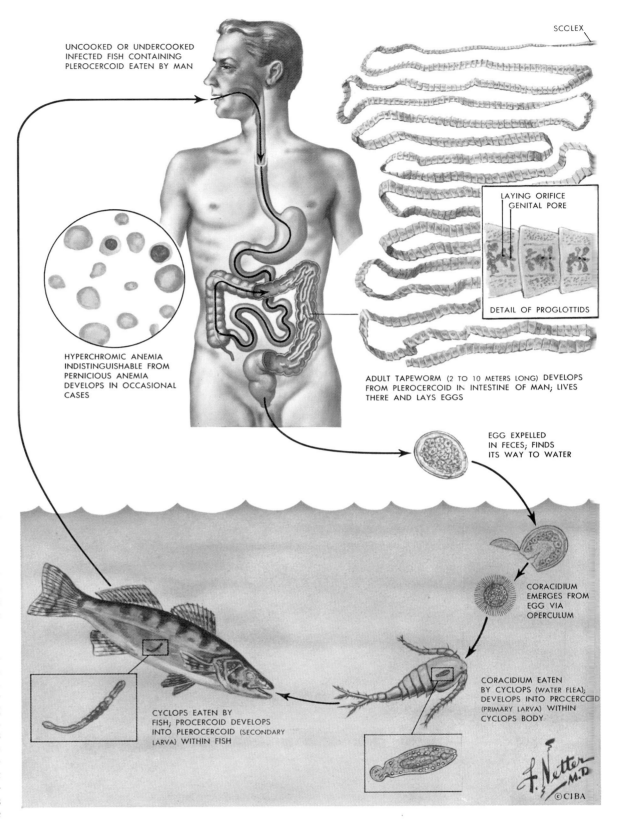

UNCOOKED OR UNDERCOOKED INFECTED FISH CONTAINING PLEROCERCOID EATEN BY MAN

SCCLEX

LAYING ORIFICE GENITAL PORE

DETAIL OF PROGLOTTIDS

HYPERCHROMIC ANEMIA INDISTINGUISHABLE FROM PERNICIOUS ANEMIA DEVELOPS IN OCCASIONAL CASES

ADULT TAPEWORM (2 TO 10 METERS LONG) DEVELOPS FROM PLEROCERCOID IN INTESTINE OF MAN; LIVES THERE AND LAYS EGGS

EGG EXPELLED IN FECES; FINDS ITS WAY TO WATER

CORACIDIUM EMERGES FROM EGG VIA OPERCULUM

CORACIDIUM EATEN BY CYCLOPS (WATER FLEA); DEVELOPS INTO PROCERCOID (PRIMARY LARVA) WITHIN CYCLOPS BODY

CYCLOPS EATEN BY FISH; PROCERCOID DEVELOPS INTO PLEROCERCOID (SECONDARY LARVA) WITHIN FISH

in the water. If it is to develop further, it must be swallowed by a suitable first intermediate host, usually a crustacean of the genus *Cyclops* or Diaptomus. In these crustaceans the coracidium metamorphoses within 2 to 3 weeks into a *procercoid* larva, which is a spindle-shaped organism (about 500 microns in size) having a cephalic invagination and a posterior spherical appendage provided with hooklets. When the infested crustacean is ingested by a suitable species of *fresh-water fish* (pike, eel, salmon, trout, perch, pickerel and many other food fish), the procercoid larva penetrates the viscera, muscles and connective tissues and develops within 1 to 4 weeks into an elongated, wormlike *plerocercoid* or sparganum larva, measuring from 10 to 20 mm. in length and from 2 to 3 mm. in breadth. When a raw or insufficiently cooked infested fish is eaten by man or another susceptible host, the plerocercoid larva attaches itself

to the mucosa of the small intestine and grows, in about 3 weeks, into an adult D. latum.

Many cases of diphyllobothriasis remain subclinical. Some, however, present a variety of clinical manifestations, including abdominal pain, diarrhea, loss of weight, asthenia, nervousness, anorexia or exaggerated appetite. The mass of tangled proglottids, especially when more than one parasite is harbored, may produce intestinal obstruction. Occasionally, D. latum infestation is associated with *macrocytic, hyperchromic anemia,* usually referred to as bothriocephalus anemia. The mechanism by which this pernicious-type anemia is produced is not yet fully understood; it is likely that, for its occurrence, other factors in addition to the presence of the tapeworm are required. The diagnosis of diphyllobothriasis is made by demonstration of the characteristic eggs in the feces (see page 184).

HELMINTHS AND PROTOZOA INFESTING THE HUMAN INTESTINE

Helminths discussed in the preceding pages are responsible for the overwhelming majority of all intestinal helminthic infestations in man. However, a few other worms may be encountered with lesser frequency. Several species of hermaphroditic intestinal flukes are found in human populations with special food habits. *Fasciolopsis buski,* a fleshy, elongated-ovoid trematode flatworm, living in the small intestine of the host, is a common parasite in the pig and in man in certain parts of eastern Asia. Its ovoid operculate eggs, about 135 microns long, are discharged in the feces and hatch in water. Miracidia that escape from them penetrate appropriate snails, pass through different evolutional stages and emerge again as cercariae, which then encyst on water caltrops (Trapa nataus, T. bispinosa, T. bicornis), water chestnut (Eleocharis tuberosa), lotus, water bamboo and other aquatic vegetation. Man acquires the parasite by eating the infested plants. In the small intestine, the flukes, attached to the mucosa, produce inflammatory reaction and ulcers, and give rise to dysentery; in heavy infestations the large number of parasites may produce intestinal obstruction, while absorption of their metabolic products may cause toxemic symptoms with edema and even ascites. *Echinostoma* ilocanum is found as a parasite in man in the Philippines, Java and Celebes. The adult fluke, measuring 2.5 to 6.5 mm., inhabits the small intestine of the dog, field rat and man. The eggs are discharged in the feces. The life cycle of this worm involves two different intermediate mollusc hosts; the man acquires the infestation by eating the second intermediate host raw or insufficiently cooked. This parasite apparently causes little or no intestinal damage. *Heterophyes heterophyes* is a parasite in man, the cat, dog, fox and probably other fish-eating mammals (chiefly in Egypt, Palestine and the Far East). This fluke (1 to 2 mm. long) lives in the small intestine of the definitive host. Eggs are passed in the feces; upon reaching water and being ingested by appropriate species of snails, they hatch; miracidia pass through various developmental stages and emerge again as cercariae that penetrate under the scales of various species of fresh-water fish, where they encyst. The definitive host becomes infested by the parasite by eating raw or insufficiently cooked infested fish. The adult flukes may produce a mild inflammatory reaction at the attachment sites; intestinal symptoms occur only in heavy infestations. Cases

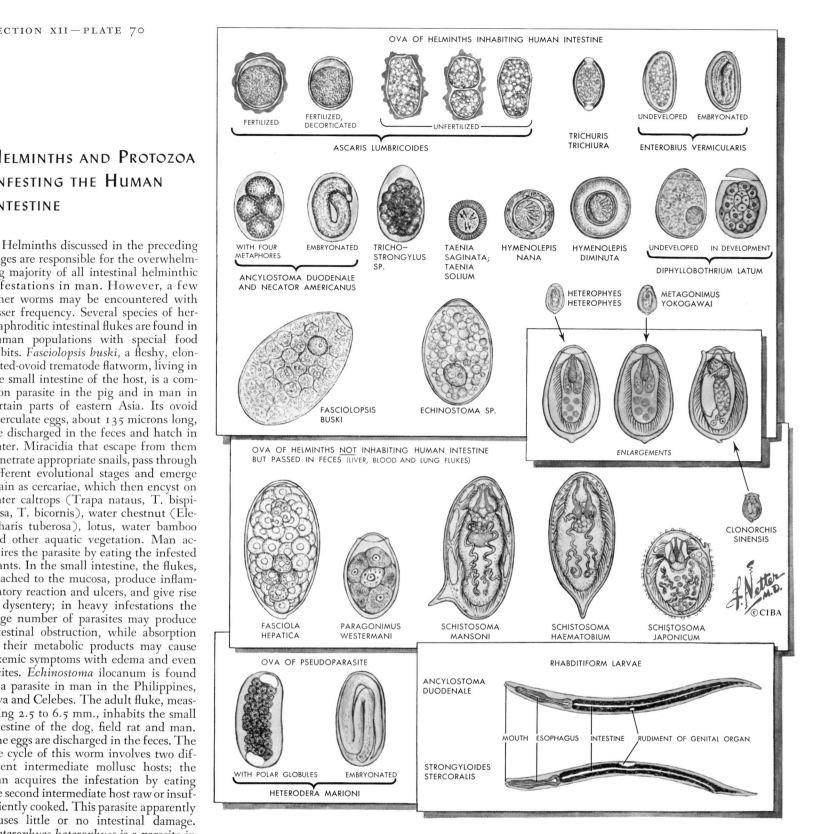

are on record in which ova of H. heterophyes, filtered through the intestinal wall, were carried to the heart and brain, where they produced tissue damage. *Metagonimus yokogawai,* a parasite resembling H. heterophyes, infests man, dog, cat, hog, pelican and probably other fish-eating mammals and birds; it is found chiefly in the Far East, but also in Spain, the Balkan States and Palestine. The life cycle of this parasite is similar to that of H. heterophyes, except in the identity of the intermediate snail and fish hosts; its pathogenicity is also similar. Besides the mentioned flukes, a great number of other intestinal helminths that act as parasites in animals may, incidentally, also infest human beings. The different species of the nematode genus *Trichostrongylus,* parasitic in ruminants, are reported with increasing frequency in man. The same applies also to *Hymenolepis diminuta,* the rat tapeworm.

Intestinal helminthic infestations, though eventually suspected on the ground of clinical symptoms or blood eosinophilia, are ultimately always diagnosed by the recovery of ova, larvae, adult parasites or parts of them (proglottids) in the feces, scrapings from anal or peri-anal regions, gastric or duodenal aspirates and, eventually, in other body fluids or tissues. For parasitologic feces examination, many different methods are used. The most simple is direct microscopic examination of fecal material spread thinly on a slide. For detection of light infestations, a number of concentration methods consisting of sedimentation, flotation and centrifugalization have been described. The search for parasitic eggs in anal and peri-anal regions is indicated mostly when enterobiasis or taeniasis is suspected. Many methods and devices for obtaining material from anal and peri-anal areas have been

(Continued on page 185)

HELMINTHS AND PROTOZOA INFESTING THE HUMAN INTESTINE

(Continued from page 184)

described. Of all common helminthic infestations, *strongyloidiasis* (see page 178) is the only one in which normally rhabditiform larvae and not ova are found in freshly voided feces; they can be differentiated from those of *hookworms* (see page 179) (found only in stools that have stood for some time before examination) chiefly by a shorter buccal vestibule and larger rudimental genital organs. In individuals infested with liver, blood or lung flukes, the eggs of these parasites, discharged via the intestine or (in the lung-fluke parasitism) reaching the intestine with the swallowed sputum, can be found in the feces. The ova of some phytoparasitic nematodes, particularly *Heterodera marioni* (radicicola), inhabiting roots and stems of many edible plants, may also be observed in the human feces, having been ingested with infested vegetables and set free in the intestine, through which they pass undamaged.

The human intestine may be invaded not only by helminthic but also by protozoan parasites. *Entamoeba histolytica* is the most important of them (see pages 155 and 156). Other species of amoebae that live in the large intestine of man include *Entamoeba coli, Endolimax nana, Dientamoeba fragilis* and *Iodamoeba bütschlii*. With the possible exception of D. fragilis, they are not pathogenic and would be of very little consequence if it were not for the danger of confusion between them and E. histolytica. They do not invade intestinal tissues, but otherwise their life cycle is similar to that of E. histolytica. In the feces they appear as trophozoites or, more commonly, as cysts. Only D. fragilis is not known to form cysts, and, since trophozoites usually perish soon after leaving the body, their transmission from host to host has not yet been adequately explained. The *trophozoites* of intestinal amoebae can be identified and differentiated by their size, motility, form of pseudopodia, endoplastic inclusions and nuclear structure. The characteristics by which the cysts can be differentiated concern the size, shape, number of nuclei and their structure, chromatoid bodies, glycogen vacuoles and the presence or absence of a cyst wall. The only known pathogenic ciliate parasite in man is *Balantidium coli*. This large protozoon (usually 50 to 100 microns in length) inhabits the large intestine of pigs, monkeys and human beings. The *trophozoites* are actively motile and have oval bodies covered with short, delicate cilia. The granular endoplasm contains two contractile and several food vacuoles, a kidney-shaped macronucleus and

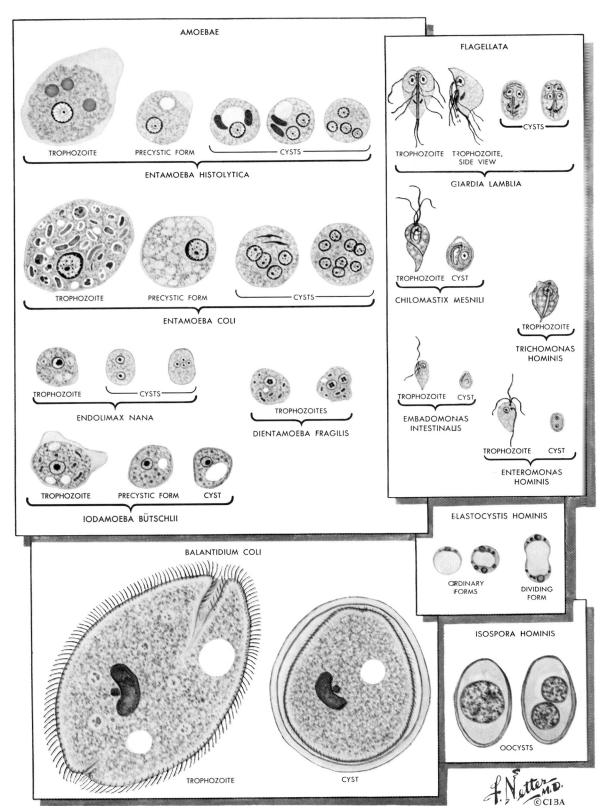

a micronucleus. The *cysts* are spherical or oval in shape and have a double-outlined wall that encloses a clearly differentiated balantidium. In older cysts, however, the outline of the organism is lost, and all structures except granular cytoplasm, macronucleus and a contractile vacuole disappear. B. coli may invade the intestinal tissues and produce ulcerations similar to those caused by E. histolytica. The majority of individuals suffering from balantidiasis have only diarrhea or are symptom-free. Only a small number of patients develop severe dysentery which may end fatally.

The flagellate protozoa that can be found in the human intestine include *Giardia lamblia, Chilomastix mesnili, Trichomonas hominis, Embadomonas intestinalis* and *Enteromonas hominis*. With the exception of T. hominis, which is not known to form cysts, their life cycle includes a trophozoite and a

cystic stage. The intestinal flagellates do not invade the tissues, and their pathogenicity is still a matter of dispute. With the possible exception of Giardia lamblia (believed to produce recurrent diarrhea), they are probably harmless to man. The coccidium *Isospora hominis*, although widely distributed, is a relatively uncommon parasite in man. Its life cycle has not yet been demonstrated, and only oocysts, passed in the feces, are known. This parasite is able to produce self-limited diarrhea. *Blastocystis hominis*, a yeastlike organism belonging to the blastomycetes, is a common and harmless inhabitant of the human intestine (in contrast to infections with B. dermatitidis and B. brasiliensis, which cause serious diseases of the skin, lungs and other organs); it is important only because it may be mistaken for a protozoan cyst.

The diagnosis of intestinal protozoan infestations is usually made by microscopic examination of the feces.

Section XIII

DISEASES AND INJURIES OF THE ABDOMINAL CAVITY

by

FRANK H. NETTER, M.D.

in collaboration with

MICHAEL E. De BAKEY, M.D.
Plates 9-14

SAMUEL H. KLEIN, M.D.
and

ARTHUR H. AUFSES, Jr., M.D.
Plates 1-4

MITJA POLAK, M.D.
Plates 5-7

SHEPPARD SIEGAL, M.D.
Plate 8

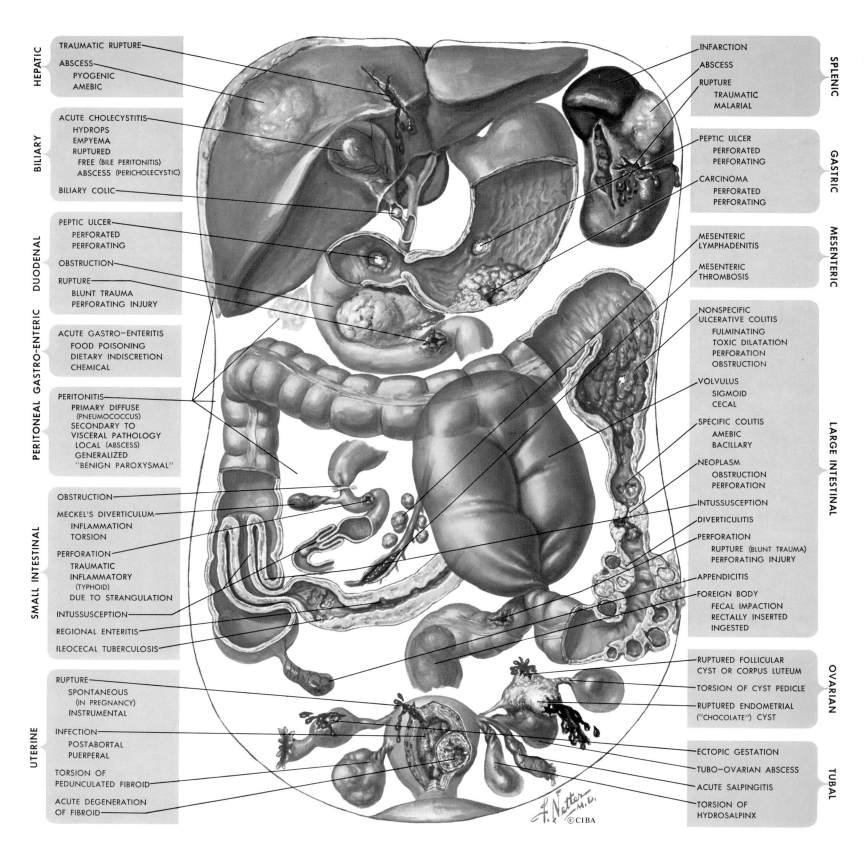

HEPATIC
TRAUMATIC RUPTURE
ABSCESS
 PYOGENIC
 AMEBIC

BILIARY
ACUTE CHOLECYSTITIS
 HYDROPS
 EMPYEMA
 RUPTURED
  FREE (BILE PERITONITIS)
  ABSCESS (PERICHOLECYSTIC)
BILIARY COLIC

DUODENAL
PEPTIC ULCER
 PERFORATED
 PERFORATING
OBSTRUCTION
RUPTURE
 BLUNT TRAUMA
 PERFORATING INJURY

PERITONEAL GASTRO-ENTERIC
ACUTE GASTRO-ENTERITIS
 FOOD POISONING
 DIETARY INDISCRETION
 CHEMICAL
PERITONITIS
 PRIMARY DIFFUSE
  (PNEUMOCOCCUS)
 SECONDARY TO
 VISCERAL PATHOLOGY
 LOCAL (ABSCESS)
 GENERALIZED
 "BENIGN PAROXYSMAL"

SMALL INTESTINAL
OBSTRUCTION
MECKEL'S DIVERTICULUM
 INFLAMMATION
 TORSION
PERFORATION
 TRAUMATIC
 INFLAMMATORY
 (TYPHOID)
 DUE TO STRANGULATION
INTUSSUSCEPTION
REGIONAL ENTERITIS
ILEOCECAL TUBERCULOSIS

UTERINE
RUPTURE
 SPONTANEOUS
 (IN PREGNANCY)
 INSTRUMENTAL
INFECTION
 POSTABORTAL
 PUERPERAL
TORSION OF
 PEDUNCULATED FIBROID
ACUTE DEGENERATION
 OF FIBROID

SPLENIC
INFARCTION
ABSCESS
RUPTURE
 TRAUMATIC
 MALARIAL

GASTRIC
PEPTIC ULCER
 PERFORATED
 PERFORATING
CARCINOMA
 PERFORATED
 PERFORATING

MESENTERIC
MESENTERIC
 LYMPHADENITIS
MESENTERIC
 THROMBOSIS

LARGE INTESTINAL
NONSPECIFIC
ULCERATIVE COLITIS
 FULMINATING
 TOXIC DILATATION
 PERFORATION
 OBSTRUCTION
VOLVULUS
 SIGMOID
 CECAL
SPECIFIC COLITIS
 AMEBIC
 BACILLARY
NEOPLASM
 OBSTRUCTION
 PERFORATION
INTUSSUSCEPTION
DIVERTICULITIS
PERFORATION
 RUPTURE (BLUNT TRAUMA)
 PERFORATING INJURY
APPENDICITIS
FOREIGN BODY
 FECAL IMPACTION
 RECTALLY INSERTED
 INGESTED

OVARIAN
RUPTURED FOLLICULAR
 CYST OR CORPUS LUTEUM
TORSION OF CYST PEDICLE
RUPTURED ENDOMETRIAL
 ("CHOCOLATE") CYST

TUBAL
ECTOPIC GESTATION
TUBO-OVARIAN ABSCESS
ACUTE SALPINGITIS
TORSION OF
 HYDROSALPINX

F. Netter M.D.
©CIBA

THE "ACUTE ABDOMEN"

An acute abdominal condition, usually described by the term "acute abdomen", must be assumed to be present when a patient complains of abdominal pain which persists for more than a few hours and is associated with tenderness or other evidence of inflammatory reaction or visceral dysfunction. The diagnosis of the cause of acute abdominal conditions remains one of the most difficult problems in medicine. Many pathologic processes, both intra-abdominal and extra-abdominal, may account for the symptom. An accurate history and thorough physical examination, and proper laboratory examinations help to differentiate the variety of causes.

Pain in the right upper quadrant may originate from cardiac, pulmonary, gastro-intestinal and renal conditions. Evidence of cardiac failure may implicate the heart; a pleuritic type of pain, cough, sputum and auscultatory findings over the right lower lobe point to disease above the diaphragm. A prodromal period of nausea and anorexia, followed by pain, jaundice and enlargement of the liver, suggests hepatitis, which must be differentiated from acute cholecystitis presenting colicky pain and a tender, globular mass in the right upper quadrant. Urinalysis showing red and/or white blood cells will suggest pyelonephritis or renal stone, whereas glycosuria and ketonuria may be the first positive evidence that the pain is a clinical facet of diabetic acidosis. Unquestionably, the most difficult area in which to make a diagnosis is the right lower quadrant

in the female. Though persistent pain in this region should be considered as due to appendicitis, until proved otherwise, one must keep in mind that a twisted, ruptured or bleeding ovarian cyst, a pelvic inflammatory process or a twisted pedunculated fibroid may cause identical symptoms. The situation is simplified only by the fact that in all these lesions surgery is indicated, provided that systemic and renal diseases have been excluded. With pain and tenderness on the left side, a tumor or diverticulitis must enter into the differential diagnosis. Needless to point out, intestinal obstruction, whatever the cause may be (see pages 190 and 191), may start its clinical appearance with the signs and symptoms of an "acute abdomen". A patient with an abdominal scar from previous surgery, who complains

(Continued on page 189)

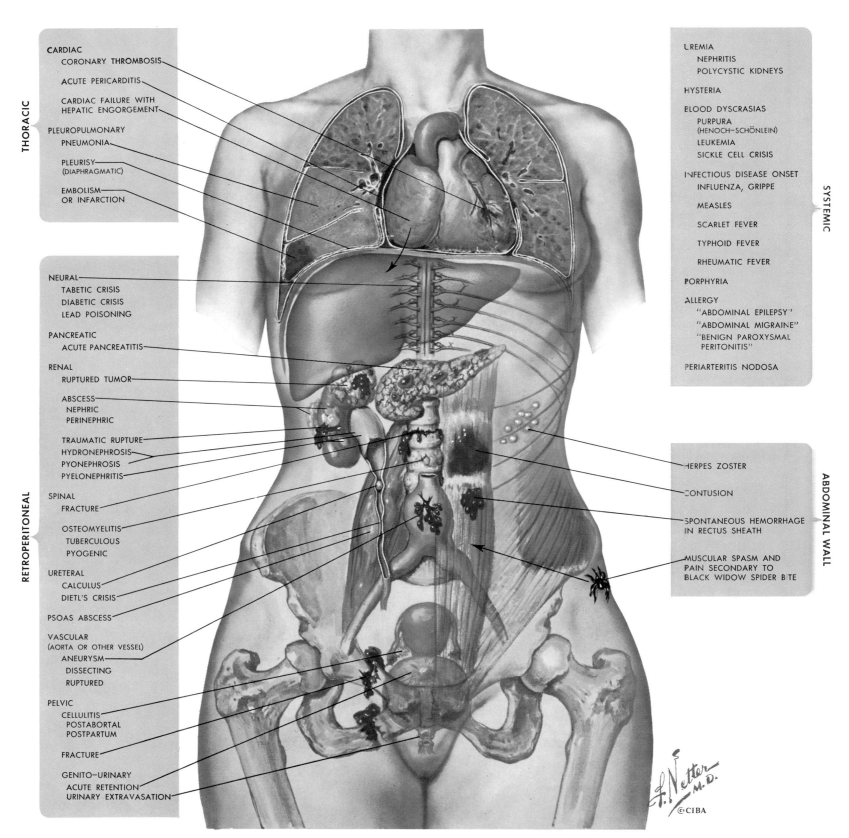

SECTION XIII — PLATE 2

THE "ACUTE ABDOMEN"

(Continued from page 188)

of cramps and vomiting, must be assumed to have intestinal obstruction until proved otherwise.

Although the location of pain usually fixes the site of a disease process, it must be borne in mind that pain may appear at a distance from the pathologic process. Appendicitis frequently begins with epigastric or peri-umbilical pain before localizing in the right lower quadrant; perforated peptic ulcer, acute cholecystitis and pancreatitis may manifest themselves with lower abdominal pain because of extravasation of inflammatory exudate down the lumbar gutter. Rebound tenderness, the most significant if not truly pathognomonic sign of peritoneal inflam-mation, is, in almost all patients, an indication of the need for surgical intervention, unless the peritoneal reaction can be shown to be due to a systemic disease (e.g., benign paroxysmal perito-nitis [see page 196] or sickle cell crisis).

A peritoneal tap performed with a fine needle may yield considerable information. Clear fluid is obtained in the presence of an early peritoneal response to an inflammatory process. The process has progressed if leukocytes and bacteria are found in a turbid fluid. Sanguineous fluid with a positive amylase reaction points to an acute hem-orrhagic pancreatitis, whereas a frankly bloody fluid must be attributed to trauma, a ruptured spleen or liver, mesenteric vascular occlusion, a ruptured or twisted and infarcted ovarian cyst or ectopic pregnancy.

With any doubt about the abdominal diag-nosis, a scout film of the abdomen and a chest roentgenogram should be made. The latter will exclude or ascertain pneumonia, pulmonary infarction, congestive heart failure, pericardial effusion as well as fractured ribs, all conditions which can present the clinical picture of an acute abdomen. On the abdominal or chest film, free air under the diaphragm is pathognomonic of a perforated viscus. Opaque calculi may be visible and lead to a diagnosis of cholecystitis, renal lithiasis or even gallstone ileus. In cases of injury manifesting paralytic ileus, roentgen examina-tion may disclose fracture of a vertebra or the pelvis. Localized ileus (the "sentinel loop") may be seen in pancreatitis, appendicitis or mesen-teric infarction. Volvulus of the sigmoid or cecum (see pages 132 and 133) presents a characteristic roentgen appearance.

189

ALIMENTARY TRACT OBSTRUCTION

Any organic or functional condition which primarily or indirectly impedes the normal propulsion of luminal contents from the esophageal inlet to the anus should be considered an obstruction of the alimentary tract, the pathophysiologic sequelae of which have been explained on page 101. In the newborn a variety of congenital anomalies (esophageal, intestinal, anal atresias, colonic malrotation, volvulus of the midgut, meconium ileus, aganglionic megacolon) resulting in obstruction are discussed on pages 112 to 124. Other causes of mechanical interference of intestinal function in early infancy include incarceration in an internal or external (inguinal) hernia (see page 214), congenital peritoneal bands, intestinal duplications, volvulus due to mesenteric cysts and annular pancreas (see CIBA COLLECTION, Vol. 3/III, page 141), though the latter may not become clinically manifest until adult life or in the aged.

Those esophageal diseases which interfere with the normal passage of fluids and solids through the gullet (illustrated in the uppermost row) are dealt with on pages 138, 142, 144, 145, 149, 150 and 154 to 156 of Part I of this volume of the CIBA COLLECTION. Fibrotic narrowing has also been observed after anastomotic or plastic procedures at the lower end of the esophagus. Too tight closure of the hiatus in the repair of sliding esophageal hiatus hernia results in compression obstruction at this point. Extraluminal pressure on the esophagus by a tumor mass or visceral abnormality in the neck or mediastinum will lead to the same results.

Gastric obstruction may be brought about by the accumulation in the stomach of ingested material such as hair (trichobezoar) or fruit or vegetable fibers (phytobezoar), by a spastic or cicatricial occlusion related to pre- or postpyloric peptic ulcer (see CIBA COLLECTION, Vol. 3/I, page 174) or by the growth of a malignant neoplasm (see ibidem, pages 182 and 183). Obstruction of the duodenum by extraluminal compression may occur as in the "superior mesenteric artery syndrome", by pressure and/or invasion by carcinoma of the head of the pancreas or neoplastic lymphadenopathy in the small bowel mesentery or transverse mesocolon.

Of the wide variety of conditions which may initiate obstruction of the

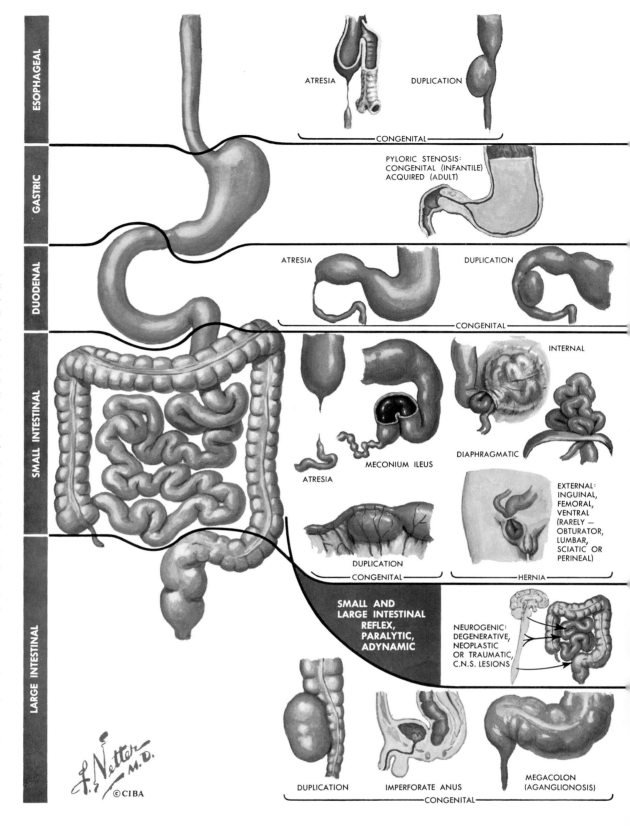

small intestine, the most common is incarceration of a loop of small bowel in an inguinal or femoral hernia. On occasion, incarceration occurs in an internal hernia, or a bowel segment may become caught in the ring of a congenital, traumatic or surgical defect in the diaphragm. A foreign body, either ingested orally or consisting of a large biliary calculus (see CIBA COLLECTION, Vol. 3/III, page 132), may by impaction result in obstruction, which has also been reported as a consequence of an accumulation of parasitic worms (see page 176). Mechanical obstruction of the small intestine may furthermore be produced by intussusception (see page 134) and by compression, torsion and/or angulation of one or more bowel loops. The various etiologic mechanisms which may be involved include recent or old postoperative adhesions, congenital peritoneal bands, metastatic tumor implants, Meckel's diverticulum (see page 127) and

plastic or adhesive peritonitis (tuberculosis, talc granuloma) (see page 194). On occasion, primary neoplasms (see pages 163 to 165) of the small intestine (carcinoma, lymphosarcoma, Hodgkin's granuloma) may cause obstructive manifestations. Varying degrees of small bowel obstruction may be the result of segmental fibrotic stricture formation, as in regional ileitis or jejunitis, or in a bowel loop that has become stenosed as the result of healing following localized infarction sustained in hernial incarceration or mesenteric vascular occlusion. Finally, iatrogenic intestinal obstruction may occur on occasion (anastomotic stenosis, torsion or angulation, or anastomosis of incorrect loops) as the result of faulty surgical technique.

Cancer of the large intestine constitutes the most frequent mechanism of obstruction of this viscus. Occlusion occurs more commonly in those areas where the bowel lumen tends to be of smaller caliber. On

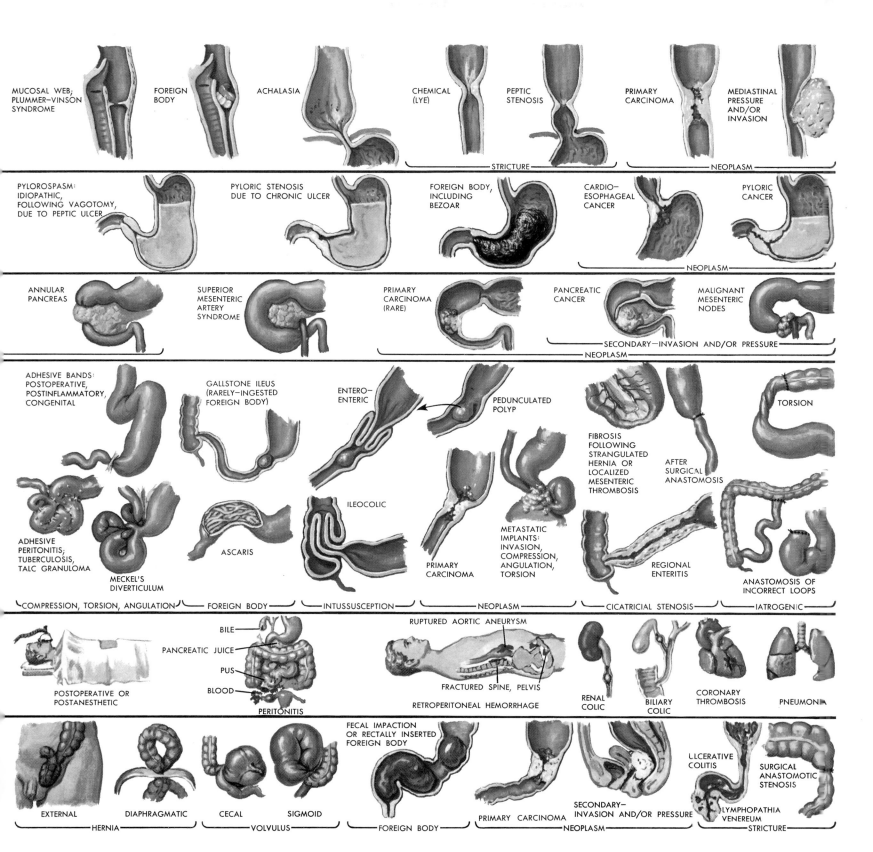

MUCOSAL WEB; PLUMMER-VINSON SYNDROME — FOREIGN BODY — ACHALASIA — CHEMICAL (LYE) — PEPTIC STENOSIS — PRIMARY CARCINOMA — MEDIASTINAL PRESSURE AND/OR INVASION

STRICTURE — NEOPLASM

PYLOROSPASM: IDIOPATHIC, FOLLOWING VAGOTOMY, DUE TO PEPTIC ULCER — PYLORIC STENOSIS DUE TO CHRONIC ULCER — FOREIGN BODY, INCLUDING BEZOAR — CARDIO-ESOPHAGEAL CANCER — PYLORIC CANCER

NEOPLASM

ANNULAR PANCREAS — SUPERIOR MESENTERIC ARTERY SYNDROME — PRIMARY CARCINOMA (RARE) — PANCREATIC CANCER — MALIGNANT MESENTERIC NODES

SECONDARY—INVASION AND/OR PRESSURE

NEOPLASM

ADHESIVE BANDS: POSTOPERATIVE, POSTINFLAMMATORY, CONGENITAL — GALLSTONE ILEUS (RARELY—INGESTED FOREIGN BODY) — ENTERO-ENTERIC — PEDUNCULATED POLYP — FIBROSIS FOLLOWING STRANGULATED HERNIA OR LOCALIZED MESENTERIC THROMBOSIS — AFTER SURGICAL ANASTOMOSIS — TORSION

ADHESIVE PERITONITIS; TUBERCULOSIS, TALC GRANULOMA — MECKEL'S DIVERTICULUM — ASCARIS — ILEOCOLIC — PRIMARY CARCINOMA — METASTATIC IMPLANTS: INVASION, COMPRESSION, ANGULATION, TORSION — REGIONAL ENTERITIS — ANASTOMOSIS OF INCORRECT LOOPS

COMPRESSION, TORSION, ANGULATION — FOREIGN BODY — INTUSSUSCEPTION — NEOPLASM — CICATRICIAL STENOSIS — IATROGENIC

POSTOPERATIVE OR POSTANESTHETIC — BILE — PANCREATIC JUICE — PUS — BLOOD — PERITONITIS — RUPTURED AORTIC ANEURYSM — FRACTURED SPINE, PELVIS — RETROPERITONEAL HEMORRHAGE — RENAL COLIC — BILIARY COLIC — CORONARY THROMBOSIS — PNEUMONIA

EXTERNAL — DIAPHRAGMATIC — CECAL — SIGMOID — FECAL IMPACTION OR RECTALLY INSERTED FOREIGN BODY — PRIMARY CARCINOMA — SECONDARY—INVASION AND/OR PRESSURE — ULCERATIVE COLITIS — LYMPHOPATHIA VENEREUM — SURGICAL ANASTOMOTIC STENOSIS

HERNIA — VOLVULUS — FOREIGN BODY — NEOPLASM — STRICTURE

occasion one may see a volvulus of the right colon if it has a long mesentery. Fecal impaction causing obstruction occurs not infrequently in the aged, as does also sigmoid colon volvulus. A large foreign body inserted per rectum may obstruct the lumen (perversion, psychosis).

Strictures of the colon may be the result of cicatricial fibrosis (granulomatous ileocolitis or colitis, nonspecific ulcerative colitis [see pages 147 and 148]), diverticulitis (see page 131) or lymphopathia venereum (see page 174) or they may occur as a postoperative complication (anastomotic stricture, posthemorrhoidectomy). Extraluminal compression, usually by pelvic tumors (primary or metastatic), rarely by pelvic inflammatory exudate or abscess formation, may obstruct the lower bowel at the level of the rectosigmoid or the rectum.

Nonmechanical impairment of intestinal motor function has been descriptively termed "reflex, adynamic or paralytic ileus" (see page 101). As a complication of various causative clinical conditions, the patient presents the syndrome of gastric retention, constipation and failure to pass flatus, abdominal distention, a "silent abdomen" and the roentgen findings of dilatation of the small and large intestine with gas and accumulated fluid. "Ileus" may be encountered in patients suffering from various lesions of the central nervous system. Intestinal atony may follow surgical anesthesia and/or the trauma of intra-abdominal surgical manipulation, extensive rib fractures or blunt abdominal trauma (immersion blast injury). Other clinical conditions in which ileus has been said to occur as a "reflex" phenomenon include renal or biliary colic, pneumonia,

torsion infarction of ovarian cyst, coronary thrombosis and retroperitoneal hemorrhage (incident to fracture of the spine or pelvis, dissecting aortic aneurysm, urinary extravasation, rupture of the kidney).

So-called "paralytic or adynamic" ileus occurs most often with purulent peritonitis (due to perforated appendicitis, perforation of a hollow viscus, pelvic inflammatory disease, leakage or dehiscence of an intestinal suture line, wound evisceration, etc.). Ileus may follow the intraperitoneal extravasation of gastric or duodenal contents (perforated peptic ulcer), pancreatic juice (acute hemorrhagic pancreatitis), bile (perforated gallbladder, bile leakage from liver or bile ducts) and blood (postoperative hemorrhage, rupture of liver, spleen, Graafian follicle, ectopic gestation or "chocolate" cyst of the ovary).

MESENTERIC VASCULAR OCCLUSION

Either mesenteric artery thrombosis or embolism or venous thrombosis may produce hemorrhagic infarction of the intestine. The extent of the resultant pathologic changes, the rate of tissue damage and the severity of the clinical picture are dependent upon the nature and location of the vascular occlusion. In general, the arterial blockade tends to be located in the main superior mesenteric artery, causing rapid and extensive hemorrhagic infarction of the small bowel and right colon. Associated closure of the inferior mesenteric artery affects the left colon as well. Mesenteric venous thrombosis more commonly involves the proximal and mid-small bowel in segmental or patchy distribution. The colon is usually not affected.

In both the arterial and the venous types of mesenteric occlusion, the resultant engorgement of the bowel wall (hemorrhagic infarction) eventuates in loss of tissue viability and in gangrene. Extravasation of blood takes place into the lumen of the bowel, and sanguineous serous fluid accumulates also in the peritoneal cavity. Purulent peritonitis (see page 193) may finally supervene, owing to a necrotic perforation of the bowel or to the passage of intestinal bacteria into the peritoneal cavity through the devitalized bowel wall.

Mesenteric arterial thrombosis is usually observed in patients in the older age group and occurs secondarily to arteriosclerotic vascular changes. An embolism, on the other hand, may originate in the left auricle or its appendage in a patient with rheumatic cardiac disease and auricular fibrillation, or in the left ventricle following an acute myocardial infarction. Paradoxical embolism, from a peripheral phlebitic focus, may occur through a patent foramen ovale (Kirschner).

The clinical picture of mesenteric arterial occlusion includes sudden onset of abdominal pain and prostration, rapid development of abdominal distention, a tender abdominal mass and shock. Vomiting, hematemesis and/or melena may occur. A marked leukocytosis is present, and a diagnostic abdominal tap yields bloody peritoneal fluid. Death may occur within 2 or 3 days as a result of shock and peritonitis. Early diagnosis and surgical intervention are therefore impera-

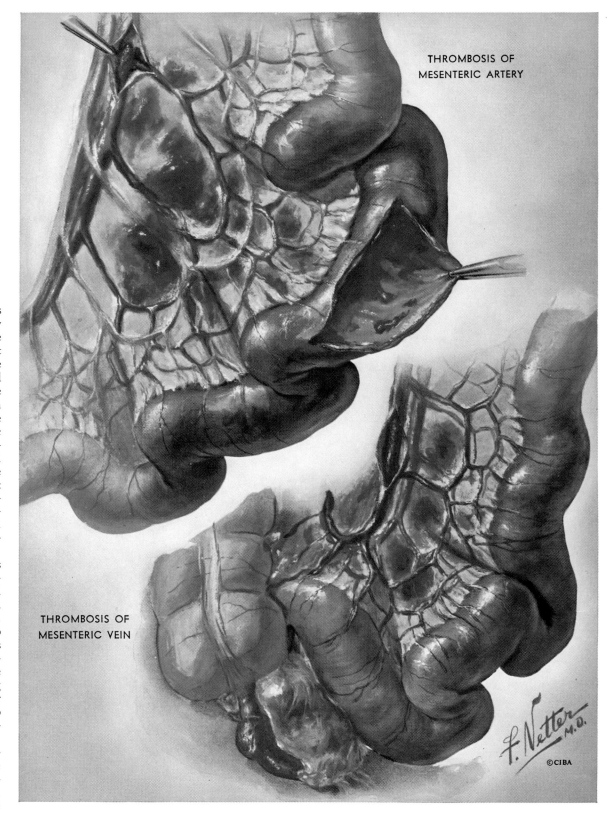

THROMBOSIS OF MESENTERIC ARTERY

THROMBOSIS OF MESENTERIC VEIN

tive. In contrast to the arterial occlusions, mesenteric venous thrombosis does not produce nearly so clear-cut a clinical picture. The etiology may be obscure, thrombosis occurring without apparent antecedent cause. Early or late after splenectomy, thrombosis of the splenic vein may extend to involve the portal and mesenteric veins. Mesenteric venous thrombosis may also follow intra-abdominal infections or may take place in association with thrombotic hematologic disorders such as polycythemia vera or postsplenectomy thrombocythemia. Because the thrombotic process in the mesenteric veins is more slowly progressive, the symptoms of pain, nausea and vomiting may be present for several days before the involved bowel becomes frankly gangrenous and the signs and symptoms of peritonitis become manifest. Emergency surgical therapy is then clearly indicated. At operation, the bowel adjoining the infarcted segment may be found to be markedly thickened and congested. Engorgement of retroperitoneal vessels may often be observed, representing collateral circulation. A striking feature may be a marked thickening of the small bowel mesentery in the areas of mesenteric thrombosis due to edema and ecchymosis. Pulsatile arterial blood flow is seen when the mesentery is cut across, while "toothpaste-like" clots are extruded from the veins.

The prognosis in mesenteric venous thrombosis is more favorable than in arterial occlusion but is nevertheless serious since further thrombosis and infarction may occur. Anticoagulant therapy may be helpful postoperatively in preventing secondary venous thrombosis. It is of interest that instances have been reported, verified at autopsy, in which mesenteric venous thrombosis caused fatal intestinal bleeding without the occurrence of hemorrhagic infarction of the bowel.

ACUTE PERITONITIS

Acute peritonitis may be caused by numerous species of pathogenic bacteria of which the more common ones are B. coli, streptococci, enterococci, staphylococci, diphtheroids, Cl. welchii, gonococci and pneumococci. The organisms frequently belong not to a single but to more than one species. They reach the peritoneum (1) from the exterior by *penetrating wounds* of the abdominal wall (trauma, surgery), (2) from an infectious process in an abdominal organ *via the lymphatics* or ostia of the *Fallopian tubes*, (3) by *rupture of a viscus* and (4) from a distant organ *via the blood stream*. The germs of the intestinal flora usually come from the alimentary tract, whereas streptococci and staphylococci are more commonly introduced from without. Gonococcal peritonitis occurs almost exclusively in females as a complication of gonorrheal salpingitis (see CIBA COLLECTION, Vol. 2, pages 181 and 184); it is usually confined to the pelvis. A form of gonococcal peritonitis localized in the upper right abdominal quadrant is characterized by the appearance of thin fibrin bands ("violin strings") between the anterior surface of the liver, the diaphragm and the anterior abdominal wall and, clinically, by severe acute pain in this region (Fitz-Hugh-Curtis syndrome). Pneumococcal peritonitis may develop as a complication of a pneumococcal infection elsewhere in the body (pneumonia, empyema, otitis, etc.), but it may occur also as a primary disease; as such, it is observed mostly in female children between the ages of 3 and 7 years, and it is believed that the pneumococci reach the peritoneum from the genital tract through the Fallopian tubes.

The course of a peritonitis is determined by the quality and the quantity both of the injurious agents and of the body defenses. The infection may remain localized and walled-in by the adhesion of adjacent structures, or it may spread and become *generalized*. The pathologic changes are those seen in inflammation of any serous membrane; the peritoneum becomes congested and, owing to the deposition of fibrin, loses its normal sheen. The exudate is serous during the earliest stages but later becomes purulent. The inflammatory process may reach the blood vessels in the mesentery, where thrombosis may develop and determine gangrene in a part of the bowel. A *localized peritonitis* in the form of an abscess may occur at the primary point of infection or at some distance from it. The commonest variety is the *periceco-appendiceal abscess* that usually develops as a complication of appendicitis (see also page 148). The pelvic abscess may also

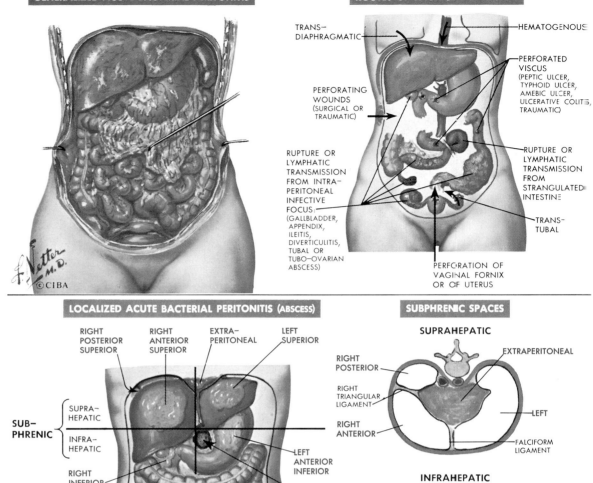

GENERALIZED ACUTE BACTERIAL PERITONITIS

ROUTES OF BACTERIAL INVASION

LOCALIZED ACUTE BACTERIAL PERITONITIS (ABSCESS)

SUBPHRENIC SPACES

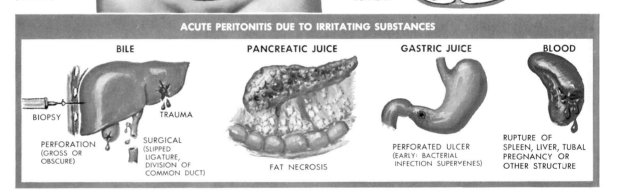

ACUTE PERITONITIS DUE TO IRRITATING SUBSTANCES

result from appendicitis, though it is more commonly due to gynecologic affections. The most important form of a localized peritonitis is, however, the *subphrenic abscess* characterized by the collection of pus in one of the subphrenic spaces. The pus usually originates in the upper abdomen, but it may also come from the right iliac fossa or even the pelvis. The most common causes of a subphrenic abscess are *gastric* or *duodenal perforation, appendicitis* and *hepatobiliary affections* (see CIBA COLLECTION, Vol. 3/III, page 131).

Acute peritonitis may result also from the entrance of *irritating substances* into the peritoneal cavity. *Bile* may escape from an injury (trauma, surgery, rupture) to the intra- or extrahepatic biliary system, but bile peritonitis may develop also without demonstrable leakage (idiopathic bile leakage), probably a perforation too small to be visually detectable. Irritat-

ing quantities of *blood* enter the cavity usually from a rupture of the spleen, tube (tubal pregnancy), liver or other structures. Pancreatic *enzymes* reach the peritoneum in the course of acute hemorrhagic pancreatitis (see ibidem, page 143), whereas the entrance of gastric juice results from gastric or duodenal perforation.

The typical symptoms of a generalized peritonitis are abdominal pain, rigidity of the abdominal musculature and vomiting; in the early stages hyperperistalsis may develop, but, as the process extends, paralysis of the intestinal tract sets in (see page 189). Both the temperature and pulse rate are elevated. The blood picture usually shows a leukocytosis. If peritonitis is due to perforation of a hollow viscus, the presence of free air or fluid may be elicited on examination. If the infection is virulent and the body defenses are poor, the disease is particularly severe and often rapidly fatal.

CHRONIC PERITONITIS

Tuberculous peritonitis, though it may occur at any age, is chiefly a disease of young adults and children. It is practically always secondary to some other focus in the body, the most frequent sources of infection being tuberculous lesions in the bowel (see pages 157 and 158), the mesenteric glands and the Fallopian tubes. In the course of a general miliary tuberculosis, the tuberculous peritonitis may occur as an acute affection; much more commonly, however, it appears as a chronic condition that manifests itself in two main forms: (1) exudative or moist and (2) plastic or dry. In the first variety the exudation is marked, and the abdominal cavity becomes filled with a thin ascitic fluid; *numerous tubercles,* about the size of a pinhead or larger, appear *on the peritoneal surfaces.* In the second variety the exudate is dense and rich in fibrin, formation of adhesions occurs most readily and the viscera become matted together; the peritoneum is studded with tubercles which, however, may be covered by deposits of fibrin; the omentum is often greatly thickened and rolled up. Caseous necrosis of tuberculous lesions may lead to formation of fistulous tracts. Both varieties may occur combined, giving rise to the so-called encysted or encapsulated form characterized by loculated collections of fluid encysted by the *dense adhesions.*

Tuberculous peritonitis may have a sudden or an insidious onset. The most common clinical manifestations are a diffuse or localized abdominal pain of variable intensity and abdominal distention due to ascites; in the dry form, however, the effusion may be small and difficult to demonstrate. Other symptoms include fever, nausea and vomiting, constipation or diarrhea, and, of course, general constitutional symptoms that usually accompany a tuberculous infection. Physical examination of the abdomen may reveal signs of fluid, a diffuse or localized tenderness and, eventually, intra-abdominal masses. Ascitic fluid obtained by paracentesis may be clear, cloudy, lemon-yellow or bloody, and, in case of erosion of the mesenteric lymphatic system, chylous; the specific gravity ranges from 1.005 to 1.035; its cellular picture shows, in the very early stages, the predominance of polymorph neutrophils which, however, are gradually replaced by lymphocytes and monocytes. Tubercle bacilli may eventually be isolated from the ascitic fluid by culture and guinea-pig inoculation. The most useful procedure for diagnosis of

TUBERCULOUS PERITONITIS: PERITONEUM STUDDED WITH TUBERCLES AND CONGESTED; SEROFIBRINOUS EXUDATE; NUMEROUS ADHESIONS BETWEEN ABDOMINAL WALL AND VISCERA

X-RAY: ARTIFICIAL PNEUMOPERITONEUM; ENCYSTED TUBERCULOUS PERITONITIS

PERITONEOSCOPIC VIEW (PARIETAL PERITONEUM)

TUBERCULOUS PERITONITIS: HISTOPATHOLOGY

GRANULOMATOUS PERITONITIS DUE TO CAUSES OTHER THAN TUBERCULOSIS

FOREIGN-BODY GRANULOMA

SOUTH AMERICAN BLASTOMYCOSIS: GRANULOMA CONTAINING PARACOCCIDIOIDES BRASILIENSIS

SCHISTOSOMIASIS: GRANULOMA (LATE STAGE) CONTAINING OVA OF SCHISTOSOMA MANSONI

peritoneal tuberculosis is *peritoneoscopy* combined with biopsy of a tubercle.

A *chronic granulomatous peritonitis* grossly resembling that caused by tuberculosis may occur in a number of other diseases. *South American blastomycosis* and coccidioidomycosis (caused by *Paracoccidioides brasiliensis* and *Coccidioides immitis,* respectively), actinomycosis, syphilis and tularemia have been found to involve occasionally the peritoneum and produce granulomatous lesions. *Foreign substances,* such as talcum and lycopodium (used as dusting powders for surgical gloves), liquid petrolatum, X-ray contrast media and others, introduced into the peritoneal cavity at operations or during diagnostic procedures (*e.g.,* hysterosalpingography), as well as extruded gastrointestinal contents left in the abdominal cavity after operations, and contents of ruptured dermoid and other cysts may all cause a chronic inflammatory reac-

tion, with formation of adhesions and foreign-body granulomas. A similar reaction may be produced also by Enterobius vermicularis (see page 177) and *ova of schistosoma* that may, by erratic migration, reach the peritoneum.

Fibrous bands and adhesions may form in the peritoneal cavity also as a late result of an acute peritonitis or in consequence of a localized chronic peritonitis (perivisceritis) occurring over the site of an ulcerative or inflammatory lesion in the stomach, intestine, gallbladder, liver or genital organs. A fibrinous perihepatitis (sugar-icing liver) and perisplenitis may accompany liver cirrhosis and other conditions with persistent ascites. Polyserositis (Pick's or Concato's disease), a disease of still-obscure etiology, is characterized by intense fibrosis with hyalinization of the peritoneum and other serous membranes, particularly the pericardium and pleura.

CANCER OF THE PERITONEUM

Primary malignant tumors of the peritoneum (mesotheliomas or endotheliomas) are extremely rare. In contrast, secondary malignancy of the peritoneum is relatively frequent. Malignant neoplasms arising in the retroperitoneal connective, nervous or muscular tissue, as well as sarcomas and teratomas localized elsewhere in the body, may invade or set up metastases — though again rarely — in the peritoneum. The tumors that produce metastases in the peritoneum are often *carcinomas,* originating most frequently in the abdominal organs, particularly in the *ovaries* (see CIBA COLLECTION, Vol. 2, page 210), *stomach* (see ibidem, Vol. 3/1, page 185) and *large intestine.* The spread of the new growth to and in the peritoneum occurs by direct extension, by way of the blood stream or lymphatics and by dissemination of the carcinomatous cells throughout the peritoneal cavity and by implantation on the peritoneal surfaces (transcelomic metastases). Irritative effects of tumorous cells on the peritoneum and lymphatic occlusion provoke exudation. Ascites that accompanies the growth of peritoneal tumors may be serous, serofibrinous, hemorrhagic or, owing to tumorous fatty degeneration products, pseudochylous. Chylous effusion, however, is due not to serosal carcinomatosis per se but to damage of the thoracic duct or its main tributaries. Peritoneal metastases can show various forms, their gross pattern being influenced by the histologic character (imitating primary tumor), the manner of spread and the intensity and type of peritoneal reaction. Most common are *nodules* scattered over the omentum, mesentery and visceral and parietal peritoneum; the smaller ones, measuring a few millimeters in diameter, are often semitranslucent, whereas the larger ones are opaque, white, yellowish white, gray or reddish in color. When surface growth exceeds growth in depth, *plaquelike masses* develop, which vary considerably in size and have, usually, a waxy appearance. Necrotic changes in the tumorous tissue may occasionally produce ulcerlike depressions. The most prevalent cause of this type of metastasis is an ovarian papillary serous cystadenoma (see CIBA COLLECTION, Vol. 2, page 198). In the so-called *adhesive form* extensive adhesions may occur in the peritoneal cavity; they are due to organi-

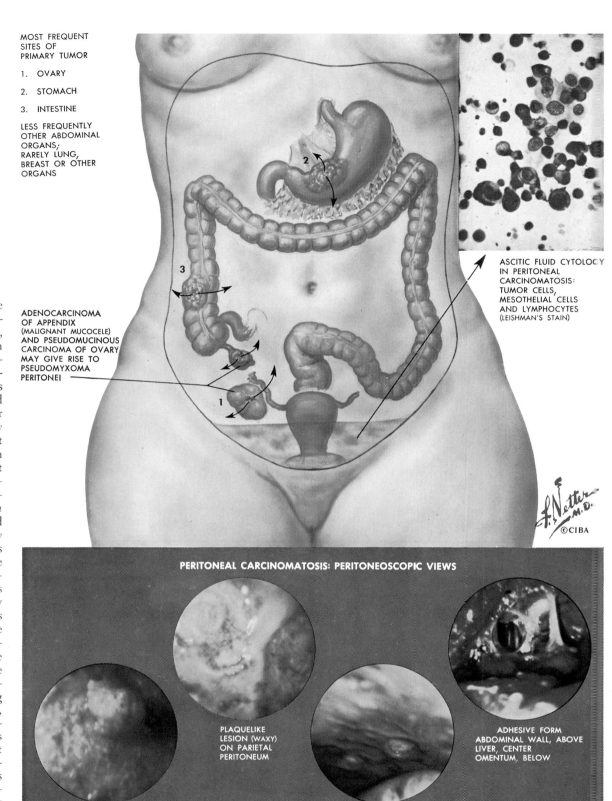

MOST FREQUENT SITES OF PRIMARY TUMOR

1. OVARY
2. STOMACH
3. INTESTINE

LESS FREQUENTLY OTHER ABDOMINAL ORGANS; RARELY LUNG, BREAST OR OTHER ORGANS

ADENOCARCINOMA OF APPENDIX (MALIGNANT MUCOCELE) AND PSEUDOMUCINOUS CARCINOMA OF OVARY MAY GIVE RISE TO PSEUDOMYXOMA PERITONEI

ASCITIC FLUID CYTOLOGY IN PERITONEAL CARCINOMATOSIS: TUMOR CELLS, MESOTHELIAL CELLS AND LYMPHOCYTES (LEISHMAN'S STAIN)

PERITONEAL CARCINOMATOSIS: PERITONEOSCOPIC VIEWS

NODULAR FORM

PLAQUELIKE LESION (WAXY) ON PARIETAL PERITONEUM

ULCERATED PLAQUES

ADHESIVE FORM ABDOMINAL WALL, ABOVE LIVER, CENTER OMENTUM, BELOW

zation of the fibrin bands produced by the dense exudate, or to confluence of the adjacent implants or to direct tumor infiltration from one organ to another. Gastric carcinoma is most prone to produce metastases, which tangle the viscera together into an inseparable scirrhous mass so that fistulas may be formed or obstruction may occur. Other types of peritoneal carcinomatosis include forms in which metastases appear as pedunculated nodules of varying size or as small cysts that may be sessile or pedunculated. The cause is usually papilliferous or cystic ovarian tumors. Metastatic implants of an appendicular adenocarcinoma or of an ovarian pseudomucinous cystadenocarcinoma (see CIBA COLLECTION, Vol. 2, pages 200 and 208) on the peritoneal surfaces may produce a condition known as *pseudomyxoma peritonei,* which is characterized by accumulation of a large quantity of gelatinous material in the peritoneal cavity.

Rupture of a nonmalignant mucocele of the appendix (see page 148) and establishment of a fistula may also lead to accumulation of mucus in the peritoneal cavity, which may be arrested by removal of the appendix.

The symptoms of peritoneal carcinomatosis are chiefly abdominal distention, due to ascites, and abdominal pain of variable intensity. Physical examination of the abdomen reveals signs of fluid and, eventually, palpable masses. In differential diagnosis all chronic peritoneal conditions (see page 194) must be considered. The best diagnostic procedure is *peritoneoscopy* (see page 110), which permits visualization of the peritoneal deposits and biopsy. The diagnosis can be made also by demonstration of *tumor cells in the ascitic fluid;* their recognition, however, is not always easy and, because of the ability of mesothelial cells to simulate carcinoma, false positive results may be obtained.

PAROXYSMAL PERITONITIS (FAMILIAL MEDITERRANEAN FEVER) AND RELATED SYNDROMES

Paroxysmal peritonitis (familial Mediterranean fever) is characterized by recurrent acute attacks of abdominal pain and fever, with physical signs indicative of peritoneal inflammation. Marked direct tenderness is invariable, rebound tenderness frequent and abdominal wall spasm occasional. Fever, usually 101 to 103 degrees, may reach 105 but need not accompany every episode. Leukocytosis, polymorphonucleosis, severe prostration, gastro-intestinal upset and constipation complete a clinical picture indistinguishable from the acute surgical abdomen. Such acute episodes usually begin in childhood or early youth and only rarely after the age of 40. Males are more frequently affected. In the beginning the attacks may occur only once or twice a year, but the intervals soon shorten and may appear as often as every week or two, sometimes with striking regularity, more often irregularly. A typical abdominal crisis may last from 1 to 4 days, during which time the patient may present the characteristic picture of acute peritonitis, with considerable abdominal distention and pain, which the patient tries to reduce to a minimum by assuming a peculiar stooped position, especially when arising from bed. It is not surprising, under these circumstances, that many patients with this disease are often operated upon under the suspicion that they suffer from acute appendicitis or cholecystitis. The attacks also may simulate an acute intestinal obstruction when X-ray studies give indication of small-bowel dilatation, though this may be excluded in the presence of diarrhea. Occasionally, the spleen may be palpable and the erythrocyte-sedimentation rate may be accelerated, most frequently during an attack, but at times persistently.

The diagnosis rests essentially on the paroxysmal character of the painful and febrile episodes. Relapsing pancreatitis (see CIBA COLLECTION, Vol. 3/III, page 144) and intermittent abdominal porphyria must be excluded by serum-amylase determination and the urine-porphobilinogen test, respectively. In women, various pelvic diseases must be considered. The attacks usually cease altogether during pregnancy. Rarely,

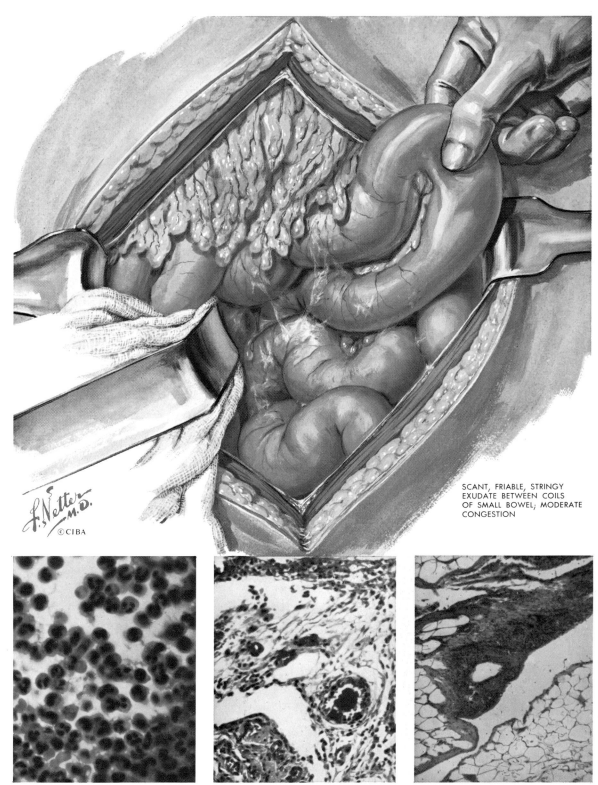

SCANT, FRIABLE, STRINGY EXUDATE BETWEEN COILS OF SMALL BOWEL; MODERATE CONGESTION

PERITONEAL EXUDATE; ACUTE PAROXYSM: INTENSE POLYMORPHONUCLEAR REACTION

PERITONEUM: CONGESTION, EDEMA AND LEUKOCYTIC INFILTRATION

OMENTUM: PERIVASCULAR AND SEPTAL POLYMORPHONUCLEAR REACTION

they may occur only in the menstrual period, in which cases it may be necessary to eliminate, by culdoscopy, reflux tubal menstruation.

The pathologic findings are those of an acute, nonspecific peritoneal inflammation, with *hyperemia* or even *edema* of the serosa and a small amount of serous or serofibrinous *exudate*. The abnormalities may be so localized as almost to escape detection. Microscopically, the exudate and the adjacent congested peritoneum or omentum show an intense *polymorphonuclear reaction* in the absence of any microorganisms. Cultures of the exudate are always sterile.

The etiology of this condition has remained an enigma. It is very probable that a genetic factor plays a major rôle, because familial occurrence is frequent and because of a peculiar predilection to this disease among people of Mediterranean descent (Jews, Armenians, Arabs and, less frequently, Italians, Greeks and Maltese). It is furthermore important that paroxysmal peritonitis is only one, though the most dramatic, phase of a more generalized disorder. Recurrent febrile paroxysms, as described above, may occur after, or may alternate with or accompany, recurrent episodes of pleuritic chest pain, repeated arthralgias, particularly of the lower extremities, or even intermittent mono-arthritis involving the larger joints. The high incidence of atopic disease, urticaria or erythema among patients with this disorder suggests a possible allergic mechanism. The disease may continue actively for as long as 50 to 70 years, though occasionally remissions may be prolonged for several years, and the attacks may become rarer or may even subside altogether in later life. The generally benign prognosis of this condition may be seriously altered by a complicating nephropathy, usually the result of amyloid deposition, to which these patients are prone.

ABDOMINAL WOUNDS I

Small Intestine

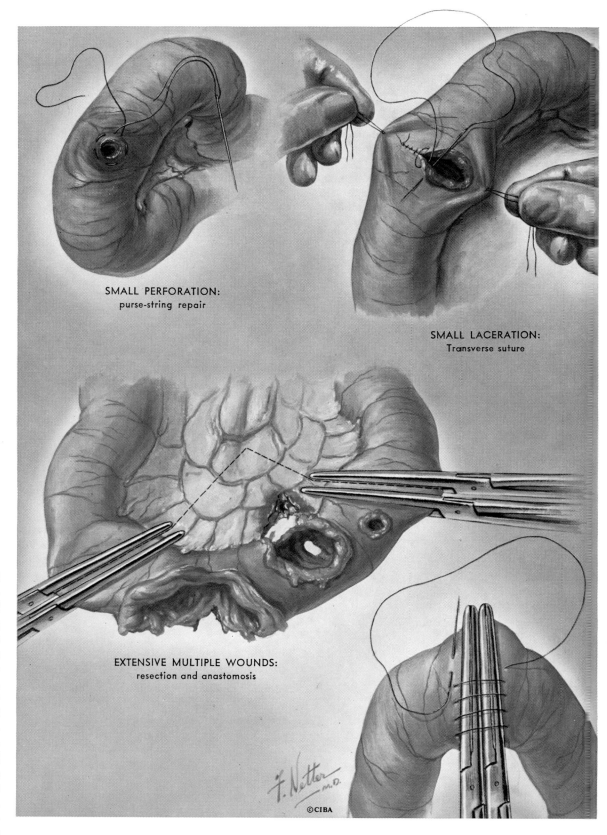

SMALL PERFORATION:
purse-string repair

SMALL LACERATION:
Transverse suture

EXTENSIVE MULTIPLE WOUNDS:
resection and anastomosis

Injuries of the small intestine demand surgical repair as early as possible. Careful inspection of the entire length of the small intestine is essential, beginning at either the ileocecal junction or at the duodenojejunal junction, whichever is the more convenient. Evisceration of large portions of the bowel should be avoided, and the inspection should be made by withdrawing and replacing lengths of about 15 to 20 cm. at a time. It is desirable to repair the injuries in each segment of bowel before replacing it and proceeding to the next part. This not only obviates further trauma but permits the surgeon to examine a sufficient length of the intestine adjacent to the perforations and thus to determine whether the perforations should be repaired individually or the segment be resected. The inspection and repair should be so thorough that re-examination is unnecessary. Practically all small perforations can be repaired by a simple purse-string suture. In small lacerated wounds, closure should be effected transverse to the long axis of the bowel in order to prevent narrowing of the lumen. Resection should be avoided as much as possible, and, even when the perforations are closely situated, individual closure is preferable if this permits adequate repair. On the other hand, if the *perforations* are *large* and are *located near each other*, if the

bowel is practically divided or if the segment is destroyed, resection should be done. Resection is also necessary in cases in which a segment of bowel is devitalized because of interference with its blood supply as a result of detachment of its mesentery or division or thrombosis of the mesenteric vessels. When resection is necessary, end-to-end anastomosis with a double row of sutures is preferred.

In dealing with *wounds of the mesentery,* the essential factors are arrest of hemorrhage and viability of the bowel. In cases in which the wound in the mesentery has not interfered with the blood supply of the intestine, hemorrhage is best controlled by individual ligation of the vessels at the torn edges. In such cases, closure of the wound by suturing is inadvisable and is best accomplished by grasping the

edges with forceps and then ligating the tissue at the tips of the approximated forceps. In the presence of a hematoma in which bleeding has apparently stopped and in which evidence of impairment of the blood supply of the nearby intestines can be excluded, nothing need be done. If, however, even a suspicion of continued bleeding remains or if the hematoma is enlarging, a search for the bleeding vessel is unavoidable.

The use of chemotherapy to control infection and of supportive measures with intravenous fluids, blood and plasma is essential to successful therapy. Physiologic rest of the bowel for the first few days postoperatively should be established by avoiding oral feedings and by instituting gastro-intestinal intubation and suction.

ABDOMINAL WOUNDS II

Mesentery

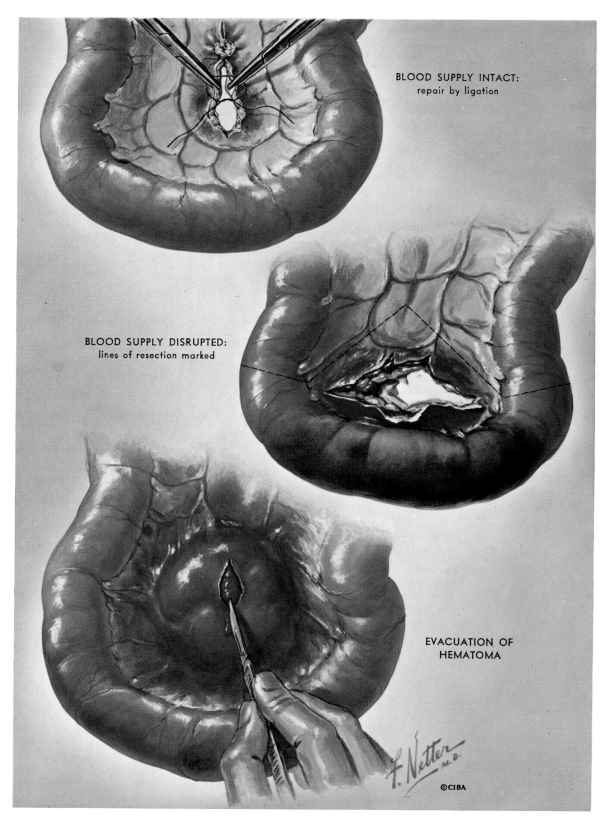

BLOOD SUPPLY INTACT:
repair by ligation

BLOOD SUPPLY DISRUPTED:
lines of resection marked

EVACUATION OF
HEMATOMA

In World War I the small intestine and its mesentery comprised 22 and 37 per cent of all abdominal injuries in the American and British forces, respectively. Other viscera which may be injured in association with wounds of the small intestine are, in the order of their frequency, the colon, stomach, bladder, liver, kidneys, rectum and spleen. The ileum (71 per cent) is most frequently involved; the jejunum (23 per cent) is next; and duodenal injuries (6 per cent) are the least frequent. In an analysis of 3,154 abdominal injuries treated by the 2nd Auxiliary Surgical Group in World War II, duodenal injuries comprised 3.7 per cent and injuries of the jejunum and ileum 37 per cent.

Because of the multiple coils of small intestine, usually more than one segment of the bowel is injured even by a single projectile. Bullets may cause contusion of the outer intestinal coat but usually produce small punctate wounds, one on each side of the bowel, with everted mucosa giving the appearance of small rosettes. In other cases, especially when the path of the bullet has approximated the long axis of the bowel, the perforations are more extensive, varying from simple slits to large gaping wounds that almost completely divide the bowel. Fragments of shells and bombs usually produce greater tissue damage with more variable and irregular wounds. Bayonet and knife wounds, which are almost non-existent in modern warfare, vary from small slits to actual division of the bowel. Lesions of the small intestine also can be produced by nonpenetrating injuries resulting from falling masonry, water blast concussions or other crushing injuries of the abdominal wall. Hemorrhage

occurs in all perforating wounds of the small intestine, the amount depending upon the extent of damage to the vessels of the mesentery.

Wounds of the mesentery, variable in type and extent, sometimes occur as independent lesions but are usually complications of intestinal wounds. They range from simple *hematomas* or *perforations* to irregular, jagged tears or *lacerations*. Their significance lies in the degree of damage to the vessels supplying the bowel. Damage to these vessels may result in hemorrhage between the leaves of the mesentery or into the retroperitoneal space with the formation of a hematoma, or into the peritoneal cavity. The mesentery may be torn in a relatively avascular area, with little hemorrhage, or it may be detached from the intestine, with consequent devitalization of this segment of bowel.

The clinical manifestations of injuries of the small

intestine depend upon the same factors mentioned in the discussion of wounds of the stomach (see CIBA COLLECTION, Vol. 3/1, page 163). Abdominal pain and evidence of peritoneal irritation, with localized or diffuse tenderness and rigidity, are common.

Among abdominal war injuries, those of the small intestine are perhaps the most important, because of their relative frequency and high mortality. In World War I the mortality was about 70 per cent, including all cases with or without operation. Injuries of the duodenum were associated with the highest mortality, 80 per cent; the jejunum was next, 78.8 per cent; and the ileum, 73 per cent. In World War II the mortality figures recorded by the 2nd Auxiliary Surgical Group were as follows: duodenum, 56.8 per cent; jejunum and ileum, 29.5 per cent. The most common causes of death are peritonitis, hemorrhage and shock.

ABDOMINAL WOUNDS III
Colon

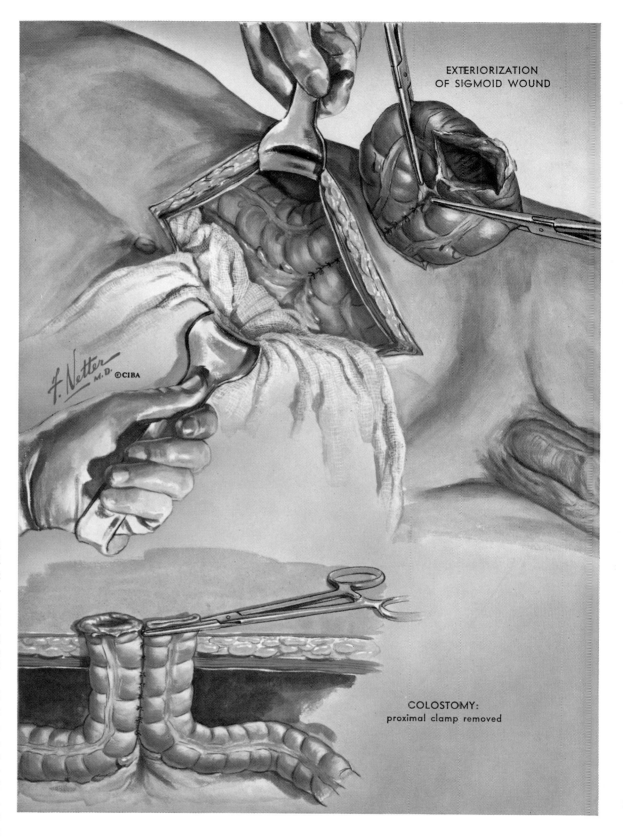

EXTERIORIZATION
OF SIGMOID WOUND

COLOSTOMY:
proximal clamp removed

Of all abdominal injuries in World War I, from 22 to 26 per cent involved the colon, and from 40 to 60 per cent were associated with injury of other viscera, according to American and British reports, respectively. In World War II the incidence of colon injuries among 3,154 abdominal injuries treated by the 2nd Auxiliary Surgical Group was 33.8 per cent.

Injuries of the colon vary from isolated bruised areas to large perforations or extensive, ragged tears, with infarction. In contradistinction to the small bowel, wounds of the colon are less liable to be multiple. Isolated bruised areas are occasionally found remote from the tract of the inflicting agent, and, in some cases, the outer coats of the bowel wall will be found ruptured and stripped back from the intact mucosal layer. Multiple lesions, when present, usually involve the flexures and pelvic colon. Small lesions involving the ascending and descending portions of the colon may be intraperitoneal or extraperitoneal and are particularly grave, because they may be easily overlooked and because of the vulnerability of the retroperitoneal tissues to anaerobic infection. Wounds of the colon are frequently associated with injuries to other viscera in the injured region.

The clinical symptoms of wounds of the colon and those of the small bowel are practically the same. Uncomplicated wounds and small perforations, espe-cially if they are extraperitoneal, may cause few early symptoms, so that thorough exploration of a suspected area is essential. Shock is usually apparent if the wound is a large one.

In general, the prognosis in wounds of the colon is grave. The total mortality ranged at approximately 59 per cent in World War I. In World War II, how-ever, this figure was reduced to about 36 per cent. In small, uncomplicated wounds involving the more distal part of the bowel, the prognosis is more favorable if spillage of semisolid fecal material is slight and if operation is performed early.

The necessity of careful exploration makes a median or paramedian incision the most desirable. A supplementary incision by lateral extension may be necessary to provide adequate exposure in wounds involving the hepatic or splenic flexures or the transverse colon. In some cases in which injury of the cecum or ascending or descending colon has been extraperitoneal with no intraperitoneal involvement, the lesion is best dealt with through a transverse flank incision which permits ready access to the posterior portion and avoids contamination of the general peritoneal cavity.

Surgical treatment consists essentially in repair by suture or in *exteriorization of the damaged segment*. Because of the extensive nature of war wounds, suture can be done in relatively few cases. However, in small tears, in simple, uncomplicated perforations or in incomplete injury of the bowel wall, suture may suffice. A double row of sutures should always be employed and, whenever possible, reinforced by

(Continued on page 200)

ABDOMINAL WOUNDS III

Colon

(Continued from page 199)

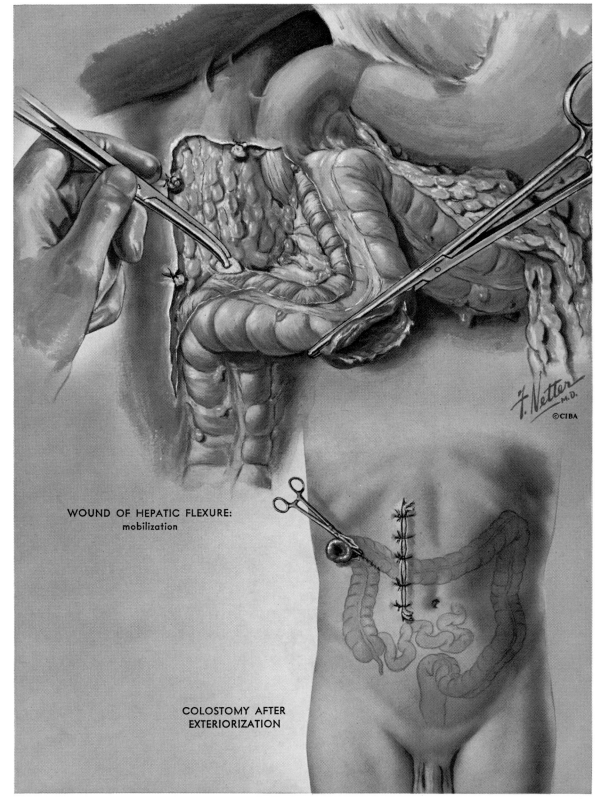

WOUND OF HEPATIC FLEXURE:
mobilization

COLOSTOMY AFTER
EXTERIORIZATION

a superimposed graft of the omentum or an appendix epiploica. If immobile parts are injured, which precludes exteriorization, repair must also be accomplished by suture. Proximal *colostomy* should always be done in these cases.

Local suture is usually inadequate, and resection of the damaged segment is necessary, because colon wounds are commonly extensive and are frequently associated with considerable contusion, infarction, hematoma and contamination in the retroperitoneal regions. Resection is best accomplished by exteriorization, a procedure which was widely employed in World War II and probably constitutes one of the most important advances in war surgery of the abdomen. The *damaged segment* is *drawn out,* usually through a separate incision, as the apex of the colonic loop, and permitted to function as a colostomy. This procedure avoids the dangers associated with resection and anastomosis, and simultaneously permits the utilization of a colostomy. The damaged colonic loop of the transverse colon is more conveniently brought out through a midline incision. Injuries of the other parts of the colon are best handled by bringing out the damaged loop through a small lateral incision either in the iliac fossae or in the hypochondriac regions. In performing *exteriorization,* it is desirable to make a long loop and approximate its limbs by suture to form a spur, because this facilitates

final closure. Mobilization is necessary in injuries of the flexures. The apex of the colonic loop is drawn through the lateral incision by means of a rubber tube passed through the mesentery and around the gut, or by forceps introduced through the lateral incision and applied to the bowel. The sutured limbs are then returned to the abdomen, leaving only the injured apex outside. It can be fixed to the abdominal wall by inserting a piece of rubber tubing or a glass rod under the apex of the loop and between the colonic loop and the skin surface, or by applying a forceps to the gut and strapping it to the skin for 24 to 48 hours. The colostomy may be allowed to function immediately or within a few hours after closure of the abdominal wall. In cases necessitating resection, exteriorization is similarly performed, except

that the damaged segment is excised between clamps, resulting in a double-barreled colostomy. The proximal clamp is removed to permit immediate functioning of the colostomy, and the distal clamp is strapped to the abdominal wall to support the two limbs and allow them to become fixed to the parietes.

For the closure of the incisions following the repair of intestinal wounds, and especially those of the large bowel in which exteriorization has been done, nonabsorbable suture material and, preferably, wire should be employed and introduced through the entire thickness of the abdominal wall as stay sutures, avoiding tension. Layered closure of the peritoneum and fascia may be done, using interrupted sutures and a strip of Vaseline® gauze laid between the skin edges.

ABDOMINAL WOUNDS IV

Rectum

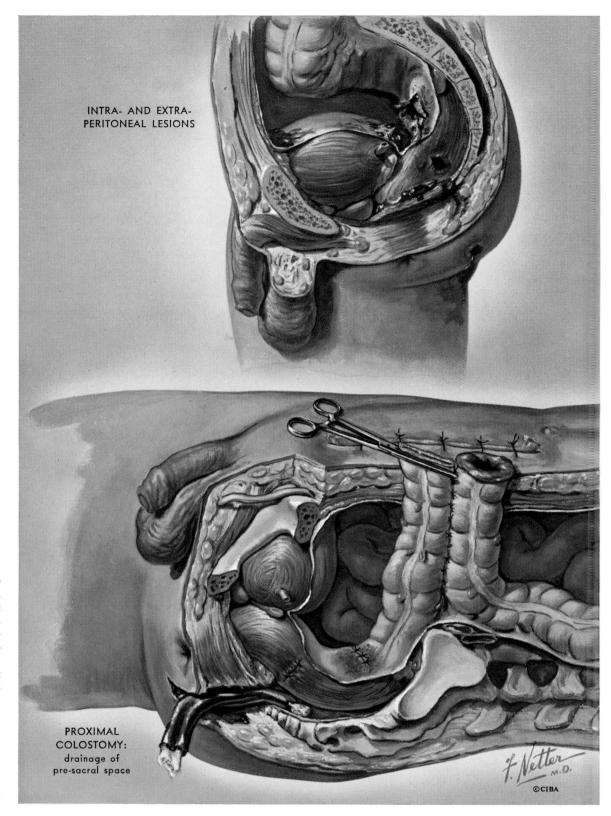

INTRA- AND EXTRA-
PERITONEAL LESIONS

PROXIMAL
COLOSTOMY:
drainage of
pre-sacral space

Injuries of the rectum occur less frequently than those of other abdominal viscera but are particularly important because of their gravity. In World War I they comprised 2.4 per cent of all abdominal injuries. In World War II the incidence of rectal injuries among abdominal injuries was 3.7 per cent. They are most often associated with lesions of the bladder, the pelvic colon and the small intestine.

Wounds of the rectum vary in type and extent. They may be extraperitoneal, intraperitoneal, or both. The lesion often consists of a small perforation, produced by a small missile or a fragment of pelvic bone, or as an extensive laceration produced by shell fragments of high explosives or land mines. The entrance wound in such injuries frequently is located posteriorly or posterolaterally in the thigh or buttocks and may deceptively suggest that the bowel has been missed. In some cases, damage to tissues externally is extensive, with tearing and laceration of the gluteal region and destruction of the anus and lower rectum. In others, the anal region remains intact, the injury being limited to the lower portion of the rectum. These cases are particularly dangerous because of infection in the extraperitoneal perirectal region. Rectal injuries are especially prone to anaerobic infection. The intraperitoneal portion of the rectum can also be injured in cases in which the missile has entered from behind or from the side. Such wounds

are not infrequently associated with fracture of the bones of the pelvis. These cases are commonly accompanied by injury of the bladder or small bowel. In addition to peritonitis, danger of infection in the presacral areolar tissue is imminent.

The signs and symptoms of rectal wounds vary with the type and extent of injury. All wounds of entrance in the buttocks and thighs should be examined for possible rectal injury, because of the great danger of retroperitoneal infection which is characterized by a severe degree of sepsis, referred to in World War I as "colon septicemia".

The mortality in World War I in wounds of the rectum was 45 per cent, but in World War II this figure was reduced to 23 per cent. Shock, fulminating infection in the retroperitoneal space and peritonitis are the most common causes of death.

The treatment of rectal injuries consists essentially

in débridement of the external wound, repairing the bowel, providing adequate drainage of the retrorectal space whenever possible, and diverting the fecal stream by temporary colostomy.

The opening in the bowel should be closed by suture whenever possible. The general peritoneal cavity must be closed off. Drainage of the retroperitoneal tissues should be effected by an incision behind the anus. Exploratory laparotomy should be done in practically all cases, and injuries to other viscera should be properly treated. Openings in the intraperitoneal portion of the rectum should be closed by suture. An inguinal *colostomy* should be done in cases in which the injury involves the lower rectum. However, if the injury involves the rectosigmoid portion of the bowel, it is apparent that subsequent reconstructive surgery will be necessary, and a transverse colostomy is desirable.

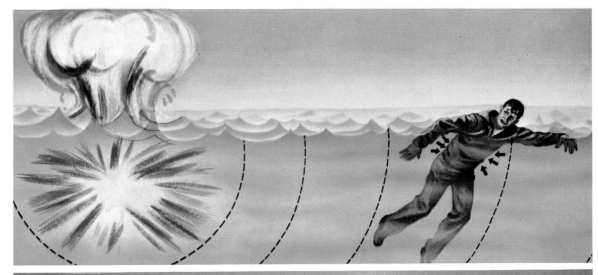

Abdominal Wounds V

Blast Injuries

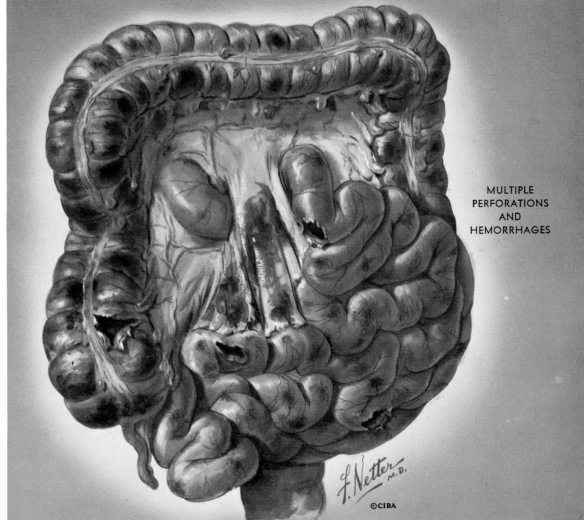

MULTIPLE
PERFORATIONS
AND
HEMORRHAGES

F. Netter M.D.

©CIBA

Immersion or "underwater" *blast injuries of the abdomen* are produced by a sudden wave of positive pressure from underwater explosions. When such waves strike men floating nearby, the intra-abdominal organs, and to some extent the intrathoracic, suffer most damage. The mechanism is not completely understood, but probably the pressure is transmitted through the body as if the tissue were water.

The size of the charge, distance from the explosion, amount of gas in the hollow viscera, and perhaps the position and the degree of submersion influence the extent and type of injury. The gastrointestinal tract injuries consist essentially of intramural hemorrhages and perforations. The former are mostly multiple and petechial and involve the submucosal and subperitoneal layers of the small intestine, especially the lower ileum and cecum. They also occur in the stomach, esophagus, colon, mesentery and omentum. Their size and shape vary widely. The larger lesions appear chiefly in the colon and, if massive, often lead to gangrene of the bowel. Bleeding also occurs in the loose areolar retroperitoneal tissue. Perforations or tears are less frequent and are more likely to involve the small intestine. They are circular or linear, with everted edges, giving a blownout appearance. Generalized or localized peritonitis often appears later.

Coincident with the explosion, the patient experiences a shocklike sensation, a griping pain, a temporary, paralyzing numbness of abdomen and legs, testicular pain or an urge to urinate or defecate. Symptoms usually have abated by the time of rescue, but severe, sharp and stabbing or colicky abdominal pain soon develops. Severe nausea, hematemesis, bloody diarrhea, diffuse abdominal tenderness and rigidity appear in cases with perforation; peritoneal irritation is pronounced, and free air can be demonstrated roentgenographically in the peritoneal cavity. Symptoms subside relatively rapidly in the absence of perforation. Evidence of blast injury of the lung can also be present.

The prognosis depends upon the extent of visceral injury; the mortality, in cases without intestinal perforation, is probably not above 10 per cent, whereas in cases with intestinal perforation, the mortality rate will be over 50 per cent. Early deaths are due to shock and late deaths to peritonitis. Associated injury of the lungs increases the gravity of the condition.

When it is fairly certain that no perforation has occurred, treatment is conservative and like that of other nonpenetrating abdominal injuries. Resuscitative measures must be instituted early, but plasma and blood transfusions should be administered cautiously in cases of lung injury. For the same reason, anesthesia is a difficult problem. Cyclopropane has been advocated, since it affords a high concentration of oxygen and is less irritating.

In case of doubt or where signs of perforation are evident, laparotomy should be done as early as possible. Exploration must be thorough, and all perforations must be closed. In extensive damage, resection is necessary. In addition to the customary postoperative measures, oxygen, continuous gastroduodenal suction and chemotherapy are important.

Section XIV

HERNIAS

by

FRANK H. NETTER, M.D.

in collaboration with

ALFRED H. IASON, M.D.
and
BEN PANSKY, Ph.D.

HERNIA I

Indirect and Direct Inguinal Hernias

Hernia (a word derived from the Greek, meaning "sprouting forth") has been defined, from the time of A. Cornelius Celsus (second century A.D.) to the most modern texts and medical dictionaries, as a protrusion of organs or parts thereof, through an abnormal opening, from their natural place in a cavity. Such a definition is unsatisfactory in that it does not cover those situations in which protruded parts have returned or have been returned, are held back by mechanical means or even have not yet protruded and only the potentiality of a protrusion may be recognized. Thus the characteristic of hernias is not the protrusion of a viscus but rather the opening through which such a protrusion may occur (Zimmerman and Anson). To designate and separate the various hernias, the medical literature, in contrast to the commonly accepted definition of hernia, quite logically uses not the protruded viscus but the location or region in which a hernia can take place and provides us with names such as diaphragmatic, abdominal, hiatal, retroperitoneal, mesenteric, paraumbilical, vaginal, etc., hernia.

Of all these locally distinct varieties, the two kinds of *inguinal hernia* are by far the most frequent (approximately four fifths) and have their highest incidence of onset in the first year of life, declining up to the time of adolescence to reach a second, though lower, peak of frequency between the ages of 16 and 20. Inguinal hernia is also at least four times as frequent in males as in females, and this fact points to an etiologic relationship, namely, to a developmental process connected with the descent of the testes (see CIBA COLLECTION, Vol. 2, page 26) in fetal life. The testes, originally intra-abdominal, retroperitoneal structures, while migrating downward to traverse the anterior abdominal wall, push ahead of themselves a fold of peritoneum, known as the *funicular process* (see Plate 2), or processus vaginalis. This process is normally obliterated during the last month of intra-uterine life, becoming a thin, solid strand of connective tissue (ligamentum vaginale). If it fails to be obliterated, *i.e.*, if it remains *partially* or *completely patent*, a peritoneal pouch or sac persists, presenting the congenital predisposing factor for an *indirect inguinal hernia*. Although this assumption

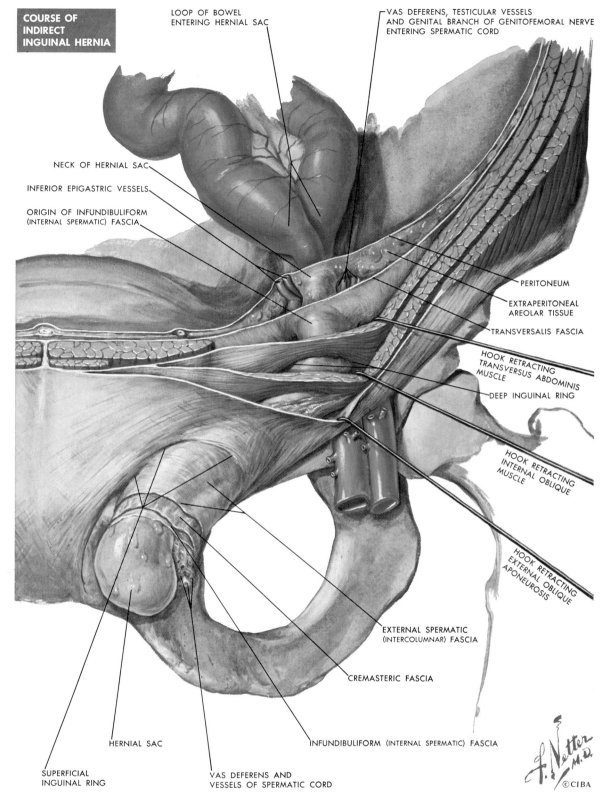

COURSE OF INDIRECT INGUINAL HERNIA

LOOP OF BOWEL ENTERING HERNIAL SAC

VAS DEFERENS, TESTICULAR VESSELS AND GENITAL BRANCH OF GENITOFEMORAL NERVE ENTERING SPERMATIC CORD

NECK OF HERNIAL SAC

INFERIOR EPIGASTRIC VESSELS

ORIGIN OF INFUNDIBULIFORM (INTERNAL SPERMATIC) FASCIA

PERITONEUM

EXTRAPERITONEAL AREOLAR TISSUE

TRANSVERSALIS FASCIA

HOOK RETRACTING TRANSVERSUS ABDOMINIS MUSCLE

DEEP INGUINAL RING

HOOK RETRACTING INTERNAL OBLIQUE MUSCLE

HOOK RETRACTING EXTERNAL OBLIQUE APONEUROSIS

EXTERNAL SPERMATIC (INTERCOLUMNAR) FASCIA

CREMASTERIC FASCIA

INFUNDIBULIFORM (INTERNAL SPERMATIC) FASCIA

HERNIAL SAC

SUPERFICIAL INGUINAL RING

VAS DEFERENS AND VESSELS OF SPERMATIC CORD

F. Netter M.D.
©CIBA

was strongly disputed some decades ago, it is now fairly generally accepted that the preformed sac in the inguinal canal is a predisposition for an indirect hernia (Zimmerman and Anson), though this should not be interpreted that the hernia itself is of congenital nature. Numerous individuals of both sexes* have been found with a patent funicular process without ever having shown any signs of a hernia. Others "acquire" a complete hernia (meaning thereby the protrusion of a viscus through the inguinal ring) only late in life.

Thus one must accept the fact that factors other than the patent funicular process play a rôle in permitting intra-abdominal structures to enter the sac. Normally, the deep (internal) inguinal ring (see also pages 17 to 19) serves as a perfect closure against the egression of any structure within the abdominal cavity. If, however, the funicular process is not obliterated completely, the sac may grow in size or may be

the object of pathologic changes resulting in damage of fascial and muscular elements and thereby lead to incompetence of the ring. Such a concept has not, however, been proved, and the more generally accepted theory is that a disparity exists between intraabdominal pressure and resistance of the fascial and muscular structures participating in the formation of the deep inguinal ring. The process responsible for the increase in abdominal pressure and enhanced tension on the wall may be a slow, steady one as in pregnancy, ascites or other space-consuming conditions, but it may also be a sudden event of traumatic

(Continued on page 205)

*The analogue of the funicular process in the female is the canal of Nuck (see CIBA COLLECTION, Vol. 2, page 91), which passes through the inguinal canal, consisting also of the remnants of a tubular peritoneal fold, which accompanies the round ligament of the uterus to its insertion in the labium majus.

HERNIA I

Indirect and Direct Inguinal Hernias

(*Continued from page 204*)

nature such as a fall, the lifting of heavy objects, etc., or repeated, intermittently occurring stresses on the wall, such as coughing, sneezing and vomiting, which exert increased pressure against a wall weakened for one reason or another.

For the understanding of the etiology, the pathology, the clinical manifestations and, particularly, the surgical repair of an indirect inguinal hernia, a profound knowledge of the anatomy of this region is indispensable. The anatomy has been illustrated and discussed on pages 17 to 19.

In acquired inguinal hernia the ring becomes dilated in time or, as in a congenital hernia, is wide enough from the very start to permit passage of the small or large intestine, the omentum or the bladder (see page 213). The size of the sac depends on its contents. It lies always anterosuperior to the spermatic cord, which contains the ductus deferens, the testicular, cremasteric and deferential vessels, the pampiniform plexus, lymphatic vessels and nerves. The narrow proximal part of the sac, which is continuous with the parietal peritoneum, is called the "neck" of the sac; the distal part is known as the "fundus". The coverings of the hernial sac are the same as those of the spermatic cord under normal conditions (see page 19). The peritoneal innermost layer is covered by areolar tissue, the internal spermatic (infundibuliform) fascia derived from the transversalis muscle and the musculofascial cremasteric layer, essentially deriving from the internal oblique muscle and aponeurosis. In moderate (more so in advanced) cases of indirect inguinal hernia, the obliqueness of the inguinal canal (see page 17) is mostly lost. With the widening of the deep (internal, abdominal) ring and the increased masses filling the canal, the two inguinal rings (deep and superficial) start to lie more and more perpendicular above each other. A medial displacement of the inferior epigastric vessels (see pages 14 and 16) is another consequence of this directional shift of the inguinal canal.

The diagnosis of an uncomplicated indirect inguinal hernia is made by inspection and palpation. Small hernias are, at times, better observed by inspection of the patient in a standing position than by palpation. This is particularly true with women and children in whom

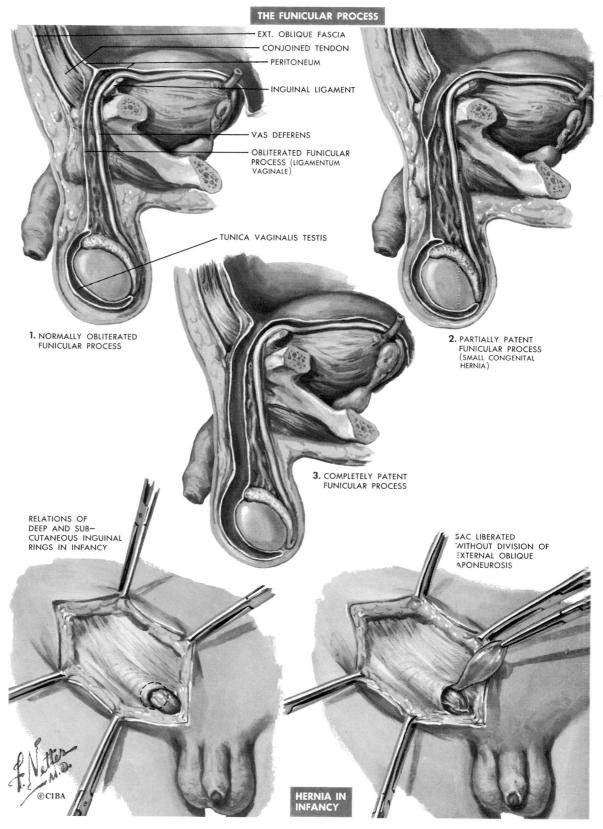

THE FUNICULAR PROCESS

EXT. OBLIQUE FASCIA
CONJOINED TENDON
PERITONEUM
INGUINAL LIGAMENT
VAS DEFERENS
OBLITERATED FUNICULAR PROCESS (LIGAMENTUM VAGINALE)
TUNICA VAGINALIS TESTIS

1. NORMALLY OBLITERATED FUNICULAR PROCESS

2. PARTIALLY PATENT FUNICULAR PROCESS (SMALL CONGENITAL HERNIA)

3. COMPLETELY PATENT FUNICULAR PROCESS

RELATIONS OF DEEP AND SUB-CUTANEOUS INGUINAL RINGS IN INFANCY

SAC LIBERATED WITHOUT DIVISION OF EXTERNAL OBLIQUE APONEUROSIS

HERNIA IN INFANCY

the expansile impulse on coughing or straining is not easily felt, owing to a varying amount of overlying fat. With a visible soft swelling in one or both inguinal regions, which increases on standing, straining or coughing and which disappears on gentle pressure or when the patient reclines, the diagnosis of an indirect hernia offers no problem, except occasionally with regard to the differentiation of the indirect type from the direct type (see below). If the herniated organ has protruded as far as the scrotum, consideration must be given to the possibility of other scrotal swellings, such as a hydrocele (see CIBA COLLECTION, Vol. 2, page 67), a varicocele (ibidem, page 68) or even testicular tumors (see ibidem, pages 84 and 85) and, in females, labial cysts, abscesses or tumors (see ibidem, pages 134, 135 and 136). The swelling may be so small that it escapes the patient's attention, or that of the mother or even a nurse in the case of an infant.

Even in adults an existing herniation may be discovered only incidentally on thorough physical examination, which always should include a search for a hernia. The histories of the patients are mostly noncontributory, although an increased incidence of hernia in families has been reported by several authors. Some patients, especially those who are middle-aged or elderly, may relate pain or discomfort in the lower abdominal quadrants, or the appearance of a swelling, with some sort of an accident or a specific event of strain, but the frequency and intensity of pain vary greatly from individual to individual. In general, however, moderate or even extensive protrusion of abdominal contents through an enlarged deep inguinal ring causes usually, except for cases with incarceration (see page 214), less discomfort than do those cases with a sudden onset.

(*Continued on page 206*)

HERNIA I

Indirect and Direct Inguinal Hernias

(Continued from page 205)

The patients should be examined in the supine as well as the erect position, first with the flat hand over the inguinal region, the finger tips resting over the superficial (subcutaneous) inguinal ring and exercising a slight pressure along the inguinal canal. Second, with the palmar surface of the hand reposing over the patient's thigh, the fifth finger should be gently pushed forward through the superficial ring invaginating the scrotal skin. The protruding abdominal tissue can thus be felt while the patient is completely relaxed. A patent but empty sac cannot be felt and diagnosed, but requesting the patient to use his abdominal musculature to increase the abdominal pressure or asking him to cough will often be helpful in discovering the functional incompetence of the deep inguinal ring and will force a part of the abdominal contents to enter the canal, so that the palpating finger feels it directly or at least feels a change or shift of the tissues within the canal. In infants the examination is naturally not so simple, and a hernia, when reduced, is hardly recognizable. Thickening of the cord at the superficial ring is said to be a reliable sign of a hernia, provided it is unilateral so that the cord on both sides can be compared (Ladd). Children with a left-sided congenital inguinal hernia have an even chance of soon revealing one on the other side. Oddly, this is not true of a right-sided hernia.

When women are concerned, the best diagnostic method consists in placing two fingers over the subcutaneous inguinal ring and palpating for an expansile impulse on coughing or, better, on a more steady increase of intra-abdominal pressure as produced by voluntary contraction of the abdominal musculature.

The treatment of choice in indirect inguinal hernia is surgical repair. A more conservative procedure, namely, the use of a truss, destined to prevent, by mechanical means, the abdominal contents from entering the inguinal canal, has been employed since ancient times and has remained in the medical armamentarium up to the twentieth century. With the development of modern surgery, with the progress made in anesthesia and postoperative care and with the avoidance of handling or of infections, however, it is generally, if not unanimously, agreed that this palliative therapy, with its inherent hazards and inconveniences to the patients, has little

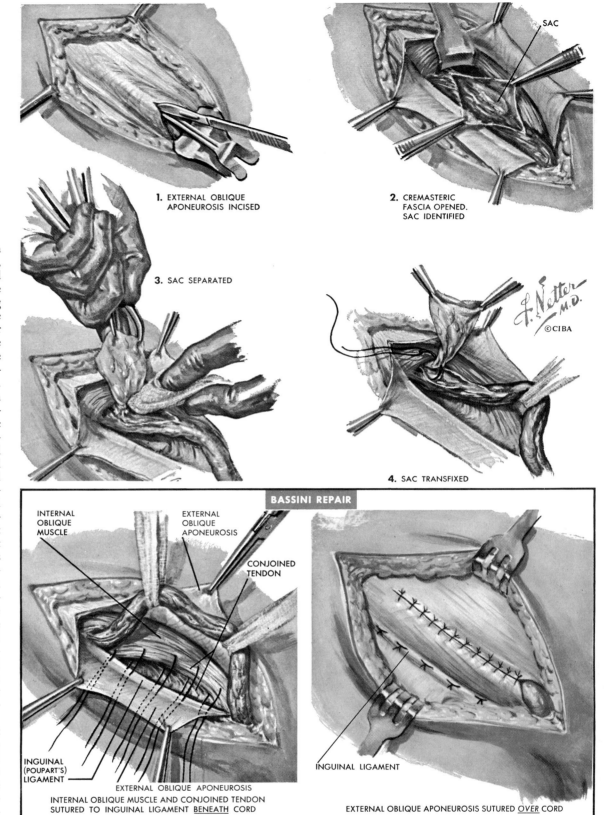

1. EXTERNAL OBLIQUE APONEUROSIS INCISED

2. CREMASTERIC FASCIA OPENED. SAC IDENTIFIED

SAC

3. SAC SEPARATED

4. SAC TRANSFIXED

BASSINI REPAIR

INTERNAL OBLIQUE MUSCLE

EXTERNAL OBLIQUE APONEUROSIS

CONJOINED TENDON

INGUINAL (POUPART'S) LIGAMENT

EXTERNAL OBLIQUE APONEUROSIS
INTERNAL OBLIQUE MUSCLE AND CONJOINED TENDON SUTURED TO INGUINAL LIGAMENT <u>BENEATH</u> CORD

INGUINAL LIGAMENT

EXTERNAL OBLIQUE APONEUROSIS SUTURED <u>OVER</u> CORD

or no advantage over the cure which, in the majority of cases, surgical repair can accomplish. A truss may, nevertheless, remain useful in cases in which for some reason (debility, old age) surgery cannot be performed. In newborns the application of a simple yarn truss for a period of 2 to 6 months is sometimes sufficient to prevent the protrusion of the abdominal contents and to allow for the spontaneous closure of a funicular process not obliterated at birth, but this method is not used much today, and surgical repair is preferred at any age.

A second nonoperative treatment of inguinal hernia, the injection of sclerosing agents, once enthusiastically advocated and practiced by some authors, has now quite generally been abandoned.

The surgical treatment of an inguinal hernia in

infants is relatively simple and can be expeditiously accomplished in 10 minutes. Many authors take the stand that the operation should be carried out as soon as the diagnosis is made, irrespective of the child's age. Ligation of the sac is all that is required, because in infants the deep inguinal ring is almost adjacent to the superficial ring, and it is not necessary to divide the external oblique aponeurosis. The canal, being extremely short, remains undisturbed during the operation, for which only a few contraindications, such as skin infections of the inguinal region, acute exanthemas, respiratory infections or a poor nutritional state, must be considered. Surgical intervention in infants is no longer purely elective but is urgently required in the presence of an extroversion

(Continued on page 207)

HERNIA I

Indirect and Direct Inguinal Hernias

(Continued from page 206)

of the urinary bladder, an undescended testis, with or without torsion (see CIBA COLLECTION, Vol. 2, page 73), or an ectopia testis. In male infants the first incision is made over the subcutaneous inguinal ring and extended laterally toward the anterosuperior iliac spine parallel with the inguinal ligament. The subcutaneous (superficial epigastric) blood vessels are ligated and divided. The aponeurosis of the external oblique muscle and the superficial ring are exposed. With the superficial (Camper's) and the deep (Scarpa's) fasciae in view, the neck of the sac can be found. The fascial investments of the cord are divided so that the thin sac, closely adherent to the superior and medial parts of the cord structures, is seen through the internal spermatic fascia. This fascia and the vas are bluntly separated from the sac down to its neck. The sac is opened, to make sure that it is empty, and is then brought down by gentle traction, twisted and transfixed as high as possible, and its redundant part is tied and amputated directly above the level of the parietal peritoneum. The stump then disappears in the peritoneal cavity. The skin is united with interrupted sutures. A small strip of gauze, immersed in collodion, is placed as a waterproof dressing. An extra layer of gauze is superimposed. In female infants with an inguinal hernia — a relative rarity — a small sac is found on the ventral aspect of the round ligament, which, at times, cannot be easily identified, so that isolation of the sac may be difficult. Otherwise, the operation proceeds along the same lines as in the male infant.

The number of operations, techniques and modifications thereof recommended for indirect hernia in the adult are legion. Modern surgery of inguinal hernias began about 70 years ago, when Bassini (in Padua, Italy) and Halsted (in Baltimore, Maryland) simultaneously and independently developed operative techniques, the fundamental principles of which were identification and excision of the persistent sac, reparation of the defective deep ring and strengthening of the posterior wall of the inguinal canal. In the *Bassini operation* (see Plate 3) an incision 8 to 10 cm. long is made parallel to the inguinal ligament (about 2 to 3 cm. above it). It extends from a point above the middle of the inguinal ligament to the spine of the os pubis. Cutting through the skin and the superficial

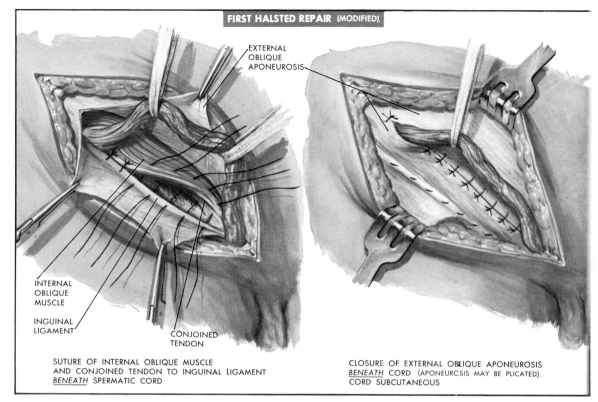

FIRST HALSTED REPAIR (MODIFIED)

SUTURE OF INTERNAL OBLIQUE MUSCLE AND CONJOINED TENDON TO INGUINAL LIGAMENT *BENEATH* SPERMATIC CORD

CLOSURE OF EXTERNAL OBLIQUE APONEUROSIS *BENEATH* CORD (APONEUROSIS MAY BE PLICATED). CORD SUBCUTANEOUS

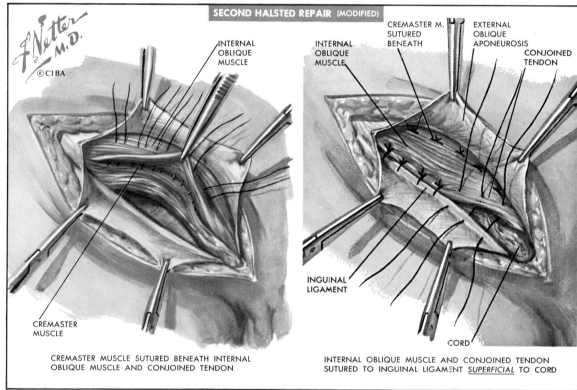

SECOND HALSTED REPAIR (MODIFIED)

CREMASTER MUSCLE SUTURED BENEATH INTERNAL OBLIQUE MUSCLE AND CONJOINED TENDON

INTERNAL OBLIQUE MUSCLE AND CONJOINED TENDON SUTURED TO INGUINAL LIGAMENT *SUPERFICIAL* TO CORD

fascia, one exposes the aponeurosis of the external oblique muscle and the subcutaneous inguinal ring, the superficial epigastric artery and vein, the superficial external pudendal artery, a branch of the superficial circumflex iliac artery (see page 36) and the corresponding veins. *Placing a grooved director in the ring* and passing it obliquely upward and laterally for about 5 cm., the *aponeurosis is split* upward (see Fig. 1, Plate 3) and laterally along the lines of its fibers. The edge of the upper flap is bluntly separated medially and upward, exposing the lateral margin of the abdominal rectus sheath. The edge of the lower flap is turned downward and laterally as far as the shelving portion of the inguinal ligament, avoiding carefully any injury to the iliohypogastric and ilio-inguinal nerves (see page 43). The *cremasteric fascia,* with the adherent, thin internal spermatic fascia, *is opened,* so that the structures of the sper-

matic cord and the hernial sac become visible (see Fig. 2, Plate 3). The sac overlies the cord and is bluntly dissected to its neck (Fig. 3, Plate 3). It is then opened and inspected to identify any contents that may be present. Omentum or bowel, if found, is replaced in the peritoneal cavity. The *sac is twisted,* and a transfixion suture is placed through and around and securely tied (see Fig. 4, Plate 3). The stump of the sac is allowed to retract into the preperitoneal space. The floor of the inguinal canal is then strengthened by stitching the conjoined tendon to the shelving portion of the inguinal ligament. For this act, several techniques have been recommended. Having reconstituted the inguinal canal, the cord, which has been kept outside the operating field during the previous procedures, is then dropped back into position, and the cut edges of the external oblique aponeurosis

(Continued on page 208)

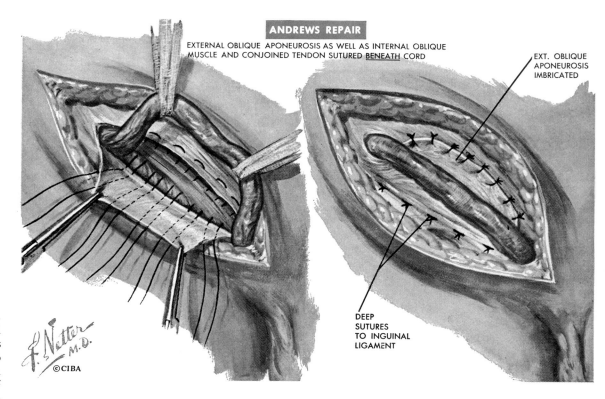

ANDREWS REPAIR

EXTERNAL OBLIQUE APONEUROSIS AS WELL AS INTERNAL OBLIQUE
MUSCLE AND CONJOINED TENDON SUTURED BENEATH CORD

EXT. OBLIQUE
APONEUROSIS
IMBRICATED

DEEP
SUTURES
TO INGUINAL
LIGAMENT

Hernia I

Indirect and Direct Inguinal Hernias

(*Continued from page 207*)

are approximated and sutured over it. The superficial fascia and skin are closed in the usual manner. The inadequacies of the Bassini repair can be attributed to the laceration and strangulation which follow the suturing of muscle fibers of the conjoined tendon, which is essentially a muscular structure and is brought into an abnormal position by being stitched to the inguinal ligament. The "tendon" may return later to its normal position, producing a gap in the posterior wall of the canal. Furthermore, the muscle fibers may separate, permitting a direct inguinal hernia to develop at the site of the new aperture.

The *operation* described independently *by Halsted* (see Plate 4) was practically identical with the Bassini technique, except that, in order to make the cord thinner, several veins of the pampiniform plexus were excised, and the aponeurosis of the external oblique muscle was sutured beneath the cord instead of over it. Later, Halsted abandoned the practice of excising the veins and subsequently devised another procedure, in which the cremaster muscle was sutured beneath the internal oblique muscle and the conjoined tendon to the inguinal ligament over the cord. This technique has, however, fallen into disuse, and the term "Halsted operation" now generally denotes a procedure in which not only the internal oblique muscle and conjoined tendon but the external oblique aponeurosis as well are sutured beneath the cord, and the latter comes to lie subcutaneously.

Using the *"Andrews repair"*, which may be considered a modification of the "Halsted operation", the internal oblique muscle and the conjoined tendon are sutured, together with the superior flap of the external oblique aponeurosis, to the shelving edge of the inguinal ligament by a single row of mattress sutures. The lower flap of the external oblique aponeurosis is then imbricated beneath the cord.

Another of the many modifications of the basic Bassini or Halsted operation is the one more recently advocated by McVay and Anson. In this technique the pectineal (Cooper's) ligament (see page 19), instead of the inguinal liga-

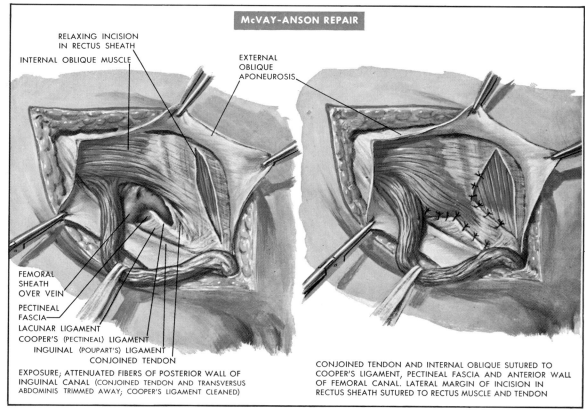

McVAY-ANSON REPAIR

RELAXING INCISION
IN RECTUS SHEATH

INTERNAL OBLIQUE MUSCLE

EXTERNAL
OBLIQUE
APONEUROSIS

FEMORAL
SHEATH
OVER VEIN

PECTINEAL
FASCIA

LACUNAR LIGAMENT

COOPER'S (PECTINEAL) LIGAMENT

INGUINAL (POUPART'S) LIGAMENT

CONJOINED TENDON

EXPOSURE; ATTENUATED FIBERS OF POSTERIOR WALL OF
INGUINAL CANAL (CONJOINED TENDON AND TRANSVERSUS
ABDOMINIS TRIMMED AWAY; COOPER'S LIGAMENT CLEANED)

CONJOINED TENDON AND INTERNAL OBLIQUE SUTURED TO
COOPER'S LIGAMENT, PECTINEAL FASCIA AND ANTERIOR WALL
OF FEMORAL CANAL. LATERAL MARGIN OF INCISION IN
RECTUS SHEATH SUTURED TO RECTUS MUSCLE AND TENDON

ment, is utilized as the principal anchoring line for the internal oblique muscle and the conjoined tendon. The attenuated fibers of the conjoined tendon are removed in this operation, and its remaining parts as well as the internal oblique and transversus abdominis muscles are sutured to the lacunar ligament and the pectineal fascia (see pages 14 and 19), the suture line actually being carried onto the anterior wall of the femoral sheath (carefully avoiding any injury to the femoral vein). A relaxing incision is made in the anterior wall of the rectus sheath. The external oblique aponeurosis is then closed over the cord. This technique has been widely accepted, its advocates pointing out that it fits in better with the anatomic situation, that it affords a more effective and secure closure of the inguinal canal and — most important of all — that the results are better, with a lower incidence of recurrence.

The *direct inguinal hernia* has an etiologic and pathologic background quite different from that of the indirect oblique inguinal hernia. Rare in children, the direct type, in the vast majority of instances, is observed at from 40 to 50 years of age, with a strong preponderance in males. Thus, although considered an acquired disease, it nevertheless must be traced back to a congenital condition characterized by a poorly developed musculofascial wall in the lowermost portion of the internal oblique muscle, where the fibers, instead of coursing obliquely, are arranged more transversely. Furthermore, partly as a result of the transverse course of the fibers, the conjoined tendon is attached to the sheath of the rectus muscle at a variable distance above the pubic crest. The predisposing factor of a direct hernia is thereby assumed to be a deficient protection of the inguinal (Hessel-

(*Continued on page 209*)

Hernia I

Indirect and Direct Inguinal Hernias

(Continued from page 208)

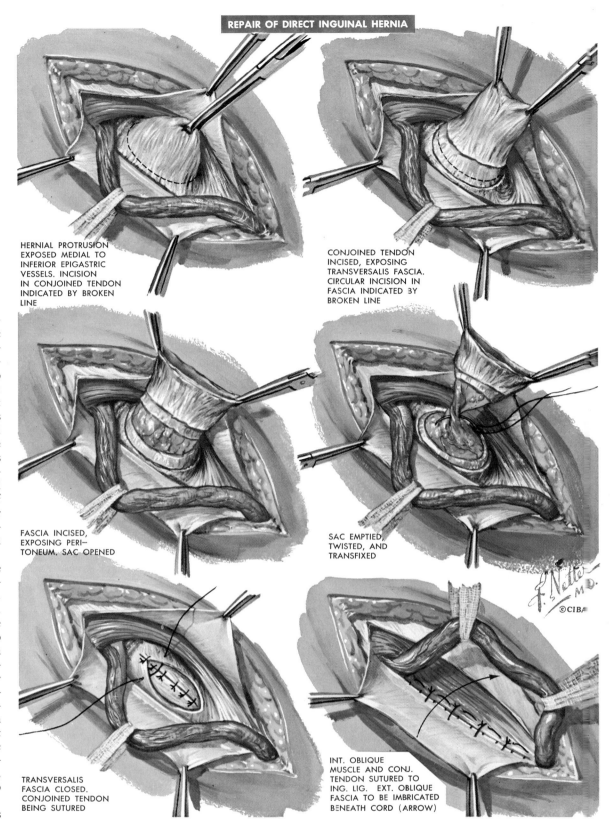

HERNIAL PROTRUSION EXPOSED MEDIAL TO INFERIOR EPIGASTRIC VESSELS. INCISION IN CONJOINED TENDON INDICATED BY BROKEN LINE

CONJOINED TENDON INCISED, EXPOSING TRANSVERSALIS FASCIA. CIRCULAR INCISION IN FASCIA INDICATED BY BROKEN LINE

FASCIA INCISED, EXPOSING PERI-TONEUM. SAC OPENED

SAC EMPTIED, TWISTED, AND TRANSFIXED

TRANSVERSALIS FASCIA CLOSED. CONJOINED TENDON BEING SUTURED

INT. OBLIQUE MUSCLE AND CONJ. TENDON SUTURED TO ING. LIG. EXT. OBLIQUE FASCIA TO BE IMBRICATED BENEATH CORD (ARROW)

bach's) triangle (see page 16), particularly of its lateral angle. The characteristic anatomic feature of a direct inguinal hernia is that it protrudes medial to the inferior epigastric vessels instead of lateral to them, as with the indirect hernia. In other words, the direct hernia does not pass through the deep ring but bulges through the posterior wall of the inguinal canal. The precipitating causes may be laborious and/or prolonged strenuous occupations in the erect position that produce a great increase in intra-abdominal pressure, or a material enlargement of the abdominal contents, as in obesity or ascites, or a progressive atrophy of abdominal muscles owing to advanced age or a wasting disease.

The clinical manifestations of the direct inguinal hernia are even less noticeable than are those of the indirect type. The onset is insidious and asymptomatic. The patient, upon viewing himself in the mirror, or the physician, incidental to a general checkup, becomes aware of a more or less painless swelling in the inguinal area. The mass is reduced instantly when the patient lies down and can reappear in the recumbent position on straining, or on arising. With an increase in size, though this is uncommon, the direct inguinal hernia remains in the area above the inguinal ligament, expanding medially, in contrast to the indirect variety, which, as a rule, enlarges downward into the scrotum.

The protrusion only rarely emerges from the subcutaneous ring and usually remains small and incomplete. The globular mass is found close to the lateral border of the os pubis, the spermatic cord resting superficially and laterally upon the protrusion. With the hernia reduced, the same maneuver outlined for the diagnosis of indirect hernia (see above) is carried out to ascertain the presence or absence of the direct hernia and the tips of two fingers, placed firmly over the inguinal canal medial to the deep ring, are used to establish an expansile impulse when the patient is requested to make a straining effort. If the impulse is felt by the index finger as coming from the floor of the canal, pushing the finger outward, instead of being felt on the tip of the fifth finger as coming from above down-

ward, the hernia is likely to be of the direct type.

The objective of the surgical treatment is to close the defect at the inguinal triangle. Here, again, several techniques have been recommended. The one described and depicted (Iason repair) has given satisfactory results. An incision is made along the long axis of the protrusion and is carried over the superficial inguinal ring far enough to give clear exposure of the pubic tubercle. The external oblique aponeurosis is divided in such fashion as to expedite the preparation of a large lower flap for subsequent imbrication. The spermatic cord structures are separated, isolated and retracted. A circular incision is made through the attenuated fibers of the conjoined tendon after the sac has been drawn outward under gentle traction. Similarly, the transversalis fascia, which then comes into view, is severed by a circular circumcision, whereupon the peritoneal sac, freed from the spermatic

cord, is opened for inspection. If the bladder interferes with complete mobilization, it is separated from the sac by blunt dissection, and a bladder diverticulum (see page 213), if present, is removed, and the resultant bladder defect is closed. Twisting the sac, transfixing it at its base and removing it, the transversalis or internal spermatic fascia is then sewed overlappingly and interruptedly over the sac stump. The suture of the conjoined tendon to the inguinal ligament or to the pectineal ligament is carried out with interrupted strands, and the external oblique aponeurosis is doubly closed (imbricated), either under or over the cord. If the pectineal ligament is used as the anchoring structure, its dangerous proximity to the femoral vessels must always be borne in mind. It may be necessary to utilize a flap of the anterior rectus sheath to reinforce the inguinal canal if the musculofascial structures are too weak.

PSOAS MAJOR MUSCLE
ANTERIOR SUPERIOR ILIAC SPINE
ILIACUS MUSCLE
ILIAC FASCIA
OBTURATOR ARTERY
EXTERNAL ILIAC ARTERY AND VEIN
INFERIOR EPIGASTRIC ARTERY AND VEIN
ROUND LIGAMENT
INGUINAL LIGAMENT
FEMORAL RING
LACUNAR (GIMBERNAT'S) LIGAMENT
COOPER'S LIGAMENT
SUPERIOR PUBIC RAMUS
FOSSA OVALIS COVERED BY CRIBRIFORM FASCIA
FALCIFORM MARGIN
SUPERFICIAL EPIGASTRIC VEIN
LONG SAPHENOUS VEIN
SUPERFICIAL EXTERNAL PUDENDAL VEIN
PUBIC TUBERCLE

F. Netter M.D.
©CIBA

Hernia II

Femoral Hernia

A protrusion of parts of abdominal viscus or of peritoneal fatty tissue through the femoral ring is termed *femoral hernia*. Its incidence is far lower than that of the inguinal hernia. It is very seldom seen in children and is more common in women than in men (ratio 3:1). The right side is affected twice as frequently as is the left. Little is known about its etiology. Few authors maintain that a femoral hernia originates from a preformed congenital sac. In view of the fact that predisposing peritoneal diverticula have been found at autopsy in adults and very seldom in infants and children, and also that far more parous than nonparous women develop a femoral hernia, it seems more probable that it is an acquired condition, in which an increased intra-abdominal pressure is an important etiologic factor. The protruding structures, pushing ahead their peritoneal covering and adherent tissue (mostly fat tissue), descend almost vertically behind and beneath the inguinal ligament and through the femoral ring (see page 19). This ring presents the superior margin of the normally only potential space, known as the "femoral canal", which is in reality the most medial portion of the venous compartment of the femoral sheath (see pages 14 and 19), *i.e.*, anteriorly a downward prolongation of the transversalis fascia over the femoral vessels and posteriorly a continuation of the pectineal fascia deriving from the iliac fascia. Medially, these two fascial layers are adherent to each other and, as they descend, they blend with the adventitia of the vessels, so that the sheath assumes a "funnellike" configuration around the vessels. Just below the inguinal ligament, the femoral sheath (and its most medial portion, the femoral canal) lies under cover of the fascia lata, except in the region of the *fossa ovalis* where the cover consists of the much weaker cribriform fascia. An advancing femoral hernia,

COURSE OF HERNIAL SAC THROUGH FEMORAL RING, FEMORAL CANAL, AND FOSSA OVALIS

SAC TURNED UPWARD OVER INGUINAL LIGAMENT ALONG SUPERFICIAL EPIGASTRIC VEIN

BILOCULAR SAC DUE TO ABERRANT OBTURATOR ARTERY

after having entered the femoral ring, opens up the femoral canal, *displacing and narrowing the femoral vein*. The hernial sac usually emerges through the fossa ovalis, pushing the cribriform fascia ahead of it. The *sac may then turn upward* and may even extend to the region in front of or above the inguinal ligament by following the *superficial epigastric vessels* (see pages 36 and 37), or the sac may turn medially toward or into the scrotum or labium majus, respectively. Laterally, the sac may pass over the femoral vessels or may descend downward along the saphenous vein. The neck, however, remains always below the inguinal ligament and lateral to the pubic tubercle, and the fundus of the sac lies usually in the medial part of Scarpa's triangle (trigonum femorale). A rather surprising number of varieties, some indeed very rare, have been described. The *sac may rest on the femoral sheath* anterior to the femoral

vessels (prevascular hernia) or may descend behind the vessels (retrovascular hernia). The sac may become divided at the femoral ring, one part following the normal route, another being directed toward the obturator foramen. A *femoral hernia* may also become *bilocular* by virtue of an aberrant obturator artery. It also has been observed that a direct inguinal hernia may shift to the femoral region instead of descending into the scrotum (cruro-scrotal hernia), thus simulating a femoral hernia.

Femoral hernias can be easily overlooked if small, but when part of the intestine is contained in the sac, pain is likely to be severe in the extreme. Strangulation occurs with great frequency. The diagnosis can usually be made upon finding a soft tumor at the femoral fossa and by ascertaining the location of the tumor below the inguinal ligament and lateral to the

(Continued on page 211)

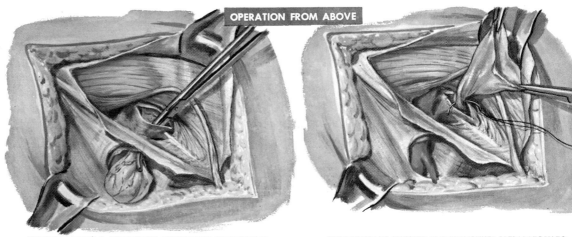

OPERATION FROM ABOVE

LIBERATION OF SAC: CONVERSION OF FEMORAL TO INGUINAL
HERNIA THROUGH INCISION IN TRANSVERSALIS FASCIA

SAC DRAWN UP, TWISTED AND TRANSFIXED PREPARATORY TO
LIGATION AND EXCISION

HERNIA II

Femoral Hernia

(Continued from page 210)

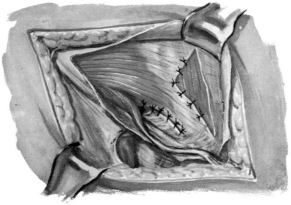

INTERNAL OBLIQUE MUSCLE AND CONJOINED TENDON SUTURED
TO COOPER'S (PECTINEAL) LIGAMENT AND PECTINEAL FASCIA

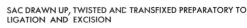
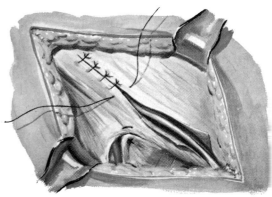

CLOSURE OF EXTERNAL OBLIQUE APONEUROSIS *OVER* ROUND
LIGAMENT OR CORD. INGUINAL LIGAMENT SUTURED TO
PECTINEAL FASCIA

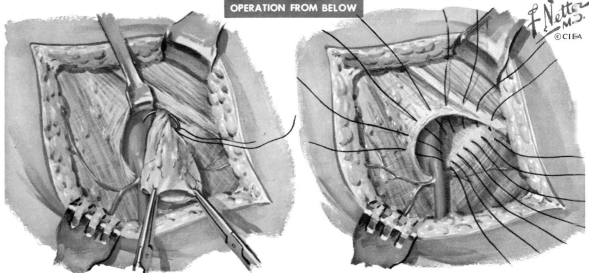

OPERATION FROM BELOW

SAC FREED, OPENED, EMPTIED, TWISTED AND
TRANSFIXED HIGH UP

BASSINI'S CLOSURE OF FEMORAL CANAL

pubic tubercle. Difficulties in the differential diagnosis may arise if the hernial sac has turned upward over the inguinal ligament along the superficial epigastric vein. In diagnosing a femoral hernia, reducible or not, one must exclude also inguinal adenitis, lipoma, varicosities of the saphenous vein, psoas abscess, obturator hernia, hydrocele of the femoral sac, hydatid cysts, dermoid cysts and other processes, which can produce a local, soft and fluctuant swelling. The omentum and small bowel are the most frequently herniated structures, but the presence of an appendix, usually inflamed, or of a Meckel's diverticulum, or of a portion of the bladder (type of sliding hernia; see page 212), ureter or broad ligament has also been observed.

The treatment of a femoral hernia is surgical. Conservative therapy by mechanical means is of little or no avail. A variety of surgical procedures have been devised, indicating that none of them is completely and absolutely satisfactory for all cases. In the main, *two avenues of approach,* the *"high"* or inguinal and the *"low"* or femoral, are available. The end results of the two approaches are about equally successful, but comparisons are difficult, even assuming that the degree of experience of the authors who used the two techniques was the same. It can, however, be stated that the frequency of recurrences is higher with the femoral than with the inguinal hernias.

With the patient in the Trendelenburg position, the "high" operation is started by making an incision 8 to 10 cm. long, parallel to and directly above the inguinal ligament. The lower flap is retracted downward and the upper flap is elevated, so that the environs of the inguinal canal and the hernial sac can be completely cleared from the adherent tissues. By incision of the aponeurosis of the external oblique muscle, the inguinal canal is exposed, and by dissecting

the flaps backward the conjoined tendon, the cremaster muscle and the spermatic cord (or round ligament, respectively) are brought into view. After elevating the latter structure an incision 2 cm. long, through the transversalis fascia, opens the posterior wall of the inguinal canal. A blunt, curved clamp, inserted through this opening, is passed downward superficially and medially to the sac behind the inguinal ligament, and the fundus of the sac is drawn upward, twisted and transfixed as high as possible, the redundant parts being excised. The inguinal canal is then taken care of according to one of the procedures described for the repair of an indirect inguinal hernia (see pages 206 to 208). The opening of the femoral ring is closed by interrupted sutures running from the lower margin of the inguinal to the pectineal ligament and fascia.

In the "low" operation, with which the femoral

ring and canal are closed directly, an incision 8 to 10 cm. long (proportionate to the size of the tumor) is made over the tumor and carried mesial to the femoral blood vessels. The falciform margin of the fascia lata (lateral margin of the fossa ovalis) and the femoral sheath are thus exposed. The sac is freed from properitoneal fat up to the femoral ring and is opened. Its contents, if any, are reduced. The sac is then drawn down and twisted, bringing parietal peritoneum into view. A transfixion ligature is placed at the base of the neck, and the sac is excised. The femoral "canal" is closed by approximation of the inguinal ligament and the falciform margin of the fossa ovalis to the pectineal fascia medial to the femoral vein. The *"Bassini closure"* utilizes a number of interrupted sutures to accomplish this. The sutures are carried close to the femoral vein, but care must be exercised to avoid injuries to that vessel.

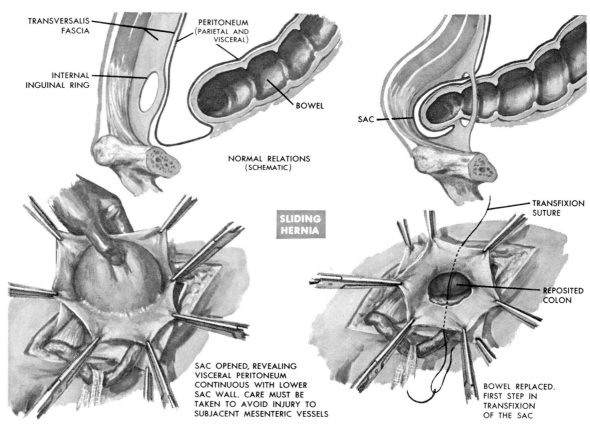

TRANSVERSALIS FASCIA

PERITONEUM (PARIETAL AND VISCERAL)

INTERNAL INGUINAL RING

BOWEL

SAC

NORMAL RELATIONS (SCHEMATIC)

SLIDING HERNIA

TRANSFIXION SUTURE

REPOSITED COLON

SAC OPENED, REVEALING VISCERAL PERITONEUM CONTINUOUS WITH LOWER SAC WALL. CARE MUST BE TAKEN TO AVOID INJURY TO SUBJACENT MESENTERIC VESSELS

BOWEL REPLACED. FIRST STEP IN TRANSFIXION OF THE SAC

HERNIA III

Special Forms and Complications of Inguinal and Femoral Hernias

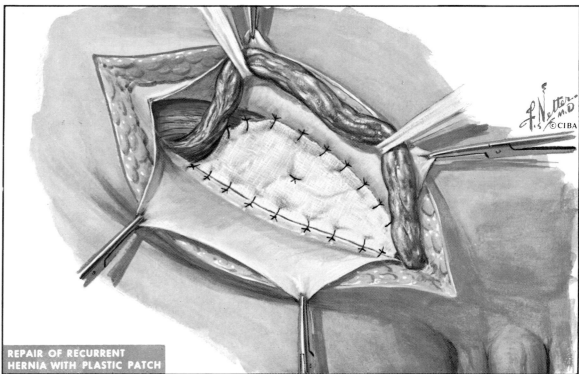

REPAIR OF RECURRENT HERNIA WITH PLASTIC PATCH

A special form of hernia has been termed "*sliding hernia*" ("en glissade"). The protruding structure in this variety of hernia is a partially extraperitoneal viscus such as cecum or colon, or, occasionally, bladder. The most probable mechanism producing such a situation is a partial detachment of the parietal peritoneum from the underlying structure, permitting the parietal peritoneum to "slide" on top of the viscus and its visceral serosa through the hernial opening. The herniated viscus is thus only partially enclosed in the sac, since the posterior margin of the sac is reflected onto the viscus itself to form the visceral peritoneum thereof. It should, however, be realized that the majority of herniations involving the colon are not of the sliding variety. In most instances the large bowel in a hernial sac is entirely covered with peritoneum and is, therefore, freely movable and readily reducible unless adhesions are present. The procedures recommended to repair this "sliding" type of hernia vary less than for the indirect or direct hernia. The peritoneal protrusion, including the contiguous bowel, is drawn into the wound. The sac is opened, and the herniated intestine is freely mobilized by dividing its peritoneal attachment to the peritoneal wall of the sac, carefully avoiding injury to subjacent vessels. When the colon is replaced in the peritoneal cavity, the neck of the sac is obliterated by approximating it to

the transversalis fascia below. The remainder of the operation corresponds to the Andrews or McVay-Anson hernioplasty (see page 208).

The *bladder may herniate* (see Plate 10) through the internal deep inguinal ring as an indirect inguinal hernia or it may pass medial to the deep inferior epigastric vessels as a direct hernia. The protruding part of the bladder may be enclosed in a peritoneal fold (*intraperitoneal indirect* or *direct hernia*), or the peritoneal fold may only partly accompany the protruding organ, lying above it (*direct or indirect paraperitoneal hernia*). These latter forms are in reality "sliding" hernias. A portion of the bladder not covered by peritoneum may herniate, usually by the direct pathway (*extraperitoneal hernia*). Finally, a peritoneal hernial sac may form, entering the inguinal canal through the deep ring, while the bladder, usually an extraperitoneal part, protrudes medial to the inferior epi-

gastric vessels ("*pantaloon*" or saddlebag *hernia*), the vessels, so to speak, forming the "crotch" of the pantaloon. The bladder may enter the hernial sac by becoming adherent to the lateral aspect of the medial wall of the sac, so that the bladder forms one of the sac's covers, particularly in massive hernias. The history presented by patients with bladder protrusion is usually that of a long-standing, large, irreducible hernia, which diminishes or disappears after urination. Besides bladder, the sac often contains intestine and/or omentum. Operation of a bladder hernia involves special techniques, beginning with a rather wide suprapubic incision. If the hernia is of moderate size, it has been customary merely to plicate the redundant part, but, in view of the frequent recurrences in this variety of hernia, it seems advisable to excise the diverticular protrusion and to close the

(Continued on page 213)

INTERNAL RING
TRANSVERSALIS FASCIA
PARIETAL
VISCERAL } PERITONEUM
BLADDER
INFERIOR EPIGASTRIC ARTERY
SPACE OF RETZIUS

INTRAPERITONEAL (INDIRECT)

INTRAPERITONEAL (DIRECT)

PARAPERITONEAL (DIRECT)

PARAPERITONEAL (INDIRECT)

EXTRAPERITONEAL

PANTALOON

HERNIA III

Special Forms and Complications of Inguinal and Femoral Hernias

(*Continued from page 212*)

BLADDER PROTRUSION HAS BEEN RESECTED. OPENING IN BLADDER IS BEING CLOSED WITH CONNELL SUTURE

RE-ENFORCEMENT OF BLADDER WALL WITH INTERRUPTED LEMBERT SUTURES

aperture with a Connell suture, reinforcing it with interrupted Lembert sutures. The remainder of the operation is then the same as with any other direct hernia. A concurrent indirect hernia is treated as indicated above. The preoperative insertion of a catheter into the bladder is important if any suspicion exists that the bladder participates in the contents of the hernial sac.

In the statistical reports of various authors, much has been written about the problem of *recurrent inguinal hernia,* the incidence of which varies from 2 to 20 per cent after operations of indirect hernia and from 4 to 33 per cent in the case of direct inguinal hernia (Zimmerman and Anson). One of the factors responsible for these operative failures is the time at which the operation is performed. The age of the patient and the duration of the hernia undoubtedly have a determining influence on the final results. The advantages of early operation cannot be overlooked and should be made clear to those patients who try for years to put off or delay a surgical intervention. Error in selecting the proper kind of surgical procedure in the repair of a particular kind of hernia, or in the erroneous application of surgical principles in effecting the repair, faulty postoperative care and, in particular, infection may be causes of hernial recurrence, which, even in the best of hands and with every possible care, cannot always

be avoided. The direct causes in an individual case may lie in an incomplete resection of the sac, an inadequate reconstruction of the canal, a residual hiatus in the transversalis fascia or misplacement of the spermatic cord, in insufficient hemostasis, wound infections or simply inherent inadequacy of the musculofascial support. The first step in the treatment of recurrent hernia is a careful presurgical examination and evaluation of the situation, taking into account the type of hernia, location, size, relationship to the cord, etc. The objective of the operation is to replace missing or weak tissue, as soon as practicable, by *fascial transplants* (see Plate 9) or by a patch of some type of mesh. Plastic materials have recently been developed and have proved to be most effective for this purpose. It may be mentioned here that these materials (plastic gauze patch, tantalum and fascia) have been found useful not only in recurrent hernias but

also in primary operations when an extensive defect is encountered or when the tissues are weak and attenuated and will, in all probability, not withstand the strain produced by the operative approximations.

If the sac and the contents of a hernia cannot be replaced within the peritoneal cavity, the hernia is termed an "irreducible" or *"incarcerated hernia"* (see Plate 11). The irreducibility may be caused by a great variety of factors, such as fat deposition of herniated structures (omentum, mesentery), occlusion of the lumen of the herniated intestine, obstruction of its blood supply, obstruction, angulation, compression or torsion of intestinal loops caught in the sac or accumulation of gas. Under favorable circumstances and/or aided by palliative treatment (complete bed rest, hot compresses) an incarcerated hernia may clear away, but surgical intervention is clearly indicated

(*Continued on page 214*)

HERNIA III

Special Forms and Complications of Inguinal and Femoral Hernias

(Continued from page 213)

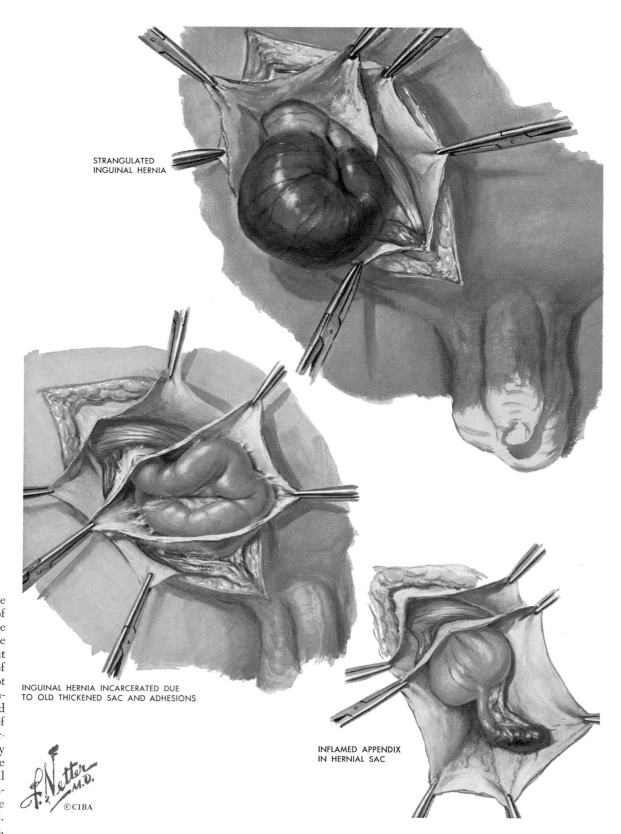

STRANGULATED
INGUINAL HERNIA

INGUINAL HERNIA INCARCERATED DUE
TO OLD THICKENED SAC AND ADHESIONS

INFLAMED APPENDIX
IN HERNIAL SAC

when the situation does not improve within a few hours. The diagnosis of strangulation, *i.e.*, obstruction of the blood supply of a herniated viscus, the onset of which may be very sudden but may also begin slowly with a variety of abdominal discomforts, is usually not difficult. A sharp pain over the very tender hernial area, as well as pain referred to the umbilicus, is present. Vomiting of gastric contents begins early, but its character soon changes to bilious and finally to fecal. All signs and symptoms of acute circulatory collapse, as observed in all more or less suddenly developing abdominal disasters ("acute abdomen", see page 188), develop with surprising speed. Surgical intervention is, in such cases, urgently required. The first operative steps are the same as in nonstrangulated hernias. If the constriction with the ring in open view cannot be relieved digitally, the constricting ring is divided with the knife; this is done laterally in the case of an indirect hernia, to avoid the deep epigastric vessels, and medially, in the case of a direct or femoral hernia, to circumvent the same vessels (or the femoral vessels, respectively). Next, it must be determined whether the herniated intestinal loop is viable or not, and that is one of the most difficult decisions a surgeon faces. Depending on whether the incarcerated loop is still viable (return of red color, restoration of elasticity, firmness and shiny appearance) or has lost its

vitality (black, green or yellowish patches, loss of peritoneal luster, flabby consistency), one may permit the loop to return into the peritoneal cavity or must resect it, and perform an end-to-end anastomosis or an exteriorization. The choice of the anastomosing technique, as well as the question whether the patient is to leave the operating room with a fistula, is for the surgeon to decide at the operating table.

Situations the same as, or very similar to, those found with strangulated hernias arise when the sac or its *contents* or parts thereof become *inflamed*, or when, as a result of prolonged or violent reduction attempts or severe pressure of a poorly applied truss, a loop has ruptured, or when torsion of the omentum has taken place.

A rare condition called "reduction en masse" (displaced hernia) comes into existence when the contents of the hernial sac return to the peritoneal cavity

with the sac, the neck of which is so small and unable to dilate that the intestinal loop cannot retreat. Other complications arise when the sac's contents become inflamed, as may happen especially with the appendix vermiformis, with a Meckel's diverticulum (see page 128) or when only a part of the intestinal wall (partial enterocele, sometimes called Littré's hernia [see page 216]) gets caught in the sac. Needless to say, these phenomena are only seldom diagnosed preoperatively. The same holds true for another variety of hernia, namely, the "hernia in W", or Maydl's hernia (see also page 216), which develops when the sac contains two intestinal loops, the connecting portion between them being left in the peritoneal cavity and becoming squeezed, strangulated (retrograde strangulation) and, finally, gangrenous as a result of a narrow neck and the pressure exercised upon the loops where they enter and leave the sac.

Hernia IV

Ventral Hernia

Strictly speaking, the inguinal hernias are those of the ventral abdominal wall, but, because of their frequency and special characteristics, they are regarded as entities in themselves and are therefore not included under the general term *"ventral hernia"*, which comprises *hernias at the linea alba, at the umbilicus* and *at the semilunar line* (Spigelian hernia). For some reasons the umbilical hernias are, by some authors (Watson), also excluded from the ventral group. Hernia of the linea alba is uncommon but not extremely rare, its incidence having been estimated at 0.4 to 1 per cent of all hernias. It appears more often in men than in women. Usually located above the umbilicus (but occurring also below) just to the left or right of the midline, it is also referred to as "epigastric hernia". Protruding, probably as a result of a weakness in the fascial wall, where ventral cutaneous blood vessels emerge (see pages 36 and 37), these hernias rarely have a peritoneal sac and rarely contain any viscus. At the right of the midline, they usually contain fat of the falciform ligament (see page 16) and at the left properitoneal fat or a properitoneal lipoma. Most epigastric hernias are symptom-free and are discovered only upon routine physical examination. Occasionally, they may cause colicky pain, a "dragging" sensation in the epigastrium, nausea, dyspepsia and even vomiting. In children, epigastric hernias tend to close spontaneously with age. Operative repair is effected by removal of fat, ligation of the neighboring vessels and suture or imbrication of the fascial layers.

Umbilical hernias are found in children up to the age of 3 years, from which time on they become rare but show another maximum of incidence at about 40 years of age. An omphalocele (see page 125) must be differentiated from an infantile umbilical hernia; since the viscera in that condition never entered the abdomen, the omphalocele is not a typical hernia. Often first noticed when the infant raises the intra-abdominal pressure upon crying, causing a protrusion of a bit of intestine, the umbilical hernias are usually small and disappear spontaneously by the third year, sometimes requiring the aid of adhesive strapping. In adults these hernias may also be small; however, they may attain a larger size and cause a variety of symptoms, particularly when a peritoneal sac contains omentum and/or viscera. Large hernias may become irreducible and incarcerated. When small, the umbilical hernias in adults can be controlled by suitable support, but larger ones require operation (opening and emptying of the sac, resection of fat or omentum, imbrication of

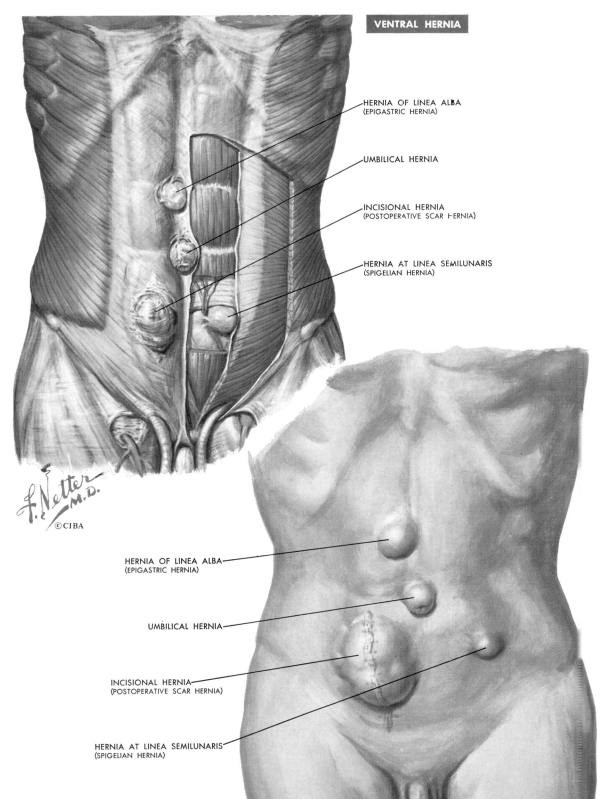

VENTRAL HERNIA

HERNIA OF LINEA ALBA
(EPIGASTRIC HERNIA)

UMBILICAL HERNIA

INCISIONAL HERNIA
(POSTOPERATIVE SCAR HERNIA)

HERNIA AT LINEA SEMILUNARIS
(SPIGELIAN HERNIA)

HERNIA OF LINEA ALBA
(EPIGASTRIC HERNIA)

UMBILICAL HERNIA

INCISIONAL HERNIA
(POSTOPERATIVE SCAR HERNIA)

HERNIA AT LINEA SEMILUNARIS
(SPIGELIAN HERNIA)

fascial layers and, occasionally, use of a plastic patch).

Sometimes, and generally during middle life, with an equal incidence of the sexes, a *hernia* may appear at the *linea semilunaris* (described by Spigel; cf. page 10) and usually close to the point at which this line and the linea semicircularis join and where the inferior epigastric vessels pierce the posterior wall of the rectus sheath (see pages 14, 16, 36 and 37). This hernia, called Spigelian hernia, always has a peritoneal sac, with an overlying lipoma, but seldom reaches more than 2 to 3 cm. in diameter. This type is assumed to be acquired and develops slowly. The symptoms and the surgical repair are similar to those of an umbilical hernia. (Strictly speaking, a direct inguinal hernia is also a hernia in the linea semilunaris.)

The so-called *incisional hernia* appears at the site of a previous laparotomy, the wound of which has not healed per primam. Infection, obesity, postopera-

tional strain, inadequate suture material and nerve injury are some of the etiologic factors of these hernias, which are first in frequency of all ventral hernias. The operative repair must be adapted to the individual case (excision of the scar, aponeurotic imbrication and, if necessary, use of a plastic patch).

A diastasis of the rectus abdominis muscles cannot be considered a true hernia. It comes about by a stretching or widening of the linea alba and is seen shortly after birth as a bulge sometimes extending from the xyphoid process to the umbilicus. It also occurs in adults, mostly in multiparous middle-aged women. In infants the diastasis disappears with development and growth. In adults this condition mostly produces no symptoms, but when it does, and a properly fitted belt does not help, an operation, similar to those recommended for ventral hernia, must be performed.

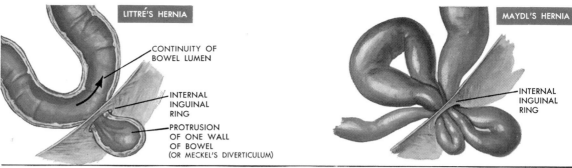

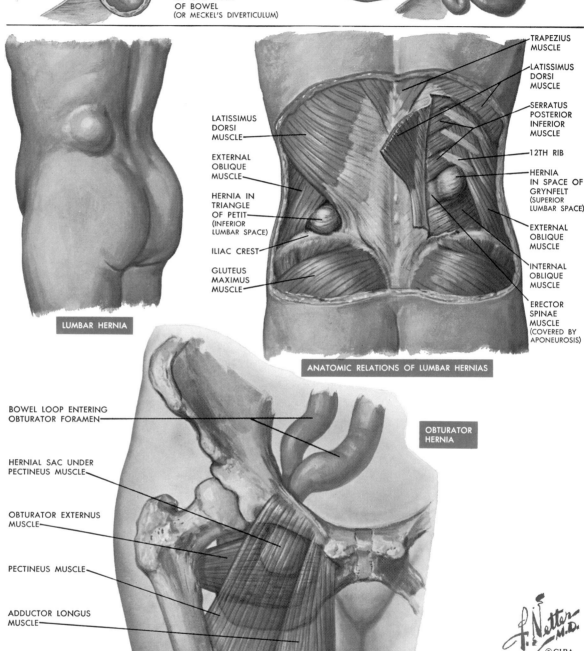

Hernia V

Lumbar and Obturator Hernias

Unusual are hernias which appear in the loin, where two weak spaces offer themselves as openings for protrusions of intra-abdominal structures. The lower of these is the *"inferior lumbar space"* or *"Petit's triangle"* (see page 15), which is bordered laterally (just above the iliac crest) by the posterior margin of the external oblique and medially by the latissimus dorsi muscles. The other, the *"superior lumbar space"*, also known as *"Grynfelt's"* or *"Grynfelt-Lesshaft's triangle"*, is bounded above by the twelfth rib and the serratus posterior inferior muscle, medially by the erector spinae muscle and inferolaterally by the internal oblique muscle. The *lumbar hernias* protruding through these spaces have, as a rule, a sac which consists of peritoneum or of extraperitoneal tissue and which may contain fat, omentum, mesentery, large or small intestine or the kidney, the latter, of course, without any peritoneal investment. The protrusion lies behind a heavy layer of fat or muscle, and, in most cases, a bulge, over which an impulse can be felt on coughing, is the principal or only symptom and sign. Occasionally, the patient complains of pain in the loin, or of nausea. The hernia, usually easily reducible, may become irreducible, but strangulation is only a very rare event. A supporting abdominal belt is sometimes all that is needed as treatment, except when dragging pain, nausea, etc., necessitate a surgical repair (emptying and excision of the sac, approximation and suturing of the fascial and muscular structures, if need be with the aid of a plastic patch).

On occasion, a hernia may develop through the obturator foramen alongside the obturator vessels and nerve (see page 16). The *obturator hernia* consists usually of a peritoneal sac and may contain small or large intestine, appendix, omentum, bladder, ovary, Fallopian tube or

uterus. The sac may pass completely through the foramen and come to lie upon the obturator externus covered by the pectineus muscle. In some instances it may pass between the fasciculi of the obturator externus muscle or may insinuate itself between the layers of the obturator membrane. Needless to say, in view of the depth at which it lies, the diagnosis of an obturator hernia is extremely difficult. A slight bulge may or may not be noticeable as a tender, tense mass in the upper obturator region, *i.e.,* the upper, inner part of the femoral (Scarpa's) triangle, when the patient is in the dorsal position with the thigh flexed, adducted and rotated outward so as to relax the pectineus, adductor longus and obturator internus muscles. Pain, characterized by its distribution along the obturator nerve and known as Howship-Romberg sign, is pathognomonic of an obturator hernia but is by no means invariably present. Pain may extend as a dull

ache down the medial aspect of the thigh to the knee or below it. Rectal or vaginal examination sometimes makes possible palpation of the neck of the sac. It is obvious that the hernia must be fairly large to be felt by means of any examination. Gastro-intestinal symptoms (nausea, vomiting, colicky pain, constipation) rarely appear before complications arise, *i.e.,* when strangulation occurs, which, with an obturator hernia, is a relatively frequent event. The differential diagnosis must take into consideration inguinal adenitis, psoas abscess, obturator neuritis, diseases of the hip joint, internal, perineal and femoral hernias and other causes of intestinal obstruction (see pages 190 and 191). For the operation of obturator hernias, the abdominal, femoral (obturator) and inguinal routes have been described. The first of these seems to be preferred because of the frequent necessity for an intestinal resection.

HERNIA VI
Sciatic and Perineal Hernias

GLUTEUS MAXIMUS
GLUTEUS MEDIUS
SUPERIOR GLUTEAL ARTERY
GLUTEUS MINIMUS
HERNIAL SAC EMERGING ABOVE PIRIFORMIS MUSCLE
PIRIFORMIS MUSCLE
HERNIAL SAC EMERGING BELOW PIRIFORMIS MUSCLE
INTERNAL PUDENDAL VESSELS AND PUDENDAL NERVE
GREATER TROCHANTER OF FEMUR
OBTURATOR INTERNUS TENDON
INFERIOR GLUTEAL ARTERY
SCIATIC NERVE
SACROTUBEROUS LIGAMENT
ISCHIAL TUBEROSITY

ANATOMIC RELATIONS OF SCIATIC HERNIAS

SCIATIC HERNIA

LABIAL HERNIA RESEMBLING CYST OF BARTHOLIN'S GLAND

ISCHIOCAVERNOSUS MUSCLE
BULBOCAVERNOSUS MUSCLE
UROGENITAL DIAPHRAGM

ANTERIOR PERINEAL (LABIAL) HERNIAS
PUBOCOCCYGEUS } LEVATOR ANI
ILIOCOCCYGEUS } MUSCLE
GLUTEUS MAXIMUS MUSCLE
POSTERIOR PERINEAL HERNIAS (INTO ISCHIORECTAL FOSSA)
COCCYGEUS MUSCLE
SACROTUBEROUS AND SACROSPINOUS LIGAMENTS (CUT AWAY)

ANATOMIC RELATIONS OF PERINEAL HERNIAS

The diagnosis of a *sciatic hernia* is as difficult as is that of an obturator hernia, unless it is rather large and bulges into the thigh. These hernias pass through the greater or, much less frequently, through the lesser sciatic notch (see page 11). In the first instance, lying above the ischial spine and the sacrospinous ligament (see page 63), the hernia may emerge either with the superior gluteal artery above the piriform muscle or with the inferior gluteal and internal pudendal vessels and sciatic nerve below the last-named muscle. In any event the hernia passes downward and presents under the lower border of the gluteus maximus muscle in the posteromedial aspect of the thigh. The patients occasionally complain of pain, the distribution of which fits the distributional pattern of the great sciatic nerve. Lipoma, gluteal aneurysm or abscess must enter into the differential diagnosis. Strangulation of the hernial contents occurs frequently and may be the cause of intestinal obstruction. The surgical repair of a sciatic hernia is performed preferably by means of the abdominal route, although a sciatic and a combined approach have also been described.

Perineal hernias escape through the structures forming the floor of the pelvis (see pages 22 and 63). The *anterior variety* of perineal hernias, also known as pudendal or *labial hernias*, which seem to occur exclusively in women, may pass through the urogenital diaphragm and present in the middle of the labium majus, where they resemble the appearance of a cyst of Bartholin's gland (see CIBA COLLECTION, Vol. 2, page 134). They also may emerge just behind the medial part of the urogenital diaphragm and present in the posterior part of the labium near the fourchette. The *posterior perineal hernias* may escape between the subdivisions of the levator ani muscle, between the fasciculi of that muscle or between the levator ani and coccygeus muscles, and in both sexes may enter the ischiorectal fossa (see page 32) to present ultimately below the margin of the gluteus maximus muscle and thus may resemble a sciatic hernia (see above). Perineal hernias usually have a peritoneal sac containing omentum, a loop of the large or small gut or other viscera. These hernias must be differentiated from cysts and tumors of the vulva (see CIBA COLLECTION, Vol. 2, pages 134 to 136) in the case of the anterior variety, and from anorectal abscesses (see page 173) of or tumors growing through the ischiorectal space. The perineal hernias are usually reducible but may occasionally become strangulated. For their repair an abdominal or a combined perineal and abdominal approach has been recommended.

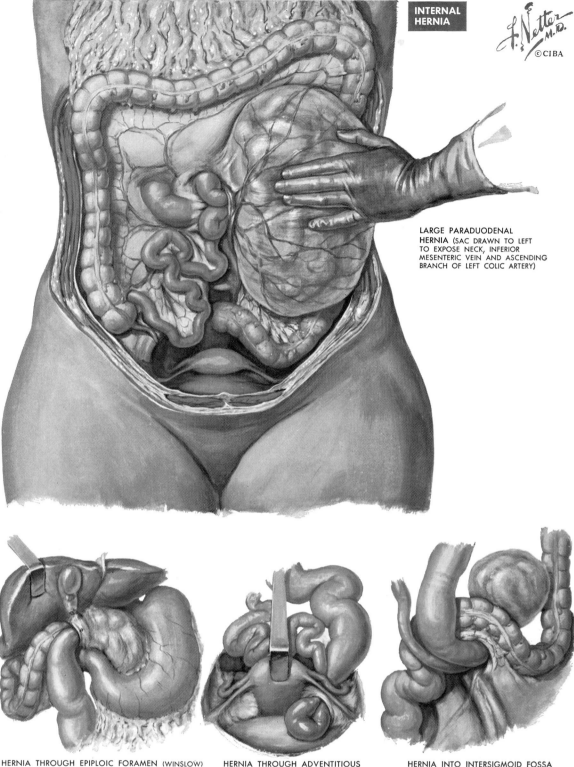

INTERNAL
HERNIA

LARGE PARADUODENAL
HERNIA (SAC DRAWN TO LEFT
TO EXPOSE NECK, INFERIOR
MESENTERIC VEIN AND ASCENDING
BRANCH OF LEFT COLIC ARTERY)

HERNIA VII

Internal Hernia

HERNIA THROUGH EPIPLOIC FORAMEN (WINSLOW)
INTO LESSER PERITONEAL SAC (OMENTAL BURSA)

HERNIA THROUGH ADVENTITIOUS
OPENING IN BROAD LIGAMENT

HERNIA INTO INTERSIGMOID FOSSA

Intra-abdominal structures, essentially a loop of the small intestine, may enter a normal or adventitious peritoneal fossa or orifice and thus form an *internal hernia*. Though this type of hernia is extremely rare, much has been speculated about its origin. The theories proposed to explain the etiology of an internal hernia agree only in so far as all the authors (Andrews, Batson, Burnham, Callander, Estrada, Hansmann and Morton, Miller and Wakefield) assume some sort of abnormal development in fetal life, such as a defect in the mesentery, irregularities during rotation of the midgut (see pages 4 to 6), etc. The common classification of internal hernia follows the anatomic distribution and thus separates (1) paraduodenal, (2) pericecal and (3) intersigmoid hernia. The most important of the fossae which give rise to internal herniation are those in the vicinity of the duodenojejunal junction (superior and inferior duodenal, paraduodenal and mesentericoparietal fossae [see CIBA COLLECTION, Vol. 3/1, page 51]), the epiploic (Winslow's) foramen (see pages 24 and 27), the intersigmoid fossa (see page 54), the fossae at the ileocecal junction and the appendix (see page 51) and an abnormal pocket or adventitious opening in the broad ligament or in the transverse mesocolon.

Very rarely is any internal hernia diagnosed preoperatively, regardless of its location. It may be suspected when signs of intestinal obstruction set in and when a mass in the corresponding region can be palpated. A remarkable feature of an internal hernia is that it may remain asymptomatic during lifetime. In several instances they have been reported as an autopsy finding, the individual never having complained of abdominal discomfort.

In operating on these hernias when they are discovered at a laparotomy, it is important to bear in mind that, in practically every case of internal hernia, a major blood vessel courses across the anterior margin of its neck. It is thus dangerous to incise the neck of the sac, so that it may be preferable to open its wall beyond the neck and to decompress the gut in order to make its reduction possible.

REFERENCES

Section VIII

	PLATE NUMBER
AREY, L. B.: *Developmental Anatomy*, W. B. Saunders Company, Philadelphia, 1954.	1-6
CRELIN, E. S.: *An unusual ectopia cordis in a human stillborn infant*, Yale J. Biol. Med., 30:38, 1957.	2
——: *Eventration of abdominal viscera and other uncommon anomalies in newborn infant*, Anat. Rec., 115:485, 1953.	1-6
HAMILTON, W., BOYD AND MOSSMANN: *Human Embryology*, W. Heffer and Sons Ltd., Cambridge, 1952.	1-6
KEIBEL, F., AND MALT: *Manual of Human Embryology*, Vols. I and II, J. B. Lippincott Company, Philadelphia, 1910 and 1912.	1-6
PATTEN, B. M.: *Human Embryology*, Blakiston Company, New York, 1946.	1-6
POTTER, E. L.: *Pathology of the Fetus and Newborn*, Year Book Publishers, Chicago, 1952.	1-6

Section IX

ADACHI, B.: *Das Arteriensystem der Japaner*, Kenyusha Druckanstalt, Tokyo, 1928.	25, 26
——: *Venensystem der Japaner*, Kenyusha Druckanstalt, Tokyo, 1940.	27, 28
ALBARRAN, J.: *Médicine Operatoire des Voies Urinaires*, Masson et Cie., Paris, 1909.	25
ANSON, B. J., BEATON AND McVAY: *Anatomy of inguinal and hypogastric regions of the abdominal wall*, Anat. Rec., 70:211, 1938.	7
——, CAULDWELL, PICK AND BEATON: *Anatomy of the pararenal system of veins, with comments on renal arteries*, J. Urol., 60:714, 1948.	28
——, ——, AND ——: *Blood supply of kidney, suprarenal gland and associated structures*, Surg. Gynec. Obstet., 84:313, 1947.	28
——, MORGAN AND McVAY: *Anatomy of hernial regions; inguinal hernia*, Surg. Gynec. Obstet., 89:417, 1949.	8-10
—— AND KURTH: *Common variations in the renal blood supply*, Surg. Gynec. Obstet., 100:157, 1955.	27, 28
BATSON, O. V.: *Function of the vertebral veins and their rôle in spread of metastases*, Ann. Surg., 112:138, 1940.	28
——: *Rôle of the vertebral veins in metastatic processes*, Ann. intern. Med., 16:38, 1942.	28
——: *Vertebral vein system*, Caldwell lecture, 1956, Amer. J. Roentgenol., 78:195, 1957.	28
CHANDLER, S. B., AND SCHADEWALD: *Studies on the inguinal region; conjoined aponeurosis versus conjoined tendon*, Anat. Rec., 89:339, 1944.	8-10
CHOUKÉ, K. S.: *Constitution of sheath of rectus abdominis muscle*, Anat. Rec., 61:341, 1935.	4, 5
COLLIS, J. L., SATCHWELL AND ABRAMS: *Nerve supply to the crura of the diaphragm*, Thorax, 9:22, 1954.	12, 30
COUINAND, C.: *Le Foie. Etudes Anatomiques et Chirurgicales*, Masson et Cie., Paris, 1957.	27

Section IX (continued)

	PLATE NUMBER
COURTNEY, H.: *Abscesses of the deep perirectal spaces, their significance, diagnosis and treatment*, N. Y. St. J. Med., 47:2552, 1947.	21-23
CUNEO, B., AND VEAU: *De la significance morphologique des aponeuroses perivesicales*, J. Anat. (Paris), 35:235, 1899.	23
CUNNINGHAM, D. J.: *Textbook of Anatomy*, J. C. Brash, ed., Oxford University Press, New York, 1951.	1-10
CURTIS, A. H., ANSON AND BEATON: *Anatomy of subperitoneal tissues and ligamentous structures in relation to surgery of the female pelvic viscera*, Surg. Gynec. Obstet., 70:643, 1940.	21
DOUGLASS, B. E., BAGGENSTOSS AND HOLLINSHEAD: *The anatomy of the portal vein and its tributaries*, Surg. Gynec. Obstet., 91:562, 1950.	27
FAGARASANU, I.: *Recherches anatomiques sur la veine rénale gauche et ses collatérales; leurs rapports avec la pathogénie du varicocèle essentiel et des varices du ligament large*, Ann. d'anat. path., 15:9, 1938.	28
GALLAUDAT, B. B.: *A Description of the Planes of Fascia of the Human Body with Special Reference to the Fascia of the Abdomen*, Columbia University Press, New York, 1931.	3-10
GILLOT, C., AND HUREAU: *Les anastomoses porto-caves et cavo-caves de la loge sousphrénique gauche. Etude anatomique et physio-pathologique*, J. Chir. (Paris), 79:578, 1960.	28
GOFF, B. H.: *Histological study of the perivaginal fascia in nullipara*, Surg. Gynec. Obstet., 52:32, 1931.	21
GOLIGHER, J. C., LEACOCK AND BROSSY: *The surgical anatomy of the anal canal*, Brit. J. Surg., 43:51, 1955.	21-24
GORSCH, R. V.: *Anorectal fistula; anatomical considerations and treatment*, Amer. J. Surg., 32:302, 1936.	24
——: *Proctologic Anatomy*, Williams & Wilkins Company, Baltimore, 1955.	21-24
——: *Proctologic considerations of the perineopelvic spaces*, Amer. J. Surg., 85:556, 1953.	21-24
GOSS, C. M.: *Gray's Anatomy of the Human Body*, Lea & Febiger, Philadelphia, 1959.	1-20
GRANT, J. C. B.: *Atlas of Anatomy*, Williams & Wilkins Company, Baltimore, 1956.	1-10
GREIG, H. W., ANSON AND COLEMAN: *The inferior phrenic artery*, Quart. Bull. Northw. Univ. med. Sch., 25:345, 1951.	25
HAMMOND, G., YGLESIAS AND DAVIS: *Urachus, its anatomy and associated fasciae*, Anat. Rec., 80:271, 1941.	7
HEALEY, J. E., JR.: *Clinical anatomic aspects of radical hepatic surgery*, J. int. Coll. Surg., 22:542, 1954.	28
—— AND SCHROY: *Anatomy of the biliary ducts within the human liver; analysis of the prevailing pattern of branchings and the major variations of the biliary ducts*, Arch. Surg., 66:599, 1953.	28

Section IX (continued)

	PLATE NUMBER
HOLLINSHEAD, W. H.: *Some variations and anomalies of the vascular system in the abdomen*, Surg. Clin. N. Amer., 35:1123, 1955.	27, 28
HUGHES, A.: *Abnormal arrangement of arteries in the region of the kidney and suprarenal body*, J. Anat. Physiol. (London), 26:305, 1892.	25
JDANOW, D. A.: *Anatomie du canal thoracique et des principaux collecteurs lymphatiques du tronc chez l'homme*, Acta anat. (Basel), 37:20, 1959.	29
JONASSAN, O., LONG, ROBERTS, McGREW AND McDONALD: *Cancer cells in the circulating blood during operative management of genitourinary tumor*, J. Urol. (Baltimore), 85:1, 1961.	28
MASSOPUST, L. C., AND GARDNER: *Infrared photographic studies of the superficial thoracic veins in the females*, Surg. Gynec. Obstet., 91:717, 1950.	27
MERKLIN, R. J., AND MICHELS: *The variant renal and suprarenal blood supply with data on the inferior phrenic, ureteral and gonadal arteries*, J. int. Coll. Surg., 29:41, 1958.	25
MICHELS, N. A.: *Variational anatomy of the hepatic, cystic and retroduodenal arteries*, A.M.A. Arch. Surg., 66:20, 1953.	25
MORRIS, H.: *Morris' Human Anatomy*, ed. by Schaeffer, Blakiston Company, New York, 1953.	1-20
NOTKOVICH, H.: *Variations of the testicular and ovarian arteries in relation to the renal pedicle*, Surg. Gynec. Obstet., 103:487, 1956.	28
SAPPEY, P.: Cited by Couinand.	27
STRAUSS, L. H.: *Beitrag zur motorischten Innervation des Zwerchfelles beim Menschen und bei Tieren*, Z. ges. exp. Med., 86:244, 1933.	34
TANIGUCHI, T.: *Beitrag zur Topographie der grossen Aste der Bauchaorta*, Folia anat. jap., 9:201, 1930.	25
TOBIN, C. E., AND BENJAMIN: *Anatomic and clinical re-evaluation of Camper's, Scarpa's and Colles' fasciae*, Surg. Gynec. Obstet., 88:545, 1949.	3, 4, 8, 9
—— AND BENJAMIN: *Anatomical and surgical restudy of Denonvilliers' fascia*, Surg. Gynec. Obstet., 80:373, 1945.	23
TOREK, F.: *First successful resection of a thoracic portion of the esophagus*, J. Amer. med. Ass., 60:1533, 1913.	25
UHLENHUTH, E.: *Problems in the Anatomy of the Pelvis*, J. B. Lippincott Company, Philadelphia, 1953.	21-24
——: *The rectogenital septum*, Surg. Gynec. Obstet., 86:148, 1948.	21, 22
——, WOLFE, SMITH AND MIDDLETON: *Fasciae and subperitoneal fascial spaces of male pelvic cavity*, Bull. Sch. Med. Maryland, 36:60, 1951.	22-24
WARWICK, R., AND MITCHELL: *The phrenic nucleus of the macaque*, J. comp. Neurol., 105:553, 1956.	34

Section X

	PLATE NUMBER

ABEL, A. L.: *Pecten; pecten band: pectenosis and pectenotomy,* Lancet, 1:714, 1932.   11, 12

ADACHI, B.: *Das Arteriensystem der Japaner,* Kenyusha Druckanstalt, Tokyo, 1928.   18-24

——: *Venensystem der Japaner,* Kenyusha Druckanstalt, Tokyo, 1940.   25-27

ANSON, B. J., AND MADDOCK: *Callander's Surgical Anatomy,* W. B. Saunders Company, Philadelphia, 1958.   5, 6, 11-27

—— AND McVAY: *Topographical positions and mutual relations of visceral branches of abdominal aorta,* Anat. Rec., 67:7, 1936.   18, 21, 22

ASHLEY, F. L., AND ANSON: *The pelvic autonomic nerves in the male,* Surg. Gynec. Obstet., 82:598, 1946.   30

AUERBACH, L.: *Fernere vorläufige Mittheilung über den Nervenapparat des Darmes,* Virchows Arch. path. Anatomie, 30:457, 1864.   31

BACON, H. E.: *Histology and embryology of the anorectal line,* Trans. Amer. proctol. Soc., 33:144, 1932.   13

—— AND SMITH: *Arterial supply of distal colon pertinent to abdominoperineal proctosigmoidectomy, with preservation of sphincter mechanism,* Ann. Surg., 127:28, 1948.   24

BALICE, G.: *L'anatomia chirurgica dell'arteria mesenterica inferiore ed il punto del Sudeck,* G. ital. Chir., 5:1, 1949.   24

BERRY, R. J. A.: *Die Anatomie des Coecum,* Anat. Anz., 10:401, 1895.   5, 6

BLAISDELL, P. C.: *Pathogenesis of anal fissure and implications as to treatment,* Surg. Gynec. Obstet., 65:672, 1937.   13 15

BROSSY, J. J.: *Anatomy and surgery of anal fissure; with special reference to internal sphincterotomy,* Ann. Surg., 144:991, 1956.   12-16

BÜHLER, A.: *Ueber eine Anastomose zwischen den Stämmen der Arteria coeliaca und der arteria mesenterica superior,* Morph. Jb., 32:185, 1904.   21

CAUDWELL, E. W., AND ANSON: *The visceral branches of the abdominal aorta. Topographical relationships,* Amer. J. Anat., 73:27, 1943.   18-21

COURTNEY, H.: *Abscesses of deep perirectal spaces; their significance, diagnosis and treatment,* N. Y. St. J. Med., 47:2552, 1947.   15, 16

DALTON, A. J.: *Electron micrography of epithelial cells of gastrointestinal tract and pancreas,* Amer. J. Anat., 89:109, 1951.   4

——, KAHLER AND LLOYD: *Structure of free surface of series of epithelial cell types in mouse as revealed by electron microscope,* Anat. Rec., 111:67, 1951.   4

DI DIO, L. J. A.: *Anatomo-Fisiologia do Piloro ileo-ceco-colica no homem,* Actas das Primeiras Jornadas Interuniversitarias Argentinas de Gastroenterologia, Rosario, 1954.   6

——: *Dados anatomicos sôbre o "piloro" ileo-ceco-colico. (Com observação direta in vivo de "papila" ileo-ceco-colica.) (English summary)* Thesis, Fac. Med., Univ. de São Paulo, 1952.   6

——: *Personal communication,* April, 1960.   26

Section X (continued)

	PLATE NUMBER

—— AND CARRIL: *Observações sôbre o mecanismo do piloro ileo-ceco-colico em individuo vivo com a papila ileo-ceco-colica exteriorizada* (English summary), An. Fac. Med. Minas Gerais (Brasil), 15:19, 1955.   6

DOGIEL, A. S.: *Ueber den Bau der Ganglien in den Geflechten des Darmes und der Gallenblase der Menschen und der Säugetiere,* Arch. Anat. Physiol. (Leipzig) Anat. Abt., 130, 1899.   31

DOUGLASS, B. E., BAGGENSTOSS AND HOLLINSHEAD: *Anatomy of portal vein and its tributaries,* Surg. Gynec. Obstet., 91:562, 1950.   25, 26

DRUMMOND, H.: *The arterial supply of the rectum and pelvic colon,* Brit. J. Surg., 1: 677, 1913.   21, 24

EISENHAMMER, S.: *The internal anal sphincter and the anorectal abscess,* Surg. Gynec. Obstet., 103:501, 1956.   13

——: *The internal anal sphincter; its surgical importance,* S. Afr. med. J., 27:266, 1953.   12, 14

ELZE, C.: *3rd ed. of Hermann Braus, Anatomie des Menschen,* 2nd Vol., page 266, Springer Verlag, Berlin, 1956.   3

FINE, J., AND LAWES: *On the muscle-fibers of the anal submucosa, with special reference to the pecten band,* Brit. J. Surg., 27:723, 1940.   12-14

FLEISCHNER, F. G., AND BERNSTEIN: *Roentgen-anatomical studies of normal ileocecal valve,* Radiology, 54:43, 1950.   6

GOLIGHER, J. C.: *Adequacy of marginal blood supply to left colon after high ligation of inferior mesenteric artery during excision of rectum,* Brit. J. Surg., 41:351, 1954.   24

——, LEACOCK AND BROSSY: *The surgical anatomy of the anal canal,* Brit. J. Surg., 43:51, 1955.   11-16

GORSCH, R. V.: *Proctologic Anatomy,* Williams & Wilkins Company, Baltimore, 1955.   10-16, 27

GRANGER, B., AND BAKER: *Electron microscope investigation of striated border of intestinal epithelium,* Anat. Rec., 107: 423, 1950.   4

HARSHA, W. T.: *Retrocecal appendix; its diagnosis and surgical approach,* Surg. Gynec. Obstet., 74:180, 1942.   7

HERMANN, G., AND DESFOSSES: *Sur la muquense de la region cloacle du rectum,* C. R. Acad. Sci. (Paris), 90:1301, 1880.   11

HILL, C. J.: *A contribution to our knowledge of the enteric plexus,* Phil. Trans. B., 215: 355, 1947.   31

HILL, M. R., SHRYOCK AND REBELL: *Rôle of anal glands in pathogenesis of anorectal disease,* J. Amer. med. Ass., 121:742, 1943.   12, 13

HILLER, R. I.: *Anal anatomy with reference to white line of Hilton and pecten of Stroud,* Ann. Surg., 102:81, 1935.   27

HOLL, M.: *Die Muskeln und Fascien des Beckenausgangs in Handbuch der Anatomie des Menschen,* Bd. 7, Teil 2, Abt. 2, G. Fischer, Jena, 1897.   11, 14, 15

HUGHES, E. S. R.: *Surgical anatomy of anal canal,* Aust. N. Z. J. Surg., 26:48, 1956.   11-16

Section X (continued)

	PLATE NUMBER

IRWIN, D. A.: *The anatomy of Auerbach's plexus,* Amer. J. Anat., 49:141, 1931.   31

KOELLIKER, A.: *Nachweis eines besonderen Baues der Cylinderzellen des Dünndarms, der zur Fettresorption in Bezug zu stehen scheint,* Verh. phys.-med. Ges. Würzb., 6:253, 1855.   3, 4

KORNBLITH, P. L., AND SIDDHARTH: Unpublished data. (Anatomy Department of Jefferson Medical College, Philadelphia.)   18, 20, 22

KUNTZ, A.: *On the occurrence of reflex arcs in the myenteric and submucous plexuses,* Anat. Rec., 24:193, 1922.   31

LANNON, J., AND WELLER: *The parasympathetic supply of the distal colon,* Brit. J. Surg., 34:373, 1947.   33, 34

LUDWIG, E., AND RICHTERICH: *Morphologische und histochemische Untersuchungen am Stäbchensaum der Darmepithelzelle,* Acta anat., 21:168, 1954.   4

MAGOUN, H. W.: *Descending connections from the hypothalamus;* page 270 in *The Hypothalamus and Central Levels of Autonomic Function,* Williams & Wilkins Company, Baltimore, 1940.   30

MARBURY, W. B.: *Retroperitoneal (retrocolic) appendix,* Ann. Surg., 107:819, 1938.   5

MAYO, C. W.: *Blood supply of the colon,* Surg. Clin. N. Amer., 35:1117, 1955.   18

MEISSNER, G.: *Ueber die Nerven der Darmwand,* Z. rat. Med., 8:364, 1857.   30-33

MEYLING, H. A.: *Structure and significance of the peripheral extension of the autonomic nervous system,* J. comp. Neurol., 99:495, 1953.   30

MICHELS, N. A.: *Blood supply and anatomy of the upper abdominal organs, with a descriptive atlas,* J. B. Lippincott Company, Philadelphia, 1955.   18, 19, 26

MILLIGAN, E. T. C.: *The surgical anatomy and disorders of the perianal space,* Proc. roy. Soc. Med., 36:365, 1943.   11-16

—— AND MORGAN: *Surgical anatomy of the anal canal, with special reference to anorectal fistulae,* Lancet, 2:1150, Nov. 24, 1934; 1213, Dec. 1, 1934.   11-16

MITCHELL, G. A. G.: *Anatomy of the Autonomic Nervous System,* E. & S. Livingstone, Edinburgh, 1956.   30

——: *Cardiovascular Innervation,* E. & S. Livingstone, Edinburgh, 1956.   30

MORGAN, C. N.: *Surgical anatomy of ischiorectal space,* Proc. roy. Soc. Med., 42:189, 1949.   11-16

—— AND GRIFFITHS: *High ligation of the inferior mesenteric artery during operations for carcinoma of the distal colon and rectum,* Surg. Gynec. Obstet., 108:641, 1959.   20, 24

—— AND THOMPSON: *Surgical anatomy of anal canal with special reference to surgical importance of internal sphincter and conjoined longitudinal muscle,* Ann. roy. Coll. Surg. Engl., 19:88, 1956.   14-16

NOER, R. J.: *Hemorrhage as a complication of diverticulitis,* Ann. Surg., 141:674, 1955.   22, 23

PALAY, S. L., AND KARLIN: *An electron microscopic study of the intestinal villus,* J. biophys. biochem. Cytol., 5:363, 1959.   4

Section X (continued)

PLATE NUMBER

Parks, A. G.: *Note on anatomy of anal canal*, Proc. roy. Soc. Med., 47:997, 1954. — 11-15

Patzelt, V.: *Der Darm; in Handbuch der mikroskopischen Anatomie des Menschen* (von Möllendorff, ed.), J. Springer, Berlin, 1936. — 2, 3

Quénu, L., Chabrol and Herelemont: *Le colon, ses variations, ses artères*, C. R. Ass. Anat.; XLI. Réunion, 1954. — 19-21

Rankin, F. W., and Learmonth: *The present status of the treatment of Hirschsprung's disease*, Amer. J. Surg., 15:219, 1932. — 33

Reuther, T. F.: *Valves and anastomoses of hemorrhoidal and related veins*, Amer. J. Surg., 49:326, 1940. — 27

Robillard, G. L., and Shapiro: *Variational anatomy of middle colic artery; its significance in gastric and colonic surgery*, J. int. Coll. Surg., 10:157, 1947. — 18, 20, 24

Shah, M. A., and Shah: *Arterial supply of vermiform appendix*, Anat. Rec., 95:457, 1946. — 22

Siddharth, P., and Kornblith: Unpublished reports from Anatomy Department, Jefferson Medical College, Philadelphia. — 19

Sonneland, J., Anson and Beaton: *Surgical anatomy of the arterial supply to the colon from the superior mesenteric artery based upon a study of 600 specimens*, Surg. Gynec. Obstet., 106:385, 1958. — 20

Steward, J. A., and Rankin: *Blood supply of large intestine; its surgical considerations*, Arch. Surg., 26:843, 1933. — 20, 21

Sudeck, P.: *Ueber die Gefässversorgung des Mastdarmes in Hinsicht auf die operative Gangrän*, Münch. med. Wschr., 54:1314, 1907. — 24

Tandler, J.: *Das Gefäss-System in Lehrbuch der systematischen Anatomie*, Vogel, Leipzig, 1936. — 18, 21

Taniguchi, T.: *Beitrag zur Topographie der grossen Aste der Bauchaorta*, Folia anat. jap., 9:201, 1930. — 22

Tucker, C. C., and Hellwig: *Histopathology of the anal crypts*, Trans. Amer. proctol. Soc., 34:47, 1933, and Surg. Gynec. Obstet., 58:145, 1934. — 12, 13

Turell, R.: *Diseases of the Colon and Anorectum*, W. B. Saunders Company, Philadelphia, 1959. — 23, 24

White, J. C., Smithwick and Simeone: *The Autonomic Nervous System*, H. Kimpton, London, 1952. — 30, 32 34

Wolfer, J. A., Beaton and Anson: *Volvulus of cecum; anatomical factors in its etiology*, Surg. Gynec. Obstet., 74:882, 1942. — 5

Zetterqvist, H.: *The ultrastructural organization of the columnar absorbing cells of mouse jejunum*, Karolinska Institutet, Stockholm, Aktiebolaget (Godvil), 1956. — 4

Section XI

Adlersberg, D.: *The Malabsorption Syndrome*, Grune & Stratton, Inc., New York, 1957. — 22

Alvarez, W. C.: *An Introduction to Gastroenterology*, Paul B. Hoeber, Inc., New York, 1948. — 1-3

Section XI (continued)

PLATE NUMBER

——: *The Mechanics of the Digestive Tract*, Paul B. Hoeber, Inc., New York, 1928. — 1-3

Babkin, B. P.: *Secretory Mechanism of the Digestive Glands*, Paul B. Hoeber, Inc., New York, 1944. — 6-9

Bayliss, W. M., and Starling: *Mechanism of pancreatic secretion*, J. Physiol., 28:325, 1902. — 10

—— and ——: *The movements and innervation of the large intestine*, J. Physiol., 26:106, 1900. — 3

—— and ——: *The movements and innervation of the small intestine*, J. Physiol., 26:125, 1901. — 1-3

Beckman, H.: *Drugs: Their Nature, Action and Use*, W. B. Saunders Company, Philadelphia, 1958. — 19

Benedict, E. B.: *Endoscopy as Related to Diseases of Bronchus, Esophagus, Stomach and Peritoneal Cavity*, Williams & Wilkins Company, Baltimore, 1951. — 26

Bergström, S., and Borgström: *Some aspects of the intestinal absorption of fats* in *Progress in the Chemistry of Fats and Other Lipids*, Vol. 3, Holman, R. T., ed., Pergamon Press, London, 1955. — 8

Bloor, W. R.: *Fat transport in animal body*, Physiol. Rev., 19:557, 1939. — 8

Bockus, H. L.: *Gastro-enterology*, W. B. Saunders Company, Philadelphia, 1946. — 12, 13

Breitenecker, R.: *Fatal gastro-intestinal hemorrhage due to chronic relapsing pancreatitis; report of two cases, one with abscess and one with pseudocyst formation*, New Engl. J. Med., 260:1167, 1959. — 18

Brick, I. B., and Jeghers: *Gastro-intestinal hemorrhage (excluding peptic ulcer and esophageal varices)*, New Engl. J. Med., 253:458, 511 and 555, 1955. — 18

Cannon, W. B.: *The Mechanical Factors of Digestion*, Longmans, Green & Company, Inc., New York, 1911. — 1-3

Cantor, M. O., and Reynolds: *Gastrointestinal Obstruction*, Williams & Wilkins Company, Baltimore, 1957. — 17

Caroli, J., Ricordeau and Fourès: *La laparoscopie simple et combinée; son importance dans le diagnostic des maladies hépato-biliaires*, Sem. Hôp. Paris, 30:1671, 1954. — 26

Clausen, S. W.: *Absorption of Vitamin A and its storage in tissues*, Harvey Lect., 38:199, 1943. — 8

Comarr, A. E.: *Bowel regulation for patients with spinal cord injury*, J. Amer. med. Ass., 167:18, 1958. — 12

Copp, D. H.: *Calcium and phosphorus metabolism*, Amer. J. Med., 22:275, 1957. — 8

Di Dio, L. J. A.: *Dados anatomicos sôbre o "piloro" ileo-ceco-colico (Con observação direta in vivo de "papila" ileo-ceco-colica)*, Irmaos Canton, São Paulo, Brasil, 1952. — 2

Dreiling, D. A., and Hollander: *Studies in pancreatic function; statistical study of pancreatic secretion following secretin in patients without pancreatic disease*, Gastroenterology, 15:620, 1950. — 10

Duffy, B. J., Jr., and Turner: *The differential diagnosis of intestinal malabsorption with I^{131}- fat and fatty acid*, Ann. intern. Med., 48:1, 1958. — 22

Section XI (continued)

PLATE NUMBER

Duncan, G. G.: *Diseases of Metabolism*, W. B. Saunders Company, Philadelphia, 1959. — 8, 12, 13

Edkins, J. S.: *On the chemical mechanism of gastric secretion*, Proc. roy. Soc. B, 76:376, 1905. — 10

Finlay, J. M., and Wightman: *The xylose tolerance test as a measure of the intestinal absorption of carbohydrate in sprue*, Ann. intern. Med., 49:1332, 1958. — 22, 23

Florey, H. W., and Harding: *Nature of hormone controlling Brunner's glands*, Quart. J. exper. Physiol., 25:329, 1935. — 10

——, Wright and Jennings: *The secretions of the intestine*, Physiol. Rev., 21:36, 1941. — 6

Fowler, D., and Cook: *Diagnostic significance of d-xylose excretion test*, Gut, 1:67, 1960. — 22 23

Frazer, A. C.: *Fat absorption and its disorders*, Brit. med. Bull., 14:212, 1958. — 8

——: *Fat absorption and its relationship to fat metabolism*, Physiol. Rev., 20:561, 1940. — 8

——: *Physiology of Fat Absorption in Modern Trends in Gastroenterology* (page 477), Jones, F. Avery, ed., Butterworth & Co., Ltd., London, 1952. — 8

——: *The absorption of triglyceride fat from the intestine*, Physiol. Rev., 26:103, 1946. — 8

——: *Transport of lipid through cell membranes*, Symp. Soc. exp. Biol., 8:490, 1954. — 8

Gaston, E. A.: *Physiological basis for preservation of fecal continence after resection of rectum*, J. Amer. med. Ass., 146:1486, 1951. — 13, 14 21

Goligher, J. C.: *The functional results after sphincter-saving resections of the rectum*, Ann. roy. Coll. Surg. Engl., 8:421, 1951. — 20 21

Goodman, L., and Gilman: *The Pharmacological Basis of Therapeutics*, Macmillan Company, New York, 1955. — 19

Grace, W. J., Wolf and Wolff: *The Human Colon. An Experimental Study Based on Direct Observations on Four Fistulous Subjects*, Paul B. Hoeber, Inc., New York, 1951. — 13, 20 21

Greengard, H.: *Hormones of the gastrointestinal tract* in *Hormones, Physiology, Chemistry and Applications*, Pincus and Thimann, ed., Acad. Press, New York, 1948. — 10

Grossmann, M. I.: *Gastrointestinal hormones*, Physiol. Rev., 30:33, 1950. — 10

—— and Jordan: *The radio-iodinated triolein test for steatorrhea*, Gastroenterology, 34:892, 1958. — 22

——, Robertson and Ivy: *Proof for hormonal mechanism for gastric secretion; humoral transmission of distention stimulus*, Amer. J. Physiol., 153:1, 1948. — 10

Harper, A. A., and Raper: *Pancreozymin, stimulant of secretion of pancreatic enzymes in extracts of small intestine*, J. Physiol., 102:115, 1943. — 10

Henning, N., Demling and Gigglberger: *Ueber die laparoskopische Cholezysto-Cholangiographie*, Münch. med. Wschr., 94:829, 1952. — 26

——, Schoen and Fahsold: *Untersuchungen über die Fettresorption beim*

221

Section XI (continued)

	PLATE NUMBER

Menschen, Dtsch. med. Wschr., 85:777, 1960.   22, 23

HERTZ, A. F.: *The passage of food along the human alimentary canal,* Guy's Hosp. Rep., 61:389, 1957.   1-3

HUNTER, F., AND PREVATT: *Diagnostic methods in intestinal malabsorption,* Amer. J. med. Sci., 236:81, 1958.   22, 23

HURST, A. F.: *Constipation and Allied Disorders,* Frowde, London, 1919.   4, 5

INGRAHAM, R. C., AND VISSCHER: *Further studies on intestinal absorption with performance of osmotic work,* Amer. J. Physiol., 121:771, 1938.   6-8

IVY, A. C., AND FARRELL: *Proof of a humoral mechanism; new procedure for study of gastric physiology,* Amer. J. Physiol., 74:639, 1925.   10

——, OLDBERG, LUETH AND KLOSTER: *Studies on a hormone mechanism for gallbladder contraction and evacuation,* Amer. J. Physiol., 90:398, 1929.   10

JACOBAEUS, H. C.: *Ueber die Möglichkeit die Zystoskopie bei Untersuchung seroser Höhlungen anzuwenden,* Münch. med. Wschr., 57:2090, 1910.   26

JACOBS, M. H.: *Permeability,* Ann. Rev. Physiol., 1:1, 1939.   6-8

JANOWITZ, H. O.: *Quantitative tests of gastro-intestinal function,* Amer. J. Med., 13:465, 1952.   22, 23

KALK, H., BRÜHL AND BURGMANN: *Leitfaden der Laparoskopie und Gastroskopie,* Georg Thieme, Stuttgart, 1951.   26

KELLING, G.: *Ueber Oesophagoskopie, Gastroskopie und Kölioskopie,* Münch. med. Wschr., 49:21, 1902.   26

LENNANDER, K. G.: *Observations on the sensitivity of the abdominal cavity,* Translat. by A. E. Barker, John Bale Sons and Danielson, Ltd., London, 1903.   11

LIM, R. K. S.: *Observations on mechanism of inhibition of gastric function by fat,* Quart. J. exp. Physiol., 23:263, 1933.   10, 12

LIVINGSTON, E. M.: *A Clinical Study of the Abdominal Cavity and Peritoneum,* Paul B. Hoeber, Inc., New York, 1932.   11

MACKAY, A., AND PAGE: *Hematemesis associated with hemobilia; report of a case due to an intrahepatic-artery aneurysm, with survival,* New Engl. J. Med., 260:468, 1959.   18

MICHEL, M. L., JR., KNAPP AND DAVIDSON: *Acute intestinal obstruction,* Surgery, 28:90, 1950.   17

NASSET, E. S.: *Enterocrinin, a hormone which excites glands of small intestine,* Amer. J. Physiol., 121:481, 1938.   10

NORDYKE, R. A.: *Analyses of blood and fecal radioactivity methods in the detection of steatorrhea,* J. Lab. clin. Med., in press.   22, 23

PETERS, J. P.: *Carbohydrate Metabolism* in *Clinical Physiology,* page 16, Grollman, A., ed., Blakiston Division, McGraw-Hill Book Co., Inc., New York, 1957.   7

——: *Protein Metabolism* in *Clinical Physiology,* page 115, Grollman, A., ed., Blakiston Division, McGraw-Hill Book Co., Inc., New York, 1957.   6

POTTENGER, F. M.: *Symptoms of Visceral Diseases. A Study of the Vegetative Nervous System in Its Relationship to Clinical Medicine,* C. V. Mosby Company, St. Louis, 1944.   4, 11

PULLEN, R. L.: *Medical Diagnosis,* W. B. Saunders Company, Philadelphia, 1950.   23, 24

RENDICH, R. A., AND HARRINGTON: *The Roentgen kymography of the normal colon; defecation in man,* Amer. J. Roentgenol., 40:173, 1938.   4, 5

RUFFIN, J. M., KEEVER AND CHEARS, JR.: *Use of radioactive labeled lipids in study of intestinal absorption,* Med. Clin. N. Amer., 41:1575, 1957.   22

——, ——, ——, SHINGLETON, BAYLISS, ISLEY AND SAUNDERS: *Further observations on the use of I[131] labeled lipids in the study of diseases of the gastro-intestinal tract,* Gastroenterology, 34:484, 1958.   22

SMYTHE, C., OSBORNE, ZAMCHECK, RICHARDS AND MADISON: *Bleeding from the upper gastro-intestinal tract,* New Engl. J. Med., 256:441, 1957.   18

SOBEL, A. E.: *The problem of absorption and transportation of fat-soluble vitamins,* Vitam. and Horm., 10:47, 1952.   8

SPENCER, R. P.: *The Intestinal Tract. Structure, Function and Pathology in Terms of the Basic Sciences,* Charles C Thomas, Publisher, Springfield, Ill., 1960.   6-8

STILL, E. U.: *Secretin,* Physiol. Rev., 11:328, 1931.   10

SWELL, L., TROUT, JR., HOPPER, FIELD, JR., AND TREADWELL: *Mechanism of cholesterol absorption,* J. biol. Chem., 232:1, 1958.   8

TODD, T. W.: *Behaviour Patterns in Alimentary Canal,* Williams & Wilkins Company, Baltimore, 1933.   1-3

VERZAR, F., AND McDOUGALL: *Absorption from the Intestine,* Longmans, Green & Company, Inc., New York, 1936.   8

VISSCHER, M. B.: *Transport of water and electrolyte across intestinal epithelia* in *Metabolic Aspects of Transport Across Cell Membranes,* Chapter 4, page 57, Murphy, Q. R., ed., University of Wisconsin Press, Madison, 1957.   8

VON KOKAS, E., AND LUDANY: *Relation between "Villikinine" and the absorption of glucose from the intestine,* Quart. J. exp. Physiol., 28:15, 1938.   10

WANGENSTEEN, O. H.: *Intestinal Obstructions,* Charles C Thomas, Publisher, Springfield, Ill., 1955.   17

WESTPHAL, K.: *Die Defäkation,* in Bethe, Bergmann, Embden, Ellinger: *Handbuch der normalen und pathologischen Physiologie,* Vol. 3, page 472, Julius Springer, Berlin, 1927.   4, 5

Section XII

ADLERSBERG, D.: *Primary malabsorption syndrome; past, present and future,* Am. J. dig. Dis., 4:8, 1959.   24, 25

——: *Symposium on the malabsorption syndrome; introduction,* J. Mt. Sinai Hosp., 24:177, 1957.   24, 25

AITKEN, J.: *Remnants of the vitello-intestinal duct; a clinical analysis of 88 cases,* Arch. Dis. Childh., 28:1, 1953.   16, 17

Section XII (continued)

ALDRICH, E. M., MORTON AND PARKER: *Intestinal obstruction resulting from malrotation of the intestine,* Ann. Surg., 141:765, 1955.   2

ALLEN, A. W., DONALDSON, SNIFFEN AND GOODALE: *Primary malignant lymphoma of gastro-intestinal tract,* Ann. Surg., 140:428, 1954.   49

ALLINGHAM, H.: *Piles: the importance of recognising the varieties as determining the selection of treatment* in Coll. Papers of St. Mark's Hospital, London, page 82, H. K. Lewis & Company, Ltd., London, 1935.   56

ALTCHEK, M. P., AND SUMMER: *Ulcerative colitis complicated by cologastric fistula,* Gastroenterology, 33:823, 1957.   31

ANDERSEN, D. H., AND DI SANT' AGNESE: *Idiopathic celiac disease; mode of onset and diagnosis,* Pediatrics, 11:207, 1953.   24, 25

ANDERSON, H. H., BOSTICK AND JOHNSTONE: *Amebiasis: Pathology, Diagnosis and Chemotherapy,* Charles C Thomas, Publisher, Springfield, Ill., 1953.   41, 42

ANDERSON, J. A., ZIEGLER AND DOEDEN: *Banana feeding and urinary excretion of 5-β-hydroxyindolacetic acid,* Science, 127:236, 1958.   51

ANDERSON, W. A. D., ED.: *Pathology,* C. V. Mosby Company, St. Louis, 1948.   15-23, 26, 28-55

ANDRESEN, A. F. R.: *Allergic manifestations in gastrointestinal tract,* Gastroenterology, 23:20, 1953.   27

AREY, L. B.: *Developmental Anatomy,* W. B. Saunders Company, Philadelphia, 1954.   1-4

ARMAS-CRUZ, R., PERALTA, FUENZALIDA, COZZI, PARROCHIA, RUFIN, DAVILA AND ARTIGAS: *A clinical evaluation of intestinal amebiasis* in *Proceedings of the World Congress of Gastroenterology, Washington, 1958,* Vol. 2, page 759, Williams & Wilkins Company, Baltimore, 1959.   41, 42

ARNHEIM, E. E.: *Surgical complications of congenital anomalies of the umbilical region,* Surg. Gynec. Obstet., 91:71, 1950.   14

ARNOLD, L.: *Experimental method for the study of bacterial flora and the hydrogen-ion concentration of the gastro-intestinal tract,* Arch. Path. Lab. Med., 1:839, 1926.   27

ARNOUS, J., AND PARNAUD: *La Petite Chirurgie des Fistules Anales,* Masson et Cie., Paris, 1954.   59

ARONSSON, H.: *Anorectal infections and sequelae, especially fistulae and incontinence; clinical study of pathogenesis, prognosis, treatment and complications,* Acta chir. scand. (suppl. 135), 96:1, 1948.   59

ASCHOFF, L.: *Die Wurmfortsatz-Entzündung; eine pathologisch-histologische und pathogenetische Studie,* G. Fischer, Jena, 1908.   34

ASH, J. E., AND SPITZ: *Pathology of Tropical Diseases,* W. B. Saunders Company, Philadelphia, 1945.   24, 25, 40-42, 65

AYREY, F.: *Outbreaks of sprue during Burma campaign,* Trans. roy. Soc. trop. med. Hyg., 41:377, 1947.   24, 25

BACON, H. E.: *Anus, Rectum, Sigmoid Colon: Diagnosis and Treatment,* J. B. Lippincott Company, Philadelphia, 1949.   20, 22, 30, 32, 33, 53-55, 56, 59

Section XII (continued)	PLATE NUMBER

—— AND BROAD: *Pathogenesis of adenomatous polyps in relation to malignancy of large bowel*, Rev. Gastroent., 15:284, 1948. 53-55

——, LOWELL AND TRIMPI: *Villous papillomas of colon and rectum; study of 28 cases with end results of treatment over 5-year period*, Surgery, 35:77, 1954. 58

—— AND McGREGOR: *Multiple primary malignant tumors of the colon; report of 141 cases*, J. int. Coll. Surg., 28:618, 1957. 53

BADENOCH, J., BEDFORD AND EVANS: *Massive diverticulosis of the small intestine with steatorrhea and megaloblastic anemia*, Quart. J. Med., 24:321, 1955. 24

BAGLIETTO, L. A.: *Fisura anal*, El Ateneo, Buenos Aires, 1942. 58

BANKS, R. W.: *Amebiasis and amebic dysentery*, in *Gastro-enterology*, Bockus, H. L., ed., Vol. 2, page 615, W. B. Saunders Company, Philadelphia and London, 1944. 41, 42

BARBOSA, J. DE C.: *Cancer do colon e do reto*, in *Colopatias*, Mendes, F., ed., page 15, Livraria Atheneu, S. A., Rio de Janeiro, 1959. 53-55

BASSLER, A.: *Diseases and Disorders of the Colon*, Charles C Thomas, Publisher, Springfield, Ill., 1957. 52

BAUMGÄRTEL, T.: *Klinische Darmbakteriologie für die ärztliche Praxis*, Georg Thieme, Stuttgart, 1954. 27

BENNETT, T. I., HUNTER AND VAUGHAN: *Idiopathic steatorrhea (Gee's disease); nutritional disturbance associated with tetany, osteomalacia, and anaemia*, Quart. J. Med., 1:603, 1932. 24, 25

BENSAUDE, A.: *L'évolution cancéreuse des tumeurs bénignes du rectum; son importance pour la prophylaxie du cancer rectum*, Masson et Cie., Paris, 1937. 58

BERCOVITZ, Z.: *Studies in cellular exudates of bowel discharges; diagnostic significance of cellular exudate studies in chronic bowel disorders*, Ann. intern. Med., 14:1323, 1941. 41, 42

BEYER, W.: *Die Therapie der Hämorrhoiden*, Münch. med. Wschr., 101:1466, 1959. 56

BILL, A. H., AND JOHNSON: *Failure of migration of the rectal opening as the cause for most cases of imperforate anus*, Surg. Gynec. Obstet., 106:643, 1958. 4

BJERKELUND, C. J.: *Symptomatic sprue*, Acta med. scand., 137:130, 1950. 24, 25

BLACK-SCHAFFER, B.: *Tinctoral demonstration of a glycoprotein in Whipple's disease*, Proc. Soc. exp. Biol., 72:225, 1949. 26

BOCKUS, H. L., ED.: *Gastroenterology*, W. B. Saunders Company, Philadelphia, 1944. 15-55

——, TUMEN AND KORNBLUM: *Diffuse primary tuberculous enterocolitis; a report of two cases*, Ann. intern. Med., 13:1461, 1940. 43-45

BODIAN, M., STEPHENS AND WARD: *Hirschsprung's disease*, Lancet, 1:19, 1950. 7-9

BOLES, R. S., AND GERSHON-COHEN: *Intestinal tuberculosis; pathologic and roentgenologic observations*, J. Amer. med. Ass., 103:1841, 1934. 43-45

BONORINO-UDAONDO, C., RAMOS MEJÍA AND D'ALOTTO, EDS.: *Colitis Ulcerosas Graves Inespecíficas*, Lopez & Etchegoyen, Buenos Aires, 1952. 31

BRAILSFORD, J. F.: *Cysticercus cellulosae; its radiographic detection in musculature and central nervous system*, Brit. J. Radiol., 14:79, 1941. 67

BREMER, J. L.: *Diverticula and duplications of intestinal tract*, Arch. Path. (Chicago), 38:132, 1944. 15

BROOKE, M. M.: *Laboratory regimens for diagnosis of intestinal amebiasis by gastroenterologists*, in *Proceedings of the World Congress of Gastroenterology, Washington, 1958*, Vol. 2, page 754, Williams & Wilkins Company, Baltimore, 1959. 41, 42

BROTTO, W.: *Aspectos neurológicos da cisticercose*, Arch. Neuro-psiquiat. (S. Paulo), 5:258, 1947. 67

BROWN, A. J.: *Vascular tumors of the intestine*, Surg. Gynec. Obstet., 39:191, 1924. 47

BROWNE, D.: *Some congenital deformities of the rectum, anus, vagina and urethra*, Ann. roy. Coll. Surg. Engl., 8:173, 1951. 4

BUCHMAN, E., KULLMAN AND MARGONIS: *Evaluation of complement fixation test in amebiasis*, Gastroenterology, 21:391, 1952. 41, 42

BUCKSTEIN, J.: *Digestive Tract in Roentgenology*, J. B. Lippincott Company, Philadelphia, 1953. 46-48

BURKE, H. E., AND ARONOVITCH: *Intestinal tuberculosis*, Canad. med. Ass. J., 45:21, 1941. 43-45

BURNS, F. J.: *Papillomas of colon and rectum*, Amer. J. Surg., 80:97, 1950. 58

CARVALHO, A. A.: *Anemia ancilostomótica na criança; aspectos de sua etiopatogenia*, Tese- Fac. Med. São Paulo, 1956. 65

CASE, J. T.: *Diverticula of small intestine, other than Meckel's diverticulum*, J. Amer. med. Ass., 75:1463, 1920. 18

CHANDLER, A. C.: *Introduction to Parasitology with Special Reference to the Parasites of Man*, John Wiley & Sons, Inc., New York, 1955. 61-71

——: *Species of hymenolepis as human parasites*, J. Amer. med. Ass., 78:636, 1922. 68

CHÉRIGIÉ, E., HILLEMAND, PROUX AND BOURDON: *La tuberculose de l'intestin grêle et de la région iléocaecale*, Sem. Hôp. Paris, 31:1373, 1955. 43-45

——, ——, —— AND ——: *L'intestin grêle normal et pathologique (étude clinique et radiologique)*, Expansion Scientifique Française, Paris, 1957. 18, 23, 26, 35-51

—— AND PROUX: *Forme pseudo-tumorale de la maladie de Crohn*, Arch. Mal. Appar. dig., 48:207, 1959. 28, 29

CHERRY, J. W., AND HILL: *Leiomyoma of the jejunum; a neoplasm imitating the symptoms of duodenal ulcer*, A. M. A. Arch. Surg., 62:580, 1951. 46, 47

CHRISTOPHER, F.: *Hemangioma of the ileum*, Ann. Surg., 116:945, 1942. 47

COLE, W. H.: *Congenital malformations of the intestinal tract and bile ducts in infancy and childhood*, Arch. Surg., 23:820, 1931. 1-13

COLEMAN, S. T., AND ECKERT: *Preservation of rectum in familial polyposis of the colon and rectum*, A. M. A. Arch. Surg., 73:635, 1956. 52

COLEY, B. L.: *Tuberculosis of Meckel's diverticulum associated with tuberculous appendix*, Arch. Surg., 11:519, 1925. 16, 17

COLLINS, E. N.: *Diagnosis and clinical course of regional enteritis*, J. Amer. med. Ass., 165:2042, 1957. 28, 29

COMFORT, M. W.: *Submucous lipomata of the gastro-intestinal tract; report of twenty-eight cases*, Surg. Gynec. Obstet., 52:101, 1931. 47

—— AND WOLLAEGER: *Nontropical sprue; pathologic physiology, diagnosis, and therapy*, A. M. A. Arch. intern. Med., 98:807, 1956. 24, 25

COMPTON, A., AND SAID: *Laboratory diagnosis of typhoid infections*, Lancet, 2:580, 1933. 37

CONNELL, A. M., ROWLANDS AND WILCOX: *Serotonin, bananas and diarrhea*, Gut, 1:44, 1960. 51

COSTA, S. DE M.: *Adenomatose familiar entero-cólica*, Rev. med. e cir. São Paulo, 11:507, 1951. 52

COUNSELL, P. B., AND DUKES: *Association of chronic ulcerative colitis and carcinoma of rectum and colon*, Brit. J. Surg., 39:485, 1952. 53

COUTINHO, J. O., CROCE, CAMPOS, AMATO AND FONSECA: *Contribuição para o conhecimento da estrongiloidíase humana em São Paulo*, Folia clin. et biol., 20 (3):141, 1953; 21 (1):19, 1954; 21 (2):93, 1954. 64

COWAN, K.: *Public health aspects of food poisoning*, Proc. Nutr. Soc., 16:136, 1957. 38, 39

CRAIG, C. F.: *Laboratory Diagnosis of Protozoan Diseases*, Lea & Febiger, Philadelphia, 1948. 70, 71

——: *The Etiology, Diagnosis and Treatment of Amebiasis*, Williams & Wilkins Company, Baltimore, 1944. 41, 42

—— AND FAUST: *Clinical Parasitology*, Lea & Febiger, Philadelphia, 1955. 61-71

CRAM, E. B.: *Studies on oxyuriasis*, Amer. J. Dis. Child., 65:46, 1943. 63

CROHN, B. B.: *Life history of regional ileitis*, Gastroenterologia (Basel), 89:352, 1958. 28, 29

——: *Regional ileitis: ileojejunitis, combined ileocolitis*, Amer. J. Gastroent., 31:536, 1959. 28, 29

——, GINZBURG AND OPPENHEIMER: *Regional ileitis; a pathologic and clinical entity*, J. Amer. med. Ass., 99:1323, 1932. 28, 29

CRUZ, W. O.: *Hookworm anemia, deficiency disease* in *Proceed. Fourth Internat. Congress on Tropical Medicine and Malaria, Washington, 1948*, Volume 2, page 1045. 65

CULLEN, T. S.: *Diseases of the Umbilicus*, W. B. Saunders Company, Philadelphia, 1916. 14

CUTAIT, D. E.: *Retocolite ulcerativa inespecífica; tratamento cirúrgico* in *Colopatias*, page 133, Mendes, F., ed., Livraria Atheneu, S. A., Rio de Janeiro, 1959. 53

—— AND FIGLIOLINI: *Tumores intestinais*, in *Atualização Terapêutica*, page 133, Livraria Luso-Espanhola, Belo Horizonte, 1958. 53

——, PEREIRA, PONTES, PONTES, MONZIONE, SIMONSEN AND SILVA: *Adenomatose familiar múltipla do intestino grosso*, Rev. paul. Med., 43:27, 1953. 52, 53

Section XII (continued)   PLATE NUMBER

Dack, G. M.: *Food Poisoning,* University of Chicago Press, Chicago, 1956.   38, 39

Daffner, J. E., and Brown: *Regional enteritis; clinical aspects and diagnosis in 100 patients,* Ann. intern. Med., 49:580, 1958.   28, 29

Darling, R. C., and Welch: *Tumors of the small intestine,* New Engl. J. Med., 260: 397, 1959.   46-51

da Silva, R. R.: *Fistulas ano-retais e seu problema cirurgico,* Arch. Cirurg. clín. exp., 7:510, 1943.   59

Davis, A. A.: *Hypertrophic intestinal tuberculosis,* Surg. Gynec. Obstet., 56:907, 1933.   44

DeBhattachary, S. N., and Sarkar: *A study of the pathogenicity of strains of bacterium coli from acute and chronic enteritis,* J. Path. Bact., 71:201, 1956.   27

Demartial, L., Viollet, Loubet and Madeline: *Volumineux schwannome du grêle,* Arch. Mal. Appar. dig., 45:449, 1956.   46, 47

de Miranda, M. P.: *Colopatias funcionais,* in *Colopatias,* page 293, Mendes, F., ed., Livraria Atheneu, Rio de Janeiro, 1959.   27

de Morais, R. Gomes: *Contribuição para o estudo do Strongyloides stercoralis e da estrongyloidose no Brasil,* Rev. Serv. espec. saúde púb., 1:507, 1947/48.   64

Dengler, H.: *Atypisches Carcinoidsyndrom mit vermehrter Aüsscheidung von 5-Hydroxyindolessigsäure bei Pankrearcarcinom,* Klin. Wschr., 37:1245, 1959.   51

Desjaques, R., Revol, Creyssel, Costaz and Dumas: *Schwannome de l'intestin grêle a symptomatologie anémique,* Lyon chir., 51:97, 1956.   46, 47

Dick, A. P.: *Association of jejunal diverticulosis and steatorrhea,* Brit. med. J., 1:145, 1955.   24

Dicke, W. K., Weijers and van de Kamer: *Coeliac disease; presence in wheat of factor having deleterious effect in cases of coeliac disease,* Acta paediat., 42:34, 1953.   25

Dittrich, J. K.: *Neue Anschauungen über die Pathogenese der Zöliakie,* Z. ärztl. Fortdild., 52:802, 1958.   25

do Amaral, A. D. F.: *Diagnóstico da teníase pelo processo do raspador anal,* Rev. Hosp. Clín. Fac. Med. S. Paulo, 10:284, 1955.   67

——, Pontes and Pires: *Amebíase; estudo etiopatogênico, clínico, terapêutico e epidemiológico,* Rossolillo, São Paulo, 1947.   41, 42

Dormandy, T. L.: *Gastrointestinal polyposis with mucocutaneous pigmentation (Peutz-Jeghers syndrome),* New Engl. J. Med., 256:1093, 1141 and 1186, 1957.   48

—— and Edwards: *Peutz's syndrome,* Gastroenterologia (Basel), 86:456, 1956.   48

Drueck, C. J.: *Anal cryptitis,* Amer. J. dig. Dis., 6:450, 1939.   58

——: *Pruritus Ani,* Medical Observer Press, Chicago, 1938.   58

Dukes, C. E.: *Cancer control in familial polyposis of the colon,* Dis. Colon Rectum, 1:413, 1958.   52

——: *Etiology of cancer of the colon and rectum,* Dis. Colon Rectum, 2:27, 1959.   55, 58

——: *Explanation of difference between papilloma and adenoma of rectum,* Proc. roy. Soc. Med., 40:829, 1947.   58

——: *Familial intestinal polyposis,* Ann. Eugen. (Lond.), 17:1, 1952.   52

Dunphy, J. E., and Pikula: *Rectal prolapse,* in *Diseases of the Colon and Anorectum,* page 169, Turell, R., ed., W. B. Saunders Company, Philadelphia, 1959.   57

Edwards, H. C.: *Diverticulosis of the small intestine,* Ann. Surg., 103:320, 1936.   18

Ehrenpreis, T.: *Megacolon in the newborn; a clinical and roentgenological study with special regard to the pathogenesis,* Acta chir. scand., 94:1, 1946.   7, 8

Elsdon-Dew, R.: *Factors influencing the pathogenicity of Entamoeba histolytica,* in *Proceedings of the World Congress of Gastroenterology, Washington, 1958,* Volume 2, page 770, Williams & Wilkins Company, Baltimore, 1959.   41, 42

Engel, G. L.: *Studies of ulcerative colitis; nature of psychologic processes,* Amer. J. Med., 19:231, 1955.   31

Enquist, I. F., and State: *Rectal and colonic polyps,* Surgery, 32:696, 1952.   58

Erspamer, V., and Asero: *Identification of enteramine, the specific hormone of enterochromaffin cell system, as 5-hydroxytryptamine,* Nature (Lond.), 169:800, 1952.   51

Falkinburg, L. W., and Kay: *Intestinal polyposis with oral pigmentation (Peutz-Jeghers Syndrome); report of a case with review,* J. Pediat., 54:162, 1959.   48

Farnan, P.: *Whipple's disease: the clinical aspects,* Quart. J. Med., 28:163, 1959.   26

Faulkner, J. W., and Dockerty: *Lymphosarcoma of small intestine,* Surg. Gynec. Obstet., 95:76, 1952.   49, 50

Faust, E. C.: *Algunos conceptos modernos sobre el diagnóstico y tratamiento de la amebiasis,* Rev. méd. Chile, 78:493, 1950.   41, 42

——: *Experimental studies on human and primate species of Strongyloides; development of Strongyloides in experimental host,* Amer. J. Hyg., 18:114, 1933.   64

—— and De Groat: *Internal autoinfection in human strongyloidiasis,* Amer. J. trop. Med., 20:359, 1940.   64

——, Sawitz, Tobie, Odom, Peres and Lincicome: *Comparative efficiency of various technics for diagnosis of protozoa and helminths in feces,* J. Parasit., 25:241, 1939.   41, 42, 70, 71

Felsen, J.: *Bacillary Dysentery, Colitis and Enteritis,* W. B. Saunders Company, Philadelphia, 1945.   40

—— and Wolarsky: *Acute and chronic bacillary dysentery and chronic ulcerative colitis,* J. Amer. med. Ass., 153:1069, 1953.   40

Ferreira, J. M.: *Febre tifóide,* Rev. med. (São Paulo), 38:181, 1954.   35-37

Feyrter, F.: *Zur Frage der Stoffwechselvorgänge im Gelbe-Zellen-Organ und Karzinoid des Magen-Darmschlauches,* Wien. klin. Wschr., 71:727, 1959.   51

Floyd, T. M., Blagg and Kader: *Studies in shigellosis; observations on incidence and etiology of diarrheal disease in Egyptian adults,* Amer. J. trop. Med., 5:812, 1956.   40

Foster, A. O., and Landsberg: *Nature and cause of hookworm anemia,* Amer. J. Hyg., 20:259, 1934.   65

Frazer, A. C.: *Fat metabolism and sprue syndrome,* Brit. med. J., 2:769, 1949.   24, 25

——: in *Tropical Sprue; Studies of U. S. Army's Sprue Team in Puerto Rico;* Crosby, W. A., ed., Walter Reed Army Institute of Research, Medical Science Bull., No. 5, 1959.   24, 25

——, French and Thompson: *Radiographic studies showing induction of segmentation pattern in small intestine in normal human subjects,* Brit. J. Radiol., 22:123, 1949.   24, 25

Fredericq, P.: *Colicins,* Annual Rev. Microbiol., 11:7, 1957.   27

French, J. M., Gaddie and Smith: *Tropical sprue; a study of seven cases and their response to combined chemotherapy,* Quart. J. Med., 25:333, 1956.   24, 25

——, Hawkins and Smith: *The effect of a wheat-gluten-free diet in adult idiopathic steatorrhea,* Quart. J. Med., 26:481, 1957.   24, 25

Fülleborn, F.: *Ueber die Entwicklung von Trichozephalus im Wirte,* Arch. Schiffsu. Tropenhyg., 27:413, 1923.   61

Gandin, J.: *Les neurinomes solitaires de l'intestin grêle,* J. Chir., 72:867, 1956.   47

Gee, S.: *On the coeliac affection,* St. Bart's Hosp. Rep., 24:17, 1888.   24, 25

Gellman, D. D.: *Diverticulosis of the small intestine with steatorrhea and megaloblastic anemia,* Lancet, 2:873, 1956.   18

Gennari, R., and Sega: *Tubercolosi iperplastica stenosante dell' ileo terminale,* Arch. ital. Mal. Appar. dig., 20:16, 1954.   43

Gentry, R. W., Dockerty and Clagett: *Vascular malformations and vascular tumors of the gastrointestinal tract,* Int. Abstr. Surg., 88:281, 1949.   47

Gilbert, A. E., and Wise: *Adenocarcinoma of the small intestine,* Amer. J. Surg., 96: 54, 1958.   49-51

Ginsberg, R. S., and Ivy: *Etiology of ulcerative colitis; analytical review of literature,* Gastroenterology, 7:67, 1946.   30, 31

Girges, R.: *Pathogenic factors in ascariasis,* Amer. J. trop. Med., 37:209, 1934.   62

Glover, D. M., and Hamann: *Intestinal obstruction in newborn due to congenital anomalies,* Ohio St. med. J., 36:833, 1940.   1-14

Golden, T., and Stout: *Smooth muscle tumors of the gastro-intestinal tract and retroperitoneal tissues,* Surg. Gynec. Obstet., 73:784, 1941.   47

Goodpasture, E. W.: *Concerning pathogenesis of typhoid fever,* Amer. J. Path., 13:175, 1937.   35

Goodsall, D. H., cit. by Edwards, F. S.: *Fistula-in-ano; why is operative interference so often ineffectual?* in *Coll. Papers of St. Mark's Hospital,* page 138, H. K. Lewis & Co., Ltd., London, 1935.   59

Gordon, H.: *Appendical oxyuriasis and appendicitis, based on study of 26,051 appendixes,* Arch. Path., 16:177, 1933.   63

Gorsch, R. V.: *Anorectal fistula,* Rev. Gastroent., 19:640, 1952.   59

Gradwohl, R. B. H., and Kourí: *Clinical Laboratory Methods and Diagnosis,* Volume 3, Fourth edition, C. V. Mosby Company, St. Louis, 1948.   61-71

Section XII (continued)

PLATE NUMBER

GREEN, P. A., WOLLAEGER, SCUDAMORE AND POWER: *Nontropical sprue. Functional efficiency of small intestine after prolonged use of gluten-free diet*, J. Amer. med. Ass., 171:2157, 1959. — 24, 25

GRELL, K. G.: *Protozoologie*, Julius Springer, Berlin, 1956. — 61-71

GROB, MAX: *Patologia Quirurgica Infantil*, Editorial Científico Médico, Barcelona, 1958. — 15

GROSS, R. E.: *The Surgery of Infancy and Childhood*, W. B. Saunders Company, Philadelphia, 1953. — 1-6, 9, 14

GUREVITCH, J., AND DELIGHTISH: *Survival time of Entamoeba histolytica in feces*, Harefuah, 32:60, 1947. — 41, 42

HABER, J. J.: *Meckel's diverticulum; review of literature and analytical study of 23 cases with particular emphasis on bowel obstruction*, Amer. J. Surg., 73:468, 1947. — 16, 17

HADFIELD, G.: *Primary histological lesion of regional ileitis*, Lancet, 2:773, 1939. — 28, 29

HARDY, A. V., AND WATT: *Studies of acute diarrheal diseases; epidemiology*, Publ. Hlth. Rep. (Wash.), 63:363, 1948. — 40

HARKINS, H. N.: *Intussusception due to invaginated Meckel's diverticulum; report of two cases with a study of 160 cases collected from the literature*, Ann. Surg., 98:1070, 1933. — 16, 17

HEDINGER, C., AND GLOOR: *Metastasiernende Dünndarmkarzinoide, Tricuspidalklappenveränderungen und Pulmonalstenose — ein neues Syndrom*, Schweiz. med. Wschr., 84:942, 1954. — 51

—— AND LABHART: *Gewebehormone* in *Klinik der inneren Sekretion*, Labhart, A., ed., page 952, Springer-Verlag, Berlin, Göttingen, Heidelberg, 1957. — 51

HELWIG, E. B.: *Adenomas and the pathogenesis of cancer of the colon and rectum*, Dis. Colon Rectum, 2:5, 1959. — 53, 54

——: *Evolution of adenomas of large intestine and their relation to carcinoma*, Surg. Gynec. Obstet., 84:36, 1947. — 53, 54

HENDRIX, J. P., BLACK-SCHAFFER, WITHERS AND HANDLER: *Whipple's intestinal lipodystrophy; report of 4 cases and discussion of possible pathogenic factors*, Arch. intern. Med., 85:91, 1950. — 26

HERTER, C. A.: *On Infantilism from Chronic Intestinal Infection*, Macmillan Company, New York, 1908. — 24, 25

HEUBNER, O.: *Ueber schwere Verdauungsinsuffizienz beim Kinde jenseits des Säuglingsalter*, Jb. Kinderheilk., 70:667, 1909. — 24, 25

HIGGINS, A. R., AND FLOYD: *Studies in shigellosis; general considerations, locale of studies, and methods*, Amer. J. trop. Med., 4:263, 1955. — 40

HILL, F. A., AND JANELLI: *Malignant tumors originating in Meckel's diverticulum; case report of leiomyosarcoma and review of literature*, Amer. J. Surg., 85:525, 1953. — 17

HILLEMAND, P., BENSAUDE AND LOYGUE: *Les maladies de l'anus et du canal anal*, page 43, Masson et Cie., Paris, 1955. — 56-60

—— AND CHÉRIGIÉ: *La maladie de Crohn; etude critique et clinico-radiologique*, Rev. Prat. (Paris), 9:1208, 1959. — 28, 29

Section XII (continued)

PLATE NUMBER

HIMES, H. W., AND ADLERSBERG: *Pathologic changes in the small bowel in idiopathic sprue: biopsy and autopsy findings*, Gastroenterology, 35:142, 1958. — 24, 25

HIRSCHSPRUNG: *Stuhlträgheit Neugeborener in Folge von Dilatation und Hypertrophie des Colon*, Jb. Kinderheilk., 27:1, 1887. — 7

HOBBS, B. C., SMITH, OAKLEY, WARRACK AND CRUICKSHANK: *Clostridium welchii food poisoning*, J. Hyg., 51:75, 1953. — 38, 39

HODGES, P. C.: *Roentgen examination of colon*, J. Amer. med. Ass., 153:1417, 1953. — 53-55

HOLDEN, W. D., AND COLE: *Familial polyposis of the colon and rectum*, in *Diseases of the Colon and Anorectum*, Volume 1, page 375, Turell, R., ed., W. B. Saunders Company, Philadelphia, 1959. — 52

HOLMES, W. H., AND STARR: *Nutritional disturbance in adults resembling celiac disease and sprue*, J. Amer. med. Ass., 92:975, 1929. — 24, 25

HOON, J. R., DOCKERTY AND PEMBERTON: *Ileocecal tuberculosis including a comparison of this disease with nonspecific enterocolitis and noncaseous tuberculated enterocolitis*, Int. Abstr. Surg., 60:417, 1950. — 43, 44

HORMAECHE, E., SURRACO, PELUFFO AND ALEPPO: *Causes of infantile summer diarrhea*, Amer. J. Dis. Child., 66:539, 1943. — 40

HOTTINGER, A.: *Enterale Allergie Immunität und Zoeliakie*, Dtsch. med. Wschr., 84:1717, 1959. — 27

HOWIE, J. W. *The bacteriology of food poisoning*, Proc. Nutr. Soc., 16:141, 1957. — 38, 39

HUNTER, F. M., AND PREVATT: *Diagnostic methods in intestinal malabsorption*, Amer. J. med. Sci., 236:81, 1958. — 24, 25

ISLER, P., AND HEDINGER: *Metastasierendes Dünndarmcarcinoid mit schweren, vorwiegend das rechte Herz betreffenden Klappenfehlern und Pulmonalstenose — ein eigenartiger Symptomenkomplex*, Schweiz. med. Wschr., 83:4, 1953. — 51

JACOBS, A. H.: *Enterobiasis in children; incidence, symptomatology, and diagnosis, with simplified Scotch cellulose tape technique*, J. Pediat., 21:497, 1942. — 63

JANBON, M., AND BERTRAND: *Sarcoidose de l'intestin grêle; ses rapports avec l'ileite régionale de Crohn*, Presse méd., 66:1491, 1958. — 28, 29

JAWETZ, E., MELNICK AND ADELBERG: *Review of Medical Microbiology*, Lange Medical Publications, Los Altos, 1960. — 40

JEGHERS, H.: *Pigmentation of the skin*, New Engl. J. Med., 231:88, 122 and 181, 1944. — 48

——, McKUSICK AND KATZ: *Generalized intestinal polyposis and melanin spots of the oral mucosa, lips and digits; a syndrome of diagnostic significance*, New Engl. J. Med., 241:993 and 1031, 1949. — 48

KAIJSER, R.: *Ueber Hämangiome des Tractus gastro-intestinalis*, Arch. klin. Chir., 187:351, 1936. — 47

KANTOR, J. L.: *Regional (terminal) ileitis: its roentgen diagnosis*, J. Amer. med. Ass., 103:2016, 1934. — 28, 29

Section XII (continued)

PLATE NUMBER

KEANE, J. F.: *Hemorrhoidal pathologic conditions: incidence of recurrence*, J. int. Coll. Surg., 28:440, 1957. — 55

KELLER, A. E., CASPARIS AND LEATHERS: *Clinical study of ascariasis*, J. Amer. med. Ass., 97:302, 1931. — 62

KERN, F., JR., ALMY, ABBOT AND BOGDONOFF: *Motility of distal colon in nonspecific ulcerative colitis*, Gastroenterology, 19:492, 1951. — 30, 31

KEYES, E. L.: *Squamous-cell carcinoma of anus and rectum*, Surg. Clin. N. Amer., 24:1151, 1944. — 53, 55

KIRSNER, J. E.: *Current concepts of the medical management of ulcerative colitis*, J. Amer. med. Ass., 169:433, 1959. — 30, 31

KIRTLAND, H. B.: *Patent omphalomesenteric duct*, A. M. A. Arch. Surg., 63:706, 1951. — 13

KRAINICK, H. G.: *Der schädliche Weizenmehleffekt und das Zöliakieproblem*, Dtsch. med. Wschr., 83:1607, 1958. — 24, 25

KREIS, H. A.: *Studies on genus Strongyloides (nematodes)*, Am. J. Hyg., 16:450, 1932. — 64

KYLE, L. H., McKAY AND SPARLING: *Strongyloidiasis*, Ann. intern. Med., 29:1014, 1948. — 64

LAKE, M., NICKEL AND ANDRUS: *Possible rôle of pancreatic enzymes in etiology of ulcerative colitis*, Gastroenterology, 17:409, 1951. — 31

LANGER, B., AND THOMSON: *Hirschsprung's disease; nine years' experience at the Hospital for Sick Children, Toronto*, Canad. J. Surg., 2:123, 1959. — 79

LECH-JUNIOR: *Cisticercose ocular*, Arq. Inst. Penido Burnier (Campinas), 8:13, 1949. — 67

LECHNER, G. W., AND CONNOLLY: *Benign neoplasms of the small intestine, with a report of three bleeding benign tumors of the jejunum*, J. Amer. med. Ass., 169:2003, 1959. — 46, 47

LEHMENSICK, R.: *Unser Ascaris (Ascaris lumbricoides Linné, 1758)*, CIBA Symposium (Basel), 8:59, 1960. — 62

LEHMKUHL, H.: *Ein Fall von gleichmässigem diffusem Lymphosarkom des Dünndarms*, Virchow's Arch. path. Anat., 264:39, 1927. — 49

LEWIS, F. T., AND THYNG: *The regular occurrence of intestinal diverticula in embryos of the pig, rabbit and man*, Amer. J. Anat., 7:505, 1907 — 15

LIEBERMAN, W.: *Syphilis of the rectum*, Rev. Gast., 18:67, 1951. — 60

LLOYD-DAVIES, O. V.: *Lithotomy — Trendelenburg position for resection of rectum and lower pelvic colon*, Lancet, 2:74, 1939. — 32, 33

LOCKHART-MUMMERY, H. E.: *The Colon*, in *Textbook of British Surgery*, Volume I, page 403, Souttar, H., and Goligher, ed., W. Heinemann Med. Books Ltd., London, 1956. — 20, 32, 33

——, DUKES AND BUSSEY: *Surgical treatment of familial polyposis of colon*, Brit. J. Surg., 43:476, 1956. — 52

LOCKHART-MUMMERY, J. P.: *Diseases of the Rectum and Colon and Their Surgical Treatment*, William Wood and Company, Baltimore, 1934. — 19-22, 30-33, 52-55

—— AND DUKES: *Familial adenomatosis of colon and rectum; its relationship to cancer*, Lancet, 2:586, 1939.   52

LOCKWOOD, A. L.: *Diverticula of stomach and small intestine*, J. Amer. med. Ass., 98:961, 1932.   18

LONGINO, L. A., WOOLLEY AND GROSS: *Esophageal replacement in infants and children, with use of a segment of colon*, J. Amer. med. Ass., 171:1187, 1959.   10, 11

LOWER, W. E.: *Intussusception in adults due to the invagination of a Meckel's diverticulum*, Ann. Surg., 82:436, 1925.   23

LUMB, G., AND PROTHEROE: *The early lesions in ulcerative colitis*, Gastroenterology, 33:457, 1957.   30, 31

LYONS, A. S., AND GARLOCK: *Relationship of ulcerative colitis to carcinoma*, Gastroenterology, 18:170, 1951.   53-55

MACDONALD, R. A.: *A study of 356 carcinoids of the gastrointestinal tract; report of four new cases of the carcinoid syndrome*, Amer. J. Med., 21:867, 1956.   51

MAGUIRE, C. H.: *Discussion of Aldrich's and Wilson's presentations*, Ann. Surg., 141:788, 1955.   1, 4-6, 12-14

MANSON, P.: *Notes on sprue*, Medical report; China Imp. Maritime Customs, Shanghai, 1879-1888.   24, 25

MANSON-BAHR, P., ED.: *Manson's Tropical Diseases*, Cassell and Company, London, 1954.   24, 25, 40-42

——: *The Dysenteric Disorders*, Cassell and Company, London, 1939.   40, 42

MARTEL, W., AND HODGES: *The small intestine in Whipple's disease*, Amer. J. Roentgenol., 81:623, 1959.   26

MARTINEZ PRADO, G.: *Diarreas crónicas del adulto*, Sem. med. (B. Aires), 112:490, 1958.   27

MASSON, P.: *Carcinoids (argentaffin-cell tumors) and nerve hyperplasia of appendicular mucosa*, Amer. J. Path., 4:181, 1928.   51

MATT, J. G., AND TIMPONE: *Peptic ulcer of Meckel's diverticulum; case report and review of the literature*, Amer. J. Surg., 47:612, 1940.   17

MAY, C. C.: *Cystic Fibrosis of the Pancreas in Infants and Children*, Charles C Thomas, Publisher, Springfield, Ill., 1954.   3

MAYO, C. W., DEWEERD AND JACKMAN: *Diffuse familial polyposis of colon*, Surg. Gynec. Obstet., 93:87, 1951.   52

MCHARDY, G. G., FRYE, FAUST, BROOKE, ELSDON-DEW AND ARMAS-CRUZ: *Panel: Intestinal infestations*, in *Proceedings of the World Congress of Gastroenterology, Washington, 1958*, Volume 2, page 774, Williams & Wilkins Company, Baltimore, 1959.   41, 42

MCKEOWN, T., MACMAHON AND RECORD: *Investigation of 69 cases of exomphalos*, Amer. J. hum. Genet., 5:168, 1953.   14

MCKITTRICK, L. S., AND WHEELOCK: *Carcinoma of the Colon*, Charles C Thomas, Publisher, Springfield, Ill., 1954.   53

MEYER, K. F.: *The status of botulism as a world health problem*, Bull. Wld Hlth Org., 15:281, 1956.   38, 39

MEYERS, S. G., RUBLE AND ASHLEY: *The clinical course of regional ileitis*, Amer. J. dig. Dis., 4:341, 1959.   28, 29

MICHAEL, P.: *Tuberculosis of Meckel's diverticulum*, Arch. Surg., 25:1152, 1932.   17

—— AND BELL: *Primary adenocarcinoma arising in a Meckel's diverticulum*, Surg. Gynec. Obstet., 54:95, 1932.   17

MICHALANY, J., FERRAZ AND PEREIRA: *Sindrome de Peutz; lentiginose bucal e polipose do intestino delgado de caráter familiar*, Rev. paul. Med., 47:446, 1955.   48

MINZ, B.: *Rôle of Humoral Agents in Nervous Activity*, Charles C Thomas, Publisher, Springfield, Ill., 1955.   27

MOHLER, D. N.: *Evaluation of the urine test for serotonin metabolites*, J. Amer. med. Ass., 163:1138, 1957.   51

MONAGHAN, J. F.: *Ulcerative colitis*, in *Gastro-enterology*, Volume 2, page 549, Bockus, H. L., ed., W. B. Saunders Company, Philadelphia, 1944.   30, 31

MONNET, P., AND NICOLLE: *Evolution endémo-épidémique, des infections a Escherichia coli spécifique (0.111 B_4, 0.26 B_6, 0.55 B_5) dans un hôpital Lyonnais d'enfants de 1954 à mars 1956*, Pédiatrie, 11:725, 1956.   27

MOORE, T. C.: *Omphalomesenteric duct anomalies*, Surg. Gynec. Obstet., 103:569, 1956.   16, 17

MORGAN, C. N.: *Surgical anatomy of ischiorectal space*, Proc. roy. Soc. Med., 42:189, 1949.   59

NEELY, J. C.: *Perforation in regional enteritis*, J. Amer. med. Ass., 174:1680, 1960.   29

NEGHME, A., BERTÍN, TAGLE, SILVA AND ARTIGAS: *Diphyllobothrium latum en Chile; primera encuesta en el Lago Colico*, Bol. chil. Parasit., 5:16, 1950.   69

——, SILVA AND ARTIGAS: *El laboratorio en el diagnóstico de la amibiasis intestinal*, Bol. chil. Parasit., 10:66, 1955.   41, 42

NELSON, C. E., BARR AND DEEB: *Carcinoma of colon in children*, Amer. J. Surg., 78:531, 1949.   53

NELSON, H., AND PIJPER: *Typhoid and paratyphoid fevers*, in *Modern Practice in Infectious Fevers*, Volume 1, page 349, Banks, H. S., ed., Butterworth & Co., Ltd., London, 1951.   35-37

NESSELROD, J. P.: *Proctology in General Practice*, page 169, W. B. Saunders Company, Philadelphia, 1950.   57

——: *Symposium on anorectal surgery; pathogenesis of common anorectal infections*, Amer. J. Surg., 88:815, 1954.   59

NEVES, D. P., CAMPANA AND BRITO: *Lipodistrofia intestinal (Moléstia de Whipple)*, Rev. Hosp. Clín. Fac. Med. S. Paulo, 13:319, 1958.   26

NISSLE, A.: *Die Dysbakterie des Dickdarms und ihre Bedeutung für die Heilkunde*, Ther. d. Gegenw., 76:119, 1935.   27

NYGAARD, K. K., AND WALTERS: *Malignant tumors of Meckel's diverticulum; report of a case of leiomyosarcoma*, Arch. Surg. (Chicago), 35:1159, 1937.   17

NYMAN, E.: *Ulcerous jejuno-ileitis with symptomatic sprue*, Acta med. scand., 134:275, 1949.   24

OSLER, W.: *On a family form of recurring epistaxis, associated with multiple telangiectases of the skin and mucous membranes*, Bull. Johns Hopk. Hosp., 12:333, 1901.   47

PASSARELLI, N.: *Retocolite ulcerative inespecifica; estudo clínico*, in *Colopatias*, page 97, Mendes, F., ed., Livraria Atheneu, S. A., Rio de Janeiro, 1959.   31

PAULINO, F., AND RODRIGUES: *Carcinoma do colon*, Rev. bras. Cir., 31:5, 1956.   53

PAULLEY, J. W.: *Ulcerative colitis; study of 173 cases*, Gastroenterology, 16:566, 1950.   31

PENFOLD, H. B.: *Signs and symptoms of Taenia saginata infestation*, Med. J. Aust., 1:531, 1937.   66

PENFOLD, W. J., PENFOLD AND PHILLIPS: *Taenia saginata; its growth and propagation*, J. Helmin., 15:41, 1937.   66

PERSSON, H.: *Meckel'sches Divertikel, durch einen Fremdkörper perforiert*, Acta chir. scand., 82:530, 1939.   17

PESHKIN, M. M.: *Allergy in children*, in *Progress in Allergy III*, page 21, Kallós, P., ed., S. Karger, Basel, 1952.   27

PESSÔA, S. B.: *Parasitologia Médica*, Livraria Editôra Guanabara, Rio de Janeiro, 1958.   61-71

PEUTZ, J. L. A.: *Over een zeer merkwaardige, gecombineerde familiaire polyposis van de slijmvliezen van den tractus intestinalis met die van de neuskeelholte en gepaard met eigenaardige pigmentaties von huiden slijmvliezen*, Ned. Maandschr. Geneesk, 10:134-146, 1921.   48

PFEIFFER, D. B., AND PATTERSON: *Congenital or hereditary polyposis of colon*, Ann. Surg., 122:606, 1945.   52

PHEAR, D. N.: *The relation between regional ileitis and sarcoidosis*, Lancet, 2:1250, 1958.   28, 29

PIEROSE, P. N.: *Hemangioma of the gastrointestinal tract*, J. Amer. med. Ass., 115:209, 1940.   47

PLUMMER, K., RUSSI, HARRIS AND CARAVATI: *Lipophagic intestinal granulomatosis (Whipple's disease); clinical and pathologic study of 34 cases, with special reference to clinical diagnosis and pathogenesis*, Arch. intern. Med., 86:280, 1950.   26

POLAK, M., AND PONTES: *Cause of postgastrectomy steatorrhea*, Gastroenterology, 30:489, 1956.   24

—— AND ——: *Diagnosis of Meckel's diverticulum by peritoneoscopy*, Gastroenterology, 38:912, 1960.   16

—— AND ——: *Ocorrencia de esteatorreia em afeccões do aparelho digestivo*, Gaz. méd. port., 8:408, 1955.   24, 28, 29

—— AND ——: *Zur Diagnostik der Steatorrhoe*, Gastroenterologia (Basel), 83:224, 1955.   24, 25

PONTES, J. F.: *Amebíase*, in *Colopatias*, page 175, Mendes, F., ed., Livraria Atheneu, S. A., Rio de Janeiro, 1959.   27

——: *Enterocolites Crônicas: Dispepsias Intestinais*, Renascença, São Paulo, 1947.   40

——, CUTAIT AND SIMONSEN: *Polipose familiar múltipla do intestino grosso*, Rev. Hosp. Clín. Fac. Med. S. Paulo, 4:43, 1949.   52

——, JAMRA AND SILVA: *Amebíase*, Melhoramentos, São Paulo, 1941.   41, 42

——, Neves and Pontes: *Enteropatias alérgicas*, in *Anais da IIª Jornada Panamericana de Gastroenterol.*, Rio de Janeiro, 1950, page 108. 27

——, Taunay, Fava and Peixoto: *Bacteriologia intestinal nas enterocolopatias crônicas; a flora bacteriana de jejuno nas enterocolopatias crônicas*, in *Anais de IIª Jornada Panamericana de Gastroenterol.*, Rio de Janeiro, 1950, page 351. 27

——, —— and Prado: *Dados sôbre a bacteriologia das enterocolites crônicas; diferentes métodos de colheita de material*, Rev. bras. Gastroent., 4:293, 1952. 27

——, Trabulsi and Campos: *Shiguelose*, in *Colopatias*, page 275, Mendes, F., ed., Livraria Atheneu, Rio de Janeiro, 1959. 40

Pontes, J. T.: *Hemorróidas*, in *Colopatias*, page 371, Mendes, F., ed., Livraria Atheneu, Rio de Janeiro, 1959. 56

Potts, W. J.: *Congenital atresia of intestine and colon*, Surg. Gynec. Obstet., 85:14, 1947. 1, 2, 4, 7

——: *Darmverschluss beim Neugeborenen*, Klin. Wschr., 35:754, 1957. 1-9

Raiford, T. S.: *Tumors of small intestine*, Arch. Surg. (Chicago), 25:122, July; 321, August 1932. 49, 50

Rainey, R.: *Association of lymphogranuloma inguinale and cancer*, Surgery, 35:221, 1954. 60

Ramos, J., Prado and Fonseca: *Enterite tuberculosa*, Rev. bras. Med., 8:389, 1942. 43-45

Rankin, F. W., and Graham: *Cancer of the Colon and Rectum; its Diagnosis and Treatment*, Charles C Thomas, Publisher, Springfield, Ill., 1945. 52, 53

Ratcliffe, J. W., Bartlett and Halsted: *Diverticulosis and acute diverticulitis of the jejunum; report of two cases*, New Engl. J. Med., 242:387, 1950. 18

Reichman, H. R.: *Multiple malignant lesions of colon*, Amer. J. Surg., 75:275, 1948. 53

Reiferscheid, M.: *Die gutartigen Tumoren des Magens und Dürndarms*, Med. Klin., 54:41, 1959. 46-48

Rhoads, C. P., Castle, Payne and Lawson: *Hookworm anemia: etiology and treatment with especial reference to iron*, Am. J. Hyg., 20:291, 1934. 65

Rhoads, J. E., Pipes and Randall: *A simultaneous abdominal and perineal approach in operations for imperforate anus with atresia of the rectum and rectosigmoid*, Ann. Surg., 127:552, 1948. 5, 6

Riggins, H. M.: *Tuberculosis of the alimentary tract*, Med. Clin. N. Amer., 26:819, 1942. 43-45

Ritchie, A. C.: *Carcinoid tumors*, Amer. J. med. Sci., 232:311, 1956. 51

River, L., Silverstein and Tope: *Benign neoplasms of the small intestine; a critical comprehensive review with reports of 20 new cases*, Int. Abstr. Surg., 102:1, 1956. 46-48

Roddy, S. R.: *Small-bowel tumors; clinical review of 34 cases*, A. M. A. Arch. Surg., 75:847, 1957. 46-50

Rosenberg, D., Vianna and Klinger: *Suboclusão intestinal por tuberculoma*, Rev. paul. Med., 54:155, 1959. 43-45

Rosenblum, A. H.: *Typhoid and paratyphoid fever in immunized subjects*, Ann. intern. Med., 31:235, 1949. 35-37

Rössle, R., and Apitz: *Atlas der Pathologischen Anatomie*, Georg Thieme, Stuttgart, 1951. 30, 31, 34, 36, 44, 52, 55

Rowe, A. H.: *Clinical Allergy due to Foods, Inhalants, Contactants, Fungi, Bacteria and Other Causes; Manifestations, Diagnosis and Treatment*, Lea & Febiger, Philadelphia, 1937. 27

——: *Elimination Diets and the Patient's Allergies; a Handbook of Allergy*, Lea & Febiger, Philadelphia, 1944. 27

——, Rowe and Uyeyama: *Allergic epigastric syndrome*, J. Allergy, 25:464, 1954. 27

——, ——, Uyeyama and Young: *Diarrhea caused by food allergy*, J. Allergy, 27:424, 1956. 27

Ruffin, J. M., and Tyor: *Steatorrhea in adults*, J. Amer. med. Ass., 172:2060, 1960. 24, 25

Russo, F. R.: *Whipple's disease; review of literature and report of two cases*, A. M. A. Arch. intern. Med., 89:600, 1952. 26

Saphra, I., and Winter: *Clinical manifestations of salmonellosis in man; an evaluation of 7779 human infections identified at the New York Salmonella Center*, New Engl. J. Med., 256:1128, 1957. 35-38

Sauer, W. G., Dearing and Flock: *Diagnosis and clinical management of functioning carcinoids*, J. Amer. med. Ass., 168:139, 1958. 51

Sawitz, W. G.: *Medical Parasitology*, McGraw-Hill Book Company, Inc., New York, 1956. 61-71

Schaetz, G.: *Beiträge zur Morphologie des Meckel'schen Divertikels (Ortsfremde Epithelformationen im Meckel)*, Beitr. path. Anat., 74:115, 1925. 16

Schneckloth, R. E., McIsaac and Page: *Serotonin metabolism in carcinoid syndrome with metastatic bronchial adenoma*, J. Amer. med. Ass., 170:1143, 1959. 51

Schreiber, H. W.: *Ueber das Pseudomyxoma peritonei ex appendice*, Bruns' Beitr. klin. Chir., 191:283, 1955. 34

Scimeca, W. B., and Dockerty: *Carcinoma of vermiform appendix: review of literature and report of case*, Proc. Mayo Clin., 30:527, 1955. 34

Scott, J. E. S., and Swenson: *Imperforate anus. Results in 63 cases and some anatomic considerations*, Ann. Surg., 150:477, 1959. 4-6

Seven, M. J.: *Mussel poisoning*, Ann. inter. Med., 48:891, 1958. 39

Shallow, T. A., Eger and Carty: *Primary malignant disease of small intestine*, Amer. J. Surg., 69:372, 1945. 49, 50

Shandalow, S. L.: *Benign tumors of the small intestine*, A. M. A. Arch. Surg., 71:761, 1955. 46-48

Sheldon, W.: *Celiac disease*, Pediatrics, 23:132, 1959. 24, 25

Shepherd, J. A.: *Angiomatous conditions of the gastro-intestinal tract*, Brit. J. Surg., 40:409, 1953. 47

Singleton, A. O., Jr., and King: *Persistent vitelline duct continuous with the appendix; case report*, Surgery, 29:278, 1951. 16

Sjoerdsma, A.: *Clinical and laboratory features of malignant carcinoid*, A. M. A. Arch. intern. Med., 102:936, 1958. 51

Sloan, W. P., Bargen and Baggenstoss: *Symposium on some complications of chronic ulcerative colitis; local complications of chronic ulcerative colitis based on study of 2,000 cases*, Proc. Mayo Clin., 25:240, 1950. 51

Smith, A. N.: *Carcinoid tumors and 5-Hydroxytryptamine*, Quart. Rev. Surg. Obstet. Gynec., 17:11, 1960. 51

Smith, D.: *Cancer of the rectum and rectosigmoid*, in *Diseases of the Digestive System*, page 727, Portis, S. A., Lea & Febiger, Philadelphia, 1944. 54, 55

Smith, F. H., and Murphy: *Carcinoid tumors*, Med. Clin. N. Amer., 44:465, 1960. 51

Smith, O. N.: *Leiomyoma of small intestine with report of case with fatal hemorrhage*, Am. J. med. Sci., 191:700, 1937. 48

Söderlund, S.: *Meckel's diverticulum in children; report of 115 cases*, Acta chir. scand., 110:261, 1956. 6

Sodri, H. A., Croce and Faria: *Tuberculose intestinal*, Rev. Hosp. Clín. Fac. Med. S. Paulo, 1 317, 1946. 43-45

Sövényi and Tiszai: *Enteritis regionalis (Crohn'sche Krankheit) im grossen Teil des Dickdarms*, Z. ärztl. Fortbild., 52:988, 1958. 28, 29

Stein, G. N., Bennett and Finkelstein: *The preoperative roentgen diagnosis of Meckel's diverticulum in adults*, Amer. J. Roentgenol., 79:815, 1958. 6

Stetten, D.: *The submucous lipoma of the gastro-intestinal tract; a report of two successfully operated cases and an analysis of the literature*, Surg. Gynec. Obstet., 9:156, 1909. 47

Stierlin, E.: *Die Radiographie in der Diagnostik der Ileozoekaltuberkulose und mancher anderer Krankheiten des Dickdarms*, Dtsch. med. Wschr., 58:1231, 1911. 44, 45

Strohl, E. L., and Diffenbaugh: *Primary tumors of the small bowel*, A. M. A. Arch. Surg., 74:709, 1957. 49, 50

Sullivan, A. J.: *Psychogenic factors in ulcerative colitis*, Amer. J. dig. Dis., 2:651, 1936. 51

Swenson, O.: *Modern treatment of Hirschsprung's disease*, J. Amer. med. Ass., 154:651, 1954. 8, 9

—— and Fisher: *Hirschsprung's disease in the newborn*, A. M. A. Arch. Surg., 79:987, 1959. 8-9

——, Neuhauser and Pickett: *New concepts of etiology, diagnosis and treatment of congenital megacolon (Hirschsprung's disease)*, Pediatrics, 4:201, 1949. 8-9

Tajes, R. V.: *Las fistulas anorrectales; conceptos clínicos y terapéuticos*, Síntesis méd., 2:2, 1958. 59

Talbot, C. H.: *Volvulus of the small intestine in adults*, Gut, 1 76, 1960. 48

Section XII (continued)

PLATE NUMBER

TAUNAY, A. DE E., PONTES, PRADO AND PEIXOTO: *Shigueloses; comparação de métodos de colheita das fezes no diagnóstico bacteriológico das enterocolites crônicas; aglutininas na enterocolite crônica,* Rev. Inst. A. Lutz (S. Paulo), 16:37, 1956. 40

TAYLOR, J.: *Bacteriology in relation to the alimentary tract,* in *Modern Trends in Gastroenterology,* page 605, Jones, F. Avery, ed., Butterworth & Co., Ltd., London, 1952. 27, 35-40

——: *Enteropathogenic Escherichia coli,* in *Recent Advances in Clinical Pathology; Series III,* page 78, Dyke, S. C., ed., J. & A. Churchill, London, 1960. 27

THAYSEN, T. E. H.: *Nontropical Sprue, a Study in Idiopathic Steatorrhea,* Oxford University Press, London, 1932. 24, 25

THOMPSON, H. R.: *Polyposis intestini,* Proc. roy. Soc. Med., 51:241, 1958. 52

THOMPSON, M. W.: *Heredity, maternal age and birth order in etiology of celiac disease,* Amer. J. hum. Genet., 3:159, 1951. 24, 25

THORSON, Å., BIÖRK, BJÖRKMAN AND WALDENSTRÖM: *Malignant carcinoid of small intestine with metastases to liver, valvular disease of right side of heart (pulmonary stenosis and tricuspid regurgitation without septal defects), peripheral vasomotor symptoms, bronchoconstriction, and unusual type of cyanosis; clinical and pathologic syndrome,* Amer. Heart J., 47:795, 1954. 51

THORSON, A. H.: *Studies on carcinoid disease,* Acta med. scand. (Suppl. 334), 161:1, 1958. 51

TODD, I. P.: *Etiological factors in the production of complete rectal prolapse,* Postgrad. med. J., 35:97, 1959. 57

TÖTTERMAN, G.: *On occurrence of pernicious tape-worm anemia in diphyllobothrium carriers,* Acta med. scand., 118:410, 1944. 69

TURELL, R.: *Venereal diseases,* in *Diseases of the Colon and Anorectum,* Volume 2, page 769, Turell, R., ed., W. B. Saunders Company, Philadelphia, 1959. 60

—— AND WILKINSON: *Adenomas of colon and rectum,* Surgery, 28:651, 1950. 58

——, KREEL AND SELEY: *The Peutz-Jeghers Syndrome. (Gastrointestinal polyposis with mucocutaneous melanin pigmentation),* Surg. Clin. N. Amer., 39:1309, 1959. 48

URBACH, E., AND GOTTLIEB: *Allergy,* Grune & Stratton, New York, 1943. 27

VACHON, A., AND LEHMANN: *Les localisations gastro-intestinales de la maladie de Recklinghausen,* Rev. lyon. Med., 1:277, 1952. 47

VAN DER BURG: *Indische Spruw (aphthae tropicae),* Ernst and Company, Batavia, 1880; transl. in Med. Rep. China Imp., Maritime Customs, 1883. 24, 25

VAN DER REIS, V.: *Die Darmbakterien des Erwachsenen und ihre klinische Bedeutung,* Ergebn. inn. Med. Kinderheilk, 27:77, 1925. 27

Section XII (continued)

PLATE NUMBER

VARELA FUENTES, B., AND RECARTE: *Resultados de la investigación de la alergia digestiva, en nuestra práctica gastroenterológica,* in *Patologia digestiva,* page 1, Varela Fuentes, B., and Capurro, eds., Espasa-Calpe, Buenos Aires, 1942. 27

VAUGHAN, W. T.: in *Practice of Allergy,* Black, J., ed., C. V. Mosby Company, St. Louis, 1948. 27

WAALKES, T. P., SJOERDSMA, CREVELING, WEISSBACH AND UDENFRIEND: *Serotonin, norepinephrine, and related compounds in bananas,* Science, 127:648, 1958. 51

WARREN, I. A., AND BERK: *The etiology of chronic nonspecific ulcerative colitis; a critical review,* Gastroenterology, 33:395, 1957. 30, 31

WARREN, K. W., AND COYLE: *Carcinoid tumors of gastrointestinal tract,* Amer. J. Surg., 82:372, 1951. 51

WARREN, S., AND LULENSKI: *Primary, solitary lymphoid tumors of gastro-intestinal tract,* Ann. Surg., 115:1, 1942. 49, 50

—— AND SOMMERS: *Pathology of regional ileitis and ulcerative colitis,* J. Amer. med. Ass., 154:189, 1954. 28, 29

WATKINSON, G., FEATHER, MARSON AND DOSSETT: *Massive jejunal diverticulosis with steatorrhea and megaloblastic anemia improved by excision of diverticula,* Brit. med. J., 2:58, 1959. 24, 25

WATSON, J. M.: *Handbook of Medical Helminthology,* Ballière, Tindall and Cox, London, 1960. 61-70

WEBER, F. P.: *Multiple hereditary developmental angiomata (telangiectases) of the skin and mucous membranes associated with recurring haemorrhages,* Lancet, 2:160, 1907. 47

WEIL, A. J., AND SAPHRA: *Salmonellae and Shigellae: Laboratory Diagnosis Correlated with Clinical Manifestations and Epidemiology,* Charles C Thomas, Publisher, Springfield, Ill., 1953. 40

WESTON, S. D., AND MARREN: *Malignant melanoma of rectum,* J. int. Coll. Surg., 17:403, 1952. 55

WHELAN, T. J., AND RAST: *Unusual lesions of the appendix,* A. M. A. Arch. Surg., 79:838, 1959. 34

WHIPPLE, G. H.: *A hitherto undescribed disease characterized anatomically by deposits of fat and fatty acids in the intestinal and mesenteric lymphatic tissues,* Bull. Johns Hopk. Hosp., 18:382, 1907. 26

WHITE, B. V., COBB AND JONES: *Mucous colitis; a psychological medical study of sixty cases,* National Research Council, Washington, 1939. 27

WILDEGANS, H.: *Tuberkulose des Darms,* Med. Klin., 52:529, 1957. 43-45

WILLIAMS, C., AND BOSHER: *Jejunal diverticulosis complicated by the development of jejuno-colic and jejuno-jejunal fistulas; report of a case,* Ann. Surg., 127:918, 1948. 18

WILSON, H., HARDY AND FARRINGER: *Intestinal obstruction. Causes and management*

Section XII (continued)

PLATE NUMBER

in infants and children, Ann. Surg., 141:778, 1955. 1-11, 14

WINKELBAUER, A.: *Ueber die chirurgischen Erkrankungen des Meckelschen Divertikels,* Wien. klin. Wschr., 42:989, 1929. 16, 17

WISSMER, B.: *Les diverticules du tube digestif, de l'estomac a l'intestin grêle,* Gastroenterologia (Basel), 89:227, 1958. 18

WOLFE, S. A., AND TESLER: *Hemorrhagic leiomyoma of small intestine, simulating giant ovarian cyst,* Amer. J. Gastroent., 30:527, 1958. 46, 47

WOLFSON, W. L., AND KAUFMAN: *Acute inflammation of Meckel's diverticulum,* Ann. Surg., 89:535, 1929. 16, 17

WOODRUFF, R., AND MCDONALD: *Benign and malignant cystic tumors of appendix,* Surg. Gynec. Obstet., 71:750, 1940. 34

WULFF, H.: *Zur Frage der peptischen Geschwüre im Meckelschen Divertikel,* Chirurg., 4:926, 1932. 16, 17

XAVIER, A.: *Contribuição ao estudo da rectite infiltrante e estenosante,* Oficinas Graficas do "Jornal do Brasil", Rio de Janeiro, 1941. 60

YEOMANS, F. C.: *Proctology; a Treatise on the Malformations, Injuries and Diseases of the Rectum, Anus and Pelvic Colon,* D. Appleton-Century, New York, 1936. 56-60

YOUMANS, W. B.: *Nervous and Neurohumoral Regulation of Intestinal Motility,* Interscience Publishers, Inc., New York, 1949. 27

ZAK, F. G.: *Aberrant pancreatic carcinoma in jejunal diverticulum,* Gastroenterology, 30:529, 1956. 18

ZANCA, P.: *Multiple hereditary cartilaginous exostoses with polyposis of colon,* U. S. armed Forces med. J., 7:116, 1956. 52

ZINSSER, H., ENDERS AND FOTHERGILL: *Immunity; Principles and Application in Medicine and Public Health,* 5th edition, Macmillan Company, New York, 1945. 35-37

ZUELZER, W. W., AND WILSON: *Functional intestinal obstruction on congenital neurogenic basis in infancy,* Am. J. Dis. Child., 75:40, 1948. 7

Section XIII

ACKERMAN, L. V.: *Tumors of the retroperitoneum, mesentery and peritoneum,* Armed Forces Inst. Path., Washington, 1954. 7

ALTHAUSEN, T. L.: *I. False "acute abdomen"; pseudoperforation of peptic ulcer. II. Henoch's purpura and abdominal allergy,* Ann. Surg., 106:62 and 242, 1937. 8

BEHMER, O. A.: *Peritonites,* Rev. Hosp. Clín. Fac. Med. S. Paulo, 10:25, 1955. 5-7

BENNETT, H. S., AND COLLINS: *Oil granuloma of peritoneum,* Gastroenterology, 20:485, 1952. 6

BOIKAN, W. S.: *Meconium peritonitis from spontaneous perforation of ileum in utero,* Arch. Path., 9:1164, 1930. 5

CARLETON, C. C.: *Mucoceles of appendix and peritoneal pseudomyxoma,* A. M. A. Arch. Path., 60:39, 1955. 7

CARLIER, P.: *Les péritonotes biliaires,* Acta chir. belg., 54:225, 1955.   5

CATTAN, R., AND MASSON: *Maládie periodique,* Bull. Soc. méd. Hôp. Paris, 67: 25-26, 1104, 1951.   8

CLEMEDSON, C. J.: *Blast Injury,* Physiol. Rev., 36:336, 1956.   14

COPE, Z.: *Early diagnosis of the Acute Abdomen,* Oxford Univ. Press, London, 1954.   1, 2

CURTIS, A. H.: *Cause of adhesions in right upper quadrant,* J. Amer. med. Ass., 94: 1221, 1930.   6

DANIEL, O.: *Differential diagnosis of malignant disease of peritoneum,* Brit. J. Surg., 39:147, 1951.   7

FITZ-HUGH, T., JR.: *Acute gonococcic perihepatitis – a new syndrome of right upper quadrant abdominal pain in young women,* Rev. Gastroent., 3:125, 1936.   5

——: *Acute gonococcic peritonitis of right upper quadrant in women,* J. Amer. med. Ass., 102:2094, 1934.   5

HARDY, J. T., AND KEIL: *Peritoneal mesothelioma: review and case report,* Amer. J. dig. Dis., 4:737, 1959.   7

HAYTHORN, S. R.: *Nodular lesions of peritoneum,* Amer. J. Path., 9:725, 1933.   6

HELLER, H., SOHAR AND SHERF: *Familial Mediterranean fever,* A. M. A. Arch. intern. Med., 102:50, 1958.   8

HILSABECK, J. R., JUDD AND WOOLNER: *Symposium on surgical aspects of cancer problem; carcinoma of vermiform appendix,* Surg. Clin. N. Amer., 31:995, 1951.   7

KIRSCHNER, P. A.: *Mesenteric vascular occlusion,* J. Mt. Sinai Hosp., 21:307, 1955.   4

LUMB, G.: *Peritoneal pseudo-tubercles in schistosomiasis,* J. Path. Bact., 67:612, 1954.   6

McCORMICK, E. J., AND RAMSEY: *Postoperative peritoneal granulomatous inflammation caused by magnesium silicate,* J. Amer. med. Ass., 116:817, 1941.   6

McLAUGHLIN, C. W., JR.: *Bile peritonitis; report of eight cases,* Ann. Surg., 115:240, 1942.   5

MEEROFF, M., TRAVERSO AND KATZ: *Peritonitis encapsulante,* Día méd., 31:2554, 1959.   6

MELENEY, F. L., HARVEY AND JERN: *Peritonitis; correlation of bacteriology of peritoneal exudate and clinical course of disease in 106 cases of peritonitis,* Arch. Surg., 22:1, 1931.   5

NORTHRUP, W. P.: *General gonococcal peritonitis in young girls under puberty; report of two cases, one simulating appendicitis, operated,* Arch. Pediat., 68:388, 1951.   5

OVERBECK, L.: *Massive Peritonealsarkomatose bei sarkomatos entartetem Uterusmyom,* Zbl. Gynäk., 75:312, 1953.   7

PRIEST, R. J., AND NIXON: *Familial recurring polyserositis: a disease entity,* Ann. intern. med., 51:1253, 1959.   8

QUER, E. A., DOCKERTY AND MAYO: *Ruptured dermoid cyst of the ovary simulating abdominal carcinomatosis: report case,* Proc. Mayo Clin., 26:489, 1951.   5

RAIA, A., BRANCO, DANTAS AND MANZIONE: *Esquistossomose peritoneal,* Rev. Cir. S. Paulo, 19:139, 1954.   6

REIMANN, H. A.: *Periodic Disease,* J. Amer. med. Ass., 136:239, 1948.   8

——, MOADIE, SEMERDJIAN AND SAHYOUN: *Periodic peritonitis; heredity and pathology,* J. Amer. med. Ass., 154:1254, 1954.   8

SCHREIBER, H. W.: *Ueber das Pseudomyxoma peritonei ex appendice,* Bruns' Beitr. klin. Chir., 191:283, 1955.   7

SIEGAL, S.: *Benign paroxysmal peritonitis,* Ann. intern. Med., 23:1, 1945.   8

——: *Benign paroxysmal peritonitis; second series,* Gastroenterology, 12:234, 1949.   8

STEINBERG, B.: *Infections of the Peritoneum,* Paul B. Hoeber, Inc., New York, 1944.   5-7

SYMMERS, W. ST. C.: *Pathology of oxyuriasis; with special reference to granulomas due to presence of Oxyuris vermicularis (Enterobius vermicularis) and its ova in tissues,* Arch. Path., 50:475, 1950.   6

TAVARES, A.: *Granulomas peritoneais de corpos estranhos,* Gaz. méd. port., 7:43, 1954.   6

WARREN, K. W.: *Acute surgical conditions of abdomen in aged and the poor risk patient,* Surg. Clin. N. Amer., 34:745, 1954.   1, 2

WILLIS, R. A.: *Pathology of Tumours,* Butterworth & Co., Ltd., London, 1948.   7

WINSLOW, D. J., AND TAYLOR: *Malignant peritoneal mesotheliomas: a clinicopathological analysis of 12 fatal cases,* Cancer, 13:127, 1960.   7

Section XIV

ANDREWS, E.: *Duodenal hernia – a misnomer,* Surg. Gynec. Obstet., 37:740, 1923.   15

—— AND BISSELL: *Direct hernia,* Surg. Gynec. Obstet., 58:753, 1934.   6

ANDREWS, E. W.: *Imbrication or lap joint method; a plastic operation for hernia,* Chicago med. Rec., 9:67, 1895.   5

ANSON, B. J., McCORMACK AND CLEVELAND: *Anatomy of hernial region; obturator hernia and general considerations,* Surg. Gynec. Obstet., 90:31, 1950.   1, 13

—— AND McVAY: *The anatomy of the inguinal and hypogastric regions of the abdominal wall,* Anat. Rec., 70:211, 1938.   1

BASSINI, E.: *Sopra 100 casi dicura radicali dell' ernia inguinale operato con metodo dell' antore,* Ital. Chir. Congress Napoli, 1888.   3

——: *Ueber die Behandlung des Leistenbruches,* Arch. klin. Chir., 40:429, 1890.   3

BATSON, O. V.: *Anatomic variations in the abdomen,* Surg. Clin. N. Amer., 35:1727, 1955.   15

BERMAN, E. F.: *Epigastric hernia; improved method of repair,* Amer. J. Surg., 68:84, 1945.   12

BIERHOFF, A., AND UNGER: *Inguinal hernia of the bladder,* Amer. J. Surg., 30:506, 1935.   9

BRYANT, A. L.: *Spiegelian hernia,* Amer. J. Surg., 73:396, 1947.   12

BURNHAM, P. J.: *Retromesocolic hernia – development and treatment,* J. int. Coll. Surg., 20:753, 1953.   15

CALLANDER, C. L., RUSK AND NEMIR: *Mechanism, symptoms, and treatment of hernia into descending mesocolon (left duodenal hernia),* Surg. Gynec. Obstet., 60:1052, 1935.   15

CELSUS, AURELIUS, CORNELIUS: *Of Medicine (De Medicina),* translated by James Greive, London, 1756.   1

COTTALORDA, J., AND ESCARRAS: *Considérations sur le diagnostic et le traitement des hernies obturatrices étranglées,* J. de Chir. (Paris), 48:22, 1936.   13

COUPER, M. W.: *Hernia,* in *Textbook of Surgery,* Moseley, H. F., ed., C. V. Mosby Company, St. Louis, 1955.   1-11

ESTRADA, R. L.: *Anomalies of intestinal rotation and fixation (including mesentericoparietal hernias),* Charles C Thomas, Publisher, Springfield, Ill., 1958.   15

GRYNFELT, J.: *Quelques mots sur la hernie lombaire,* Montpellier méd., 16:329 and 504, 1866.   13

HALSTED, W. S.: *The cure of more difficult as well as simple inguinal ruptures,* Johns Hopk. Hosp. Bull., 14:208, 1903.   4

——: *The operative treatment of hernia,* Amer. J. med. Sci., 110:13, 1895.   4

——: *The radical cure of inguinal hernia in the male,* Johns Hopk. Hosp. Bull., 4:17, 1893.   4

HANCOCK, T. H.: *Traumatic hernia in Petit's triangle,* Sth. med. J., 13:521, 1920.   13

HANSMANN, G., AND MORTON: *Intra-abdominal hernia. Report of case and review of literature,* Arch. Surg., 39:973, 1909.   15

IASON, A. H.: *Hernia,* Blakiston Company, Philadelphia, 1941.   1-15

——: *Hernia in infancy and childhood,* Amer. J. Surg., 68:287, 1945.   3, 4

——: *Recurrences following inguinal hernioplasties,* Amer. J. Surg., 27:268, 1935.   9

——: *Tantalum gauze in hernial surgery,* N. Y. med. J., 54:1621, 1954.   9

KEITH, A.: *On the origin and nature of hernia,* Brit. J. Surg., 11:455, 1923.   1

LADD, W. E.: *Hernia in infancy and childhood,* Neb. St. med. J., 26:235, 1941.   2, 3

MAHORNER, H.: *Umbilical and midline ventral herniae,* Ann. Surg., 111:979, 1940.   2

MAIER, R. L.: *The present status of injection treatment of hernia,* Ann. Surg., 122:85, 1945.   3

McVAY, C. B., AND ANSON: *Fundamental error in current methods of inguinal herniorrhaphy,* Surg. Gynec. Obstet., 74: 746, 1942.   5

—— AND ANSON: *Inguinal and femoral hernioplasty,* Surg. Gynec. Obstet., 88:473, 1949.   5

MILLER, J. M., AND WAKEFIELD: *Congenital anomalies of primary midgut loop,* Amer. J. dig. Dis., 9:383, 1942.   15

MONTAGU, M. F. A.: *A case of familial inheritance of oblique inguinal hernia,* J. Hered., 33:355, 1942.   2

Section XIV (continued)

PATRICK, W.: *Recurrent Hernia. An investigation of the causes of recurrence and the application of the principles of treatment of the primary lesion*, Brit. J. Surg., 31: 231, 1944. — Plate 9

PERRY, H. C.: *Strangulated sciatic hernia with pregnancy*, Lancet, 1:318, 1920. — Plate 14

RISHMILLER, J. H.: *Hernia through triangle of Petit*, Surg. Gynec. Obstet., 24:589, 1917. — Plate 13

RIVER, L. P.: *Spigelian hernia*, Ann. Surg., 116:405, 1942. — Plate 12

ROCHE, A. E.: *Strangulated obturator hernia*, Clin. J., 59:49, 1930. — Plate 13

Section XIV (continued)

SKINNER, H. L., AND DUNCAN: *Recurrent inguinal hernia*, Ann. Surg., 122:68, 1945. — Plate 9

SUMMERS, J. E.: *Classical herniorrhaphies of Bassini, Halsted and Ferguson*, Amer. J. Surg., 73:87, 1947. — Plate 3, 4

TURNER, W. Y.: *Lumbar hernia*, Brit. med. J., 2:389, 1917. — Plate 13

USHER, F. C., AND GANNON: *Marlex mesh, a new plastic mesh for replacing time defects*, A. M. A. Arch. Surg., 78:131, 1959. — Plate 9

WANGENSTEEN, O. H.: *Repair of recurrent and difficult hernia*, Surg. Gynec. Obstet., 59:766, 1934. — Plate 9, 10

Section XIV (continued)

WATSON, L. F.: *Hernia: Anatomy, Etiology, Symptoms, Diagnosis. Differential Diagnosis, Prognosis and Treatment*, C. V. Mosby Company, St. Louis, 1948. — Plate 2-15

WEST, L. S.: *Two pedigrees showing inherited predisposition to hernia*, J. Hered., 27: 449, 1936. — Plate 3

YEOMANS, F. C.: *Levator hernia, perineal and pudendal*, Amer. J. Surg., 43:695, 1939. — Plate 14

ZIMMERMAN, L. M., AND ANSON: *Anatomy and Surgery of Hernia*, Williams & Wilkins Company, Baltimore, 1953. — Plate 1, 3-8

—— AND LAUFMAN: *Sliding hernia*, Surg. Gynec. Obstet., 75:76, 1942. — Plate 9

243